Enhancing the Therapeutic Efficacy of Herbal Formulations

Rajesh Kumar Kesharwani
Nehru Gram Bharati (Deemed), Prayagraj, India

Raj K. Keservani
Faculty of B. Pharmacy, CSM Group of Institutions, Prayagraj, India

Anil K. Sharma
GD Goenka University, India

IGI Global
PUBLISHER of TIMELY KNOWLEDGE

A volume in the Advances in Medical Diagnosis, Treatment, and Care (AMDTC) Book Series

Published in the United States of America by
IGI Global
Medical Information Science Reference (an imprint of IGI Global)
701 E. Chocolate Avenue
Hershey PA, USA 17033
Tel: 717-533-8845
Fax: 717-533-8661
E-mail: cust@igi-global.com
Web site: http://www.igi-global.com

Library of Congress Cataloging-in-Publication Data

Names: Kesharwani, Rajesh Kumar, 1978- editor. | Keservani, Raj K., 1981- editor. | Sharma, Anil K., 1980- editor.
Title: Enhancing the therapeutic efficacy of herbal formulations / Rajesh Kumar Kesharwani, Raj K. Keservani, and Anil K. Sharma, editors.
Description: Hershey, PA : Medical Information Science Reference, [2021] | Includes bibliographical references and index. | Summary: "This book explores the preparation and use of herbal formulation in novel drug delivery systems"-- Provided by publisher.
Identifiers: LCCN 2020003266 (print) | LCCN 2020003267 (ebook) | ISBN 9781799844532 (hardcover) | ISBN 9781799844549 (ebook)
Subjects: MESH: Plant Preparations--therapeutic use | Plant Preparations--pharmacology | Phytotherapy | Drug Delivery Systems--methods
Classification: LCC RS164 (print) | LCC RS164 (ebook) | NLM QV 766 | DDC 615.3/21--dc23
LC record available at https://lccn.loc.gov/2020003266
LC ebook record available at https://lccn.loc.gov/2020003267

This book is published in the IGI Global book series Advances in Medical Diagnosis, Treatment, and Care (AMDTC) (ISSN: 2475-6628; eISSN: 2475-6636)

British Cataloguing in Publication Data
A Cataloguing in Publication record for this book is available from the British Library.

For electronic access to this publication, please contact: eresources@igi-global.com.

Advances in Medical Diagnosis, Treatment, and Care (AMDTC) Book Series

ISSN:2475-6628
EISSN:2475-6636

Mission

Advancements in medicine have prolonged the life expectancy of individuals all over the world. Once life-threatening conditions have become significantly easier to treat and even cure in many cases. Continued research in the medical field will further improve the quality of life, longevity, and wellbeing of individuals.

The **Advances in Medical Diagnosis, Treatment, and Care (AMDTC)** book series seeks to highlight publications on innovative treatment methodologies, diagnosis tools and techniques, and best practices for patient care. Comprised of comprehensive resources aimed to assist professionals in the medical field apply the latest innovations in the identification and management of medical conditions as well as patient care and interaction, the books within the AMDTC series are relevant to the research and practical needs of medical practitioners, researchers, students, and hospital administrators.

Coverage

- Patient-Centered Care
- Critical Care
- Chronic Conditions
- Disease Management
- Medical Testing
- Disease Prevention
- Internal Medicine
- Alternative Medicine
- Cancer Treatment
- Patient Interaction

IGI Global is currently accepting manuscripts for publication within this series. To submit a proposal for a volume in this series, please contact our Acquisition Editors at Acquisitions@igi-global.com or visit: http://www.igi-global.com/publish/.

The Advances in Medical Diagnosis, Treatment, and Care (AMDTC) Book Series (ISSN 2475-6628) is published by IGI Global, 701 E. Chocolate Avenue, Hershey, PA 17033-1240, USA, www.igi-global.com. This series is composed of titles available for purchase individually; each title is edited to be contextually exclusive from any other title within the series. For pricing and ordering information please visit http://www.igi-global.com/book-series/advances-medical-diagnosis-treatment-care/129618. Postmaster: Send all address changes to above address.

Titles in this Series

For a list of additional titles in this series, please visit:
http://www.igi-global.com/book-series/advances-medical-diagnosis-treatment-care/129618

Treating Endocrine and Metabolic Disorders With Herbal Medicines
Arif Hussain (Manipal Academy of Higher Education, UAE) and Shalini Behl (Manipal Academy of Higher Education, UAE)
Medical Information Science Reference • © 2021 • 489pp • H/C (ISBN: 9781799848080) • US $295.00

Handbook of Research on Advancements in Cancer Therapeutics
Sumit Kumar (National Institute of Pathology, New Delhi, India) Moshahid Alam Rizvi (Jamia Millia Islamia, India) and Saurabh Verma (National Institute of Pathology, India)
Medical Information Science Reference • © 2021 • 913pp • H/C (ISBN: 9781799865308) • US $465.00

Cases on Medical Nutrition Therapy for Gastrointestinal Disorders
Elham Abbas Aljaaly (King Abdulaziz University, Saudi Arabia) Nahlaa Abdelwahab Khalifa (King Abdulaziz University, Saudi Arabia) Rouba Khalil Naaman (King Abdulaziz University, Saudi Arabia) and Manar Abduljalil Bakhsh (King Abdulaziz University, Saudi Arabia)
Medical Information Science Reference • © 2021 • 254pp • H/C (ISBN: 9781799838029) • US $245.00

Handbook of Research on Disease Prediction Through Data Analytics and Machine Learning
Geeta Rani (Manipal University Jaipur, India) and Pradeep Kumar Tiwari (Manipal University Jaipur, India)
Medical Information Science Reference • © 2021 • 586pp • H/C (ISBN: 9781799827429) • US $395.00

Handbook of Research on Evidence-Based Perspectives on the Psychophysiology of Yoga and Its Applications
Shirley Telles (Patanjali Research Foundation, India) and Ram Kumar Gupta (Patanjali Research Foundation, India)
Medical Information Science Reference • © 2021 • 577pp • H/C (ISBN: 9781799832546) • US $345.00

New Developments in Diagnosing, Assessing, and Treating ADHD
Rejani Thudalikunnil Gopalan (Mahatma Gandhi Medical College and Hospital, India)
Medical Information Science Reference • © 2021 • 419pp • H/C (ISBN: 9781799854951) • US $265.00

Handbook of Research on Oncological and Endoscopical Dilemmas in Modern Gynecological Clinical Practice
Konstantinos Dinas (2nd Department of Obstetrics and Gynaecology, Aristotle University of Thessaloniki, Greece) Stamatios Petousis (2nd Department of Obstetrics and Gynaecology, Aristotle University of Thessaloniki, Greece) Matthias Kalder (Department of Obstetrics and Gynaecology, Philipps-University of Marburg, Germany) and George Mavromatidis (2nd Department of Obstetrics and Gynaecology, Aristotle University of Thessaloniki, Greece)
Medical Information Science Reference • © 2021 • 460pp • H/C (ISBN: 9781799842132) • US $385.00

IGI Global
PUBLISHER of TIMELY KNOWLEDGE

701 East Chocolate Avenue, Hershey, PA 17033, USA
Tel: 717-533-8845 x100 • Fax: 717-533-8661
E-Mail: cust@igi-global.com • www.igi-global.com

Table of Contents

Detailed Table of Contents

The herbal-based drugs have been getting wide attention over the last few decades. The herbal drugs have been used from the ancient times, but the dose accuracy, efficacy, and treatment was just based on symptomatic observatory. Modern research is focused on pure bioactive compound instead of crude. The researchers are trying to apply the current advanced nanotechnology-based knowledge on the herbal medicines to improve efficacy and reduces the unwanted pharmacological actions' adverse effects of the therapeutic molecules. The many novel drug delivery systems available used for the herbal bioactive molecules include polymeric micelle, injectable hydrogel, nano gel, nano emulsions, microsphere, polymeric nanoparticles, nano capsules, liposomes, phytosomes, transferosomes, dendrimer, and ethosomes. This chapter highlights the existing research and development of current standing of the of various novel formulations especially for the herbal bioactive molecules and summarizes their active ingredients, commercial formulations, route of drug administration, and pharmacological activity.

Herbal medications have restorative potential, which can be given through different advantageous medication conveyance frameworks. Utilizing the bioactive and plant extricates, the assortment of novel natural details like polymeric nanoparticles, liposomes, phytosomes, nanoemulsions, microsphere,

be accomplished by designing novel drug delivery systems (NDDS) for herbal constituents. NDDSs not only reduce the frequency of drug administration to improve patient compliance but also help to enhance the therapeutic value by dropping toxicity and enhancing the drug bioavailability. A nanotechnology is a new approach in which nano-sized drug delivery systems of herbal drugs have a prospective future for enhancing the therapeutic activity and conquer problems associated with plant medicines. Hence, the addition of the nanotechnology as an NDDS in traditional medication is essential for the treatment of more chronic diseases like cancer, diabetes, asthma, and others.

Hepatitis B is an infectious disease caused by the hepatitis B virus (HBV) which is one of the most serious public health problems in the world. Some common approved drugs bring about dose-dependent adverse effects or drug resistance. Therefore, safe and useful new HBV therapeutics are essential. Medicinal plants have particular benefits to treat HBV-infected patients. Traditional medicines have many bioactive compounds that are effective as antiviral candidates including esculetin, helioxanthin, oxymatrine, epigallocatechin-3-gallate, wogonin, alkaloids, polysaccharides, etc. In this chapter, the authors summarize the pathogenesis and protein targets for the treatment of hepatitis B disease. They also indicate several medicinal plants and isolated compounds which are used for preventing and reduce symptoms of this disease.

Flavonoids are a group of heterocyclic compounds that are well-known for their anti-cancer activity. Fruits and vegetables are the main dietary sources of flavonoids. Several mechanisms have been proposed for the effect of flavonoids to combat cancer. But before considering the flavonoids as chemotherapeutic drugs for cancer, a number of problems still need to be addressed before their therapeutic uses. Solubility may play a major role in the therapeutic efficacy of flavonoids. Bioavailability of flavonoids are also affected by several other factors. Nanotechnology is the most efficient tool to solve the problems of solubility, stability, and oral bioavailability. Nanotechnology-based drug delivery has several benefits compared to the traditional drug delivery systems. Different types of nano delivery systems are used for producing nanomedicines such as lipid-based nanomedicines, polymer-based nanomedicines, and inorganic nanoparticles. Different types of flavonoids encapsulated nanoparticles have been developed to improve their effectiveness against different types of cancer.

Phytosomes are a new approach for delivery of drugs. Phytosomes mean herbal drugs loaded in vesicles, which are available in the nano form. The phytosome offers an envelope like coating around the active moieties of drug, and due to this, the main constituent of herbal extract remains safe from degradation by bacteria and digestive secretion. It is a patented technology which is advantageous in delivering the herbal drugs. Phytosomes have better pharmacological and pharmacokinetic parameters. It is used for development of delivery system with improved bioavailability of phytoconstituents present in herbal extracts. Phytosomes are prepared by the use of phospholipids by forming the complex between phospholipids and phytoconstituent. Phytosomes have a vast scope in pharma-industries and good research space for industry, scholars, students. Phospholipids are use as carriers for water soluble and lipid soluble nutrients and natural digestive aids.

Nutraceuticals have both wholesome and therapeutic properties. In recent years, there are many research works accessible in writing which recommend the utilization of nutraceuticals in treatment of different maladies like diabetes, malignancy, Alzheimer's, etc. It is additionally demonstrated that they are protected to utilize and have potential medical advantages. Yet, the fundamental interest in building up a nutraceutical detailing is its low bio-availability, substance flimsiness, and poor bioavailability. Because of these reasons, nutraceuticals are not misused appropriately and not generally acknowledged in pharma divisions for relief and treatment. In any case, with progression in science and innovation, it is conceivable to create systems or methodologies that can be utilized to define the nutraceuticals to its greatest use. In this chapter, the authors examine different advances in methodologies and procedures accessible for building up nutraceuticals.

Gout is a complex form of arthritis which is characterized by sudden, severe attacks of pain, swelling, redness, and tenderness in the joints. Gout is a type of inflammatory arthritis that is triggered by the crystallization of uric acid within the joints and is often associated with hyperuricemia. Natural products offer many options to reduce the progress and symptoms of diseases, including gout. Natural compound structure including lignans, flavonoids, tannins, polyphenols, triterpenes, sterols, and alkaloids have anti-inflammatory, antioxidant, and XO activities. In this chapter, the authors present medicinal plants and isolated compounds which are used to prevent and reduce the pathogenesis of gout.

Foreword

It is a matter of great pleasure for me to write a foreword for this book entitled *Enhancing the Therapeutic Efficacy of Herbal Formulations.* Various traditional systems of Indian and Chinese medicine use herbal formulations. After the cracking of human genome in the beginning of this century molecular targets of different diseases have been identified in modern medicine. The herbal components reported 5000 years back are now being found to target these molecules. Multicomponent herbal formulations act synergistically, avoiding many adverse effects of single, pure active principles. Modern medicine is now using combination therapy. However, the need is to enhance the efficacy of these formulations .The ancient Indian medicinal system, Ayurveda uses the herbal preparations with accompaniments, for example, ginger, cumin water, honey, milk, tulsi extract, etc. These increase cellular uptake, protect against unwanted toxicity, deliver trace elements, have synergistic and protective effects due to buffering between various constituents. In the present book it is very aptly brought out that these herbal formulations with such additional benefits can be made more efficacious if principles of modern medicine are applied.

Novel drug delivery devices such as polymeric nanoparticles, nanocapsules, liposomes, phytosomes, nanoemulsions, microsphere, transferosomes, and ethosomes having various advantages over the traditional methods of delivery can induce improved solubility, bioavailability, reduced toxicity, controlled drug delivery and protections of plant actives from degradation.

A number of herbal constituents like flavonoids, tannins, terpenoids, alkaloids are described in the book to show enhanced therapeutic effect at same or reduced level of dose when incorporated into novel drug delivery vehicles as compared to conventional methods. There is a great potential in development of novel drug delivery systems for enhancing the efficacy of herbal drugs as it provides efficient and economical drug delivery without any side effects.

The volume highlights that the nanoparticulate drug delivery is most commonly used due to its safety, efficacy and targeted drug delivery. It also enhances the solubility and bioavailability, increases the therapeutic value and reduces the dosing frequency.

Diseases like Hepatitis B and Gout have been shown to be responding better to herbal formulations when approved drugs cause adverse effects or drug resistance. Novel approaches have also been highlighted for use of Nutraceuticals.

The present book deals with both herbal formulations and novel drug delivery systems to provide a coherent information to scientists, industrialists, researchers and other academicians with pharmaceutical and biomedical background.

All the contributing authors demonstrate an exceptional expertise in the field of medicinal research and development, and provide a global perspective on current and future advances in new drug delivery systems.

I congratulate the editors for bringing together experts in the field of naturally occurring bioactive constituents as drugs and nanodevices for drug delivery, and the authors for their excellent contributions.

Krishna Misra
Indian Institute of Information Technology, Allahabad, India

Preface

"In science the credit goes to the man who convinces the world, not to the man to whom the idea first occurs." –William Osler

"Science will never be a finished book. Any development over time reveals more and deeper difficulties" – Albert Einstein

This new volume on *Enhancing the Therapeutic Efficacy of Herbal Formulations* deals with both herbal formulations and novel drug delivery systems is to provide scattered information in gathered form to the scientist, industrialist, researchers and academicians of pharmaceutical and biomedical sciences. This book gives state of the art picture about the herbal formulation and its therapeutic efficacy with emphasis on its present, past and future. The present book is well documented and covers different applied research involved in enhancing the therapeutic efficacy of herbal formulations, nutraceuticals-an effective and safe way from microbes of marine sources; an innovative approach as self-emulsifying drug delivery system for phytoconstituents; effect of NDDS on polyherbal formulation; phytosomes as a novel approach for herbal phytoconstituents; enhancing the therapeutic efficacy of herbal formulations through novel drug delivery systems; preparing flavonoids as anticancer therapeutics in novel drug delivery system; novel approaches in herbal formulations; nanoparticulate drug delivery system: an emphasis on herbal medicines.

With high demand of herbal formulation globally, the research on these are of more concern and this volume will be valuable resource for the medical researcher, pharmaceutical manufacturers, healthcare personnel, and academician. The present book includes 12 chapters containing information about the advanced research on enhancing the therapeutic efficacy of herbal formulations with its different applications for the human welfare.

Chapter 1 entitled "Therapeutic Efficacy of Herbal Formulations Through Novel Drug Delivery Systems" authored by Arvind Singh Chandel, highlights the existing research and development of the various novel formulations especially for the herbal bioactive molecules and summarizes their active ingredients, commercial formulations and route of drug administration, pharmacological activity. Several herbal bioactive molecules such as alkaloids, glycosides, terpenoids flavonoids, tannins, etc. exhibited enhanced therapeutic and pharmacological activity at equal or less dose when it associated with a novel drug delivery formulation as compared to conventional herbal formulations.

Chapter 2, "Novel Approaches in Herbal Formulations," is well described by Bhushan R. Rane and coauthors. In this chapter authors describe that herbal medications have numerous restorative potential which can be given through different advantageous medication conveyance frameworks. Novel methodology of herbal definition has picked up the significance to diminishing harmfulness, enhancement of the viability and safety of natural medications, assurance from physical and compound degradation as well as expanding the helpful value, increasing the steadiness, expanding the pharmacological action, improved bioavailability of homegrown plans.

Chapter 3 entitled "An Innovative Approach as Self-Emulsifying Drug Delivery System for Phytoconstituents" is authored by Swati G. Talele and associates. In recent years herbal drugs flourish as the method of rehabilitation of choice in numerous parts of the world and even most of populations considered as alternative conventional medicaments. However, most of the herbal drugs shows poor solubility and bioavailability, ultimately leading to diminished efficacy and frequency of administration increased. Consequently, self-emulsifying drug delivery system has been highlighted for poor water-soluble herbal medicaments.

Chapter 4 written by Charu Gupta and co-authors, describes the marine sources as nutraceuticals under the title, "Nutraceuticals: An Effective and Safe Way From Microbes of Marine Sources." Therapeutic compounds can be derived from various natural sources like plants, animals, marine organisms and microorganisms. Although the marine biota accounts for around 50% of the total world biodiversity. But their potential as a rich source of bioactive products and their applications in both pharmaceutical and nutraceutical industries, have only recently been identified through several scientific studies. Marine biotechnology is an upcoming area that involves about the study of marine microorganisms and animals including algae, sponges, and coral as a novel source of bioactive substances that can be used in the treatment of various human diseases like cancer, anaemia, diarrhoea, obesity, diabetes, atopic dermatitis, Crohn's disease, etc. A very limited scientific data is available on bioactive potential of marine microorganisms. This chapter deals with the exploitation of microbes from marine sources as potential sources for various nutraceuticals and their possibilities for applications in variety of diseases and as functional food supplement.

Chapter 5 entitled "Effect of NDDS on Polyherbal Formulation" is well documented by Sandeep O. Waghulde and colleagues. Herbal drugs have enormous therapeutic potential which can be explored through various beneficial novel drug delivery systems. In recent time the less use of single herbal formulations due to lack of their standardization. Great advancement has been made in the uses of plant therapeutics on the development of novel herbal formulations like polymeric nanoparticles, nanocapsules, liposomes, phytosomes, nanoemulsions, microsphere, transferosomes, and ethosomes etc. These formulations having various advantages over the traditional formulations such as improved solubility and bioavailability, reduced toxicity, controlled drug delivery, protections of plant actives from degradation.

Chapter 6 entitled "Nanoparticles for the Enhancement of the Therapeutic Efficacy of Herbal Formulations" by Mohammad Irfan Ali and associates has documented the role of nanotechnology well for the herbal formulation enhancement. A number of plant constituents like flavonoids, tannins, terpenoids etc. showed enhanced therapeutic effect at similar or less dose when incorporated into novel drug delivery vesicles as compared to conventional plant extracts. Hence, there is a great potential in development of novel drug delivery system for valuable herbal drugs as it provides efficient and economical drug delivery. Also, the trend of incorporating NDDS for herbal drugs has also been adopted at industrial scale.

Chapter 7 entitled "Nanoparticulate Drug Delivery System: An Emphasis on Herbal Medicines" by Akshada Atul Bakliwal and coauthors, describes that nanotechnology is one of the leading technologies used worldwide. In this chapter, the use of various types of nanomaterials and nanocarriers are well described. The nanoparticulate drug delivery is most commonly used due to its safety, efficacy and targeted drug delivery. It also enhances the solubility and bioavailability, increases the therapeutic value and reduces the dosing frequency. Nowadays, researchers focus on development of drug delivery system using herbal medicaments using a scientific justification. But there are many challenges in this like conduction of clinical research, pharmacological and toxicological evaluation, etc. Still the herbal medicines are more preferred over the conventional medicines due to its fewer side effects. This chapter focuses on different herbal drugs which are encapsulated in different formulation of nanocarriers.

Chapter 8 entitled "Herbal Formulation and Hepatitis B" by Tung Bui Thanh and his associates. Hepatitis B is an infectious disease caused by hepatitis B virus (HBV) that is one of the most serious public health problem in the world. Despite some common approved drugs, they bring about dose-dependent adverse effects or drug resistance. Therefore, safe and useful new HBV therapeutics are absolutely essential. Medicinal plants have particularly beneficial to treat HBV-infected patients. Traditional medicines have many bioactive compounds that are potential and effective as antiviral candidates including esculetin, helioxanthin, oxymatrine, epigallocatechin-3-gallate, wogonin, alkaloids, polysaccharides, etc.

Chapter 9 entitled "Therapeutic Enhancement of Flavonoids Efficacy as Anticancer Drugs Through Novel Drug Delivery Systems" by Anamika Basu. Flavonoids are a group of heterocyclic compounds that are well-known for their anti-cancer activity. Fruits and vegetables are the main dietary sources of flavonoids. Several mechanisms have been proposed for the effect of flavonoids to combat cancer. But before considering the flavonoids as chemotherapeutic drugs for cancer, a number of problems still need to be addressed before their therapeutic uses. Solubility may play major role in the therapeutic efficacy of flavonoids. Bioavailability of flavonoids are also affected by several other factors. Different types of flavonoids encapsulated nanoparticles have been developed to improve their effectiveness against different types of cancer.

Chapter 10 entitled "Phytosomes as a Novel Approach for Herbal Phytoconstituents" is written by Shweta Gedam and coauthors. The authors have described that nowadays, the phytoconstituents have great importance and used worldwide due to its less side effects. There is necessity of suitable drug delivery for the ideal delivery of active constituents. Considering that most of the herbal medicaments have poor aqueous solubility and bioavailability, to enhance the solubility and bioavailability of herbal extract, delivery via phytosomes is an innovative approach which is utilized successfully.

Chapter 11 entitled "Novel Approaches in Nutraceuticals" by Bhushan R. Rane and coauthors. In this chapter authors describe the status of commercialized nutraceuticals to meet the requirements of human in maintenance of well-beings. This objective is impelling development in the nutraceutical market places internationally. The rising popularity of these products appears to be bound to lodge the set in the new period. Its huge advancement has solutions for the sustained pharmaceutical and medicinal agents, and many researchers believe that the same will catalyze another energizing research in domain of nutraceuticals.

Chapter 12 entitled "Medicinal Plants and Their Formulation for the Management and Treatment of Gout" is very well structured by Tung Bui Thanh. This chapter describes that there are many valuable medicinal plants which can be applied to reduce signals and towards the treatment of gout's. The main chemical compounds such as flavonoids, alkaloids have shown strong effect against gout. Therefore, it is necessary to study deeper details about medicinal plants and find new active compounds against Gout's disease.

It would be catering the needs of students and researchers encompassing the recent strategies of Herbal Formulations through novel drug delivery systems for human health. Only a few publications have dealt with these topics inclusively so far. The person has to refer numerous sources for variety of topics. Such all information will be collectively presented in our work. The book integrates a wide variety of research and theories in an attempt to reveal their diversity and capture the recent techniques employed by developers and content experts in the herbal formulation field.

Rajesh Kumar Kesharwani
Nehru Gram Bharati (Deemed), Prayagraj, India

Raj K. Keservani
Faculty of B. Pharmacy, C.S.M. Group of Institution, Prayagraj, India

Anil K. Sharma
GD Goenka University, India

Chapter 1
Therapeutic Efficacy of Herbal Formulations Through Novel Drug Delivery Systems

Arvind Kumar Singh Chandel
Council of Scientific and Industrial Research, Central Salt and Marine Chemicals Research Institute (CSIR–CSMCR), Bhavnagar, India

Nutan Bhingradiya
Council of Scientific and Industrial Research, Central Salt and Marine Chemicals Research Institute (CSIR–CSMCR), Bhavnagar, India

ABSTRACT

The herbal-based drugs have been getting wide attention over the last few decades. The herbal drugs have been used from the ancient times, but the dose accuracy, efficacy, and treatment was just based on symptomatic observatory. Modern research is focused on pure bioactive compound instead of crude. The researchers are trying to apply the current advanced nanotechnology-based knowledge on the herbal medicines to improve efficacy and reduces the unwanted pharmacological actions' adverse effects of the therapeutic molecules. The many novel drug delivery systems available used for the herbal bioactive molecules include polymeric micelle, injectable hydrogel, nano gel, nano emulsions, microsphere, polymeric nanoparticles, nano capsules, liposomes, phytosomes, transferosomes, dendrimer, and ethosomes. This chapter highlights the existing research and development of current standing of the of various novel formulations especially for the herbal bioactive molecules and summarizes their active ingredients, commercial formulations, route of drug administration, and pharmacological activity.

DOI: 10.4018/978-1-7998-4453-2.ch001

1. INTRODUCTION

Nature having all solutions for the technically developing world with evolving several health problems and diseases. Naturally available medicinal plant-based bioactive constituents are using by human beings for several centuries (Davies, 2000). From the past several decades, the researchers are focused on the development of new pharmaceutical active ingredient, in the Ayurveda medicine system, the medicine for the disease or symptom was available, but the mechanism and active ingredient dose was not very well cleared. In other words, we can say the future technology or system is embedded in their beginning or past before ancient chemists started to make silver-based tablets for all kind of diseases and infections and before pharmaceutical industries involved our cooperative health that arises billions of dollars. But in ancient times, every medicine system was depending on the plant sources; the plant being man's only chemist for ages of ailments in place of mainstream medicine (Saraf et al., 2010; Medina et al., 2014). There are several reasons for the extensive acceptance of herbal based medicine system: After the awareness of the active pharmaceutical ingredients and their pharmacological action researchers are focused in to engineer theirs pharmacological action, dose, side effects, route of administration, pharmacokinetics and pharmacodynamics correlation to understand the overall conclusion which makes the drug molecule safer, effective and patients compliance. The novel drug delivery system should possess some of the essential feathers, such as the delivery rate of the therapeutics should match the requirements and minimum therapeutic range throughout the treatment time. Besides, it should deliver the active form of the therapeutic molecule molecules at the actual site of action in a sustained and controlled manner (Sharma et al., 2006; Terreno et al., 2008).

The isolation of pure bioactive herbal molecule is a big task, because of the crude herbal having thousands of molecules from there a single desired intact active molecule isolation is a challenging task to the researchers, after that the quality, purity testing, characterization and biological evaluation of the pharmacokinetics and pharmacodynamics are required a series of analytical and biochemical lab facility required, along with experts. For every single new molecule, the isolation, characterization, and activity evaluation required separate process validation (Sharma et al., 2006; Terreno et al., 2008).

Nanotechnology is a rapidly gowning field of science because of its massive involvement in other fields of science, which makes them advance and user friendly. Nowadays the nanotechnology using almost all significant areas of science, such as agriculture, medical science, pharmaceutical science, computer science, food technology, textile technology, polymer science, chemical, and biological science. The chapter mainly discusses the use of nanotechnology in the pharmaceutical, mostly on the delivery of the various herbal active molecules (Paroha et al., 2017; Paroha et al., 2018). Today's primary concern is the pharmaceutical industries having potent drug molecules by their clinical use is limited due to their poor water solubility, protein interaction, low distribution, or their short half-life due to that they are facing a challenge in drug development. In another hand less potent pharmaceutical molecule which having good water solubility become suitable candidates for the drug development, in either case, there is every time degree of compromise between desired parameters and actual parameters taken by the manufacturers. Such type of distinguishing tradeoffs causes the production of the less active and poor quality formulation. However, the recent advances in the field of nanotechnology and pharmaceuticals achieved to solve the above-mentioned problem at a certain level, but still, this area requires a lot of effort to accomplish the goal; it has become gradually possible to overcome such type of problem. By using advanced nanotechnology techniques, it's possible to increase water solubility, the half-life of the drug molecules. The interpapillary research, such as pharmaceutical and nanotechnology, together able to solve several exiting problems, which above mentioned as one example that showing the power and possibilities of nanotechnology specially in the pharmaceutical industries (Shiet et al., 2010).

In ancient time the Ayurveda medicine system had involved in the human development and development of the existing medical system from the beginning when humans were learning about the trial and error basis their medicinal and nutritional importance to select various plants for the food and treatment of different kind of infections and diseases that information and application knowledge of various plants as herbal medicines. However, throughout the twentieth century, predominantly in the Western part of the globe are involved in the substitution of the herbal medicines by synthetic allopathic medicine system. Whereas at the present time, the allopathic medicine system the chief medicine system across the globe for the treatments of nearly all kinds of health problems and disease, the advanced allopathic and drug delivery formulations equipped with modern nanotechnology, especially in various developed countries. But still, multiple developing counties partly using their conventional medicine system because they cannot afford the costly allopathic medicines (Bonifacio et al., 2014). As per reports of the WHO, approximately 80% of peoples from developing nations partly still depend on their conventional medicines for their primary health needs (Pires et al., 2011).

The current data regarding the source of drugs or the basics of drugs shows that the maximum of the drugs molecules that are in use today are based on natural products. Combination of advance nanotechnology-based approach for delivering herbal bioactive products increased drug stability, reduces drug-protein binding, increase drug half-life, and toxic properties by gathering of drugs to the unspecified targeted extents reduces their first-pass metabolism, increase bioavailability and rise their patient acceptance due to ease in drug administration and suitability (Alexander et al., 2016; Gunasekaran et al., 2014).

The crude herbal extract possessed thousands of the organic-inorganic compounds along with their active molecules that complexity of active constituents makes it very challenging to the progress of advanced drug delivery system development for various kinds of herbal bioactive compounds (Alexander et al., 2016; Gunasekaran et al., 2014). Hence, for enhancing the drug bioavailability, half-life, and targeted delivery and dose accuracy, there have to be nanotechnology drug delivery systems that can able to overcome all above-mentioned problems which associated with conventional dosage form and defend the therapeutic molecules from the other interruptions of the body such reticuloendothelial system, low pH, and metabolism process. So, for an improved therapeutic consequence, it is essential to integrate herbal drugs based bioactive molecules in advanced nanotechnology and interdisciplinary areas-based drug delivery systems (Alexander et al., 2016; Gunasekaran et al., 2014).

Thousands of medicinal plants are well characterized by researchers. They have reported and developed a database about their full active constitutes and biological and pharmacological actions of those herbal medicinal plants. Maximum pharmacologically active plant constituents are founds into their various plant part leaf, root, stem flower, etc. extracts, such as alkaloids, tannins, flavonoids, resins, gums, oleoresin, and terpenoids, are having potent pharmacological activity, but reveal a poor water solubility, and absorption, so that are incapable of permeating plasma membranes, have less polarity high molecular weight, and exhibited poor GIT absorption and assimilation, subsequently decreases the bioavailability and efficacy of the bioactive molecules. The various research outcomes have revealed that phytochemicals show good pharmacological activity in their different type of in vitro assays. Still, those results cannot reproduce in them in-vivo experiments. To overcome above-mentioned problems, the bioactive molecules are delivered with advanced nanotechnological techniques (Holmberg et al., 2002).

2. HERBAL MEDICINE

The herbal medicine may be considered as dosage form from various part of the plant, which may be useful for treatment, diagnosis, and nutritional values for the human and animal. At the present time, whatever advanced therapeutics are available in the various medicine system, those all are closely connected to the herbal medicine system. The herbal medicines are herbal medicinal plants, which comprise as bioactive constituents such as alkaloid, essential oils, glycosides, terpenoids, gums, fatty oils, juices and many other medicinally important substances. These material basically found in the various part of the plant such as fruit, leaves, seed, bark, cork stem, root, or other parts of the plants entirely or segregated by using various separation isolation techniques such as percolation, decoction, maceration, extraction, purification, fractionation with the different solvent system, etc. (Rowland, 1999; Gullett et al., 2010; Johnson, 2007)

Alkaloids belong to the family of naturally occurring chemical compounds, which are majorly having basic nitrogen atoms. This class also covers several relevant molecules having weakly acidic and neutral characteristics. Various synthetically prepared molecules having the same structure are also named as alkaloids. Hydrogen, nitrogen, and carbon are the main constituents in alkaloids, while sulfur and oxygen are also present in alkaloids. Bromine, phosphorus, and chlorine are rarely found in it (Yan et al., 2010; Dewick et al., 2002; Bruneton, 1995).

Naturally, alkaloids are synthesized in plants, bacteria, animals, and fungi. Crude alkaloids are extracted from the source and then purified and separated by acid-base extraction. Alkaloids are common in some specific groups of flowering plant species. More significant than 3,000 types of different alkaloids have been recognized out of more than 4,000 plant varieties. Opium poppy, ergot fungus Ranunculaceae, Amaryllidaceae, and Solanaceae are some of the alkaloid-containing families. Some animal species also contain alkaloids, for example, Castor Canadensis and poison-dart frogs (Yan et al., 2010; Dewick et al., 2002; Bruneton 1995).

Alkaloids show a broad spectrum of pharmacological activities such as antiasthma (Ephedrine), antimalarial (Quinine), anticancer (Homoharringtonine), vasodilatory (vincamine), cholinomimetic (Galantamine), antiarrhythmic (Quinidine), antibacterial (Chelerythrine), analgesic (Morphine), and antihyperglycemic activities (Piperine). Out of them, several were used in ancient times and find use in modern medication. Some of the alkaloids are exhibit psychotropic effects (psilocin) and stimulant effects (cocaine, nicotine, caffeine, and theobromine). These are employed in recreational drugs or as an entheogenic ritual. Several alkaloids are toxic also (atropine and tubocurarine), the secondary herbal metabolites and their applications are described in figure (Yan et al., 2010; Dewick et al., 2002; Bruneton, 1995).

3. BIOAVAILABILITY OF HERBAL MEDICINES

Bioavailability is a very critical parameter for any pharmacologically active molecules.

The bioavailability is in the simple terms the amount of the drug administered into the body and the fraction which successfully reaches into the peripheral circulation known as bioavailability. The bioavailability of any therapeutic molecules mainly depends on their route of administration (Griffin, 2009). As per various research and investigations, the highest bioavailability can achieve by intravenous route (100%), Sublingual (100%), intramuscular (75%), Subcutaneous (75%), Oral (50%), Rectal (50%), Nasal

Figure 1. Classification of herbal medicines
(Yan et al., 2010; Dewick et al., 2002; Bruneton, 1995)

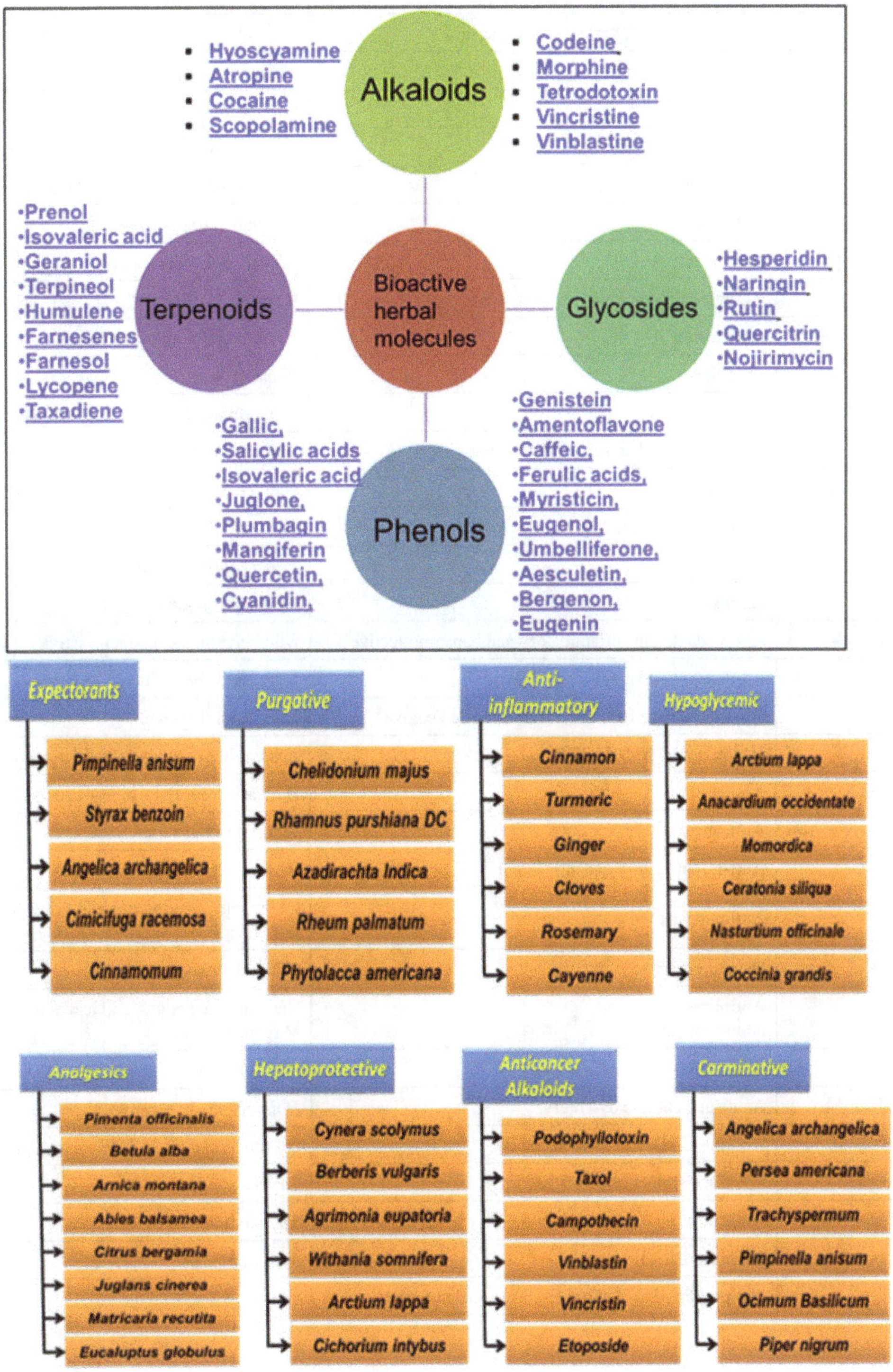

Table 1. Different types of bioactive constituents of natural products. (Subramanian et al. 2016; Kokate et al. 2003; Evans 2009).

Phytochemical	Pharmacological action	Biological source
Apigenin	Alzheimer's disease	Chamomile tea, celery,
Quercitine	Antioxidant	Quercetin
Berberine	Antidiabetic	Barberry, Turmeric, Goldenseal, Oregon grape
Luteolin	Anticancer	Green pepper, Olive oil, Celery, Peppermint
Eugenol	Antiseptic	*Eugenia Caryophyllus*
Combretastatin A-4	Anticancer	African bush-willow tree,
Hesperidin	Antihyperlipidemic, Antihypertensive, Antidiabetic	Citrus fruit
Ferulic acid	Antioxidant	Coffee, Apple, Peanut, Orange,
Visnagin	Vasodilator	*Ammi visnaga*
Ursolic acid	Antitumor	Peppermint, Rosemary, Apples, Lavender, thyme,
Ellagic acid	Antioxidant and anti-proliferative/anti-cancer	European red oak, North American white oak,
Epigallocatechin gallate	Antioxidant	Green tea, Black tea, Plums, Onions, Hazelnuts,
Curcumin	Antimicrobial, antioxidant, astringents	Turmeric
Pilocarpine	Glaucoma	*Pilocarpus cearensis*
Gallic acid	Antioxidant	Indian gooseberry
Thymoquinone	Antioxidant, anti-inflammatory and hepatoprotective	wild bergamot and Nigella sativa
Shatavarin	Antioxidant and anti-inflammatory	*Asparagus racemosus*
Emodin	Tyrosine-kinase inhibitor, antineoplastic laxative	Buckthorn, Rhubarb,
Ouabain	Inhibiting the Na^{+}/K^{+}-ATPase	*Acokanthera schimperi* and *Strophanthus gratus*
Beta-Lapachone	Anticancer	Bark and leaves of Chinese catalpa
Gambogic acid	Anticancer	Indian gamboge tree (resin)
Nobiletin	Anti-inflammatory and anti-tumor	Peels of citrus fruits
Resveratrol	Antioxidants,	Outer fruit covering of mulberries, blueberries, raspberries,
Silibinin	Hepatoprotective	Milk thistle seeds
Honokiol	Antitumorigenic, Antithrambotic	Bark and seed cones, and leaves of genus Magnolia
Noscapine	Antitussive	Poppy family
Conessine	Acute and chronic dysentery	*Holarrhena pubescens*
Hyoscyamine	Antimuscarinic	*Datura stramonium, Solanum lycopersicum*
Strychnine	Erectile dysfunction	*Strychnos nux-vomica*
Triptolide	Anticancer	Thunder god vine
Oleandrin	Toxic cardiac glycoside	*Nerium oleander*
Zerumbone	Antiproliferative, Antioxidant, Anti-inflammatory	Ginger

(80%), Transdermal (80%) (Tripathi, 2013). When any drug administrated by other than the intravenous route, a significant amount does not reach into the systemic circulation due to several factors hinders, such as hepatic first-pass metabolism, absorption of the drug-protein binding, the aqueous solubility of the therapeutic molecules, etc. The bioavailability of the phytochemicals also faces a similar situation to attain maximum bioavailability when we eat any polyphenol containing food the polyphenol influenced by several factors such as absorption in the gut, excretion by glucuronide conjugation, intestinal microbial metabolism, plasma drug kinetics, bile, urinary excretion, tissue accumulation and various steps of liver gut metabolism and other several types of metabolites in the blood circulation, serum albumin binding, cell assimilation and metabolism of the therapeutic molecules (Manach, 2001). The concentration of active constituent of the various herbal formulations in the plasma is measured by the complex bioavailability. For example, when catechin takes, it gets absorbed fast but affected by its dimerization. Flavones are exhibit slow absorption due to conjugation with disaccharides. Among the flavones, the isoflavones show the highest absorption rate. However, anthocyanins have high absorption, but their bioavailability is less among all flavonoids (Nemeth, 2003).

The bioavailability of the herbal bioactive ingredients is a well-known issue, and Numerous approaches have been established by the researchers to enhance their absorption. The chemical derivatization of the phytochemicals was applied, and compounds exhibited an enhanced bioavailability. This strategy was the mother of several other concepts, such as the screening of the suitable chemical analog the necessary. Establishment of substitute procedures in combination with previous one for the bioactive molecules with other chemically similar molecules as adjuvants encouraging the absorption of the bioactive molecules and improving the bioavailability of the phytochemicals (Khajuria et al., 1998). One of another method involves widespread in this strategy researchers work according to the molecules structure and modification and try to make the molecules which capable enhance half-life and absorption without altering the pharmacological activity of the molecules. In this research, several formulation and preparation come under this category, such as nanoparticles, micelles, liposomes, Nanoemulsions, nanogel, dendrimers, drug conjugation, microsphere or other complexes. The Phytosome® is one of the newest approaches which claims a well-defined pharmacokinetic profile without the use of any adjuvants or structural modification of the phytochemical constituents and without altering the pharmacological efficacy of the molecules.

Most of the phytochemical which consumed by the human having less bioavailability because of the rapid first metabolism and exertion with less amount of absorption, these are the key problem which is to be faced before applying these phytochemicals for the treatment of disease and as a nutrient supplement. However, the immersion of advanced nanotechnology-based drug delivery systems has established to enhance the bioavailability of the phytochemicals.

4. NANOTECHNOLOGY-BASED ADVANCED DRUG DELIVERY SYSTEMS FOR HERBAL THERAPEUTICS

The nanotechnology-based dosage forms of the active herbal biomolecules have amazing advantages, these advanced nanotechnology-based dosage forms such as nanoemulsion, polymeric micelles, liposomes, spherosomes, nanoparticles, and metal nanoparticles conjugated with the active biomolecules. These series of advanced drug delivery formulations are enhanced the bioactive molecule solubility, stability, bioavailability, tissue macrophage distribution, localization, clearance from the body, metabo-

Figure 2. List of different nanotechnology-based drug delivery system
(Awasthi et al., 2009; Lawrence et al., 2012; Chien, et al., 1991)

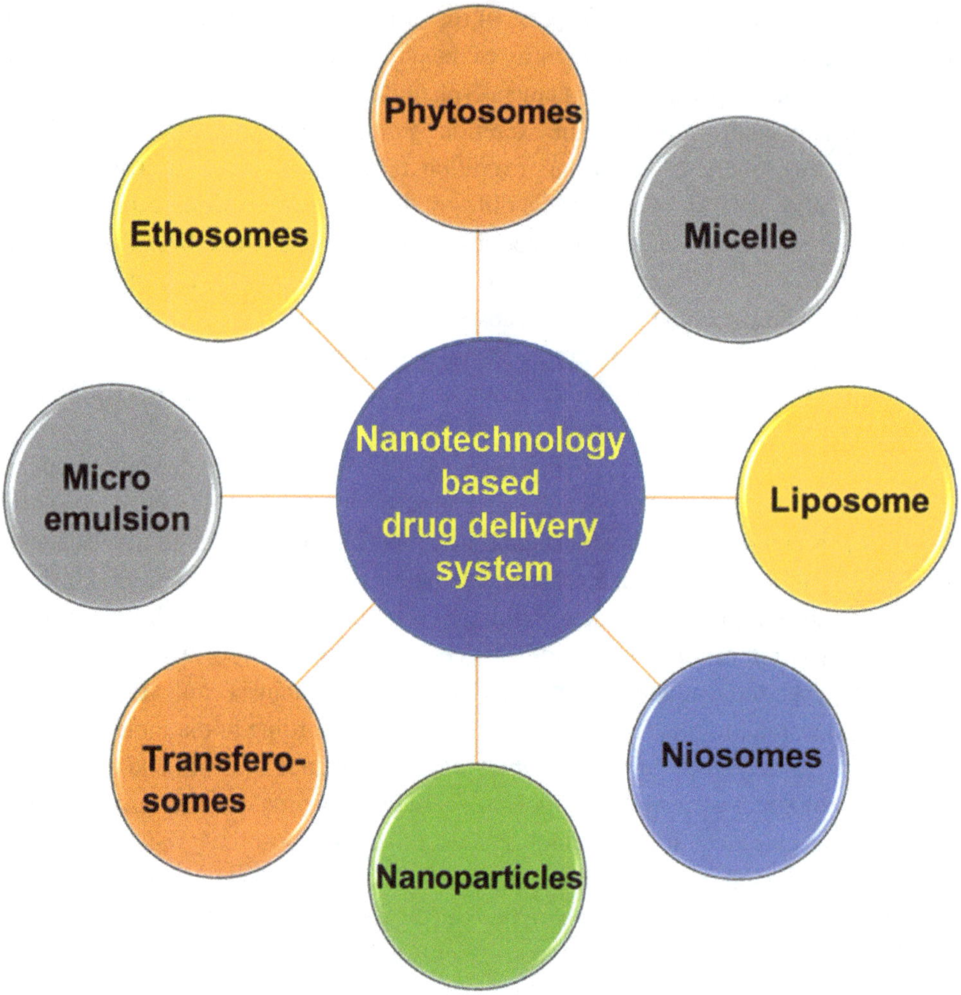

lism, prolonged-release, and minimize the toxic side effects, biomagnification, plasma protein binding, degradation of the bioactive herbal molecules. Therefore, nano-sized formulations of bioactive herbal molecules have a potential future scope for improving their pharmacological efficacy, dose minimization reducing the toxicity and overwhelming hitches related to crude herbal medicines. Liposomes, micelles, nanoparticles, which are biocompatible/biodegradable carriers these can encapsulate both types of molecules hydrophilic as well as hydrophobic ingredients (Bhattacharya et al., 2009).

The amphiphilic polymer-based nanoparticles, micelles, liposomes are deals the improved therapeutic index of several drugs, which are requires to enhanced bioavailability, tissue permeability, increases the drug concentration above the minimum inhibitory concentration, prolong and controlled release over the time, trigger release as well as minimize the side effect, and dose frequency, such as anticancer drugs. These formulations offer the site targeted drug delivery by tagging the molecular markers over the surface of the liposome, polymeric micelles and nanoparticles such as, folate, biotin, streptavidin, glucosamine, and ester and thiol linkage in the polymers; all promote the site-directed delivery which overcomes the

Figure 3. Advantages of novel drug delivery systems
(Vyas et el. 2008, Chandel et al. 2016)

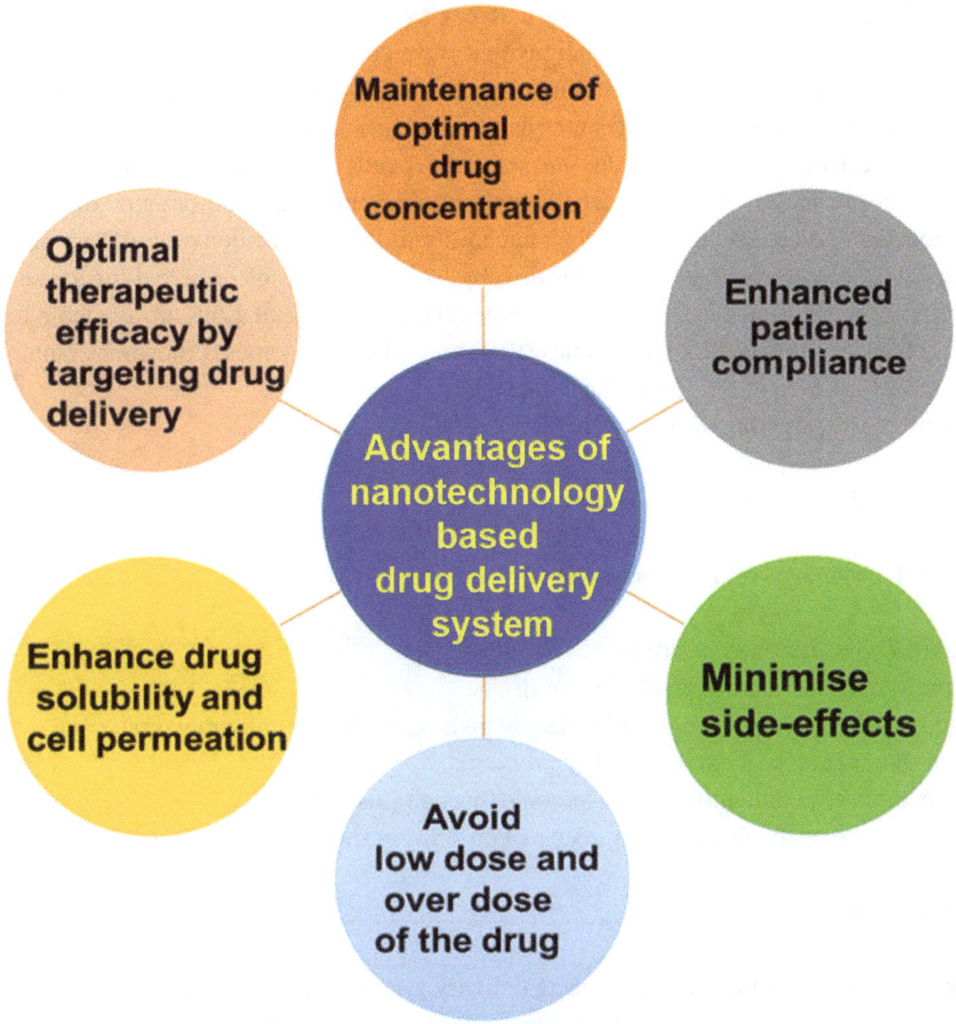

problem of the non-targeted systemic toxicity of the drugs (Awasthi et al., 2009; Lawrence et al., 2012; Chien, et al., 1991).

Nano sized advanced formulation having several other advantages like, (i) easy and tunable body clearance, which can customize according to the requirement. (ii) Use of biocompatible and biodegradable FDA approved polymeric materials. (iii) avoids the non-targeted drug delivery and minimizes the toxicity of cytotoxic drugs such as anti-cancer agents. (iv) controlled and triggered the release of the herbal bioactive therapeutics' molecules. The easy alteration pharmacokinetic properties of herbal bioactive therapeutics by varying the chemical structure of the polymers. Nanosize formulations (< 70 nm) are easily passed through the reticuloendothelial system.

Likewise, the other polymeric Nanocarriers' systems, such as dendrimers, metal nanoparticles conjugate, transferosomes, ethosomes, nano-emulsion, and neosomes, are extremely useful associations and find numerous benefits in the delivery of herbal bioactive compound delivery.

4.1 The Advanced Vesicular Delivery System

The lipid and polymer-based advanced drug delivery system, which has a vesicular structure, may define as well organized molecular associations that were containing one or more concentric bilayers fashioned as an outcome of the self-assembling of amphiphilic construction in the aqueous environment. The hydrophilic moiety makes the shell outer part of the vesicle, and the hydrophilic part is the core, the location of the drug or guest molecules entrapment depends on their chemical nature. The vesicular delivery systems are mainly important for the hydrophobic molecules and targeted delivery of drugs or herbal bioactive molecules because of their capability to localize the delivery of drug or herbal bioactive molecules at the desired site of action thereby let down drugs of or herbal bioactive molecules concentration at the additional sites in the body. Several types of formulations are available Liposomes, Emulsomes, Transferosomes, Pharmacosomes, Virosomes. Enzymosomes, Ethosomes, Sphingosomes, (Saraf, et al., 2010; Chien et al., 1991; Tacar et al., 2014)

Non- lipoidal site targeting drug carriers

1. Aquasomes 2. Ethosomes 3. Niosomes

The several advantages of the vesicular system are listed below

- Enhanced bioavailability of drugs.
- It is prolonged the circulation lifetime of drugs.
- Site-directed delivery of drugs molecules by tagging with molecular markers.
- Solved the drug stability and solubility problems.
- The toxicity of specific molecules overcome through this approach.
- Trigger release of the therapeutic molecule can achieve through this method.

4.2 Phytosomes

Phytosomes is a member of the advanced drug delivery system, which is made up phospholipid this is one of the very promising systems for the delivery of the herbal bioactive constituents.

Phytosomes shows better bioavailability because of its ability to overcome of maximum conventional drug delivery challenges, by the better pharmacokinetic and absorbance (Atmakuri et al., 2010). Over the before several decades the physiochemists are identified numerous medicinal plants which having potent pharmacological activity against the disease, but the many of the active phytoconstituents are the water-soluble in nature such alkaloids, flavonoids, glycosides, tannins, terpenoids, etc. are poorly absorbed by the GIT because of their some limitations such as high molecular weight, improper hydrophilic and lipophilic balance and many more due to that this moiety unable to diffuse across the plasma membrane, resultant of this very low bioavailability occurred. The possibility of a loss of activity during extraction and purification is also a major concern for the phytochemical drug molecules. Extracts when it takes its chances its chances orally to degrade in the gastric pH. It has been noticed by researchers the phytochemicals make complex with several substances such as other pharmacologically useful substances and enhanced bioavailability significantly, such as herbal extracts and phytochemical molecules and their individual chemical molecule. The GIT absorption of the phospholipids is also promoted by several kinds of nutrients. The Phytosome® is a type of advance dosage form with various features as mentioned above in this solid dispersion based formulation especially for the herbal chemical ingredients over a dietary class of lecithin based phospholipid matrix, and entrapment of the phytochemical basically hydrophobic, provides an amphiphilic milieu which able to prevents its self-aggregation, degradation, increase half-life, etc. Phytosomes have their specific goal to improve the drug molecules' bioavailability of poor hydrophilic, hydrophobic drug molecules and whole mechanisms like the absorption of the dietary fat molecules. The Phytosomes are the company proprietary right technology by multinational top drug and nutraceutical manufacturers. This company mainly incorporates the bioactive herbal extracts and water-soluble ingredients into phospholipid matrix to produce lipid companionable molecular complexes, named as phytosomes, for enhanced bioavailability (Bombardelli et al. 1989). For the optimization of bioavailability of the various phytochemical basically, Phytosome®s are used. The phytochemical ingredients which having high polarity or high-water solubility also cannot cross the lipid barrier of the cell membrane or other cells where formulation applied. So, the Phytosome® assists in the optimizing the molecular polarity of the ingredients and adjust according to the better absorption, so the phytochemical gets absorbed by the phytosome without any extra effort. In other words, the Phytosome® based herbal formulation is a result of the integration of the nanotechnology into the pharmaceutical science that work synergistically and upgrade the delivery system which overcomes the all conventional problems so we can say it is an advanced carrier system for poorly water-soluble and highly water-soluble phytochemical ingredients. Into the mechanism of the Phytosome® system, the poor hydrophilic bioavailable phytochemical ingredient is encored with the phospholipid, which polar in nature and develops an important portion of the micellar outermost covering layer, distinct from the liposomes system. In the liposomal system, basically, the active ingredient is situated inner side the micellar structure, which comprises phospholipids: the cell membrane made-up phospholipid and proteins. The major part is the phophospholipid. Phospholipids are working as natural digestive assistances in higher living organisms such as humans and animals and as transporters molecules for both hydrophilic and lipophilic molecules. Phospholipids are miscible in both hydrophilic and lipophilic environments and are shows well abortion and bioavailability via the oral route of delivery.

Riva et al. reported that enhanced oral absorption of quercetin by through quercetin loaded phytosome®. The food-grade lecithin used for the preparation of the phytomes and established that delivery of that the substantial enhancements in the invivo as well as in vivo experiment for the quercetin phytosome formulation as compared other quercetin-based formulation (Riva et al., 2019).

The bioavailability compared to conventional phytochemical ingredients through the Phytosomes are more as owed to their improved volume to cross the plasma membrane and eventually reached into the peripheral circulation system (Ajazuddin et al., 2010; Carini et al., 2001; Kidd et al., 1997). Several curcumin-based food supplements which are commercially available such as available are BCM-95®, Theracurmin®, Meriva®, Sabinsa's Curcumin C3 complex®, MicroActive Curcumin®. and Longvida® these products are tested clinically and exhibited better bioavailability less toxicity with antioxidative, anticancer, hepatoprotective, and apoptotic properties Alzheimer's disease, osteoarthritis, get enhancement successfully into their vascular endothelial function, and regulates gene transcription factors. (Sundaramoorthy et al., 2019.)

4.3 Ethosomes

The transdermal drug delivery system exhibited better performance in comparison to oral drug delivery system because of in this system eliminates first-pass metabolism and gastrointestinal interferences of

Figure 4. Typical structure of phytosome
(karimi et al 2015, Ajazuddin et al., 2010; Carini et al., 2001; Kidd et al., 1997)

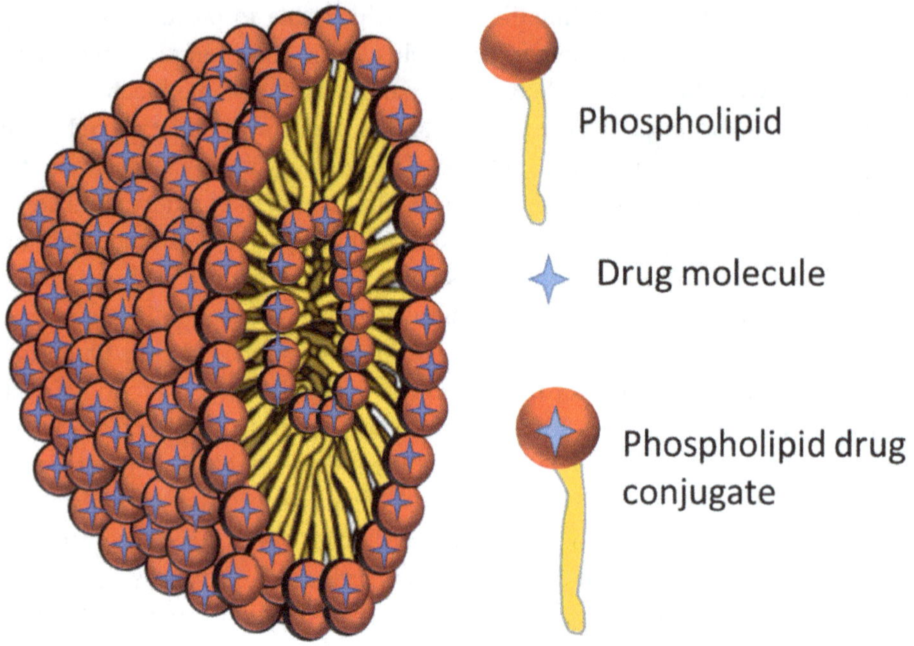

the therapeutic molecule, but then the disadvantage of TDDS is it comes across the skin stratum corneum barrier properties, this barrier layer allows only the lipophilic drugs moiety molecular weight < 500 Da can pass across to this layer. To enhance the topical route drug permeation various techniques are developed, with the application of different advanced cell membrane penetration enhancer activity, such as sonophoresis, phonophoresis iontophoresis, etc. transferosomes, liposomes, niosomes and ethosomes also have been extensively described for the enhancement of drug permeability across the various skin layer.

Chemical penetration enhancers can enhance the drug penetrability across the stratum corneum barrier layer of the skin (Touitou et al., 2000; Schreir et al., 1994).

Ethosomes are like liposomes, but these are ethanolic liposomes. In other words, ethosomes is a type of noninvasive drug delivery transporters that facilitates the drugs molecules to cross the skin stratum corneum barrier layer and allow to the drug molecules to reach into the systemic blood circulation with their intact pharmacological activity. Ethosomes are very soft, flexible vesicles structure, which is customized for improved drug delivery. The ethosomes vesicles are very important for their cellular communication and particle transportation. This formulation also capable release the drug in controlled and sustained release kinetics for a long time. Ethosomes also protects the drug molecules from cellular immune response and other cellular immune responses (Touitou et al., 1997).

The mechanism behind the ethosomal drug delivery is the well-reported. The component of the ethosome phospholipids and ethanol are act synergistically to improve the drug permeation across the stratum corneum barrier layer of the skin. Ethanol act as a softener for the cell membrane lipid bilayers

Table 2. List of reported phytosome based herbal formulations (Afrin et al., 2018)

Brand Name	Plant Active/Extracts	Botanical Source	Biological Activity
18B-Glycyrrhetinic acid Phytosome	Glycyrrhetinic acid	Root of *Glycyrrhiza glabra*	Soothing, Lenitive
Bosexil	Boswellic acids	Resin of Boswellia serrata	Soothing, Anti-photo ageing
Casperome	boswellic acids	Resin of Boswellia serrata	Joint health
Centella Asiatica selected Triterpenes Phytosome	Selected triterpenes	Leaf of *Centella asiatica*	Anti-wrinkles, Collagen repairment
Curcuvet	Curcuminoids	Rhizome of *Curcuma longa*	Antioxidants
Ginkgo biloba dimeric flavonoids Phytosome	ginkgetin	Leaf of Ginkgo biloba	Vasokinetic, Lipolytic, Phosphodiesterase inhibitor
Ginkgo biloba terpenes Phytosome	Ginkgo terpenes bilobalide, ginkgolides A, B, C, J	Leaf of Ginkgo biloba	Soothing, Lenitive
Escin ß-sitosterol Phytosome	Escin ß-sitosterol	Fruit of horse chestnut	Capillaroprotective
Ginkgoselect Phytosome Ginkgo biloba Phytosome	Ginkgo flavone glucosides, ginkgo terpenes, bilobalide and ginkgolides	Leaf of Ginkgo biloba	Antioxidant, Cognition and Vasokinetic, blood circulation enhancer
Ginseng IDB Phytosome Ginselect Phytosome	Ginseng constituents	Root of *Panax ginseng*	Adaptogen, Tonic
	Dimeric flavonoids from	Leaf of Ginkgo biloba	Cognitive enhancer
Greenselect Phytosome	Polyphenols	Leaf of green tea	Antioxidant, fat absorption inhibitor
Hawthorn phytosome	Rhamnoside and Vitexin	Flowering top of Crataegus spp.	Antioxidant and Cardioprotective,
Grape seed phytosome Leucoselect Phytosome	proanthocyanidins	Seed of *Vitis vinifera*	Antioxidant and Cardioprotective,
Meriva® Turmeric Phytosome	Curcuminoids	Seed of Curcuma longa	Anti-inflammatory
Mirtoselect phytosome	Vaccinium myrtillus	Berries of *Vaccinium myrtillus*	Prostate cancer
Proanthocyanidin A_2 Phytosome	Proanthocyanidin A2	Bark of horse chestnut	Anti-inflammatory
Quercefit	Quercetin	*Sophora japonica*	Sports nutrition, antioxidant activity
Quercevita	Quercetin	*Sophora japonica*	Soothing, lenitive, first aid for skin challenges
Rexatrol	Resveratrol	Rhizome of *Polygonum cuspidatum*	Antioxidant, Anti-ageing
Sericoside Phytosome	Sericoside	Root of *Terminalia sericea*	anti-inflammatory
Silybin Siliphos Phytosome	Silybin	Fruit of *Silybum marianum*	Antioxidant, Hepatoprotective
Sabalselect phytosome	Serenoa repens extract	*Serenoa repens*	Immune modulator
Silymarin Phytosome	Silybin-like substances	Fruit of *Silybum marianum*	Antioxidant, Hepatoprotective
Ubiqsome	coenzyme Q10	-	Cellular Energy
Virtiva	Ginkgo flavone glucosides, ginkgolides, bilobalide	Leaf of *Ginkgo biloba*	Cognitive enhancer
Vazguard – Bergamot Phytosome	Flavanols	Fruit juice of Citrus *bergamia Risso*	Healthy blood levels
Visnadex	Visnadin	*Ammi visnaga*	urolithiasis and hypertriglyceridemia

of the stratum corneum barrier layer of the epithelial cell and ethosomes works simultaneously by rearranging, altering and reducing the density cell membrane lipids bilayers. Thus, the extremely flexible and soft vesicle texture of an ethosomal preparation is preferably allowed to cross the altered structure of the stratum corneum layer of the skin and generate a Tartous path through several layers of skin and cell membrane. The therapeutic moiety release by the intimate fusion of ethosomes to the cell membranes in the deepest layer of the skin. Ethosomal drug delivery systems comprise numerous advantages, such as It's possible to deliver the high molecular weight biomacromolecules based therapeutics. The ethosomal based formulation is a passive, non-invasive method. These are applicable in the biomedical, veterinary, cosmetic pharmaceutical fields, Ethosomes are having a high degree of patient compliance because of semisolid form of ethosomal based drug is administrated (gel or cream) due to that this formulation having high degree of the patient's compliance. In the synthesis process, no involvement of non-FDA approved materials. So, we can say ethosaomal drug delivery system is very simple and easy to apply without any trend technical education as compare to the others such as sonophoresis, iontophoresis type of very complex, and tedious methods. It has enhanced drug permeation across the skin stratum corneum barrier layer (Abdulbaqi et al., 2016). This formulation is unable to release rapid bolus dose to attain instant minimum therapeutic level, while it's for controlled, sustained drug delivery for the long-time duration. Passable drug solubility in both hydrophilic and lipophilic milieus to spread into the skin microcirculation and get contact to the main systemic blood circulation. The considerable molecular weight of the therapeutic molecule limits bioavailability. It's quite expensive, so it's may not be economical. During synthesis, the yield is less. There may be chances of dermatitis skin or irritation due to excipients and penetration enhancers, which used in this formulation. The chances of ethosomes coalescence due to the evaporation of alcohol by improper capping of container (Mbah et al., 2014; Sudhakar et al., 2012).

4.4 Transferosome

The concept and term of the transferosomes comes in existence in 1991 coined by Gregor Cevc. A Transferosome is basically an artificial carrier or is an artificial vesicle that bears a resemblance to the normal cell vesicle. Therefore, it is a very promising approach for targeted and controlled herbal bioactive therapeutics delivery. Additionally, these shows stress-responsive and highly flexible, complex aggregate structure. It is an extremely deformable vesicle structure that contains a very tiny aqueous core structure surrounded by the compound lipid bilayer structure. Transferosome can cross various cellular transport barriers in a very efficient manner and then act as an herbal bioactive therapeutic molecule carrier which facilitates the targeted drug, non-invasive topical type of drug delivery, and exhibit controlled and sustained release of therapeutic agents. Transferosomes are a type of spontaneous formation of aggregates, and these structures are self-optimized, which possess extremely flexible lipid membranes, which facilitate to the therapeutic molecule's delivery either into or through the skin, which reliant on the application and route of the administration. These are flexible than the standard liposome structure and highly suitable for the topical administration. Transferosomes can overcome herbal bioactive therapeutic molecule permeation difficulties by their flexible and squeezing behavior along with the intracellular sealing lipid of the stratum corneum layer of the skin. The flexible behavior of transferosome membrane is achieved by the incorporation of suitable surface-active agents in a suitable amount that can be tailored according to the application and route of the administration. There are several advantages to the use of transferosomes, some of them listed below (Wu et al., 2019).

Transferosomes are capable of carrying a wide range of molecules such as antibiotics, antifungal, anticancer, anesthetic, analgesic, insulin, sex hormone, corticosteroids, gap junction protein, and albumin. Transferosomes able to cross from a very narrow gap from a 10-time small size gap of own size by without any deformation. These are having high loading capacity for the lipophilic molecules, about 90%. These are the very flexible structure which facilitates better penetration into the skin. They can load and deliver hydrophilic as well as the hydrophobic type of materials. These are making the depot system and release the drug molecules in a prolonged and controlled manner. Transferosomes are made-up of biocompatible, biodegradable materials, and these are delivering the therapeutic molecules at the desired size by protecting them from physical and chemical degradation and loss, also enhances

Figure 5. Typical Structure of ethosome
(Abdulbaqi et al., 2016)

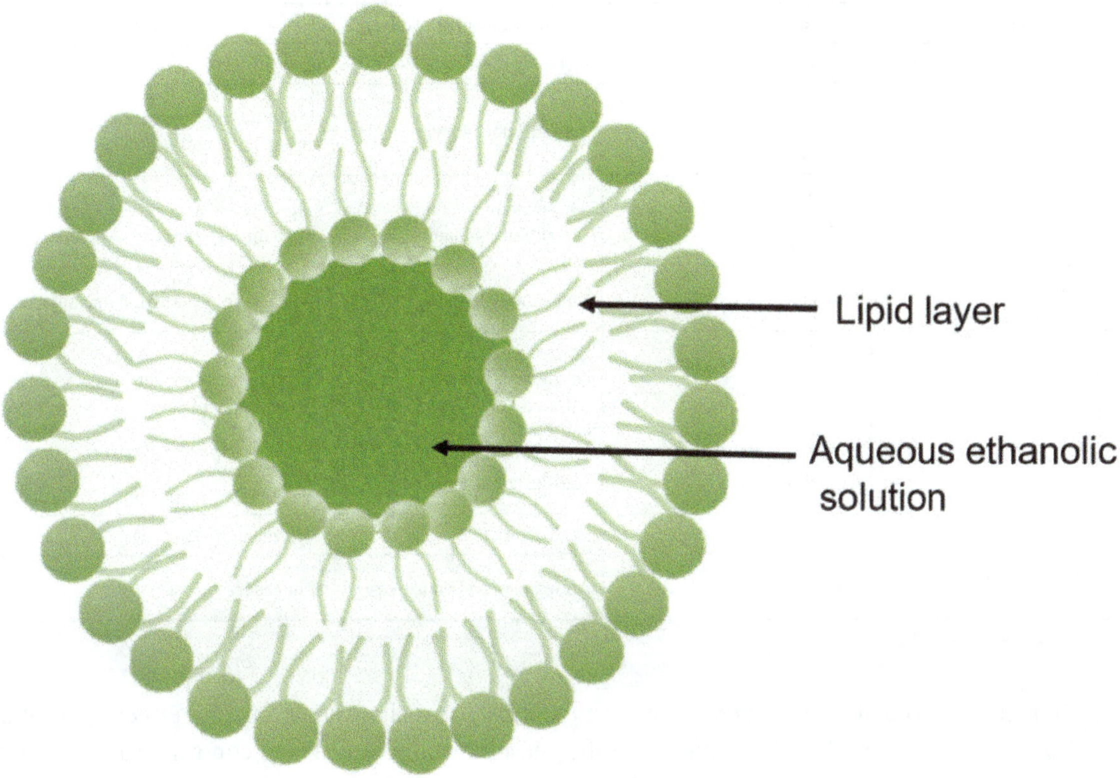

the bioavailability of the drug molecules. Researchers have used the transferosomes for the delivery of herbal drugs molecules such as the delivery of curcumin by transferosomes (Patel et al., 2009; Saraf et al., 2011), Lymph and transdermal targeting transferosomes of vincristine (Lu et al., 2007).

Recently Jiang et al., reported that transfersome-embedded oligopeptide hydrogel for topical chemotherapy of melanoma was reported with enhanced transdermal drug delivery (Jiang et al., 2018). Preparation of transferosomes of vincristine sulfate for percutaneous application (Lu et al., 2005) capsaicin-loaded transferosomes in arthritic rats (Sarwa et al., 2015). Delivery of colchicine by transferosome (Zheng et al., 2006). These reports also indicate the transferosomes are also very promising method for the delivery of the herbal bioactive molecules.

4.5 Niosome

Niosome are micro-sized polymeric structures which typically formed by the nonionic surfactant and cholesterol. It also comes under the novel drug delivery system. Generally, niosomes are designed on the combination of several non-ionic types of surfactants such as cholesterol and alkyl or dialkyl polyglycerol ether class followed by hydration in aqueous, (Buckton, 1995). Niosomes are of two types unilayer and multilayer. Niosomes are similar to plasma membrane structures. It possesses the bilayers of the surfactant. The hydrophilic layer generally faced the outer and inner layer composed of hydrophobic

Table 3. List of ethosomal based formulation (Kausar et al., 2019; Moolakkadath et al., 2019; Zang et al., 2019; Abdulbaqi et al., 2016; Fatima et al., 2014, Sebastian et al., 2012)

Botanical Name	Active Constituents	Pharmacological Activity	Application
Curcumin	Curcumin	Inflammatory	Topical Anti-Psoriatic
Glycyrrhiza glabra	Amonium Glycyrrhizinate Ethosomes	Anti-inflammatory	Enhanced drug permeation and their anti-inflammatory activity
Sophora alopecuroides	Sophora Alopecuroides ethosomes	Anti-endotoxic, anticancer and antiinflammatory	Ethosome enhances the delivery of drugs through the deep skin layer
Sesbania grandiflora	Sesbania	Ethosome Anti-microbial	Enhance Transdermal permeation
Podophyllum hexandrum	Podophyllotoxin	Purgative, antirheumatic, antiviral and antitumor	High drug loading and efficacy of the therapeutic molecule
Tripterygium wilfordi	Triptolide	Anti-inflammatory	high entrapment efficiency, good percutaneous permeability
Nigella sativa	Thymoquinone	Antibacterial	Treatment of skin acne
strawberry, persimmon, onion and apple	Fisetin	Antioxidant and anticancer	skin cancer

part. Niosomes also can load the herbal bioactive molecules in a significant amount, either hydrophilic or hydrophobic in nature. The release kinetic of the guest molecules are also in controlled and sustained also follow first-order kinetics (Ge et al., 2019; Azmin et al., 1985) The niosomal technology used for the treatment of many kind of disease, because this system used for the delivery of the drug on the targeted therapeutics, vaccines and drugs to the reticulo-endothelial system. Generally, niosomers are favorably taken up by the reticulo-endothelial system (RES). The circulating serum factors regulate the niosomes uptake this process known as opsonins; in this process niosome are marked for their clearance from the systemic blood circulation (Weissmann et al., 1975). Several body cells comprise the innate capability to recognize and fix with some precise carbohydrate determinants moiety, and this can be subjugated by niosomes to direct carrier system to cells. Niosomsl system also can change the drug metabolism, drug stability, clearance, prolonged circulation, protein binding, and half-life of a drug, thus diminishing the

Table 4. List of commercial ethosome based products (Verma et al., 2010)

Brand Name	Application	Manufactures
Cellulite EF	Enhance the fat break down and metabolism	Hampden Health, USA
Decorin cream	Anti-aging, skin repairing, skin tightening, scar and marks removal activity	Genome Cosmetics, Pennsylvania, US
Nanominox	Hair growth promotor	Sinere, Germany
Noicellex	Fat cutting effect	Novel therapeutic Technologies, Israel
Skin genuity	Cellulite treatment	Physonics, Nottingham, UK
Supravir cream	Herpes virus	Trima, Israel

Figure 6. Typical Structure of transferosome
(Patel et al., 2009; Saraf et al., 2011)

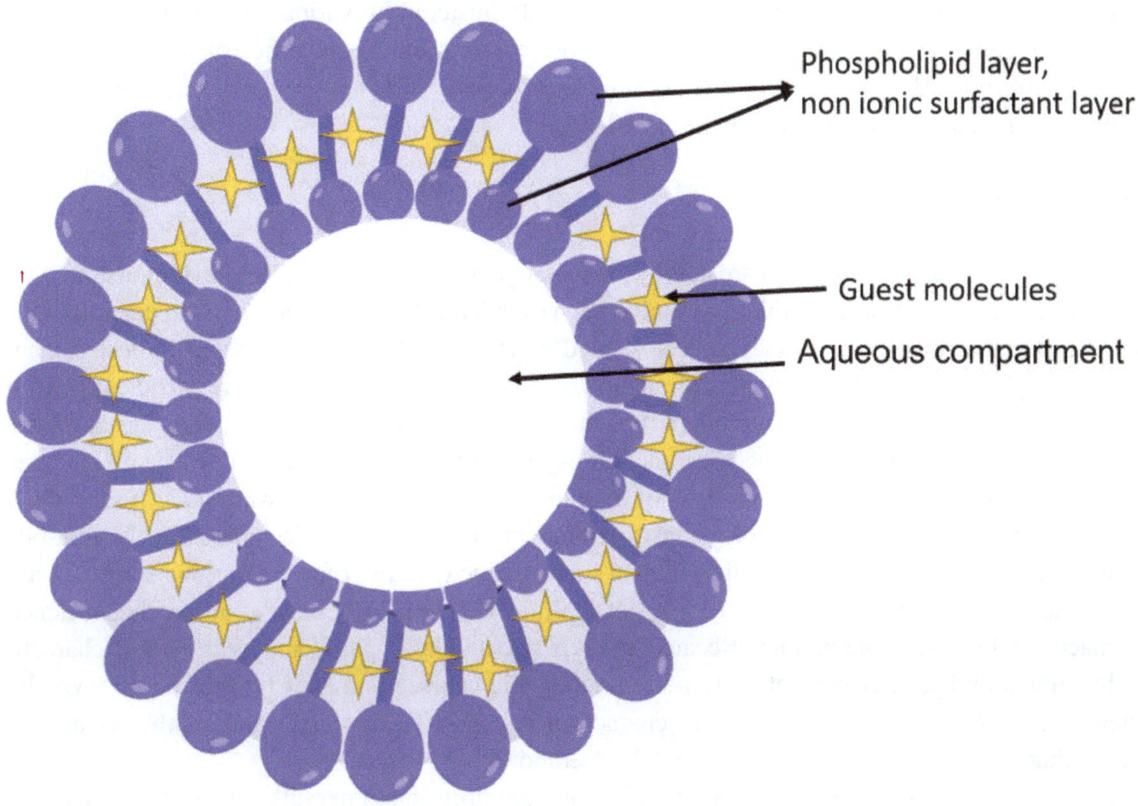

drug side effect. The localization of the Niosome vesicles also can be tuned according to the desired site in the various disease condition, and Niosome system also used for the leishmaniasis treatment in this condition the Leishmania parasite endive and leave into the macrophages (Khandare et al., 1994; Okore, et al., 2011). Ghadi et al., reported that in vivo assessment of novel hyaluronan encompassing niosomes tailor-made by Box-Behnken design to co-encapsulate curcumin and quercetin and found that better release performance comparatively to conventional niosomes based formulations. Ghadi et al., reported the higher antioxidant and anti-inflammatory effects by hyaluronan containing niosomes (Ghadi et al., 2019).

The oral peptide delivery is also facing challenges because the gastric degradation and first-pass metabolism, but sheena et al., reported that oral delivery of vasopressin by the niosomes exhibited a significantly high degree of entrapment and stability of the peptide (Sheena, et al., 1998). Many researchers successfully load and deliver herbal-based bioactive molecules. Kambe et al., reported that the delivery of nonionic surfactant-based *Gymnema sylvestre* extract-loaded niosomes for better pharmacodynamic and kinetic Performances (Kamble et al., 2013). Encapsulation of lycopene in niosomes for the treatment of cancer (Sharma et al., 2016), curcumin delivery by niosomal system for treatment of Ovarian Cancer (Xu et al., 2016) and Niosomal delivery of silymarin for hepatoprotective activity (El-Ridy et al., 2012) has been reported. Studies on a high degree of colchicine encapsulation by a niosome system (Hao et al., 2002). The niosomal system has several advantages such as Niosomes are biocompatible, biodegradable, non-toxic and non-immunogenic, having better patient compliances, and the loading capacity is high, it can load both hydrophilic as well as hydrophobic therapeutic molecules and release them in a very controlled manner. Niosomes can be administered by various routes such as topical, transdermal, parenteral, and oral, etc. with diverse dosage forms and formulations such as suspensions, powders, semisolids. These are chemically high stable formulations, so the storage of these formulations is effortless and convenient (Rahimpour et al., 2012).

4.6 Liposome

The idea of liposomes was first demarcated by Alec Bangham in the 1960s when he demonstrated the impulsive assemblage of egg lecithin into multilayer vesicular of phospholipids into the aqueous solutions (Leung et al., 2019). Liposomes, sphere-shaped vesicles, small vesicles made up cholesterol, and one or more phospholipid bilayers of phospholipids. In other words, the liposomes are particles probably in the spherical in shape that can entrap a part of the dissolution medium, in which they easily diffuse (float) into their inner body part of the liposome. Liposomes comprise numerous concentric membranes. Generally, liposomal structures are made-up of lipophilic and hydrophilic groups of polar lipids, which are characterized by having an on their construction. Liposomes are first designated in the mid-60s. Today, extensively applicable to the drug delivery and biomedical field for the various scientific disciplines, including biophysics, chemistry, physics, colloid science, biochemistry, and medical science, pharmaceutical science, and biology. Because of their size and hydrophilic and hydrophobic character and biocompatibility, hemocompatibility nonimmunogenic characters makes liposomes are favorable systems for therapeutics delivery. Liposome characteristics are differing significantly with varying their surface charge n, size, lipid composition, and the method of the formulations.

Recently Luo coworkers reported that the effect of short drug-light intervals the pharmacodynamics and pharmacokinetics of liposomal system for chemotherapy and found that chemo phototherapy anti-patient-derived pancreatic cancer xenografts tumor response based on improved drug delivery at the short drug-light interval used by the Luo and coworkers (Luo et 2019).

Polar lipid part when interacting with water forms the self-assembles which disperse into the hydrophilic medium, the hydrophilic part form shell of the liposome, and the lipophilic part forms the core of the interlayer of the liposomes system. The Liposome system is an amphiphilic system that can entrap amphiphilic, hydrophilic as well as hydrophobic therapeutic molecules and herbal based bioactive molecules. Therefore, the water-soluble drug or bioactive moiety is encapsulated in the hydrophilic compartment, and less hydrophilic or lipophilic moiety is encapsulated into the hydrophobic or lipophilic compartment of the liposomes. Liposomes typically made-up by phospholipids; this part of the liposome contributes in the altering the drug pharmacokinetics profile of therapeutics release. Liposomes have their exceptional properties that can increase the product performance by increasing their constituent solubility, intracellular uptake bioavailability, vitro and in vivo stability and changed pharmacokinetics and biodistribution of the therapeutics (Xiao et al., 2002).

The liposomes drug delivery system can improve bioavailability, biocompatibility, safety, and the therapeutic activity along with this liposome can able to minimize the drug toxicity by delivering therapeutics at the desired site of action and by controlled and sustained release of therapeutics (Abou et al., 2005). The advanced liposome systems are investigated by Massiot et al., which were photo-trigged liposome-based drug delivery systems by insertion of porphyrin group into the lipid bilayer to lipid–porphyrin conjugates of supramolecular assemblies (Massiot et al., 2019). The liposome manufacturing

Figure 7. Typical structure of noisome
(Khandare et al., 1994; Okore, et al., 2011)

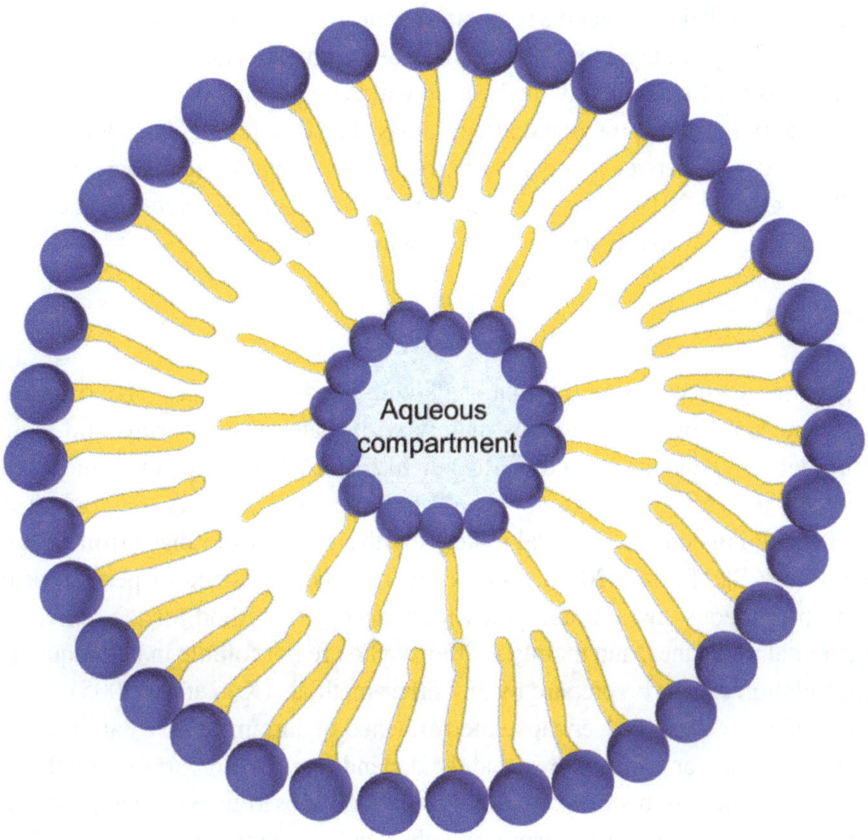

companies are Gilead Sciences, Luye Pharma, Pacira, Sun Pharmaceutical, Johnson & Johnson, Tau Group, Sigma, Sigma-Tau Group, Ipsen (Onivyde), Fudan-Zhangjiang, Kingond Pharm, CSPC, Novartis, Shanghai New Asia, Spectrum Pharmaceuticals which are main producers of liposomal drug delivery system worldwide.

The flexibility of liposome-based drug delivery carrier provides a very promising approach for the delivery of the herbal bioactive molecule's delivery of an extensive range of herbal and synthetic therapeutics and drugs through any route without concerning their solubility profile. The liposomal system also prolongs the action of drugs by a controlled releasing mechanism to the target sites of applications. There are several other characteristics which make it for promising drug carrier for herbal delivery. The distribution and release of any drug molecules not only controlled by molecules itself, whereas it's also governed by carrier molecules so that liposome can significantly affect the pharmacokinetics and pharmacodynamics profile of any drugs molecules. The liposome has fashioned a new-age drug delivery system (Rafe, 2018). The years between 1980–2000 were productive in the milieu of various advanced liposomal systems received regulatory approval for the treatment of cancer infectious diseases (Abelcet®, Ambisome®, Amphotec®), macular degeneration (Visudyne®),(Doxil®, DaunoXome®, Depocyt®, Myocet®), as well as for the control of viral infections in the form of virosomal vaccines (Epaxal® and Inflexal®).

Onpattro® is a most recently approved liposomal formulation that consists of an siRNA targeting the production of the transthyretin (TTR) protein. Vyxeos® (formerly known as CPX-351) is the first dual-drug liposomal formulation to receive regulatory approval. It contains cytarabine and daunorubicin anticancer molecules. They are used for the treatment of treatment-related or secondary acute myeloid leukemia. Onpattro® is the first, and only medication which approved for the treatment of polyneuropathy began by genetic transthyretin-mediated amyloidosis. The development of Onpattro® brings about from collaborative hard work between Alnylam Pharmaceuticals and Acuitas Therapeutics (then AlCana Technologies) (Leung et al., 2019). The numerous kinds of herbal liposome-based dosage forms have been studied by researchers who are brief in the following table.

4.7 Nanoparticles

Nanotechnology is the science of material that deals with nanoscale particle size of the materials. The pharmaceutical nanotechnology stream deals mainly with material with drugs and their applications in imaging, drug delivery, diagnostic and biosensor materials. Nowadays the nanonization of herbal bioactive ingredients is getting wide attention in the whole world. In this category of drug delivery, nanoparticle and nanoemulsion are colloidal systems with particle size ranges from 10 nm to 1000 nm (Ali and Ahmed 2018; Saraf et al., 2010). In other words, the nanosized dispersion of therapeutic or drug particles in the aqueous environment is a widely accepted method for the delivery of synthetic, water-insoluble herbal medicines, and mainly for those who are not soluble in both aqueous and organic solvents and formulation cannot be prepare by any other methods (Koo et al., 2005).

The drug molecules are dissolved, encapsulated attached or entrapped, to a nanoparticle matrix. The formation of Nanocapsules or nanospheres mainly depends on the preparation method. In the Nano capsule, the drug molecules are restricted to a hollow area enclosed by a unique polymeric membrane layer, whereas the drug molecules are uniformly and physically dispersed within the matrix systems in the nanospheres. The main goal of nanoparticle synthesis is to modifying NPs as according to dosage forms where the surface properties, particle size control, and release kinetics of herbal bioactive molecules. The nanoparticles provide the platform to achieve the site-specific targeted delivery of therapeutics and ensure their stability at delivery sites such as biomacromolecules DNA, RNA, proteins, enzymes delivery (Ali and Ahmed 2018; Manmode et al., 2009).

Patil et al., reported recently herbal nanoparticle for the treatment of many conditions like a bacterial infection, hepatotoxicity, inflammation, oxidation and chronic diseases like cancer, wound healing and found that these disease conditions can be cured by nano herbals more effectively as compared to allopathic medicines (Patil et al., 2018) The nanoparticles can be made from various materials for different applications such as Drug nanoparticles, ceramic-based nanoparticles, polymer-based nanoparticles, solid nanoparticles, albumin nanoparticles lipid-based nanoparticles, Nanoparticles, which are range between 10-100 nm particle size are reported in literature.

4.8 Emulsion

Several phytochemical active ingredients are water-insoluble or lipophilic in nature, delivery of such type of bioactive material is very challenging. The emulsion is a thermodynamically unstable system that can load lipophilic drugs and delivery. Emulsion mainly comprises the mixture of lipophilic material(oil), surfactant, and water after mechanical shaking or homogenization forms a transparent isotropic solu-

Figure 8. Typical structure of liposome. Xiao et al., 2002

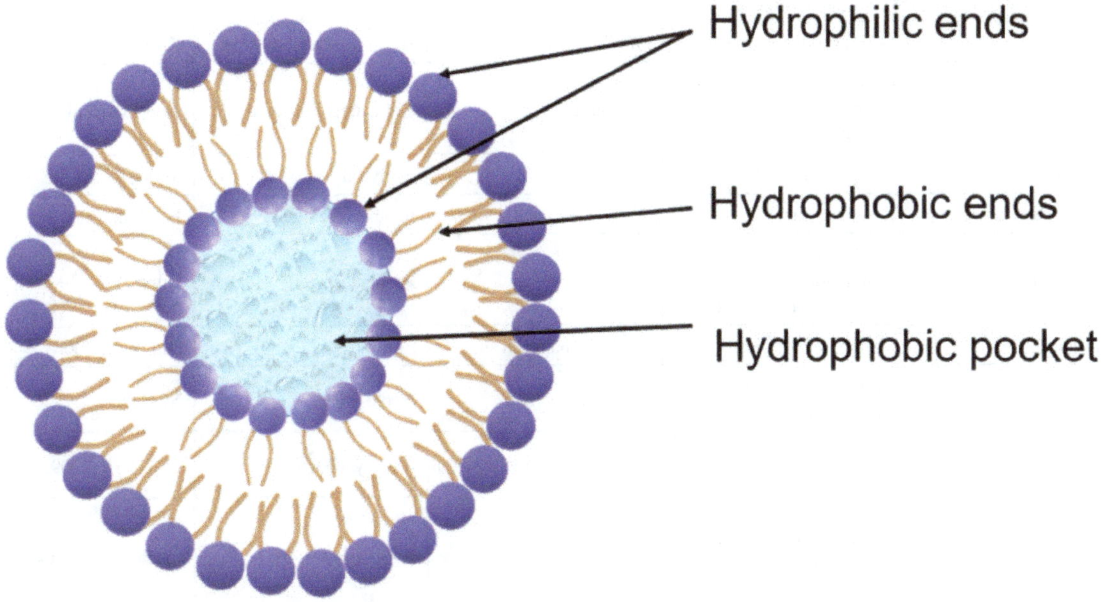

tion. It is a nonhomogenous dispersion system developed by two types of liquids that are incapable of dissolving each other in this system, one phase disperses or continuous, and another is form droplets (Zhang et al., .2006).

Usually, the emulsion system is assembled by the water phase, oil phase, co-surfactant, and surface-active agents. The appearance and morphology of a typical emulsion are translucent to transparent. The droplet size of the emulsion ranges (0.1-1000 nm) based on the size it's categorized (0.1–100 μm), micro-emulsion (Nanoemulsions) (10–100 nm), sub-micro-emulsion (lipid emulsion) (100–600 nm). Generally, emulsions are used as in-vivo targeted drug delivery because they have an affinity towards the lymph. In addition, the emulsions are used for sustained and controlled release of the therapeutics because the drug moiety resides into the inner core part that not directly into the body fluid (Lu et al., 2005).

The lipophilic drug formulations prepared into the O/W/O or O/W emulsion system, while hydrophilic drugs formulations developed into the W/O or W/O/W emulsion system. At the time of assimilation, the oil droplets are phagocytosed by the macrophages or hepatocytes and released loaded drugs. The loading capacity of the emulsion is also high; it can be easily administered by intravenous or intramuscular injection, and the particle size of the emulsion has also affected the target distribution. Apart from this, emulsion also enhances the herbal medicine stability and protects them from hydrolytic degradation. The emulsion system also facilitates the penetration, bioavailability, distribution and avoided bitter taste and gastric irritation of various of the phytomedicine (Wadhwa, et al., 2012).

Table 5. List of reported herbal liposomal formulations

Active Ingredients	Application of Formulation	Administration Route	Biological Activity	Reference
Silymarin	Enhanced bioavailability	Oral	Hepatoprotective	Samaligy et al., 2006
Quercetin	Enhanced BBB penetration and dose redution	Intranasal	Anticancer Antioxidant	Aroonsri et al., 2008
Artemisia	Improved penetration	In-vitro	Antiviral	Sinico, et al., 2005
Ampelopsin liposome	Ampelopsin	In-vitro	Increase efficiency	He et al., 2008
Curcumin	Enhanced systemic circulation with entrapment efficiency	In-vitro	Anticancer	Hong et al., 2008
Garlicin	Improved efficiency	Inhalation	Lungs	Gui et al., 2008
Rutin and Quercetin	Enhanced binding of flavonoids and Hb	Intravenous	Hemoglobin	Xi et al., 2007
Usnea acid	Prolonged release and enhanced solubility	In-vitro	Antimycobacterial	Lira et al., 2009
Colchicine	Sustained drug release enhances skin accumulation, and increased site specificity	Topical	Antigout	Godin et al., 2004
Catechins	Increased skin permeation	Transdermal	Antioxidant and chemo preventive	Fang et al., 2006
Docetaxel	with BBB targeting CNS delivery	Intravenous	Anticancer	Pattani et al., 2015
Breviscapin	Prolonged delivery of breviscapine	Intramuscular	Cardiovascular diseases	Zhong et al., 2005
Ampelopsin	Anti-cancer	Intravenous	Anti-cancer	Wen et al., 2010
Capsaicin	Prolong action, permeation enhancement	Topical	Analgesic	Hong et al., 2008
Morphine sulphate, DepoDur	Enhanced efficacy	Epidural	Pain	Fan and Zhang, 2013
Nux vomica	Improved stability	Invitro	Analgesic Anti-neoplastic, and Anti inflammatory	Rane and Prabhakar 2010
Paclitaxel	pH sensitive and enhanced encapsulation efficiency	Invitro	Anti-cancer	Priprem et al., 2008
Psoralen	Enhanced Bioavailability	Topical	Psoriasis treatment	Pattani et al., 2015
Puerarin	Enhanced efficacy	Oral	Antioxidant and anti hypercholesterolemic	Xi et al., 2007
Topotecan	Enhanced efficacy	Intravenous	Advanced solid tumor	Fan and Zhang 2013
Vinorelbine	Enhanced efficacy	Intravenous	Breast, colon and lung cancers	Fan and Zhang 2013
Vincristine	Enhanced Bioavailability	Intravenous	MDR cancer	Pattani et al., 2015
Wogonin	Prolong duration of action	Invitro	Anti-cancer	Chen et al., 2009

Table 6. List of reported herbal nanoparticle (NP) based formulation

Formulations	Applications	Biological activity	Active ingredients	Reference
NP of Cuscuta chinensis	Enhanced water solubility,	Antioxidant and Hepatoprotective	Flavonoids and lignans	Feng-Lin, et al., 2008
Nanocapsules of Artemisinin	Sustained release	Anticancer	Artemisinin	Chen et al., 2009
NPs of Triptolide	Improved drug permeation by skin layers	Anti-inflammatory	Triptolide	Zhinan et al., 2003
NPs of Radix salvia miltiorrhiza	Enhanced bioavailability	Coronary heart diseases Angina pectoris, and myocardial infarction	R. salvia miltiorrhiza	Su et al., 2008
Triptolide-loaded solid lipid NPs	Diminishing the toxicity	Anti-inflammatory	Triptolide	Zhinan et al., 2005
Taxel-loaded NPs	Improved bioavailability and prolonged release	Anticancer	Taxel	Fu, et al., (2006),
NPs of Ginkgo biloba	Enhanced blood flow in cerebral area and metabolism	Activation of brain function	Ginkgo biloba extract	Shimada 2008
NPs of curcuminoids	Extended release	Antioxidant and Anticancer	Curcuminoids	Upadhyaya et al., 2009; Mukerjee, and Vishwanatha, 2009; Kesharwani et al., 2015;)
Glycyrrhizic acid-loaded NPs	Enhanced bioavailability	Antihypertensive and Anti-inflammatory,	Glycyrrhizic acid	J. Hou and Zhou (2008),
Naringenin-loaded nanoparticles	Enhanced the release of NAR and enhanced its solubility	Hepatoprotective	Naringenin	Feng-Lin et al., 2009

4.8.1 Nanoemulsion

Nanoemulsion is a type of emulsion, can also load and release the herbal bioactive molecules in a controlled manner, the size range is 70-100 nm, the transparent appearance of nanoemulsion due to their small size, and sedimentation and creaming prevent by Brownian motion, so the life span of the nanoemulsion is higher than normal emulsion. In contrast to nanoemulsions, microemulsions, can be diluted with water or buffer without changing their droplet size distribution.Nanoemulsion are thermodynamically steady system in which the two immiscible liquid (hydrophilic and hydrophobic) are blended to form a single-phase by the use of the little volume of a suitable surfactant. Another technique for the preparation of nanoemulsion is high speed and pressure homogenization: piston homogenizer and high-speed pressure homogenizer produces nanoemulsion of minimal particle size up to 1 nm and this apparatus uses high pressure with a positive displacement pump (1000-20000 psi). During this process, the product formed through the mixing chamber, which contains the small microchannel. The final product drives through the microchannel on to the impingement resulting in the formation of thermodynamically very stable nanoemulsion loaded with an herbal bioactive molecule (Jain et al., 2014; Mujoriya et al., 2011).

The Nanoemulsion is a type of emulsion with an average particle size less than 500 nm; these are oil-in-water (O/W), water-in-oil (W/O) dispersion stabilized by suitable stabilizers. Clear transparent to

Table 7. List of reported herbal emulsion-based formulation

Formulation	Applications	Biological activity	Active ingredients	Reference
Submicron emulsion of Docetaxel	Prolonged circulation time	Anticancer	Docetaxel	Li et al., 2007
Emulsion of Zedoary essential oil	Enhanced aqueous dispersibility and stability	Anticancer hepatoprotective and anti-bacterial	Zedoary turmeric oil	Zhao, et al., 2010
Triptolide micro-emulsion	Improved drug penetration through skin layers by skin hydration	Anti-inflammatory	Triptolide	Zhinan, et al., 2003
Nanoemulsion of Silybin	Prolonged release formulation	Hepatoprotective	Silybin	Song et al., 2005
Nanoemulsion of Berberine	Enhanced drug absorption and circulation time	Anticancer	Berberine	Gui et al., 2007
Micro-emulsion of Quercetin	Improved stratum corneum and epidermis penetration	Antioxidant	Quercetin	Vicentini, et al., 2008

hazy, the appearance of the nanoemulsion is due to stable and small droplet size. Nanoemulsion can be utilized in several other dosage forms such as cream, gel, spray, aerosol, liquid, etc. this can be administered by several routes such as intravenous, intramuscular, nasal, oral, ocular, peritoneal, pulmonary, etc. (Singh et al., 2017). The first nanoemulsion was prepared in 1940; it can be made by three types such as water-in-oil (W/O), oil-in-water (O/W), and a discontinuous phase. The surfactant used for the preparation of nanoemulsion should be USFDA approved. Nanoemulsions have higher drug or therapeutics solubilization capacity than other micellar dispersions, and it's also possessed more excellent kinetic stability than the coarse type of emulsions such as type of emulsion generally use in cosmetics and pesticide industry (Yukuyama et al., 2016; Wang et al., 2007). Nanoemulsion is also used for the delivery of phytomedicine, and this exhibits the controlled and sustained release of therapeutics and protects the herbal bioactive molecules from hydrolysis and degradation.

The evaluation of microemulsion in the following parameter:

U.V. Spectrometer: Loading and release capacity of a microemulsion of the herbal bioactive molecule can be evaluated through the UV and the transparent appearance of the microemulsion formulation may determine by computing percentage light transmission across the emulsion sample.

Dynamic Light Scattering (DLS): The droplet size and distribution analysis.

Zeta-Potential: Charge base stability and interaction analysis, Viscosity.

Transmission Electron microscopy (TEM): Surface morphology and size analysis can be performed through TEM. Stability Studies: The optimized nanoemulsion store for the 6 months at three different temperature ranges such as room temperature, elevated temperature (20 - 50 oC) and refrigerating condition (50 - 20 oC), through the visual inspection the shelf life of the stored microemulsion can be estimated by observing their phase septation and transparency.

4.8.2 Microemulsion

Microemulsions are also the type of emulsion these are thermodynamically stable system; microemulsion can be defined as a uni-phase system comprising oil, water, and an amphiphile(s), these significantly vary from conventional emulsion formulations by their several physical characteristics such as small particle

Table 8. List of reported herbal nanoemulsion based formulation

Biological source	Applications	Biological activity	Active ingredients	Reference
Berberis vulgaris	Enhanced absorption and residence time	Anticancer	Berberine	Sun and Ouyang 2007
Curcuma zedoaria	Enhanced oral bioavailability, stability and dispersibility,	Hepato-protection anti-bacterial and anticancer	β-elemene	He and Tang 2005
Colchicum autumnale	Enhanced bioavailability	Anti-gout	Colchicine	Shen et al., 2011
Genista tinctoria	Improved skin permeation	Anticancer	Genistein	Silva et al., 2009
Silibum marianum	Enhanced therapeutic efficacy and solubility	Hepato-protective	Silymarin	Song et al., 2005
Sophora alopencerides	Improved percutaneous permeability	Anti-inflammatory, anti-bacterial, and anti-virus	Matrine	Cao et al., 2007

size, low viscosity, transparency, the particle size range is <100–200 nm. Microemulsions are possessed numerous different microstructures that may be similar to conventional emulsion formulations. Though microemulsions are thermodynamic stable, system but emulsion droplets may get coalescence and such phenomenon leading to phase separation in the emulsion system. The droplets of the microemulsion get fussed to each other, known as the consequence reason behind this phenomenon is very low interfacial tension between the two opposite water and oil phases. The use of surfactants and cosurfactants can be prevented from such type of problem by reducing the interfacial tension of two different phages. The spontaneous formation of microemulsions are without the use of any high high-shear pressure; the formulation procedure is free from any excipient. The ultra-stable microemulsions guaranteed a long shelf-life—furthermore, microemulsions against the phase separation over a broad temperature range and other physical conditions.

4.9 Herbal Drug Bioconjugates

The bioconjugate system is a process through which bioactive molecules attached chemically with some polymers biopolymers nanoparticle or other carrier molecules.

This approach used when bioactive molecules are having some limitations such as less bioavailability, solubility, distribution, half-life, clearance, etc. Several natural bioactive constituents are water-insoluble that limits their application as drugs, such as curcumin, polyphenol, many alkaloids, glycosides, terpenoids, essential oils many other classes of bioactive molecules can be conjugated with suitable polymers for overcoming the above-mentioned various challenges.

Many researchers are already working in this area, such as Manju and Srinivasan has developed the curcumin and hyaluronic acid conjugate, and the report enhanced its aqueous solubility and stability of the curcumin (Manju et al., 2011). Preclinical study of a Folate-Vinca Alkaloid Conjugate reported by Reddy and workers (Reddy et al., .2007), Hyoscyamus polyamines conjugates (Biondi et al., 2000). Nicotine conjugate with a vaccine for the reduction of nicotine distribution to Brain (Pentel et al., 2000). Capsaicin silver nanoparticles conjugates for the study of their kinetics, characterization, and biocompat-

Table 9. List of reported herbal micro emulsion-based formulation

Biological source	Applications	Biological activity	Active ingredients	Reference
Azadirachita indica	Low toxicity	Acricidal, Antifungal, Antibacterial	Neem oil	Sun and Ouyang 2007
Ligusticum Wallichii	Increased permeation rate	Inhibit platelet aggregation and Lower blood levels	Ligustrazine Phosphate	Cui et al., 2011
Pilocarpus Jaborandi	Enhanced ocular retention time,	Glaucoma treatment	Pilocarpine	Chan et al., 2007
Psoralea Corylifolia	Improved skin penetration	Treatment of psoriasis	Bavchi oil	Ali et al., 2008
Radix puerariae	Increase bioavailability	Cardio and cerebrovascular disease	Puerarin	Yu and, Zhai 2006
Tripterygium wilfordii	Enhance the penetration by increase hydration	Anti-inflammatory	Triptolide	Chen et al., 2004
Taxus brevifolia	Prolonged release	Anticancer	Docetaxol	Ling et al., 2007

ibility (Amruthraj et al., .2015). Colchicine glycopeptide dendrimer conjugates for targeting cancer cells (Johansson et al., 2010). Dextran-Polyalcohol-Camptothecin Conjugate for anticancer activity (Inoue et al., 2004). Water-soluble poly-(l-glutamic acid)–Gly-camptothecin conjugates for improved stability and efficacy in vivo (Singer et al., 2001). Ding and coworkers reported albumin–hesperidin bioconjugate for protein vector function and conformation (Ding et al., 2012). Wu et al., reported recently the berberine nanoparticles of chitosan/fucoidan-taurine conjugate for the treatment of defective tight junction barrier of intestinal epithelia (Wu et al., .2014). Quercetin hyaluronic acid conjugates for modulation of binding to human serum albumin and LDL oxidation (Janisch et al., 2004; Pang et al., .2014). Paclitaxel encapsulated hyaluronic acid nanoparticles for targeted cancer therapy (Thomas et al., 2015; Wang et al., 2014). Glycyrrhizic acid conjugates with α-D-glucosamine and some glycosylamines for antiviral activity (Kondratenko et al., 2004). Ginkgolic acid conjugates for anxiolytic activity (Satyan et al. 1998) and many more bioactive herbal constituents based bioconjugates are reported earlier, these conjugates facilitate in the enhancement of solubility, bioavailability, distribution, clearance and self-life of the bioactive moiety during application as drug for treating the various disease conditions.

4.10 Microsphere

Microencapsulation is a promising drug delivery technology in this process the various bioactive molecules are encapsulated with a polymeric material that targets delivery by control release of bioactive molecules. The microsphere is a novel drug delivery system; it is a small spherical shape particle in micrometer the size range (1 μm to 1000 μm). These micro drug carriers can be made by various types of polymeric materials such as Polyethylene microspheres, Glass microsphere, etc. Microsphere drug-delivery systems are used commercially, and several marketed products are available for herbal bioactive molecules, small molecules, and biopharmaceuticals. The conventional microencapsulation technology for herbal and other therapeutics microencapsulation comprises emulsification in a particularly designed homogenizer. But in current technologies enable adequate dispersion, the ability to easily scale up to commercial production is a significant hurdle. In this system, drug molecules are homogeneously dispersed into the polymeric matrix. There are various techniques for the preparation of the microsphere, such as double emulsion technique, single emulsion technique, Polymerization techniques, spray congealing and spray drying phase separation coacervation technique, and solvent extraction technique are generally used (Scarfato et al., 2008; Chao et al., 2010).

Generally, first-order release kinetics follow this system, and release mechanism is diffusion and dissolution. Many herbal bioactive compounds are delivered by this formulation. Some are listed in the below table.

4.11 Dendrimer

A dendrimer is a hyperbranched polymeric structure; in other words, dendrimers-are highly branched star-shaped nanosized polymeric material. The size range of the dendrimers is 1-10 nm; it increases in a very fixed manner. Dendrimers are comprising three fundamental parts a central core (core), an internal part of the dendritic structure (branching), and an external surface with various functional groups. By merging these segments, it is possible to acquire dendritic structure with different molecular shapes and sizes, with ideal (externally shielded) space in biological science pharmaceutical science and biomedical science applications (Banker et al., 1996). The core part of the dendrimer imparts exclusive properties to internal size, loading, and releases capacity of the dendrimers. However, the terminal groups on the dendrimer surface facilitate various physicochemical properties such as chelating ability and solubility (Grayson et al., 2001). Hyperbranched polymers are polydisperse macromolecular structure with a dendritic structure and are synthesized by low-cost polymerization methods. In current since last decades, it has been got wide attention in the fields of pharmaceutical technology and nanotechnology, such as herbal bioactive molecule delivery and nanoscale catalysts, gene transfer, light-collecting compounds, standard substances for measuring molecular weight and size, photoreactive materials, and rheology control agents. There are several advantages of the dendrimer such as its very suitable for targeted delivery of therapeutics controlled and sustained drug delivery of poor water-soluble bioactive molecules, its ability to bypass the acid environment of the stomach and hence the avoiding the discrepancy due to effect of gastric secretions (Frechet et al., .2001). Several articles are published on dendrimers recently; many of them are used for delivering the herbal bioactive compounds; Mollazade et al., reported the polymeric dendrimers for curcumin delivery to inhibit the cancer cell proliferation (Mollazade et al., .2013).

Basically, there are three methods used for the drug delivery through the dendrimer first is a drug is adhered with the outer surface of the dendrimer to form dendrimer prodrugs second here the dendrimer acts as a unimolecular micelle by loading a therapeutic molecule and form dendrimer drug complex or (i.e., host-guest) supramolecular assembly. The third is a drug that is conjugated to the outer surface functional groups via ionic interactions (Zhang et al., 2010). Gupta et al., reported recently the covalently conjugated berberine to amine-terminated G4 PAMAM dendrimers (Gupta et al., 2017).

5. FUTURE PROSPECTIVE OF NOVEL DRUG DELIVERY FOR HERBAL BIOACTIVE MOLECULES

Today the world population are choosing for herbal base medication more as compare to another conventional system as treatment of disease as well as nutraceuticals for their improved therapeutic efficacy and minimum adverse effects dose, dose frequency, so there is an obligation to develop a smart and

Table 10. List of reported herbal microsphere-based formulation

Active Constituent of plant	Application	Biological Activity	Reference
Camptothecin	Dose reduction	Anti-cancer	Natrajan et al., 2010
Ginsenosides	Solubility and stability improvement	Anti-cancer	Xiao et al., 2008
Piper sarmentosumn	Easy for industrial scale up	Antidiabetic	Xiao et al., 2008
Quercetin	Anti-inflammatory and antioxidant	Permeation enhanced	Garg et al., 2010
Rutin	Site specific delivery to brain vascular systems and heart	Antioxidant	Lieberman et al., 1998
Silymarin	Sustained release of medicament Improved patient compliance	Hepatoprotective	Lachman et al., 1996

advanced drug delivery system with several upgradations such as stability, enhanced bioavailability, the half-life of drug, targeted delivery for an herbal bioactive molecule. The advanced drug delivery offers safe and effective delivery of therapeutics, as well as raising the faith and confidence into the peoples for the herbal-based therapeutics and their newer drug delivery systems due to that the market value of the herbal-based therapeutic and nutritional formulations are getting peaks. Numerous other nanotechnology-based techniques can be used for enhancing the efficacy bioavailability site targeting of herbal bioactive. Such as sublingual delivery of herbal bioactive molecules for the quick action of the drug, and it's also overcome the first pass metabolism issue, which is the leading problem of the herbal-based formulation. The drug delivery through the mucus membrane by mucoadhesive drug delivery system also having several advantages improved bioavailability, targeted delivery, and minimize the dose, toxicity, and adverse reactions. An injectable hydrogel system with herbal bioactive molecules can be injected for local and sustained delivery of the therapeutics. Floating tablet-based drug delivery avoids the degradation of the drug into the gastric pH and improved absorption in the upper gastrointestinal tract.

CONCLUSION

Various herbal bioactive molecules are obtained from the plant kingdom and possesses numerous pharmacological activities against different kind of pathophysiological abnormalities or illness. The bioactive molecules cannot be used directly as therapeutic molecules because of certain physiochemical limitations such as solubility, permeability, delivery, first-pass metabolism, molecular size, acid degradation, hydrophilic-lipophilic valence, etc. these limitations can be overcome through using novel drug delivery system. Lipid solubility, large molecular size, bioactive molecules get degraded in the gastric environment. These types of barriers limit the pharmacological activity of the therapeutics. They are using modern nanotechnology-based techniques with pharmaceutical science. It is possible to overcome the above-mentioned problems. The novel drug delivery systems directed to improved bioavailability of herbal bioactive molecules by increasing the solubility and permeability as well as a decrease in side effects. Several herbal bioactive molecules such as alkaloids, glycosides, terpenoids flavonoids, tannins, etc. exhibited enhanced therapeutic and pharmacological activity at equal or less dose when it associated with a novel drug delivery formulation as compared to conventional herbal formulations. Therefore,

Figure 9. Typical structure of the dendrimer
(Zhang et al., 2010, Banker et al., 1996)

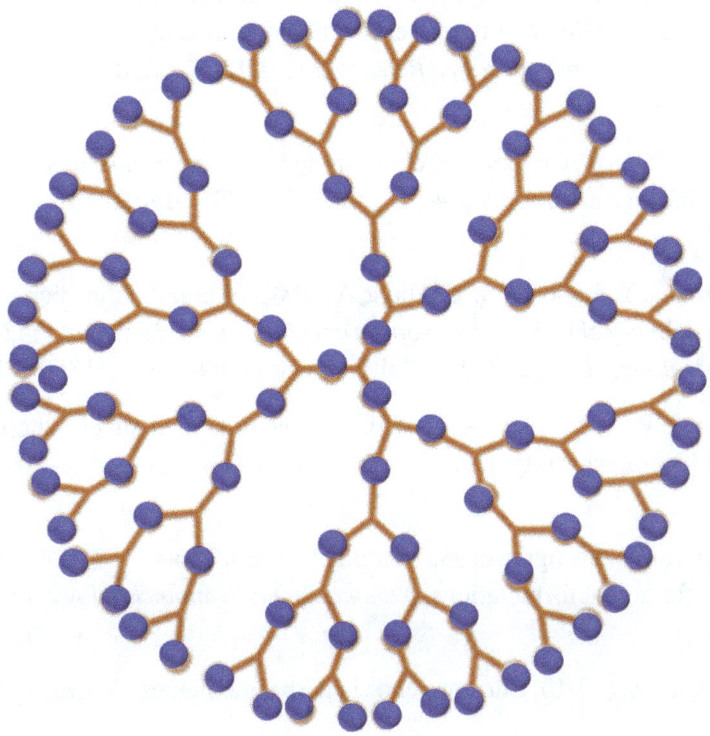

there is potential gap area is available for the further research and development for the development of nanotechnology associated smart and advanced drug delivery formulations for the valuable herbal bioactive molecule as it offers effective and inexpensive formulations, and the trends of combining novel drug delivery systems for herbal bioactive molecules have also been accepted at industrial scale-up of the production.

REFERENCES

Abdulbaqi, I. M., Darwis, Y., Khan, N. A. K., Assi, R. A., & Khan, A. A. (2016). Ethosomal nanocarriers: The impact of constituents and formulation techniques on ethosomal properties, in vivo studies, and clinical trials. *International Journal of Nanomedicine*, •••, 11.

Abou El Wafa, A. A., Mursi, N. M., & El-Shaboury, K. M. (2003). *A pharmaceutical study on certain ocular drug delivery systems* (Doctoral dissertation). Cairo University, Cairo, Egypt.

Afrin, S., Jahan, I., Hasan, A. N., & Deepa, K. N. (2018). Novel Approaches of Herbal Drug Delivery. *Journal of Pharmaceutical Research International*, *21*(5), 1–11. doi:10.9734/JPRI/2018/39143

Ajazuddin Saraf, S. (2010). Applications of novel drug delivery system for herbal formulations. *Fitoterapia, 81*(7), 680–689. doi:10.1016/j.fitote.2010.05.001 PMID:20471457

Alexander, A., Patel, R. J., Saraf, S., & Saraf, S. (2016). Recent expansion of pharmaceutical nanotechnologies and targeting strategies in the field of phytopharmaceuticals for the delivery of herbal extracts and bioactives. *Journal of Controlled Release, 241*, 110–124. doi:10.1016/j.jconrel.2016.09.017 PMID:27663228

Ali, A., & Ahmed, S. (2018). A review on chitosan and its nanocomposites in drug delivery. *International Journal of Biological Macromolecules, 109*, 273–286. doi:10.1016/j.ijbiomac.2017.12.078 PMID:29248555

Ali, J., Akhtar, N., Sultana, Y., Baboota, S., & Ahuja, A. (2008). Antipsoriatic microemulsion gel formulations for topical drug delivery of babchi oil (Psoralea corylifolia). *Methods and Findings in Experimental and Clinical Pharmacology, 30*(4), 277–285. doi:10.1358/mf.2008.30.4.1185802 PMID:18773122

Amruthraj, N. J., Raj, J. P. P., & Lebel, A. (2015). Capsaicin-capped silver nanoparticles: Its kinetics, characterization and biocompatibility assay. *Applied Nanoscience, 5*(4), 403–409. doi:10.100713204-014-0330-5

Aroonsri, P., Jintanaporn, W., Saengrawee, S., Wathita, P., & Supaporn, M. (2008). Applications of novel drug delivery system for herbal formulations. *Nanomedicine; Nanotechnology, Biology, and Medicine, 4*, 70–78.

Atmakuri, L. R., & Dathi, S. (2010). Current trends in herbal medicines. *Journal of Pharmacy Research, 3*(1), 109–113.

Awasthi, R., Kulkarni, G. T., & Pawar, V. K. (2011). Phytosomes: An approach to increase the bioavailability of plant extracts. *International Journal of Pharmacy and Pharmaceutical Sciences, 3*(2), 1–3.

Azmin, M. N., Florence, A. T., Handjani-Vila, R. M., Stuart, J. F. B., Vanlerberghe, G., & Whittaker, J. S. (1985). The effect of non-ionic surfactant vesicle (niosome) entrapment on the absorption and distribution of methotrexate in mice. *The Journal of Pharmacy and Pharmacology, 37*(4), 237–242. doi:10.1111/j.2042-7158.1985.tb05051.x PMID:2860220

Banker, G. S., Lieberman, H. A., & Rieger, M. M. (Eds.). (1996). Pharmaceutical dosage forms: disperse systems. Academic Press.

Barragan-Montero, V., Winum, J. Y., Molès, J. P., Juan, E., Clavel, C., & Montero, J. L. (2005). Synthesis and properties of isocannabinoid and cholesterol derivatized rhamnosurfactants: Application to liposomal targeting of keratinocytes and skin. *European Journal of Medicinal Chemistry, 40*(10), 1022–1029. doi:10.1016/j.ejmech.2005.04.009 PMID:15950324

Biondi, S., Fornalé, S., Oksman-Caldentey, K. M., Eeva, M., Agostani, S., & Bagni, N. (2000). Jasmonates induce over-accumulation of methylputrescine and conjugated polyamines in Hyoscyamus muticus L. root cultures. *Plant Cell Reports, 19*(7), 691–697. doi:10.1007002999900178 PMID:30754807

Bombardelli, E., & Curri, S. B., Della Loggia, R., Del Negro, P., Gariboldi, P., & Tubaro, A. (1989). Complexes between phospholipids and vegetal derivates of biological interest. *Fitoterapia, 60*, 1–9.

Bonifacio, B. V., da Silva, P. B., dos Santos Ramos, M. A., Negri, K. M. S., Bauab, T. M., & Chorilli, M. (2014). Nanotechnology-based drug delivery systems and herbal medicines: A review. *International Journal of Nanomedicine*, *9*, 1. PMID:24363556

Bruneton, J. (1995). *Pharmacognosy, phytochemistry, medicinal plants*. Lavoisier publishing.

Buckton, G. (1995). Harwood. Interfacial phenomena in Drug Delivery and Targeting. Academic Publishers.

Cammidge, A. (2003). Dendrimers and other dendritic polymers. John Wiley and Sons Ltd.

Carini, M., Aldini, G., Rossoni, G., Morazzoni, P., & Facino, R. M. (2001). Complexation of Ginkgo biloba extract with phosphatidylcholine improves cardioprotective activity and increases the plasma antioxidant capacity in the rat. *Planta Medica*, *67*(04), 326–330. doi:10.1055-2001-14313 PMID:11458448

Chan, J., El Maghraby, G. M., Craig, J. P., & Alany, R. G. (2007). Phase transition water-in-oil microemulsions as ocular drug delivery systems: In vitro and in vivo evaluation. *International Journal of Pharmaceutics*, *328*(1), 65–71. doi:10.1016/j.ijpharm.2006.10.004 PMID:17092668

Chanchal, D., & Swarnlata, S. (2008). Novel approaches in herbal cosmetics. *Journal of Cosmetic Dermatology*, *7*(2), 89–95. doi:10.1111/j.1473-2165.2008.00369.x PMID:18482010

Chandel, A. K. S., Kumar, C. U., & Jewrajka, S. K. (2016). Effect of polyethylene glycol on properties and drug encapsulation–release performance of biodegradable/cytocompatible agarose–polyethylene glycol–polycaprolactone amphiphilic co-network gels. *ACS Applied Materials & Interfaces*, *8*(5), 3182–3192. doi:10.1021/acsami.5b10675 PMID:26760672

Chao, P., Deshmukh, M., Kutscher, H. L., Gao, D., Rajan, S. S., Hu, P., Laskin, D. L., Stein, S., & Sinko, P. J. (2010). Pulmonary targeting microparticulate camptothecin delivery system: Anti-cancer evaluation in a rat orthotopic lung cancer model. *Anti-Cancer Drugs*, *21*(1), 65–76. doi:10.1097/CAD.0b013e328332a322 PMID:19966540

Chen, H., Chang, X., Weng, T., Zhao, X., Gao, Z., Yang, Y., Xu, H., & Yang, X. (2004). A study of microemulsion systems for transdermal delivery of triptolide. *Journal of Controlled Release*, *98*(3), 427–436. doi:10.1016/j.jconrel.2004.06.001 PMID:15312998

Chen, Y., Lin, X., Park, H., & Greever, R. (2009). Study of artemisinin nanocapsules as anticancer drug delivery systems. *Nanomedicine; Nanotechnology, Biology, and Medicine*, *5*(3), 316–322. doi:10.1016/j.nano.2008.12.005 PMID:19523432

Chien, Y. (1991). *Novel drug delivery systems*. CRC Press. doi:10.1201/9780367805456

Cui, Y., Li, L., Gu, J., Zhang, T., & Zhang, L. (2011). Investigation of microemulsion system for transdermal delivery of ligustrazine phosphate. *African Journal of Pharmacy and Pharmacology*, *5*(14), 1674–1681. doi:10.5897/AJPP11.138

Davies, G. (2000). *Timetables of Medicine*. Black Dog & Leventhal.

Dewick, P. M. (2002). *Medicinal natural products: a biosynthetic approach*. John Wiley & Sons.

Ding, F., Diao, J. X., Sun, Y., & Sun, Y. (2012). Bioevaluation of human serum albumin–hesperidin bioconjugate: Insight into protein vector function and conformation. *Journal of Agricultural and Food Chemistry*, *60*(29), 7218–7228. doi:10.1021/jf300424w PMID:22702966

El-Ridy, M. S., Badawi, A. A., Safar, M. M., & Mohsen, A. M. (2012). Niosomes as a novel pharmaceutical formulation encapsulating the hepatoprotective drug silymarin. *International Journal of Pharmacy and Pharmaceutical Sciences*, *4*(1), 549–559.

Evans, W. C. (2009). *Trease and Evans Pharmacognosy* (International Edition). E-Book. Elsevier Health Sciences.

Fahao, C., Wuqing, O., & Yanping, W. (2007). Study of preparation of matrin nanoemulsion and its anti-oxidation on mice. *Journal of Northwest Sci-Tech University of Agriculture and Forestry.*

Fan, Y., & Zhang, Q. (2013). Development of liposomal formulations: From concept to clinical investigations. *Asian Journal of Pharmaceutical Sciences, 8*(2), 81-87.

Fang, J. Y., Hwang, T. L., Huang, Y. L., & Fang, C. L. (2006). Enhancement of the transdermal delivery of catechins by liposomes incorporating anionic surfactants and ethanol. *International Journal of Pharmaceutics*, *310*(1-2), 131–138. doi:10.1016/j.ijpharm.2005.12.004 PMID:16413711

Fatima Grace, X., Rahul Raj, S., Reshma, I., Sandeep, T., Shanmuganathan, S., & Chamundeeswari, D. (2014). Herbal ethosomes-A novel approach in herbal drug technology. *American Journal of Ethnomedicine*, *1*(4), 226–230.

Feng-Lin, Y., Tzu-Hui, W., Liang-Tzung, L., Thau-Ming, C., & Chun-Ching, L. (2009). Preparation of naringenin nanoparticles. *Pharmaceutical Research*, *26*(4), 893–902. PMID:19034626

Fu, R. Q., He, F. C., Meng, D. S., & Chen, L. (2006). Taxol PLA nanoparticles. *ACTA Academiae medicinae militaris tertiae, 28*, 1573-1574.

Garg, R., & Gupta, G. D. (2010). Gastroretentive floating microspheres of silymarin: Preparation and in vitro evaluation. *Tropical Journal of Pharmaceutical Research*, *9*(1). Advance online publication. doi:10.4314/tjpr.v9i1.52037

Ge, X., Wei, M., He, S., & Yuan, W. E. (2019). Advances of Non-Ionic Surfactant Vesicles (Niosomes) and Their Application in Drug Delivery. *Pharmaceutics*, *11*(2), 55. doi:10.3390/pharmaceutics11020055 PMID:30700021

Ghadi, Z. S., Dinarvand, R., Asemi, N., Amiri, F. T., & Ebrahimnejad, P. (2019). Preparation, characterization and in vivo evaluation of novel hyaluronan containing niosomes tailored by Box-Behnken design to co-encapsulate curcumin and quercetin. *European Journal of Pharmaceutical Sciences*, *130*, 234–246. doi:10.1016/j.ejps.2019.01.035 PMID:30711688

Girhepunje, K., Pal, R., Gevariya, H., Behera, A., & Thirumoorthy, N. (2010). Ethosomes: A novel vesicular carrier for enhanced dermal delivery of Ciclopiroxolamine. *Der Pharmacia Lettre*, *2*(1), 360–367.

Godin, B., & Touitou, E. (2004). Mechanism of bacitracin permeation enhancement through the skin and cellular membranes from an ethosomal carrier. *Journal of Controlled Release*, *94*(2-3), 365–379. doi:10.1016/j.jconrel.2003.10.014 PMID:14744487

Grayson, S. M., & Frechet, J. M. (2001). Convergent dendrons and dendrimers: From synthesis to applications. *Chemical Reviews*, *101*(12), 3819–3868. doi:10.1021/cr990116h PMID:11740922

Griffin, J. P., & O'Grady, J. (Eds.). (2006). *The textbook of pharmaceutical medicine*. Blackwell.

Gui, S. Y., Wu, L., Peng, D. Y., Liu, Q. Y., Yin, B. P., & Shen, J. Z. (2008). Preparation and evaluation of a microemulsion for oral delivery of berberine. *Die Pharmazie-An International Journal of Pharmaceutical Sciences*, *63*(7), 516–519. PMID:18717486

Gullett, N. P., Amin, A. R., Bayraktar, S., Pezzuto, J. M., Shin, D. M., Khuri, F. R., ... Kucuk, O. (2010, June). Cancer prevention with natural compounds. *Seminars in Oncology*, *37*(3), 258–281. doi:10.1053/j.seminoncol.2010.06.014 PMID:20709209

Gunasekaran, T., Haile, T., Nigusse, T., & Dhanaraju, M. D. (2014). Nanotechnology: An effective tool for enhancing bioavailability and bioactivity of phytomedicine. *Asian Pacific Journal of Tropical Biomedicine*, *4*, S1–S7. doi:10.12980/APJTB.4.2014C980 PMID:25183064

Gupta, L., Sharma, A. K., Gothwal, A., Khan, M. S., Khinchi, M. P., Qayum, A., Singh, S. K., & Gupta, U. (2017). Dendrimer encapsulated and conjugated delivery of berberine: A novel approach mitigating toxicity and improving in vivo pharmacokinetics. *International Journal of Pharmaceutics*, *528*(1-2), 88–99. doi:10.1016/j.ijpharm.2017.04.073 PMID:28533175

Hao, Y., Zhao, F., Li, N., Yang, Y., & Li, K. A. (2002). Studies on a high encapsulation of colchicine by a niosome system. *International Journal of Pharmaceutics*, *244*(1-2), 73–80. doi:10.1016/S0378-5173(02)00301-0 PMID:12204566

He, H. B., & Tang, X. (2005). Preparation of zedoary oil nano-emulsion and the influence factors on its preparation process. *Journal of Shenyang Pharmaceutical University*, *3*, 164–186. http://www.indena.com/pdf/phytosome_int.pdf

He, Z. F., Liu, D. Y., Zeng, S., & Ye, J. T. (2008). Study on preparation of ampelopsin liposomes. Zhongguo Zhong yao za zhi Zhongguo zhongyao zazhi. *Zhongguo Zhongyao Zazhi*, *33*(1), 27–30. PMID:18338614

Holmberg, K., Shah, D. O., & Schwuger, M. J. (2002). *Handbook of applied surface and colloid chemistry* (Vol. 1). John Wiley & Sons.

Hong, W., Chen, D. W., Zhao, X. L., Qiao, M. X., & Hu, H. Y. (2008). Preparation and study in vitro of long-circulating nanoliposomes of curcumin. Zhongguo Zhong yao za zhi, Zhongguo zhongyao zazhi. *Zhongguo Zhongyao Zazhi*, *33*(8), 889–892. PMID:18619344

Hou, J., & Zhou, S. (2003). Formulation and preparation of glycyrrhizic acid solid lipid nanoparticles. *Journal of Third Military Medical University*, (11).

Inoue, K., Kumazawa, E., Kuga, H., Susaki, H., Masubuchi, N., & Kajimura, T. (2004). *CM-dextran-polyalcohol-camptothecin conjugate. In Polymer Drugs in the Clinical Stage*. Springer.

Jain, S., Jain, V., & Mahajan, S. C. (2014). Lipid based vesicular drug delivery systems. *Advances in Pharmaceutics*.

Janisch, K. M., Williamson, G., Needs, P., & Plumb, G. W. (2004). Properties of quercetin conjugates: Modulation of LDL oxidation and binding to human serum albumin. *Free Radical Research, 38*(8), 877–884. doi:10.1080/10715760410001728415 PMID:15493462

Jiang, T., Wang, T., Li, T., Ma, Y., Shen, S., He, B., & Mo, R. (2018). Enhanced Transdermal Drug Delivery by Transfersome-Embedded Oligopeptide Hydrogel for Topical Chemotherapy of Melanoma. *ACS Nano, 12*(10), 9693–9701. doi:10.1021/acsnano.8b03800 PMID:30183253

Johansson, E. M., Dubois, J., Darbre, T., & Reymond, J. L. (2010). Glycopeptide dendrimer colchicine conjugates targeting cancer cells. *Bioorganic & Medicinal Chemistry, 18*(17), 6589–6597. doi:10.1016/j.bmc.2010.04.026 PMID:20674369

Johnson, I. T. (2007). Phytochemicals and cancer. *The Proceedings of the Nutrition Society, 66*(2), 207–215. doi:10.1017/S0029665107005459 PMID:17466103

Kamble, B., Talreja, S., Gupta, A., Patil, D., Pathak, D., Moothedath, I., & Duraiswamy, B. (2013). Development and biological evaluation of Gymnema sylvestre extract-loaded nonionic surfactant-based niosomes. *Nanomedicine (London), 8*(8), 1295–1305. doi:10.2217/nnm.12.162 PMID:23259778

Karimi, N., Ghanbarzadeh, B., Hamishehkar, H., Keyvani, F., Pezeshki, A., & Gholian, M. M. (2015). Phytosome and liposome: the beneficial encapsulation systems in drug delivery and food application. *Applied Food Biotechnology,* 17-27.

Kausar, H., Mujeeb, M., Ahad, A., Moolakkadath, T., Aqil, M., Ahmad, A., & Akhter, M. H. (2019). Optimization of ethosomes for topical thymoquinone delivery for the treatment of skin acne. *Journal of Drug Delivery Science and Technology, 49*, 177–187. doi:10.1016/j.jddst.2018.11.016

Kesharwani, R. K., Srivastava, V., Singh, P., Rizvi, S. I., Adeppa, K., & Misra, K. (2015). A novel approach for overcoming drug resistance in breast cancer chemotherapy by targeting new synthetic curcumin analogues against Aldehyde Dehydrogenase 1 (ALDH1A1) and Glycogen Synthase Kinase-3 β (GSK-3β). *Applied Biochemistry and Biotechnology, 176*(7), 1996–2017. doi:10.100712010-015-1696-x PMID:26113217

Khajuria, A., Zutshi, U., & Bedi, K. L. (1998). Permeability characteristics of piperine on oral absorption-an active alkaloid from peppers and a bioavailability enhancer. *Indian Journal of Experimental Biology, 36*, 46–50. PMID:9536651

Khandare, J. N., Madhavi, G., & Tamhankar, B. M. (1994). Niosomes-novel drug Delivery system. *Eastern Pharmacist, 37*, 61–61.

Kidd, P. M. (1997). Glutathione: Systemic protectant against oxidative and free radical damage. *Alternative Medicine Review, 2*(3), 155–176.

Kokate, C. K., Purohit, A. P., & Gokhale, S. B. (2003). *Textbook of Pharmacognosy*. Nirali Prakashan.

Kondratenko, R. M., Baltina, L. A., Mustafina, S. R., Vasil'eva, E. V., Pompei, R., Deidda, D., Plyasunova, O. A., Pokrovskii, A. G., & Tolstikov, G. A. (2004). The Synthesis and antiviral activity of glycyrrhizic acid conjugates with α-d-glucosamine and some glycosylamines. *Russian Journal of Bioorganic Chemistry, 30*(3), 275–282. doi:10.1023/B:RUBI.0000030135.97089.37 PMID:15344661

Koo, O. M., Rubinstein, I., & Onyuksel, H. (2005). Role of nanotechnology in targeted drug delivery and imaging: A concise review. *Nanomedicine; Nanotechnology, Biology, and Medicine*, *1*(3), 193–212. doi:10.1016/j.nano.2005.06.004 PMID:17292079

Lawrence, M. J., & Rees, G. D. (2012). Microemulsion-based media as novel drug delivery systems. *Advanced Drug Delivery Reviews*, *64*, 175–193. doi:10.1016/j.addr.2012.09.018 PMID:11104900

Leung, A. W., Amador, C., Wang, L. C., Mody, U. V., & Bally, M. B. (2019). What Drives Innovation: The Canadian Touch on Liposomal Therapeutics. *Pharmaceutics*, *11*(3), 124. doi:10.3390/pharmaceutics11030124 PMID:30884782

Li, L., Wang, D. K., Li, L. S., Jia, J., Chang, D., & Ai, L. (2007). Preparation of docetaxel submicron emulsion for intravenous administration. *Journal of Shenyang Pharmaceutical University*, *12*, 736–739.

Lira, M. C., Ferraz, M. S., da Silva, D. G., Cortes, M. E., Teixeira, K. I., Caetano, N. P., ... Santos-Magalhaes, N. S. (2009). Inclusion complex of usnic acid with β-cyclodextrin: Characterization and nanoencapsulation into liposomes. *Journal of Inclusion Phenomena and Macrocyclic Chemistry*, *64*(3-4), 215–224. doi:10.100710847-009-9554-5

Lu, M. F., Cheng, Y. Q., Li, L. J., & Wu, J. J. (2005). Progress of study on passive targeting of drug delivery system. *Mater Rev*, *19*(9), 108–110.

Lu, Y., Hou, S. X., Chen, T., Sun, Y. Y., Yang, B. X., & Yuan, Z. Y. (2005). Preparation of transfersomes of vincristine sulfate and study on its prcutaneous penetration. Zhongguo Zhong yao za zhi, Zhongguo zhongyao zazhi. *Zhongguo Zhongyao Zazhi*, *30*(12), 900–903. PMID:16124605

Lu, Y., Hou, S. X., Zhang, L. K., Li, Y., He, J. Y., & Guo, D. D. (2007). Transdermal and lymph targeting transfersomes of vincristine. *Yao Xue Xue Bao*, *42*(10), 1097–1101. PMID:18229621

Luo, D., Carter, K. A., Molins, E. A., Straubinger, N. L., Geng, J., Shao, S., Jusko, W. J., Straubinger, R. M., & Lovell, J. F. (2019). Pharmacokinetics and pharmacodynamics of liposomal chemophototherapy with short drug-light intervals. *Journal of Controlled Release*, *297*, 39–47. doi:10.1016/j.jconrel.2019.01.030 PMID:30684512

Manju, S., & Sreenivasan, K. (2011). Conjugation of curcumin onto hyaluronic acid enhances its aqueous solubility and stability. *Journal of Colloid and Interface Science*, *359*(1), 318–325. doi:10.1016/j.jcis.2011.03.071 PMID:21492865

Manmode, A. S., Sakarkar, D. M., & Mahajan, N. M. (2009). Nanoparticles-tremendous therapeutic potential: A review. *International Journal of Pharm Tech Research*, *1*(4), 1020–1027.

Massiot, J., Rosilio, V., & Makky, A. (2019). Photo-triggerable liposomal drug delivery systems: From simple porphyrin insertion in the lipid bilayer towards supramolecular assemblies of lipid–porphyrin conjugates. *Journal of Materials Chemistry. B, Materials for Biology and Medicine*, *7*(11), 1805–1823. doi:10.1039/C9TB00015A PMID:32255044

Mbah, C. C., Builders, P. F., & Attama, A. A. (2014). Nanovesicular carriers as alternative drug delivery systems: Ethosomes in focus. *Expert Opinion on Drug Delivery*, *11*(1), 45–59. doi:10.1517/17425247.2013.860130 PMID:24294974

Medina, O. P., Zhu, Y., & Kairemo, K. (2004). Targeted liposomal drug delivery in cancer. *Current Pharmaceutical Design*, *10*(24), 2981–2989. doi:10.2174/1381612043383467 PMID:15379663

Mei, Z., Chen, H., Weng, T., Yang, Y., & Yang, X. (2003). Solid lipid nanoparticle and microemulsion for topical delivery of triptolide. *European Journal of Pharmaceutics and Biopharmaceutics*, *56*(2), 189–196. doi:10.1016/S0939-6411(03)00067-5 PMID:12957632

Mei, Z., Li, X., Wu, Q., Hu, S., & Yang, X. (2005). The research on the anti-inflammatory activity and hepatotoxicity of triptolide-loaded solid lipid nanoparticle. *Pharmacological Research*, *51*(4), 345–351. doi:10.1016/j.phrs.2004.10.007 PMID:15683748

Mollazade, M., Nejati-Koshki, K., Akbarzadeh, A., Zarghami, N., Nasiri, M., Jahanban-Esfahlan, R., & Alibakhshi, A. (2013). PAMAM dendrimers augment inhibitory effects of curcumin on cancer cell proliferation: Possible inhibition of telomerase. *Asian Pacific Journal of Cancer Prevention*, *14*(11), 6925–6928. doi:10.7314/APJCP.2013.14.11.6925 PMID:24377627

Moolakkadath, T., Aqil, M., Ahad, A., Imam, S. S., Praveen, A., Sultana, Y., Mujeeb, M., & Iqbal, Z. (2019). Fisetin loaded binary ethosomes for management of skin cancer by dermal application on UV exposed mice. *International Journal of Pharmaceutics*, *560*, 78–91. doi:10.1016/j.ijpharm.2019.01.067 PMID:30742987

Mujoriya, R. Z., Dhamande, K., & Bodla, R. B. (2011). Niosomal drug delivery system—A review. *Int J Appl Pharm*, *3*(3), 7–10.

Mujoriya, R. Z., Dhamande, K., & Bodla, R. B. (2011). Niosomal drug delivery system—A review. *International Journal of Applied Pharmaceutics*, *3*(3), 7–10.

Mukerjee, A., & Vishwanatha, J. K. (2009). Formulation, characterization and evaluation of curcumin loaded PLGA nanospheres for cancer therapy. *Anticancer Research*, *29*(10), 3867–3875. PMID:19846921

Natrajan, V., Madhan, B., & Sehgal, P. (2010). Formulation and evalution of qucertin polycaprolactone microsphere for the treatment of Rheumatoid arthritis. *J Pharm Sophora Alopecuroides Sci*, *100*, 195-205.

Okore, V. C., Attama, A. A., Ofokansi, K. C., Esimone, C. O., & Onuigbo, E. B. (2011). Formulation and evaluation of niosomes. *Indian Journal of Pharmaceutical Sciences*, *73*(3), 323. PMID:22457561

Pang, X., Lu, Z., Du, H., Yang, X., & Zhai, G. (2014). Hyaluronic acid-quercetin conjugate micelles: Synthesis, characterization, in vitro and in vivo evaluation. *Colloids and Surfaces. B, Biointerfaces*, *123*, 778–786. doi:10.1016/j.colsurfb.2014.10.025 PMID:25454664

Paroha, S., Chandel, A. K. S., & Dubey, R. D. (2017). *Nanotechnology Delivery Systems of Coenzyme Q10: Pharmacokinetic and Clinical Implications. In Nanoscience in Food and Agriculture 4*. Springer.

Paroha, S., Chandel, A. K. S., & Dubey, R. D. (2018). Nanosystems for drug delivery of coenzyme Q10. *Environmental Chemistry Letters*, *16*(1), 71–77. doi:10.100710311-017-0664-9

Patel, R., Singh, S. K., Singh, S., Sheth, N. R., & Gendle, R. (2009). Development and characterization of curcumin loaded transfersome for transdermal delivery. *Journal of Pharmaceutical Sciences and Research*, *1*(4), 71.

Patil, R. Y., Patil, S. A., Chivate, N. D., & Patil, Y. N. (2018). Herbal Drug Nanoparticles: Advancements in Herbal Treatment. *Research Journal of Pharmacy and Technology*, *11*(1), 421–426. doi:10.5958/0974-360X.2018.00078.1

Pattni, B. S., Chupin, V. V., & Torchilin, V. P. (2015). New developments in liposomal drug delivery. *Chemical Reviews*, *115*(19), 10938–10966. doi:10.1021/acs.chemrev.5b00046 PMID:26010257

Pentel, P. R., Malin, D. H., Ennifar, S., Hieda, Y., Keyler, D. E., Lake, J. R., ... Naso, R. (2000). A nicotine conjugate vaccine reduces nicotine distribution to brain and attenuates its behavioral and cardiovascular effects in rats. *Pharmacology, Biochemistry, and Behavior*, *65*(1), 191–198. doi:10.1016/S0091-3057(99)00206-3 PMID:10638653

Pires, A. M., & Araújo, P. S. (2012). Percepção de risco e conceitos sobre plantas medicinais, fitoterápicos e medicamentos alopáticos entre gestantes. *Revista baiana de saúde pública*, *35*(2), 320.

Priprem, A., Watanatorn, J., Sutthiparinyanont, S., Phachonpai, W., & Muchimapura, S. (2008). Anxiety and cognitive effects of quercetin liposomes in rats. *Nanomedicine; Nanotechnology, Biology, and Medicine*, *4*(1), 70–78. doi:10.1016/j.nano.2007.12.001 PMID:18249157

Rafe, M. R. (2018). Liposomal Drug Delivery Systems Have Opened a New Window in Pharmaceutical Sciences: A Literature-based Review. *Asian Journal of Pharmaceutics*, *11*(04).

Rahimpour, Y., & Hamishehkar, H. (2012). Niosomes as carrier in dermal drug delivery. In *Recent Advances in Novel Drug Carrier Systems*. IntechOpen. doi:10.5772/51729

Rane, S., & Prabhakar, B. (2009). Formulation and Evaluation of pH-Sensitive, Long circulating Liposomes for Paclitaxel Delivery. *International Journal of Pharm Tech Research*, *1*, 914–917.

Reddy, J. A., Dorton, R., Westrick, E., Dawson, A., Smith, T., Xu, L. C., Vetzel, M., Kleindl, P., Vlahov, I. R., & Leamon, C. P. (2007). Preclinical evaluation of EC145, a folate-vinca alkaloid conjugate. *Cancer Research*, *67*(9), 4434–4442. doi:10.1158/0008-5472.CAN-07-0033 PMID:17483358

Riva, A., Ronchi, M., Petrangolini, G., Bosisio, S., & Allegrini, P. (2019). Improved Oral Absorption of Quercetin from Quercetin Phytosome®, a New Delivery System Based on Food Grade Lecithin. *European Journal of Drug Metabolism and Pharmacokinetics*, *44*(2), 169–177. doi:10.100713318-018-0517-3 PMID:30328058

Rowland, I. (1999). Optimal nutrition: Fibre and phytochemicals. *The Proceedings of the Nutrition Society*, *58*(2), 415–419. doi:10.1017/S0029665199000543 PMID:10466185

Saraf, S. (2010). Applications of novel drug delivery system for herbal formulations. *Fitoterapia*, *81*(7), 680–689. doi:10.1016/j.fitote.2010.05.001 PMID:20471457

Saraf, S., Jeswani, G., Kaur, C. D., & Saraf, S. (2011). Development of novel herbal cosmetic cream with Curcuma longa extract loaded transfersomes for antiwrinkle effect. *The Journal of Pharmacy and Pharmacology*, *5*(8), 1054–1062.

Sarwa, K. K., Mazumder, B., Rudrapal, M., & Verma, V. K. (2015). Potential of capsaicin-loaded transfersomes in arthritic rats. *Drug Delivery*, *22*(5), 638–646. doi:10.3109/10717544.2013.871601 PMID:24471764

Satyan, K. S., Jaiswal, A. K., Ghosal, S., & Bhattacharya, S. K. (1998). Anxiolytic activity of ginkgolic acid conjugates from Indian Ginkgo biloba. *Psychopharmacology, 136*(2), 148–152. doi:10.1007002130050550 PMID:9551771

Scarfato, P., Avallone, E., Iannelli, P., Aquino, R. P., Lauro, M. R., Rossi, A., & Acierno, D. (2008). Quercetin microspheres by solvent evaporation: Preparation, characterization and release behavior. *Journal of Applied Polymer Science, 109*(5), 2994–3001. doi:10.1002/app.28365

Schreier, H., & Bouwstra, J. (1994). Liposomes and niosomes as topical drug carriers: Dermal and transdermal drug delivery. *Journal of Controlled Release, 30*(1), 1–15. doi:10.1016/0168-3659(94)90039-6

Sebastian, M., Ninan, N., & Haghi, A. K. (Eds.). (2012). *Nanomedicine and drug delivery*. CRC Press. doi:10.1201/b13119

Sharma, G., Anabousi, S., Ehrhardt, C., & Ravi Kumar, M. N. V. (2006). Liposomes as targeted drug delivery systems in the treatment of breast cancer. *Journal of Drug Targeting, 14*(5), 301–310. doi:10.1080/10611860600809112 PMID:16882550

Sharma, P. K., Saxena, P., Jaswanth, A., Chalamaiah, M., Tekade, K. R., & Balasubramaniam, A. (2016). Novel encapsulation of lycopene in niosomes and assessment of its anticancer activity. *Journal of Bioequivalence & Bioavailability, 8*(5), 224–232.

Sheena, I. P., Singh, U. V., Kamath, R., Devi, P. U., & Udupa, N. (1998). Niosomal withaferin A with better antitumor efficacy. *Indian Journal of Pharmaceutical Sciences, 60*(1), 45–48.

Shen, Q., Wang, Y., & Zhang, Y. (2011). Improvement of colchicine oral bioavailability by incorporating eugenol in the nanoemulsion as an oil excipient and enhancer. *International Journal of Nanomedicine, 6*, 1237. doi:10.2147/IJN.S20903 PMID:21753875

Shi, J., Votruba, A. R., Farokhzad, O. C., & Langer, R. (2010). Nanotechnology in drug delivery and tissue engineering: From discovery to applications. *Nano Letters, 10*(9), 3223–3230. doi:10.1021/nl102184c PMID:20726522

Shimada, S. (2008). Composition comprising nanoparticle Ginkgo biloba extract with the effect of brain function activation IPC8 Class-AA61K914FI, USPC Class-424489.

Silva, A. P., Nunes, B. R., De Oliveira, M. C., Koester, L. S., Mayorga, P., Bassani, V. L., & Teixeira, H. F. (2009). Development of topical nanoemulsions containing the isoflavone genistein. Die Pharmazie-An. *International Journal of Pharma Sciences, 64*(1), 32–35. PMID:19216228

Singer, J. W., Bhatt, R., Tulinsky, J., Buhler, K. R., Heasley, E., Klein, P., & de Vries, P. (2001). Water-soluble poly-(l-glutamic acid)–Gly-camptothecin conjugates enhance camptothecin stability and efficacy in vivo. *Journal of Controlled Release, 74*(1-3), 243–247. doi:10.1016/S0168-3659(01)00323-6 PMID:11489501

Singh, Y., Meher, J. G., Raval, K., Khan, F. A., Chaurasia, M., Jain, N. K., & Chourasia, M. K. (2017). Nanoemulsion: Concepts, development and applications in drug delivery. *Journal of Controlled Release, 252*, 28–49. doi:10.1016/j.jconrel.2017.03.008 PMID:28279798

Sinico, C., De Logu, A., Lai, F., Valenti, D., Manconi, M., Loy, G., Bonsignore, L., & Fadda, A. M. (2005). Liposomal incorporation of Artemisia arborescens L. essential oil and in vitro antiviral activity. *European Journal of Pharmaceutics and Biopharmaceutics*, *59*(1), 161–168. doi:10.1016/j.ejpb.2004.06.005 PMID:15567314

Song, Y., Ping, Q., & Wu, Z. (2005). Preparation of silybin nanoemulsion and its pharmacokinetics in rabbits. *Zhongguo Yaoke Daxue Xuebao*, *36*(5), 427.

Sri, S. N., Thiagarajan, R., Manikandan, R., & Arumugam, M. (2019). Curcumin-Based Food Supplements: Challenges and Future Prospects. In Nonvitamin and Nonmineral Nutritional Supplements. Academic Press.

Su, Y. L., Fu, Z. Y., Zhang, J. Y., Wang, W. M., Wang, H., Wang, Y. C., & Zhang, Q. J. (2008). Microencapsulation of Radix salvia miltiorrhiza nanoparticles by spray-drying. *Powder Technology*, *184*(1), 114–121. doi:10.1016/j.powtec.2007.08.014

Subramanian, A. P., Jaganathan, S. K., Manikandan, A., Pandiaraj, K. N., Gomathi, N., & Supriyanto, E. (2016). Recent trends in nano-based drug delivery systems for efficient delivery of phytochemicals in chemotherapy. *RSC Advances*, *6*(54), 48294–48314. doi:10.1039/C6RA07802H

Sudhakar, C. K., Upadhyay, N., Verma, A., Jain, A., Charyulu, R. N., & Jain, S. (2015). Nanomedicine and tissue engineering. In *Nanotechnology Applications for Tissue Engineering* (pp. 1–19). William Andrew Publishing. doi:10.1016/B978-0-323-32889-0.00001-7

Sun, H. W., & Ouyang, W. Q. (2007). Preparation, Quality and Safety Evaluation of Berberine Nanoemulsion for Oral Application. *Shanghai Jiaotong Daxue Xuebao. Nongye Kexueban*, 1.

Sun, H. W., & Ouyang, W. Q. (2007). The preparation of neem oil microemulsion (Azdirachta Indica) and the comparission of acaricidal time between neemoil microemulsion and other formulation in vitro. [Agric Sci]. *J Shanghai Jiao Tong Univy*, *1*, 60–65.

Tacar, O., Sriamornsak, P., & Dass, C. R. (2013). Doxorubicin: An update on anticancer molecular action, toxicity and novel drug delivery systems. *The Journal of Pharmacy and Pharmacology*, *65*(2), 157–170. doi:10.1111/j.2042-7158.2012.01567.x PMID:23278683

Terreno, E., Delli Castelli, D., Cabella, C., Dastrù, W., Sanino, A., Stancanello, J., Tei, L., & Aime, S. (2008). Paramagnetic liposomes as innovative contrast agents for magnetic resonance (MR) molecular imaging applications. *Chemistry & Biodiversity*, *5*(10), 1901–1912. doi:10.1002/cbdv.200890178 PMID:18972531

Thomas, R. G., Moon, M., Lee, S., & Jeong, Y. Y. (2015). Paclitaxel loaded hyaluronic acid nanoparticles for targeted cancer therapy: In vitro and in vivo analysis. *International Journal of Biological Macromolecules*, *72*, 510–518. doi:10.1016/j.ijbiomac.2014.08.054 PMID:25224289

Touitou, E. (2010). *Terbinafine compositions for onchomycosis treatment.* WPO Patent application WO/2010/086723.

Touitou, E., Dayan, N., Bergelson, L., Godin, B., & Eliaz, M. (2000). Ethosomes-novel vesicular carriers for enhanced delivery: Characterization and skin penetration properties. *Journal of Controlled Release, 65*(3), 403–418. doi:10.1016/S0168-3659(99)00222-9 PMID:10699298

Upadhyaya, J., Kesharwani, R. K., & Misra, K. (2009). Metabolism, Pharmacokinetics and Bioavailability of Ascorbic Acid; Synergistic Effect in presence of Tocopherols and Curcumin. *J Comput Intel Bioinform, 2*(1), 77–84.

Verma, P., & Pathak, K. (2010). Therapeutic and cosmeceutical potential of ethosomes: An overview. *Journal of Advanced Pharmaceutical Technology & Research, 1*(3), 274. doi:10.4103/0110-5558.72415 PMID:22247858

Vicentini, F. T., Simi, T. R., Del Ciampo, J. O., Wolga, N. O., Pitol, D. L., Iyomasa, M. M., Bentley, M., & Fonseca, M. J. (2008). Quercetin in w/o microemulsion: In vitro and in vivo skin penetration and efficacy against UVB-induced skin damages evaluated in vivo. *European Journal of Pharmaceutics and Biopharmaceutics, 69*(3), 948–957. doi:10.1016/j.ejpb.2008.01.012 PMID:18304790

Vyas, A., Saraf, S., & Saraf, S. (2008). Cyclodextrin based novel drug delivery systems. *Journal of Inclusion Phenomena and Macrocyclic Chemistry, 62*(1-2), 23–42. doi:10.100710847-008-9456-y

Wadhwa, J., Nair, A., & Kumria, R. (2012). Emulsion forming drug delivery system for lipophilic drugs. *Acta Poloniae Pharmaceutica, 69*(2), 179–191. PMID:22568032

Wang, L., Li, X., Zhang, G., Dong, J., & Eastoe, J. (2007). Oil-in-water nanoemulsions for pesticide formulations. *Journal of Colloid and Interface Science, 314*(1), 230–235. doi:10.1016/j.jcis.2007.04.079 PMID:17612555

Wang, X., Chen, Y., Dahmani, F. Z., Yin, L., Zhou, J., & Yao, J. (2014). Amphiphilic carboxymethyl chitosan-quercetin conjugate with P-gp inhibitory properties for oral delivery of paclitaxel. *Biomaterials, 35*(26), 7654–7665. doi:10.1016/j.biomaterials.2014.05.053 PMID:24927684

Weissmann, G., Bloomgarden, D., Kaplan, R., Cohen, C., Hoffstein, S., Collins, T., Gotlieb, A., & Nagle, D. (1975). A general method for the introduction of enzymes, by means of immunoglobulin-coated liposomes, into lysosomes of deficient cells. *Proceedings of the National Academy of Sciences of the United States of America, 72*(1), 88–92. doi:10.1073/pnas.72.1.88 PMID:1054517

Wen, Z., Liu, B., Zheng, Z., You, X., Pu, Y., & Li, Q. (2010). Preparation of liposomes entrapping essential oil from Atractylodes macrocephala Koidz by modified RESS technique. *Chemical Engineering Research & Design, 88*(8), 1102–1107. doi:10.1016/j.cherd.2010.01.020

Wu, P. S., Li, Y. S., Kuo, Y. C., Tsai, S. J. J., & Lin, C. C. (2019). Preparation and Evaluation of Novel Transfersomes Combined with the Natural Antioxidant Resveratrol. *Molecules (Basel, Switzerland), 24*(3), 600. doi:10.3390/molecules24030600 PMID:30743989

Wu, S. J., Don, T. M., Lin, C. W., & Mi, F. L. (2014). Delivery of berberine using chitosan/fucoidan-taurine conjugate nanoparticles for treatment of defective intestinal epithelial tight junction barrier. *Marine Drugs, 12*(11), 5677–5697. doi:10.3390/md12115677 PMID:25421323

Xi, J., & Guo, R. (2007). Interactions between flavonoids and hemoglobin in lecithin liposomes. *International Journal of Biological Macromolecules*, *40*(4), 305–311. doi:10.1016/j.ijbiomac.2006.08.011 PMID:16997370

Xiao, J., Shen, X., Wu, M., & Lu, R. (2002). Epidemiologic survey on the association between green tea intake and fatty liver disease. *China Public Health*, *18*, 385–387.

Xiao, L., Zhang, Y., Jianchen, X. U., & Jin, X. (1994). Preparation of floating rutin-alginate-chitosan microcapsule. *Chinese Traditional and Herbal Drugs*, (2).

Xu, Y. Q., Chen, W. R., Tsosie, J. K., Xie, X., Li, P., Wan, J. B., He, C.-W., & Chen, M. W. (2016). Niosome encapsulation of curcumin: Characterization and cytotoxic effect on ovarian cancer cells. *Journal of Nanomaterials*, *2016*, 2016. doi:10.1155/2016/6365295

Yen, F. L., Wu, T. H., Lin, L. T., Cham, T. M., & Lin, C. C. (2008). Nanoparticles formulation of Cuscuta chinensis prevents acetaminophen-induced hepatotoxicity in rats. *Food and Chemical Toxicology*, *46*(5), 1771–1777. doi:10.1016/j.fct.2008.01.021 PMID:18308443

Yu, A. H., & Zhai, G. X. (2006). Preparation and quality evaluation of puerarin microemulsion. *Chinese Journal of Pharmaceuticals*, *7*, 471-473.

Yukuyama, M. N., Ghisleni, D. D. M., Pinto, T. D. J. A., & Bou-Chacra, N. A. (2016). Nanoemulsion: Process selection and application in cosmetics–a review. *International Journal of Cosmetic Science*, *38*(1), 13–24. doi:10.1111/ics.12260 PMID:26171789

Zhang, L., Pornpattananangkul, D., Hu, C. M., & Huang, C. M. (2010). Development of nanoparticles for antimicrobial drug delivery. *Current Medicinal Chemistry*, *17*(6), 585–594. doi:10.2174/092986710790416290 PMID:20015030

Zhang, Y. (1994). Advances in research on target-oriented drug delivery system of Chinese materia medica. *Chinese Traditional and Herbal Drugs*, (5).

Zhang, Y., Xia, Q., Li, Y., He, Z., Li, Z., Guo, T., Wu, Z., & Feng, N. (2019). CD44 Assists the Topical Anti-Psoriatic Efficacy of Curcumin-Loaded Hyaluronan-Modified Ethosomes: A New Strategy for Clustering Drug in Inflammatory Skin. *Theranostics*, *9*(1), 48–64. doi:10.7150/thno.29715 PMID:30662553

Zhao, Y., Wang, C., Chow, A. H., Ren, K., Gong, T., Zhang, Z., & Zheng, Y. (2010). Self-nanoemulsifying drug delivery system (SNEDDS) for oral delivery of Zedoary essential oil: Formulation and bioavailability studies. *International Journal of Pharmaceutics*, *383*(1-2), 170–177. doi:10.1016/j.ijpharm.2009.08.035 PMID:19732813

Zheng, Y., Hou, S. X., Chen, T., & Lu, Y. (2006). Preparation and characterization of transfersomes of three drugs in vitro. Zhongguo Zhong yao za zhi, Zhongguo zhongyao zazhi. *Zhongguo Zhongyao Zazhi*, *31*(9), 728–731. PMID:17048677

Zhong, H., Deng, Y., Wang, X., & Yang, B. (2005). Multivesicular liposome formulation for the sustained delivery of breviscapine. *International Journal of Pharmaceutics*, *301*(1-2), 15–24. doi:10.1016/j.ijpharm.2005.04.001 PMID:16023316

Zhou, Y., Wei, Y., Liu, H., Zhang, G., & Wu, X. A. (2010). Preparation and in vitro evaluation of ethosomal total alkaloids of Sophora alopecuroides loaded by a transmembrane pH-gradient method. *AAPS PharmSciTech*, *11*(3), 1350–1358. doi:10.120812249-010-9509-6 PMID:20740333

Zhou, Y., Wei, Y. H., Zhang, G. Q., & Wu, X. A. (2010). Synergistic penetration of ethosomes and lipophilic prodrug on the transdermal delivery of acyclovir. *Archives of Pharmacal Research*, *33*(4), 567–574. doi:10.100712272-010-0411-2 PMID:20422366

Chapter 2
Novel Approaches in Herbal Formulations

Bhushan Rajendra Rane
https://orcid.org/0000-0002-1482-1884
Shri D.D. Vispute College of Pharmacy and Research Center, Raigad, India

Aishwarya Keshav Patil
Shri D.D. Vispute College of Pharmacy and Research Center, Raigad, India

Raj K. Keservani
Faculty of B. Pharmacy, CSM Group of Institutions, Prayagraj, India

Ashish S Jain
Shri D.D. Vispute College of Pharmacy and Research Center, Raigad, India

Rajesh Kumar Kesharwani
https://orcid.org/0000-0002-7507-9556
Nehru Gram Bharati (Deemed), India

ABSTRACT

Herbal medications have restorative potential, which can be given through different advantageous medication conveyance frameworks. Utilizing the bioactive and plant extricates, the assortment of novel natural details like polymeric nanoparticles, liposomes, phytosomes, nanoemulsions, microsphere, transfersomes, and ethosomes are accounted for. The chapter features the novel methodologies of natural detailing and condenses their strategy for planning and use of novel home-grown definition to accomplish better helpful reaction.

DOI: 10.4018/978-1-7998-4453-2.ch002

1. INTRODUCTION

1.1 Background

Since very old days herbal medications have been broadly utilized worldwide and have been used by doctors and patients for their beneficial qualities as they have fewer adverse effects when compared with allopathic drugs. Herbal drugs have complex structure of many active constituents from which all of them provide synergistic action and enhance the therapeutic value.

In development of novel herbal formulation, nano-sized dosage forms like polymeric nanoparticles, liposomes, solid lipid nanoparticles, phytosomes, transferosomes, and nanoemulsion has a number of advantages for herbal drugs, including enhancement of solubility and bioavailability, reducing toxicity, increasing the pharmacological activity, enhancement of stability, improve tissue macrophage distribution, sustained delivery as well as provide protection from physical and chemical degradation. Thus, the nano-sized novel herbal drug delivery has a potential future for enhancing the activity and overcoming problems associated with the plant medicines (Sarangi et al., 2018). For example, liposomes act as effective vehicles to deliver anti-cancer agents by increasing amount of drug at the site of tumor and decrease the accumulation of drug at site of normal tissues thereby preventing tissue toxicity effects (Bhokare et al., 2016). Phytosome is a novel technology developed by a leading manufacturer of drugs and nutraceuticals, to incorporate plant extracts or water soluble phytoconsituents into phospholipids to produce lipid compatible molecular complexes (Sachan et al., 2015). Other approaches like microspheres, nanoemulsions, polymeric nanoparticles and so forth have been proved beneficial to carry herbal drug.

***Herbal medications*:** Herbal medications mean dosage form consisting of one or more herbs or processed herbs in indicated amounts to provide specific nutritional, cosmetic benefits or other benefits meant for use to diagnose, treat and moderate infections of individual or animals (Afrin et al., 2018).

1.2 Advantages of Herbal Medications

1. Low risk of side effects: Mostly natural medications are secure for patient, having less unintended impact and fewer symptoms than customary prescription.
2. Greater effectivity: Herbal drugs are more effective for longer health complaints that don't respond well to traditional medicine. Here, example is the herbs and alternative remedies used to treat arthritis.
3. Minimal effort: Cost of natural medications is much less than prescribed medications. Research, testing and advertising increase significantly to the cost of prescription drug compare to natural medicines.
4. Broad accessibility: Herbs are accessible in wide amount. As simple herbs like chamomile and peppermint can be cultivated at home (Bhokare et al., 2016; Kharat et al.,2014).

1.3 Drawback of Herbal Medications

There are not many restrictions of herbal medications, for example,

1. Herbal medications show instability in exceedingly acidic pH, pre systemic metabolism in liver, solubility, and absorption problems, which may lead to drug levels below therapeutic concentration in the plasma, hence give less or no therapeutic effects.
2. Most of the plant actives like glycosides, tannins, flavonoids, and so forth, are polar in nature and are ineffectively absorbed due to large molecular size which may limits the absorption via passive diffusion and poor lipid solubility severely limits their ability to cross the lipid-rich biological membranes, due to which bioavailability reduced which give low therapeutic index of plant actives (Goyal et al., 2011).

2. IMPORTANCE OF NOVEL HERBAL FORMULATIONS

Herbal medicines are becoming increasingly popular in today's world because of their application to treat a variety of diseases with better therapeutic and less toxic side effects. Herbal ingredients are easily absorbed by the body. Therefore, they produce fewer side effects and provide increased absorption into the bloodstream leading to complete and effective treatment. Chemical agents are associated with side effects. The human body tends to reject certain chemical compounds. This rejection comes in the form of side effects (Devi et al., 2010). Phytopharmaceuticals are drugs that use traditional compounds derived from herbs instead of chemicals. Most active organic compounds are water-soluble molecules such as flavonoids, tannins, terpenoids, which are poorly ingested because of their sub-atomic size that can absorb due to inactive dispersion, or because of poor lipid dissolvability which reduces their ability to cross the lipid membrane (Nalla et al., 2017). Before reaching the bloodstream, many herbal supplements are stable in the pH with high acidity in the stomach and some nutrients may be linked to the liver because a large number of herbal medicines may not reach the bloodstream which is why they show minimal therapeutic effect. Nanocarriers that work with herbal remedies will carry the right amount of the drug into their environment that crosses all barriers such as stomach acidic pH, liver metabolism and increase the long-term distribution of the drug into the bloodstream due to herbal remedies (Ansari et al., 2012; Sharma et al., 2014).

2.1 Challenges in Development of Herbal Formulations

1. Bulk dosing.
2. Low bioavailability and low ingestion.
3. Require high amount of drug to produce desire effect.
4. High measure of crude material require for processing the medicine.
5. Loss of numerous species.
6. Harmful impact on nature which ultimately responsible for global warming.
7. In case of present formulations there is no target specificity (Kumar et al., 2012).

3. ADVANTAGES OF NOVEL HERBAL FORMULATION

1. Novel herbal preparationincreases the bioavailability of herbal medications.
2. Solubility enhancement.

3. Reduced toxicity.
4. Stability enhancement.
5. Give protection from physical and chemical degradation.
6. Increasing pharmacological movement.
7. Novel herbal formulations helps to reduce quantity of component with improving quality of drug effect as well as increase the efficacy and reduce the side effect of various herbal compounds.
8. Improved tissue macrophages distribution.
9. Low amount of raw materials are required to achieve the desire effect and control drug delivery to provide exact specification regarding drug dose form.
10. Novel herbal drug delivery system can carry maximum amount of drug to the site of action by crossing all barriers. Such as acidic environment of stomach, also increases prolong circulation of drug into blood due to their small particle size.
11. Reduced repeat administration and also helps to increase the therapeutic value by reducing toxicity and increase the bioavailability (Nalla et al., 2017; Mueller et al., 2000).

4. TECHNOLOGIES USED IN HERBAL FORMULATIONS

4.1 Traditional Technologies

Various routine plants generally utilized for more than 1000 years named rasayana are available in herbal preparations (Modak et al., 2007). There are a few techniques involved in obtaining the herbal extract/ bioactive phytoconstituents which depend somewhat on the specific part of the plant which is being utilized. A few techniques are used for extraction of bioactive material from traditional plant which are as follows (Dibua et al., 2011).

1. Grinding
2. Extraction
3. Soxhlet extractor.
4. Filtration
5. Fixation
6. Refining
7. Articulation
8. Enfleurage
9. Maceration with water and non-polar solvents

4.2 Traditional Techniques For Herbal Formulation

4.2.1 Infusions

Infusions are commonly used for aromatic herbs, leaves and fresh delicate plants. In this way the water simply boils and is poured over the tree. Covered and allowed to stand for 10-15 minutes, however. It can be prepared in a drinking cup by simply pouring warm water over the tree. Empty teabags are also found in some vegetable stores that are filled with herbs and then sealed with metal. The amount of vegetables and water can vary depending on the herb, the plant, and whether an herbicide or powdered medicine is used. In preparation for giving him *Ocimum gratissimum*, the new leaves of the plant are washed. In a beaker 100 ml of boiled water is added to the leaves, to ensure the indirect heat of the plant material (Dike et al., 2012).

4.2.2 Decoctions

Decoctions method is usually used for strong and fibrous plants, bark, and roots in which water soluble components are present. Plant materials are boiled for a long time to soften the wood and release active substances from the plant material. The required number of herbs is measured in a ceramic pot with an equal filling lid by adding the correct amount of cold water depending on how many cups of decoction you wish to prepare and heated to boiling. Usually one to one cup is a moderate amount of decoction, two or three times daily. Solid decoctions depend on the type of plant material used in the preparation of the decoction. Solid decoctions can be prepared by boiling the mixture for about two hours or more which is indicative of working with large pieces of bark to break it down. Decoctions method can be used for the roots of *Azadirachta Indica* (Neem) and stem in the treatment of malaria (Taylor et al., 2004).

4.2.3 Tinctures

Tincture is a water and alcohol extract which is used when active constituents of plant material are not freely soluble in water. Tinctures are used for plant materials when a larger quantity is prepared for better convenience and wanted for longer term storage. Many plant tinctures which are properly prepared can last several years or more without losing potency. The shelf life usually determines by percentage of alcohol, as more alcohol used, longer the shelf life.

4.2.4 Asava and Arishta

Asava and Arishta are traditionally use in Ayurveda which is a novel dispirited continuous hydroalcoholic extraction method. Asava and Arishta are alcoholic medicines prepared by using the herbal juice or their decoctions to undergo fermentation with the adding of sugars. Arishta are made with decoctions of herbs in hot water whereas Asavas are prepared by directly using fresh herbal juices. Due to certain superior properties Asava and Arishta are very popular forms of ayurvedic system of medications which make them extra advantageous than other medications. They are effective, edible, stable and prominently they have no side effects (Nandre et al., 2012).

4.3 Novel Techniques For Herbal Detailing

Most of the colloidal drug delivery approaches are used in the development of Herbal formulations.

4.3.1 Phytosomes

The Phospholipids-based drug delivery system has been found to promise the delivery of valuable and effective drugs (Sharma et al., 2014). Phytosomes are phytoconstituents that are dissolved in water that are converted into a complex of lipid-binding vesicles. Phytosomes are vesicular system and novel for-

Figure 1. Classification of colloidal drug delivery system (CDDS)

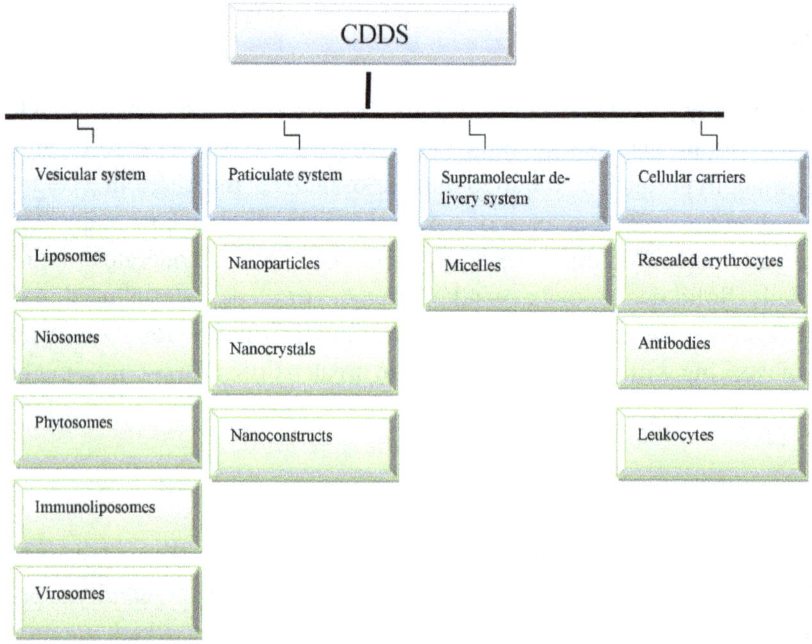

mulas containing herbal extracts (active phytoconstituents) combined with phospholipids that produce molecular arrangement (Pawar et al., 2015). Phytosomes have improved absorption characteristics and more bioavailable than conventional herbal extracts. A number of phytosomal formulations are available for the delivery of poorly lipid soluble drugs like extracts of *Ginkgo biloba*, grape seed, hawthorn, milk thistle, green tea etc. Phytosomal system prevent valuable component of herbal extract from destruction by digestive secretion and gut bacteria they show better absorption which produces better bioavailability and improved pharmacological and pharmacokinetic parameters (Joshi et al., 2008). Phytosomes applied to botanical and phytoconstituents will open new avenues to explore maximum therapeutic potential of plant substances of polar nature (Acharya et al., 2011). Some of herbal formulations in phytosomal drug delivery system were listed in Table no 1.

Table 1. Various Phytosomal Herbal Formulation

S. No.	Active ingredients	Derived from which plant	Biological Activity	Application of technology	Method of preparation	Route of administration	Reference
1	Curcumin	*Curcuma longa*	Anti-tumour, anti-oxidant and antiplatelet aggregation	Enhance anti-inflammatory activity,	Curcumin–phospholipid complexation	Oral	(Bhattacharya, 2009; Feng-Lin, 2009)
2	Green Tea	Epigallocatechin from *Thea sinensis*	Nutraceutical, Systemic antioxidant. It is best choice for protection against cancer and damage to cholesterol.	Increase in absorption	Phospholipids complexation	Oral	(Gandhi,2012)
3	Naringenin	Flavonoid obtained from *Citrus reticulata*	Antioxidant activity	Prolonged duration of action	Naringenin–phospholipid complex	Oral	(Maiti, 2006)

4.3.2 Advantages of Phytosomes

1. Phytosomes is a vesicular structure which has the ability to prevent from degradation by gut bacteria and digestive secretions.
2. It shows better stability due to the formation of chemical bonds that it forms between phytoconstituents and phosphatidyl choline molecules.
3. Targeted drug delivery of herbal is possible due to phytosomes which improves percutaneous absorption of phytoconstituents therefore can be use in cosmetics (Afrin et al., 2018).
4. It has greater therapeutic benefit because it improves the absorption profile of lipid insoluble polar phytoconstituents thus showing better bioavailability (Goyal et al., 2011).
5. There is no need to remove the unentrapped drug which is required to be removed in case of liposomes (Pandita et al., 2013; Kavitha et al., 2010).
6. It is able to permeate the hydrophilic botanical extract to be better absorbed in intestinal lumen.
7. Its dose requirement is small because it increases the absorption of active phytoconstituents.
8. Targeting to liver can be possible because appreciable drug entrapment and improvement in the solubility of bile to herbal constituents.

4.3.3 Disadvantages of Phytosomes

1. A compound can be synthesized depending on the amphiphilic nature.
2. They require superficial as well as mass drug-lipid interaction.
3. Covalent type of bond is required to restrict drug leakage.
4. Pharmacosomes are susceptible to aggregation, or hydrolysis on storage (Pandita et al., 2013).

4.4 Liposomes

Liposomes are vesicular system consisting of bilayers which form spontaneously when phospholipids are dispersed in water. In this microscopic vesicle an aqueous volume is completely enclosed by a membrane composed of lipid bilayers (Bangham et al., 1964). Liposomes have got a potential advantage in encapsulating hydrophilic as well as hydrophobic drugs and targeted delivery to site can be achieved (Kumar, 2011). Recently, a new generation of liposomes called 'stealth liposomes' has been developed.

Table 2. Herbal Formulations of Liposomes

S. No.	Active ingredient	Derived from which plant	Biological Activity	Application of technology	Method of preparation	Route of administration	Reference
1	Artemisia	*Artemisia annua*	Anti-viral activity	Increase in anti-viral activity and stability Targeting of essential oils to cells, enhance penetration into cytoplasmatic barrier	Film method and sonication	In vitro	(Fadda et al., 2005)
2	Nux vomica	*Strychnosnux-vomica*	Anti-tumour, anti-inflammatory and analgesic	Activities increase stability of formulation	Stealth liposome technique	Oral	(Chen et al., 2010)
3	Catechins	*Cacia catechu*	Antioxidant and chemopreventive	Increased permeation through skin	Rotary evaporation sonication method	Transdermal	(Ajazuddin et al., 2010)
4	Curcumin	*Curcumin longa*	Anticancer	Long-circulating with high entrapment efficiency	Ethanol injection method	In vitro	(Hong et al., 2008)
5	Breviscapine	*Erigeron breviscapus*	Cardiovascular diseases	Sustained delivery of breviscapine	Double emulsification process	Intramuscular	(Zhong et al., 2005)

Stealth liposomes have the ability to circumvent the interception by the immune systems, and therefore, it has longer half-life. Singh et al. designed Elastic Liposomes containing colchicine for its sustained drug delivery which enhanced anti gout activity (Singh, 2009). Liposomes are biocompatible, non-toxic, and biodegradable in nature; hence, it is widely used in enhancing the therapeutic efficacy of various phytoconstituents. The advantages of liposomes in herbal formulations are given below (Allen et al., 2013). A variety of herbal liposomal formulations have been summarized in Table 2

4.4.1 Advantages of Liposomes

1. Sustained release can be possible for delivery of herbal drugs.
2. Reduces peak-valley fluctuations.
3. Directed herbal medication delivery.
4. Improving the solubility and bioavailability profile of poorly soluble herbal medications.
5. Precipitation at the infusion site and in the blood, course can be avoided.
6. Phospholipids are one of the few solubilizers that are well tolerated intravenously.
7. Provide selective passive targeting to tumour tissues.
8. Increase safety and therapeutic index as well increases stability via encapsulation.
9. Site avoidance effect (Nalla et al., 2017; Fadda et al., 2005).

4.4.2 Limitations of liposomes

1. Much expensive preparations.
2. Deterioration of lipids by oxidation.
3. Settling of vesicles in suspension.

4. Drug spillage from vesicles.
5. Lack of pureness of unrefined phospholipids (Pandita et al., 2013).

4.4.3 Pro liposomes

Although liposomes has several merits for herbal delivery, they still have some demerit of instability like aggregation, sedimentation, fusion, phospholipid hydrolysis, oxidation and sterilization in large scale production .To overcome these problems a novel method is designed for liposome production namely Pro-liposomes. Pro-liposomes is a dry, free flowing particles that immediately form liposomal suspension on contact with water. This solid property of liposomes solves the stability problems of liposomes (Sachan et al., 2015).

4.4.4 Ethosomes

Ethosomes are vesicles composed of phospholipids with high concentration of ethanol. Due to High concentration of ethanol in the vesicles there is enhancement in their permeability through the skin and fluidises the lipid domain of the skin (Dayan, 2000). These carriers can penetrate deeply into the skin, delivery into deeper layers of skin and even into blood circulation (Kuma et al., 2012). Ethosomes are as novel vesicles in transdermal medication conveyance show attractive impacts of medication (Jain et al., 2011; Nikalje et al., 2012; Gupta et al., 2012). The size range may vary from tens of nanometers (nm) to microns (μ), ethosomes permeated through the skin layers more rapidly and possess significantly higher transdermal flux (Nikalje et al., 2012). Ethosomal herbal formulations are shown in Table 3.

4.4.5 Key features of ethosomes (Tiwari et al., 2016; Upadhyay et al., 2011)

1. Delivery of variety of medications.
2. Ethosomes can enhance transdermal saturation of medication through skin.
3. Ethosomes are a platform for the delivery of large amounts of diverse groups of drugs.
4. The ethosomal drug can be administered in semisolid form, resulting in improved patient compliance (Sivakranth et al., 2012).

4.5 Transfersomes

Transfersome is a highly flexible and stress-responsive, complex compound. It is a highly deformed vesicle that constitutes an aqueous core which is surrounded by a complex lipid bilayer. Transfersomes are developed to benefit from phospholipids vesicles as a transdermal drug carrier (Walve et al., 2011). The development of transfersomes has been instrumental in overcoming the problem of transit drug delivery such as failure to transport large molecules (Abdulbaqi et al., 2016). The Transfersome carrier is similar to natural skin cells, suitable for the delivery of targeted and controlled drugs (Devi et al., 2010). Transfersomes are a vesicular system that contains phospholipids as the main active ingredient of 10-25% surfactant as sodium cholate and 3-10% ethanol. Surfactants act as "edge activators," providing ultra-deformability function in the formation of the transferosome, helping them to clear holes in the stratum corneum. Some remedies for the production of transferosomes are shown in Table 4.

Table 3. Herbal Formulations of Ethosomes

S. No.	Active ingredients	Derived from which plant	Biological Activity	Application of technology	Route of administration	Reference
1	Podophyllotoxin	*Podophyllum hexandrum*	Purgative, anti-rheumatic, antiviral and antitumor	Higher entrapment efficiency	Topical	(Choudhary et al., 2014)
2	Matrine	*Sophoraflavescens*	Anti- inflammatory, anti-cancer, anti-rheumatism and anti-bacterial	Permeation enhancement and improved efficacy	Topical	(Guang et al., 2010)
3	Ammonium glycyrrhizinate	*Glycyrrhiza glabra*	Anti-inflammatory	Increase of the in vitro percutaneous permeation	Topical	(Ajazuddin et al., 2010)

4.5.1 Advantages of Transfersomes

1. They can act as a carrier for low as well as high molecular weight drugs (Walve et al., 2011).
2. Transfersomes can deform and pass through narrow constriction without measurable loss.
3. They have high entrapment efficiency, in case of the lipophilic drug near to 90%.
4. Easy to scale up, as the procedure is simple, and it avoid procedure and unnecessary use or pharmaceutically unacceptable additives (Sachan et al., 2013).

4.5.2 Limitations of Transfersomes

1. Transfersomes are chemically unstable because of their predisposition to oxidative degradation.
2. Transfersomes formulations are expensive.
3. Lack of purity of natural phospholipids (Walve et al., 2011).

4.6 Niosomes

Niosomes are formed usually by non-ionic surfactant of the alkyl or diallyl polyglycerol and cholesterol. It is similar to liposomes and is advantageous than liposomes. Niosomes offer advantages like being stable as it is able to encapsulate different types of drugs, economic and are different from liposomes (Kharat et al., 2014). Liposomes face problems such as they are expensive; their ingredients such as phospholipids are chemically unstable because of their predisposition to oxidative degradation. Niosomes do not have any of these problems (Gupta et al., 2011). Several niosomes based preparation of natural medications are accounted for and summarized in the Table 5.

4.6.1 Advantages

1. Niosomes are biodegradable, biocompatible, non-poisonous and non-immunogenic.
2. Niosomes are able to encapsulate large amount of materials in a small volume of vesicles.
3. Niosomes have better patient adherence and satisfaction and also better effectiveness than conventional oily formulations.
4. Niosomes can entrap wide range of chemicals (hydrophilic, lipophilic, and amphiphilic drugs) due to its unique structure.

Table 4. Herbal Formulations of Transferosomes

Sr.No.	Active ingredient	Derived from which plant	Biological Activity	Application of technology	Route of administration	Reference
1	Capsaicin	*Capsicum annum*	Treatment of Rheumatism Capsaicin	Increased skin penetration	Topical	(Kushwaha et al., 2012)
2	Curcumin	*Curcuma longa*	Anti-inflammatory	Increase skin permeability	Topical	(Yadav et al., 2014)
3	Colchicine	*Colchicum automnale*	Treatment of Gout	Reduction in GIT side effects	Topical	(Kushwaha et al., 2012)
4	Vincristine	*Catharanthus roseus*	Anticancer	Increase entrapment efficiency and skin permeation	In vitro	(Zheng et al., 2006)

5. The characteristics of niosomes such as shape, fluidity and size can be easily controlled by changing in structural composition and method of production.
6. Niosomes can be prescribed via different administration routes such as oral, parenteral and topical, etc. with different dosage forms such as semisolids, powders, suspensions.
7. Because of chemical stability of structural composition, the storage of the niosomes is easy (Rahimpour et al., 2012).

4.6.2 Disadvantages

1. Shelf life is limited due to aggregation, leaching or hydrolysis of entrapped drug.
2. Time consuming, instable, and inefficient (Pandita et al., 2013).

4.6.3 Pro Niosomes

Pro-niosomes gel system is step forward to niosome, which can be utilized for various applications in delivery of actives at desired site (Shukla et al., 2011). Pro-niosomes are water-soluble carrier particles which are coated with surfactant and can be hydrated to form niosomal dispersion immediately before use on brief agitation in hot aqueous media (Raja et al., 2011).

4.6.4 Key Features of Pro-Niosomes

1. Pro-niosomes are more stable during storage and sterilization
2. Easy to transfer and distribution

4.7 Nanoparticle

The main purpose after designing the nanoparticle as a drug delivery system is to control particle size, surface properties and release of pharmaceutical agents. The main objective is to achieve specific drug-specific action with appropriate dosage and type of drug (Goyal et al., 2011). Nanoparticles are effective

Table 5. Herbal formulations of niosomes

S. No.	Active ingredient	Derived from which plant	Biological Activity	Application of technology	Route of administration	Reference
1	Colchicine	*Colchicum autumnase*	Rheumatic complaints	Prolonged release profile	Topical	(Joshi et al., 2014)
2	Silymarin	*Silybummarianum*	Treat liver and gall bladder disorders	Increase drug bioavailability	Oral	(Rahimpour et al., 2012)

drug delivery systems. Nanoparticles are particles of size of submicron with a range of about 10 to 1000 nm. In recent years, polymeric nanoparticles have attracted much attention as drug delivery devices. Nanoparticles also tend to have unpredictable visual properties as they are small enough to bind their electrons and produce quantum effects. For example, gold nanoparticles from deep red to black in solution (Mamillapalli et al., 2016). The different types of herbal nanoparticle are summarized in Table 6.

4.7.1 Advantages

1. Nanoparticles are small in size than microspheres and liposome's due to which they can easily pass through the sinusoidal spaces in the bone marrow and spleen as compared to other systems with long circulation time.
2. Nanoparticles increases stability of herbal drug and proteins against enzymatic degradation
3. They offer a significant improvement over traditional intravenous (IV) methods of administration in terms of efficiency and effectiveness also reduces the toxicity of liver.
4. The nanoparticulate system of herbal formulation shows advantage, as its solubility is increased and the herbal drug can reach the target site, as compared to other systems (Chaturvedi, 2011)
5. Nanoparticles can also reach the choice of formulations which promote the drugs through the biological barriers and increase the bioavailability of drugs.

4.7.2 Limitations

1. They tend to aggregate due to high surface and energy.
2. It has immunogenicity.
3. Expensive.
4. Poor targeting.

4.7.3 Solid Lipid Nanoparticles (SLNs)

SLNs are used as other substances that carry common colloids such as emulsions (Schwarz et al., 1994). Basically, SLNs are a solid lipid base with a monolayer phospholipid shell. Many drugs or diagnoses can be detected by SLNs, especially lipophilic ingredients. This nano system offers benefits such as inclusion stability, controlled kinetics extraction, tolerance, and labile protection. SLNs are prepared by various methods such as homogenization and micro-emulsion rapid heating that stimulates ultrasonication and method distribution only (Chih-hung et al., 2017). Lipids exhibit lipophilic drug adherence and

Table 6. Herbal Formulations of Nanoparticles

S. No.	Active ingredients	Derived from which plant	Biological Activity	Application of technology	Method of preparation	Route of administration	Reference
1	Paclitaxel	Derived from the bark of the Pacific yew tree *Taxusbrevifolia*	Anti-tumour activity	Show sustained release	Emulsion solvent evaporation method	In vitro	(Fang et al., 2008)
2	Berberine	*Berberis vulgaris*	Anti-neoplastic activity	H. pylori growth inhibition	Ionic gelation method	In vitro	(Chang et al., 2011)
3	Naringenin-	*citrus reticulata*	Hepatoprotective	Improved the release of NAR and improved its solubility	Nanoprecipitation method	Oral	(Ajazuddin et al., 2010)
4	Triptolide	Diterpenoid triepoxide obtained from Chinese medicine *Tripterygium Wilfondii*Hook F	Anti-inflammatory	Enhance the penetration of drugs through the stratum corneum by increased hydration	Emulsification-ultrasound	Topical	(Zhinan et al., 2003)

increase the efficacy of drug capture and loading in SLNs (Gande et al., 2007). The different types of SLN plants are shown in Table 7.

4.7.4 Advantages of SLN Herbal Formulation

1. It provides controlled release and site-specific drug targeting.
2. Large-scale production is possible.
3. In this formulation, both lipophilic and hydrophilic drugs can be loaded.
4. Another advantage is that it is made of lipid matrix (physiological lipids), which decreases danger of chronic and acute toxicity (Yaddalapudi, 2015).

4.8 Microspheres

Microspheres are spherical particles ranging from normal particle size from 1 to 50 microns. Microspheres are classified as delegated biodegradable or non-biodegradable. Biodegradable microspheres include albumin microspheres, modified starch microspheres, gelatine microspheres, polypropylene dextran microspheres, polylactic acid microspheres, etc. biodegradable polymers are often used in the formation of microsphere matrix such as polylactic acid and copolymer for lactic acid and glycolic acid. According to current literature reports on non-biodegradable microspheres, polylactic acid is the only polymer approved for human use and is used as a controlled release agent. (Mukherjee et al., 2015). Drug treatment with small particle systems is helpful because microspheres can be incorporated or injected; they can be configured for the release profiles you want and the drug delivery specific to the site and in some cases may also provide targeted release (Parida et al., 2013). The various compositions of herbs is shown in Table 8.

Table 7. Herbal Formulations of SLNs

S. No.	Active ingredient	Derived from which plant	Biological Activity	Application of technology	Method of preparation	Route of administration	Reference
1	Curcuminoids	*Curcuma longa*	Anti-malarial activity,Anti-tumour, antioxidant and anti-inflammatory activities	Prolonged-release of the curcuminoids	Micro-emulsion technique	In vitro	(Mukerjee et al., 2009)
2	Neem oil	*Azadirachtaindica*	Anti bacterial action on acne microbes	Prolong treatment of acne	Double emulsification method	Topical	(Shaikh et al., 2013)

4.8.1 Advantages of Microsphere

1. Administration of medication via micro-particulate system is advantageous because microspheres can be ingested or injected, and they can be tailored for desired release profiles and used for site-specific delivery of drugs and in some cases can even provide organ targeted release. (Vyas et al., 2004).
2. Drug can be easily released from the formulation.
3. It can protect the specific function of drugs and can release the drugs into an outer phase for a long period.
4. Microspheres provide constant and prolonged therapeutic effect.
5. Reduces the dosing frequency and thereby improve the patient compliance.
6. They could be infused into the body because of the circular shape and littler size.
7. Better drug utilization will improve the bioavailability.
8. Microsphere morphology all owes a controllable variability in degradation and drug release.

4.8.2 Polymeric Micelles

Polymeric micelles are a popular attraction for scientists from many years of age because of their controlled properties and chemical properties. They are amphiphilic, the inner core is hydrophobic, while the outer shell is hydrophilic and is formed by combining hydrophobic and hydrophilic groups placed in water. Micelles are 20-100 nm in size and low polydispersity index. These have a low critical micellar concentration (CMC) and have high stability. Typically, a hydrophilic shell contains polyethylene oxide, polyethylene glycol. Taxol is produced by up to 40% production using PEG - poly (ortho ester) - PEG block copolymer micelle. This is made up of amphiphilic blocks that have been successfully used to deliver water-soluble drugs. The characteristic feature of micelles such as particle size, composition, drug loading, large-scale cell production, stability and release of kinetics of drugs can be enhanced by modifying the physicochemical properties of constituent block copolymers and the preparation method (Lavasanifar, 2002). Artemisinin from *Artemisia annua L.* and Curcumin from the roots of *Curcuma longa L.* are used as anti-malarial drugs, but these are less soluble drugs. Micelles composition of these sodium dodecyl sulphate drugs has led to a 25-fold increase in the solubility of these drugs. (Lapenna, 2009)

4.8.3 Emulsion

Emulsion is a biphasic system in which one phase is widely distributed in another phase in the form of minute droplets ranging from 0.1 μm to 100 μm. In an emulsion, one phase remains a liquid or aqueous

Table 8. Herbal Formulations of Microspheres

S. No.	Active ingredient	Derived from which plant	Biological Activity	Application of technology	Method of preparation	Route of administration	Reference
1	Camptothecin	Bark and stem of *Camptothecaacuminata*	Anti-cancer	Dose reduction	Oil-in-water evaporation method	Intraperitoneally and intravenously	(Ajazuddin et al., 2010; Garg et al., 2010; Paolino, 2005)
2	Quercetin	citrus fruits, apples, onions	Anti-oxidant and anti-inflammatory activity	Enhance bioavailability and sustained release the formulation	Solvent evaporation	In vitro	(Gangwar et al., 2010)
3	Zedoary oil	*Curcuma zedoaria*	Hepatoprotective	Sustained release and Higher bioavailability	Quasi-emulsion–solvent diffusion method	Oral	(You et al., 2006)
4	Rutin	*Fagopyrum esculentum*	Cardiovascular and Cerebrovascular diseases	Targeting into cardiovascular and cerebrovascular region	Complex coacervation method	In vitro	(Sanli et al., 2009)

phase, and the other phase is an oily liquid, i.e., a non-aqueous liquid. Its appearance changes to a visible liquid. The emulsion can be divided into standard emulsion [0.1-100 μm], micro-emulsion [10-100 nm], sub-micro-emulsion [100-600 nm], etc. Among them, micro-emulsion is also called nano emulsion, and sub-micro-emulsion is also called lipid emulsion (Chaturvedi, 2011). Emulsion drug delivery system is targeted or well-distributed due to proximity to the lymph. Micro-emulsions are solutions that contain nanometer droplets in a liquid that is not dispersed in a water reservoir (Shah, 2010). These types of emulsions have a high surface area and that is why they can easily penetrate the skin. It is also non-toxic and environmentally friendly and can be used in animals and for animal purposes. Nano emulsion can be prepared with advanced homogenization and microfluidization technique (Lieberman, 1998; Lachman, 1996). The different types of herbal emulsion formulations are shown in Table 9.

4.8.4 Advantages

1. It can release the drug for a long time because it is packed in the inner phase and makes direct contact with the body and other tissues.
2. As a result of the lipophilic drugs being made into o/w/o emulsion, the droplets of oil are phagocytised by macrophages and increase its concentration in liver, spleen, and kidney.
3. As the emulsion contains herbal formulation, it will increase the stability of hydrolysed formulated material and improve the penetrability of drug into skin and mucous. The new type, viz., Elemenum emulsion, is used as an anti-cancer drug and causes no harm to the heart and liver (Cui, 2007).

4.9 Transdermal Patch

Transdermal drug delivery system means a patch which is attached to the body surface. This patch is a medicated adhesive pad which is designed to release the active ingredient at a constant rate over a constant period of several hours to days after application to the skin. This system provides drug delivery at control rate, high bioavailability, easy application, sustainable action (Atram, 2014). Transdermal drug delivery systems are potentially used for the sustained delivery of the drugs up to several days or even months. The combination was used to produce the synergistic action of the drugs. The increase in

Table 9. Herbal Formulations of Emulsion

S. No.	Active ingredients	Derived from which plant	Biological Activity	Application of technology	Method of preparation	Route of administration	Reference
1	Triptolide	Diterpenoid triepoxide obtained from Chinese medicine *Tripterygium WilfondiI*Hook F	Anti-inflammatory	Enhance the penetration of drugs through the stratum corneum by increased hydration	Pressure Homogenization method	Topical	(Yin, 2009)
2	Berberine	*Berberis vulgaris*	Anticancer	More residence time in the body	Drawing ternary phase diagram	Oral	(Zhang, 2010)
3	Silybin	*Silybummarianum*	Hepatoprotective	Sustained release formulation	Emulsification method	Intramuscular	(Song, 2005; Li, 2007)
4	Quercetin	*Ginkgo biloba*	Antioxidant	Enhance penetration into stratum corneum and epidermis	High speed Homogenization method	Topical	(Sun, 2007; Fabiana, 2008)
5	Zedoary turmeric oil (self nano-emulsification)	*Curcuma zedoaria*	Hepatoprotection anticancer and anti-bacterial	Improved aqueous dispersibility, stability and oral bioavailability.	Drawing ternary phase Diagram	Oral	(Zhaoa, 2010; Lu, 2005)

the efficacy of the drug was observed with the formulation of transdermal films. Transdermal herbal formulations are shown in table 10

Transdermal system overcomes the limitation of hepatic first pass metabolism; it maintains a strong plasma level of the drug. Transdermal route has shown mild skin irritation and in vivo results have shown that cakes effectively lower blood sugar levels and have been shown to be ineffective for diabetes using modern medical methods (Bhujbal, 2011).

4.10 Implants

Implants are the polymeric devices used for controlled and sustained delivery of the drugs. These implants have fabricated using biodegradable polymer and directly placed in the body fluids/cavities (Brahmankar, 2008). The wounds and tissues were observed to be healed best and it also prevented the patient from frequent dosing (Zhao, 2002).

4.11 Bhasma as a Nano Herbal Medication Innovation

Bhasma is a metal formulation in which the metal acts as a nanocarrier for drug delivery and is widely recommended in the treatment of various chronic diseases and is taken in combination with milk, butter, honey or ghee to eliminate the harmful effects of iron and improve its allergic reactions. Such systems used traditionally to treat anemia, hepatotoxicity (Rasheed, 2012). It helps to protect the body from major free radicals, digests iron, reduces harmful acids, and helps to cleanse the intestines, liver, and kidneys (Pal, 2014). Various techniques such as the atomic force microscopy, scanning electron microscopy, transmission electron microscopy and energy dispersive spectroscopy have been used for characterization of bhasma

Table 10. Transdermal Herbal Formulations

S. No.	Active ingredients	Derived from which plant	Biological Activity	Application of technology	Method of preparation	Route of administration	Reference
1	Scopolamine	*Datura stramonium*	Prevent Motion Sickness	Improved patient compliance	Matrix diffusion	Topical	(Yadav, 2014)
2	Nicotine	*Nicotiana tabalum*	Antismoking Agent	Quit smoking	Matrix diffusion	Topical	(Yadav, 2014)

4.11 Methods for Novel Formulations

The methods most regularly utilized for the preparations are:

1. High Pressure Homogenization Technique

In this method, with high pressure of 100 to 2000 bar, lipid is pushed through a very high shear stress which results in disruption of particles down to the submicrometer or nanometer range.

For the large-scale production of nanostructured lipid carriers, lipid drug conjugate, SLNs, and parenteral emulsions high-pressure homogenization method is a very reliable and powerful technique (Mueller, 2000; Sahni, 2011; Yadav, 2011).

2. Complex Coacervation Technique

This is a spontaneous phase separation process of two liquid phases in colloidal systems, which results by the interaction of two oppositely charged polyelectrolytes upon mixing in an aqueous solution (Sahni, 2011; Yadav, 2011).

3. Co-Precipitation Method

This method is a modification of the complex coacervation which provide good dispersion stability to poorly water-soluble drugs. This method is use for the preparation of nanoscale core-shell particles (Sahni, 2011; Yadav, 2011).

4. Salting-Out Method

Salting out method is based on the solubility of a non-electrolyte in water is decreased upon addition of an electrolyte. (Sahni, 2011; Yadav, 2011).

5. Nanoprecipitation Method or Solvent Displacement Method

In this method, a decrease in the interfacial tension between the two phases, which increases the surface area with a subsequent formation of small droplets of organic solvent even without any mechanical stirring is due to interfacial deposition of a polymer after displacement of a semipolar solvent miscible with water from a lipophilic solution (Sahni, 2011; Yadav, 2011).

6. Solvent Emulsification–Diffusion Method

In this method of preparing oil-in-water (o / w) the emulsion is ready to apply a polymer-containing oil phase in the natural environment, reinforced with a liquid phase, consisting of a stabilizer, in a high shear blender, followed by a water expansion to promote disintegration, with the lines of nanoparticles (Sahni, 2011; Yadav, 2011)

7. Supercritical Liquid Techniques

A supercritical fluid (SCFs) can be a liquid or gas and used above its thermodynamic critical point of temperature and pressure. The commonly used SCFs are carbon dioxide and water. In this method submicrometric-sized and nano-sized formulations are prepared (Sahni, 2011; Yadav, 2011).

8. Self-Assembly Methods

Self-assembly is the physical process whereby physical or chemical reactions without any contribution from any external source may leads to pre-existing disordered components, atoms, or molecules organize themselves into regulated nanoscale structures (Sahni, 2011; Yadav, 2011).

5. RECENT DEVELOPMENTS

The method of nanoparticles is capable drug delivery systems which are used for the delivery of drugs in the treatment of various diseases such as cancer through reticulo endothelial system, increased stiffness and retention effect, and direct orientation of the tumor. Recently, the focus of pharmacologists has shifted the design of drug delivery systems using the scientific method. The traditional Chinese medicine of *Cuscuta chinensis* is commonly used to feed liver and kidney diseases. Nanoparticles have been found promising approach for targeting of herbal drugs. Issue with the herbal drugs is their lack of water solubility, their major constituents such as flavonoids and lignans, their oral absorption is limited (Ansari, 2012; Yadav, 2011). Recently, studies were conducted on lipophilic anti-cancer herb drugs (Cucurbitacins and Curcuminoids) as a polylactic acid nanoparticle. Work has also been done on traditional Chinese medicine in the development and demonstration of SLNs with the intended delivery and increased availability and effectiveness of Chinese medicine. In recent years, the distribution of anticancer drugs by oral route is a system of nanostructured carriers such as polymeric nanoparticles, liposomes, SLNs, polymeric micelles, nanoemulsions, etc. In addition, attention is focused on the development of oral chemotherapy in herbal oncology because the oral method provides greater potential for the delivery of cytotoxic agents (Yadav, 2011; Zhang, 2007).

6. FUTURE PROSPECTIVE

It is hoped that with the advent of research focused on this field, in the near future, large sections of synthetic drugs will be replaced by herbal remedies and health care is expected to be completely improved. Pharmaceutical companies are keen to research the use of herbal remedies. Alternative drug delivery systems have many opportunities, and several researchers are working to develop new drug delivery systems such as oral contraceptives, continuous and extended synthetic methods, mucoadhesive systems, transdermal dosage forms, microparticles, microcapsules, nanoparticles, implants etc. Herbs reduce side effects and provide alternative, natural, and cost-effective alternatives to synthetic drugs and the discovery and separation by High performance thin layer chromatography (HPTLC) has confirmed the use of herbal remedies to facilitate polyherbal formulation with complementary active ingredients.

7. CONCLUSION

The development of drugs such as Novel Herbal Drug Delivery Systems provides health professionals with a wide range of treatment options and demonstrates the delivery of the best drugs possible. The NHDDS not only smoothes the pattern of drug levels in the blood, but also provides the identification of drugs on their site and thus minimizes dose-related side effects. There is a great deal of untruth about coming up with an innovative herbal remedy delivery system as its safe, effective, simple and inexpensive delivery of the economy, can lead to overcoming the problem associated with herbal formulation leading to increased efficiency and more available by not increasing its solubility, controlled release and target.

REFERENCES

Abdulbaqi, I., Darwis, Y., Khan, N., Assi, R., & Khan, A. (2016). Ethosomal nanocarriers: The impact of constituents and formulation techniques on ethosomal properties, in vivo studies, and clinical trials. *International Journal of Nanomedicine*, *11*, 2279–2304. doi:10.2147/IJN.S105016 PMID:27307730

Acharya, N., Parihar, G., & Acharya, S. (2011). Phytosomes: Novel approach for delivering herbal extract with improved bioavailability. *Pharma Science Monitor*, *2*(1), 144–160.

Afrin, S., Jahan, I., Hasan, A., & Deepa, K. (2018). Novel approaches of herbal drug delivery. *Journal of Pharmaceutical Research International*, *21*(5), 1–11. doi:10.9734/JPRI/2018/39143

Ajazuddin, S., & Saraf, S. (2010). Applications of novel drug delivery system for herbal formulations. *Fitoterapia*, *81*(7), 680–689. doi:10.1016/j.fitote.2010.05.001 PMID:20471457

Allen, T., & Cullis, P. (2013). Liposomal drug delivery systems: From concept to clinical applications. *Advanced Drug Delivery Reviews*, *65*(1), 36–48. doi:10.1016/j.addr.2012.09.037 PMID:23036225

Ansari, S. H., Islam, F., & Sameem, M. (2012). Influence of nanotechnology on herbal drugs: A Review. *Journal of Advanced Pharmaceutical Technology & Research*, *3*(3), 142–146. doi:10.4103/2231-4040.101006 PMID:23057000

Atram, S. (2014). Recent development of herbal formulation- a novel drug delivery system. *International Ayurvedic Medical Journal, 2*, 953–958.

Bangham, A., & Horne, R. (1964). Negative staining of phospholipids and their structured modification by surface active agents as observed in the electron microscope. *Journal of Molecular Biology, 8*(5), 660–668. doi:10.1016/S0022-2836(64)80115-7 PMID:14187392

Bhardwaj, A., & Kumar, L. (2011). Colloidal drug delivery system: A future prospective for treatment of tuberculosis. *American Journal of PharmTech Research, 1*(3), 102–123.

Bhattacharya, S. (2009). Phytosomes: Emerging Strategy in Delivery of Herbal Drugs and Nutraceuticals. *Pharmacy Times, 41*, 9–12.

Bhokare, S., Dhongaonkar, C., Lahane, S., Salunke, P., Savale, V., & Thobare, M. (2016). Herbal novel drug delivery- A review. *Wjpps, 5*(6), 593–611.

Bhujbal, S., Kulkarni, P. A., Thatte, V. A., Yeola, R. R., Hadawale, S. S., Bidkar, J. S., & Providencia, C. A. (2011). A novel herbal formulation in the management of diabetes. *International Journal of Pharmaceutical Investigation, 1*(4), 222–226. doi:10.4103/2230-973X.93009 PMID:23071947

Brahmankar, D., & Jaiswal, S. (1998). Biopharmaceutics and Pharmacokinetics -A Treatise. Vallabh Prakashan, 61, 359, 362.

Chang, C., Huang, W., Lai, C., Hsu, Y., Yao, Y., Chen, T., Wu, J.-Y., Peng, S.-F., & Lin, Y.-H. (2011). Development of novel nanoparticles shelled with heparin for berberine delivery to treat Helicobacter pylori. *Acta Biomaterialia, 7*(2), 593–603. doi:10.1016/j.actbio.2010.08.028 PMID:20813208

Chaturvedi, M. & Kumar, M. (2011). Recent development in novel drug delivery systems of herbal drugs. *International Journal of Green Pharmacy*, 87-94.

Chaudhary, G., & Dewakar, K. (2014). Role of Herbs in Preventing Cancer, *Int. Res. J. Pharm, 5*(4), 264–266.

Chen, J., Chen, Z., & Wang, W. (2010). Ammonium sulphate gradient loading of brucine into liposome: Effect of phospholipid composition on entrapment efficiency and physicochemical properties in vitro. *Drug Development and Industrial Pharmacy, 36*(3), 245–253. doi:10.3109/03639040903099736 PMID:19678739

Chih-Hung, L., Chun-Han, C., Zih-Chan, L., & Jia-You, F. (2017). Recent advances in oral delivery of drugs and bioactive natural products using solid lipid nanoparticles as the carriers. *Yao Wu Shi Pin Fen Xi, 25*, 219–234. PMID:28911663

Cui, F., Wang, Y., Wang, J., Feng, L., & Ning, K. (2007). Preparation of an enteric soluble solid-state emulsion using oily drugs. *International Journal of Pharmaceutics, 338*(1-2), 152–156. doi:10.1016/j.ijpharm.2007.01.044 PMID:17349753

Dayan, N., & Touitou, E. (2000). Carriers for skin delivery of trihexyphenidyl HCl: Ethosomes vs. liposomes. *Biomaterials, 21*(18), 1879–1885. doi:10.1016/S0142-9612(00)00063-6 PMID:10919691

DeMario, M., & Ratain, M. (1998). Oral chemotherapy: Rationale and future directions. *Journal of Clinical Oncology, 16*(7), 2557–2567. doi:10.1200/JCO.1998.16.7.2557 PMID:9667278

Devi, V., Jain, N., & Valli, K. (2010). Importance of novel drug delivery systems in herbal medicines. *Pharmacognosy Reviews, 4*(7), 27–31. doi:10.4103/0973-7847.65322 PMID:22228938

Dibua, E., & Nnamani, P. (2011). Antimicrobial properties of clove, tobacco and bitter on tooth decay. *Asian Pacific Journal of Tropical Medicine, 4*(10), 412–420.

Edris, A. E. (2007). Pharmaceutical and therapeutic potentials of essential oils and their individual volatile constituents: A review. *Phytotherapy Research, 21*(4), 308–323. doi:10.1002/ptr.2072 PMID:17199238

Fabiana, T., Thais, R., Jose, O., Nilce, O., Dimitrius, L., & Mamie, M. (2008). Quercetin in w/o micro-emulsion: In vitro and in vivo skin penetration and efficacy against UVB-induced skin damages evaluated in vivo. *J PharmBiopharm, 69*, 948–957. PMID:18304790

Fadda, A., Sinico, C., Lai, F., & Logu, A. (2005). Liposomal incorporation of artemisia arborescence L. Essential oil and in vitro antiviral activity. *European Journal of Pharmaceutics and Biopharmaceutics, 59*(1), 161–168. doi:10.1016/j.ejpb.2004.06.005 PMID:15567314

Feng-Lin, Y., Tzu-Hui, W., Liang-Tzung, L., Thau-Ming, C., & Chun-Chingaa, L. (2009). Preparation of naringenin nanopartciles. *Pharmaceutical Research, 26*(4), 893–902. PMID:19034626

Gande, S., Kopparam, M., & Vobalaboina, V. (2007). Preparation characterization and in vitro and in vivo evalution of lovastatin solid lipid nanoparticle. *AAPS PharmSciTech, 8*, 1–8.

Gandhi A., Dutta A., Pal A., & Bakshi P. (2012). Recent Trends of Phytosomes for Delivering Herbal Extract with Improved Bioavailability. *Journal of Pharmacognosy and Phytochemistry, 1*(4), 6-14.

Gangwar, S., Singh, S., & Garg, G. (2010). Ethosomes: A novel tool for drug delivery through skin. *Journal of Pharmacy Research, 3*, 688–691.

Garg, R., & Gupta, G. (2010). Gastro retentive floating microspheres of Silymarin: Preparation and in vitro evaluation. *Tropical Journal ofPharmaceutical Research, 9*(1), 59–66. doi:10.4314/tjpr.v9i1.52037

Goyal, A., Kumar, S., Nagpal, M., Singh, I., & Arora, S. (2011). Potential of novel drug delivery systems for herbal drugs. *Indian J Pharm Educ Res, 45*, 225–235.

Goyal, A., Kumar, S., Nagpal, M., Singh, I., & Arora, S. (2011). Potential of novel drug delivery systems for herbal drugs. *Ind J Pharm Edu Res, 45*(3), 225–235.

Guang, C., Yu, L., & Wen, G. (2010). Preparation and anti-inflammatory activity of Triptolide ethosomes in an erythema model. *Journal ofLiposome Research, 20*(4), 297–303. doi:10.3109/08982100903544144 PMID:20102297

Gupta, N., Loona, S., & Khan, M. (2012). Ethosomes as elastic vesicles in transdermal drug delivery: An overview. *International Journal of Current Pharmaceutical Research, 3*(3), 682–687.

Gupta, S., Singh, R., Lokwani, P., Yadav, S., & Gupta, S. (2011). Vesicular system as targeted drug delivery system: An overview. *Int J Pharm Technol, 3*, 987–1021.

Hong, W., Chen, D., Zhao, X., Qiao, M., & Hu, H. (2008). Preparation and study in vitro of long-circulating nanoliposomes of curcumin. *Zhongguo Zhongyao Zazhi*, *33*, 889–892. PMID:18619344

Jain, H., Patel, J., Joshi, K., Patel, P., & Upadhyay, U. (2011). Ethosomes: A novel drug carrier. *Pharm Globale Int J Compr Pharm*, *7*, 1–4.

John, D. N., Franklin, C. K., Anthony, A. A., & Salome, A. C. (2012). Different approaches to formulation of herbal extracts/ phytopharmaceuticals/ bioactive phytoconstituents- A review. *International Journal of Pharmaceutical Sciences Review and Research*, *16*(1), 1–8.

Joshi, A., Chaturvedi, S., Kumar, V., & Pathak, A. (2008). *Phytosomes: A revolution in herbal drugs. The Pharma Review*. Kongposh Publications Pvt. Ltd.

Kavitha, D., Naga, S. J., & Panaganti, S. (2010). Pharmacosomes: An emerging vesicular system. *International Journal of Pharmaceutical Sciences Review and Research*, *5*(3), 168–171.

Kharat, A. (2014). Novel drug delivery system in herbal's. *International Journal of Pharma and Bio Sciences*, *4*(4), 910–930.

Kharat, A., & Pawar, P. (2014). Novel drug delivery system in Herbal's. *International Journal of Pharmaceutical, Chemical and Biological Sciences*, *4*(4), 910–930.

Kumar, K., & Rai, A. (2012). Miraculous therapeutic effect of herbal drug using novel drug delivery system. *IRJP*, *3*(2), 27–30.

Kumar, V., & Kesari, A. (2011). Herbosome a novel carrier for herbal drug delivery. *International Journal of Current Pharmaceutical Research*, *3*(3), 36–41.

Kushwaha, S., Rastogi, A., Rai, A., & Singh, S. (2012). Novel drug delivery system for anticancer drug: A review. *International Journal of Pharm Tech Research*, *4*(2), 542–553.

Lachman, L., Lieberman, H., & Kanig, J. (1996). *The Theory and Practice of Industrial Pharmacy* (3rd ed.). Lea & Febiger.

Lapenna, S., Bilia, A., Morris, G., & Nilsson, M. (2009). Novel artemisinin and curcumin micellar formulation: Drug solubility studies by NMR spectroscopy. *Journal of Pharmaceutical Sciences*, *98*(10), 3666–3675. doi:10.1002/jps.21685 PMID:19199296

Lavasanifar, A., Samuel, J., & Kwon, G. (2002). Poly (ethylene oxide)-block-poly (L-amino acid) micelles for drug delivery. *Advanced Drug Delivery Reviews*, *54*(2), 169–190. doi:10.1016/S0169-409X(02)00015-7 PMID:11897144

Li, L., Wang, D., Li, L., Jia, J., Chang, D., & Ai, L. (2007). Preparation of docetaxel submicron emulsion formation for intravenous administration. *Journal of Shenyang Pharmaceutical University*, *7*(12), 736–739.

Lieberman, H., Rieger, M., & Banker, G. (1998). Pharmaceutical Dosage Forms: Disperse systems. New York: Marcel Dekker Inc.

Lu, M., Cheng, Y., Li, L., & Wu, J. (2005). Progress of study on passive targeting of drug delivery system. *Mater Rev*, *19*, 108–110.

Maiti, K., Mukherjee, K., Gantait, A., Bishnu, P., & Mukherjee, P. (2006). Enhanced therapeutic potential of naringenin-phospholipid complex in rats. *The Journal of Pharmacy and Pharmacology*, *58*(9), 1227–1233. doi:10.1211/jpp.58.9.0009 PMID:16945181

Mamillapalli, V. (2016). Nanoparticles for Herbal Extracts. *Asian Journal of Pharmaceutics*, *10*(2), S54–S60.

Meena, K., Dangi, J., Samal, P., & Namdeo, K. (2011). Recent advances in microspheres manufacturing technology. *Int J Pharm Technol*, *3*, 854–893.

Modak, M., Dixit, P., Londhe, J., Ghaskadbi, S., & Devasagayam, T. P. A. (2007). Indian herbs & herbal drugs used for the treatment of diabetes. *Journal of Clinical Biochemistry and Nutrition*, *40*(3), 163–173. doi:10.3164/jcbn.40.163 PMID:18398493

Mueller, R. H., Maeder, K., & Gohla, S. (2000). Solid lipid nanoparticles (SLN) for controlled drug delivery – a review of the state of the art. *European Journal of Pharmaceutics and Biopharmaceutics*, *50*, 161–177. doi:10.1016/S0939-6411(00)00087-4 PMID:10840199

Mukerjee, A., & Vishwanatha, J. (2009). Formulation, characterization and evaluation of curcumin-loaded PLGA nanospheres for cancer therapy. *Anticancer Research*, *29*(10), 3867–3875. PMID:19846921

Mukherjee, P., Harwansh, R., & Bhattacharyya, S. (2015). Bioavailability of herbal products: approach toward improved pharmacokinetics. In Evidence-Based Validation of Herbal Medicine. Elsevier Inc. doi:10.1016/B978-0-12-800874-4.00010-6

Nalla, A., & Chinnala, K. (2017). Novel herbal drug delivery system - An overview. *World Journal of Pharmacy and Pharmaceutical Sciences*, *6*(8), 369–395. doi:10.20959/wjpps20178-9712

Nandre, B., Bakliwal, S., Rane, B., & Pawar, S. (2012). Traditional fermented formulations- Asava and arishta. *International Journal of Pharmaceutical and Biological Archives*, *3*(6), 1313–1319.

Nikalje, A., & Tiwari, S. (2012). Ethosomes: A novel tool for transdermal drug delivery. *International Journal of Current Pharmaceutical Research*, *2*(1), 1–20.

Pal, D., Sahu, C., & Haldar, A. (2014). Bhasma: The ancient Indian nanomedicine. *Journal of Advanced Pharmaceutical Technology & Research*, *5*(1), 4–12. doi:10.4103/2231-4040.126980 PMID:24696811

Pandita, A., & Sharma, P. (2013). Pharmacosomes: An Emerging Novel Vesicular Drug Delivery System for Poorly Soluble Synthetic and Herbal Drugs. *ISRN Pharmaceutics*, *2013*, 1–10. doi:10.1155/2013/348186 PMID:24106615

Paolino, D., Lucania, G., Mardente, D., Alhaique, F., & Fresta, M. (2005). Ethosomes for skin delivery of ammonium glycyrrhizinate: In vitro percutaneous permeation through human skin and in vivo anti-inflammatory activity on human volunteers. *Journal of Controlled Release*, *106*(1-2), 99–110. doi:10.1016/j.jconrel.2005.04.007 PMID:15935505

Parida, K., Panda, S., Ravanan, P., & Roy, H. (2013). Microparticles Based Drug Delivery Systems: Preparation and Application in Cancer Therapeutics. *IAAST*, *4*(3), 68–75.

Patil, P., Salunkhe, V., Magdum, C., & Mohite, S. (2016). Phytosomes: Increasing bioavailability of phytoconstituents. *International Journal of Universal Pharmacy and Bio Sciences*, *5*(4), 81–94.

Pawar, H., & Bhangale, B. (2015). Phytosome as a novel biomedicine: A microencapsulated drug delivery system. *Journal of Bioanalysis & Biomedicine*, *7*(1), 6–12.

Rahimpour, Y. & Hamishehkar, H. (2012). Niosomes as carrier in dermal drug delivery. *Recent Advances in Novel Drug Carrier Systems*, 141-164.

Raja, K., Ukken, J., Athul, P., Tamizharasi, S., & Sivakumar, T. (2011). Formulation and evaluation of maltodextrin based proniosomal drug delivery system containing antidiabetic (glipizide) drug. *International Journal of Pharm Tech Research*, *3*, 471–477.

Rasheed, A., Sravya, R. & Roja, C. (2012). A Review on standardization of herbal formulation. *International Journal of Phytotherapy*, *2*, 74-88.

Ravi, G., Chandur, V., Shabaraya, A., & Sanjay, K. (2015). Phytosomes: An advanced herbal drug delivery system. *International Journal of Pharmaceutical Research and Bio-Science*, *4*(3), 415–432.

Sachan, K., & Gupta, A. (2015). A review on nanotized herbal drugs. *International Journal of Pharmaceutical Sciences and Research*, *6*(3), 961–970.

Sachan, R., Parashar, T., Singh, S., Singh, G., Tyagi, S., Patel, C., & Gupta, A. (2013). A drug carrier transferosomes: A novel tool for transdermal drug delivery system. *International Journal of Research and Development in Pharmacy and Life Sciences*, *2*(2), 309–316.

Sahni, J., Baboota, S., & Ali, J. (2011). Promising Role of Nanopharmaceuticals in Drug Delivery. *Pharmacy Times*, *43*, 16–18.

Sanli, O., Karaca, I., & Isiklan, N. (2009). Preparation, characterization, and salicylic acid release behaviour of chitosan/poly (vinyl alcohol) blend microspheres. *Journal of Applied Polymer Science*, *111*(6), 2731–2740. doi:10.1002/app.29319

Sarangi, M., & Padhi, S. (2018). Novel herbal drug delivery system: an overview. *Arch Med Health Sci*, *6*, 171-9.

Schulz, V., Hansel, R., & Tyler, V. E. (2000). *A physicians guide to herbal medicine. In Rational phytotherapy*. Springer.

Schwarz, C., Mehnert, M., Lucks, J., & Muller, R. (1994). Solid lipid nanoparticles (SLN) for controlled drug delivery: I. Production, characterization and sterilization. *Journal of Controlled Release*, *30*(1), 83–96. doi:10.1016/0168-3659(94)90047-7

Shah, P., Halodia, D., & Shelat, P. (2010). Nanoemulsion: A pharmaceutical review. *Systematic Reviews in Pharmacy*, *1*(1), 24–32. doi:10.4103/0975-8453.59509

Sharma, G., Anabousi, S., Ehrhardt, C., & Ravi Kumar, M. (2006). Liposomes as targeted drug delivery systems in the treatment of breast cancer. *Journal of Drug Targeting*, *14*(5), 301–310. doi:10.1080/10611860600809112 PMID:16882550

Sharma, M. (2014). Applications of nanotechnology based dosage forms for delivery of herbal drugs. *Research and Reviews: Journal of Pharmaceutics and Nanotechnology, 2*(1), 23-30.

Shukla, N., & Tiwari, M. (2011). Proniosomal drug delivery systems – Clinical applications. *International Journal of Research in Pharmaceutical and Biomedical Sciences, 2*, 880–887.

Singh, H., Utreja, P., Tiwari, A., & Jain, S. (2009). Elastic Liposomal formulation for sustained delivery of colchicine: In vitro Characterization and in vivo evaluation of anti-gout activity. *AAPS, 11*(1), 54–64. doi:10.120812248-008-9078-8 PMID:19191031

Sivakranth, M., Anjuma, A., Krishnaveni, C., & Venkatesh, E. (2012). Ethosomes: A novel vesicular drug delivery system. *Int J Adv Pharm, 2*(1), 16–27.

Song, Y., Ping, Q., & Wu, Z. H. (2005). Preparation of silybin nano emulsion and its pharmacokinetics in rabbits. *J Chin Pharm Univ, 5*, 427–431.

Sun, H., & Ouyang, W. (2007). Preparation, quality and safety evaluation of berbarinenano emulsion for oral application. *Journal of Shanghai Jiaotong University, 1*, 60–65.

Taylor, L. (2004). *The healing power of rainforest herbs: A Guide to Understanding and Using Herbal Medicinals*. Square One Publishers Inc.

Tiwari, A., Mishra, M., Nayak, K., Yadav, S., & Shukla, A. (2016). Ethosomes: A novel vesicular carrier system for therapeutic applications. *IOSR Journal of Pharmacy, 6*(9), 1, 25–33.

Upadhyay, N., Mandal, S., Bhatia, L., Shailesh, S., & Chauhan, P. (2011). A review on ethosomes: An emerging approach for drug delivery through the skin. *Rec Res Sci Tec, 3*(7), 19–24.

Vijayan, V., & Shaik, A. (2013). Formulation and characterization of solid lipid nanoparticles loaded neem oil for topical treatment of acne. *Journal of Acute Disease*, 2(4), 282–286. doi:10.1016/S2221-6189(13)60144-4

Vyas, S., & Khar, R. (2004). Targeted and controlled drug delivery. *CBS Publisher and Distributors, New Delhi India, 1*, 420–445.

Walve, J., Bakliwal, S., Rane, B., & Pawar, S. (2011). Transfersomes: A surrogated carrier for transdermal drug delivery system. *International Journal of Applied Biology and Pharmaceutical Technology, 2*(1), 204–213.

Xu, H., Fang, Q., Wang, J., & Wang, P. (2008). Study on preparation of paclitaxel loaded PEG-PLGA nanoparticles in vitro experiment. *China Hospital Pharmacy Journal, 28*, 11–14.

Yadav, D., Suri, S., Choudhary, A., Sikender, M., & Hemant, N. (2011). Novel approach: Herbal remedies and natural products in pharmaceutical science as nano drug delivery systems. *Int J Pharm Tech, 3*, 3092–3116.

Yadav, M., Bhatia, V., Doshi, G., & Shastri, K. (2014). Novel techniques in herbal drug delivery systems. *International Journal of Pharmaceutical Sciences Review and Research, 28*(2), 83–89.

Yaddalapudi, S., Palla, G., & Krishnaiah, D. (2015). Solid lipid Nanoparticles. *J Compr Phar, 2*(4), 128–144. doi:10.37483/JCP.2015.2404

Yin, Y., Cui, F., Mu, C., Choi, M., Kim, J., Chung, S., Shim, C., & Kim, D. (2009). Docetaxel microemulsion for enhanced oral bioavailability: Preparation and in vitro and in vivo evaluation. *Journal of Controlled Release*, *140*(2), 86–94. doi:10.1016/j.jconrel.2009.08.015 PMID:19709639

You, J., Cui, F., Han, X., Wang, Y., Yang, L., Yu, Y., & Li, Q. (2006). Study of the preparation of sustained-release microspheres containing zedoary turmeric oil by the emulsion-solvent-diffusion method and evaluation of the self-emulsification and bioavailability of the oil colloids. *Surf B*, *48*(1), 35–41. doi:10.1016/j.colsurfb.2005.12.011 PMID:16480856

Zhang, H., Cui, Y., Zhu, S., Feng, F., & Zheng, X. (2010). Characterization and antimicrobial activity of a pharmaceutical microemulsion. *International Journal of Pharmaceutics*, *395*(1-2), 154–160. doi:10.1016/j.ijpharm.2010.05.022 PMID:20580790

Zhang, J., Hou, S., & Liu, H. (2007). Comparison of preparing two polylactide nanoparticles loaded lipophilic anti-cancer herb drug by nanoprecipitation method. *Zhongguo Zhongyao Zazhi*, *32*, 303–306. PMID:17455462

Zhao, H., Wang, K., Zhao, Y., & Pan, L. (2002). Novel sustained release implant of herbal extract using chitosan. *Biomaterials*, *23*(23), 4459–4462. doi:10.1016/S0142-9612(02)00162-X PMID:12322964

Zhaoa, Y., Wanga, C., Albert, H., Chowb, K., Gongc, T., & Zhangc, Z. (2010). Self-nano emulsifying drug delivery system (SNEDDS) for oral delivery of Zedoary essential oil: Formulation and bioavailability studies. *International Journal of Pharmaceutics*, *383*(1–2), 170–177. doi:10.1016/j.ijpharm.2009.08.035 PMID:19732813

Zhinan, M., Huabing, C., Ting, W., Yajiang, Y., & Xiangliang, Y. (2003). Solid lipid nanoparticle and microemulsion for topical delivery of triptolide. *European Journal of Pharmaceutics and Biopharmaceutics*, *56*(2), 189–196. doi:10.1016/S0939-6411(03)00067-5 PMID:12957632

Zhong, H., Deng, Y., Wang, X., & Yang, B. (2005). Multivesicular liposome formulation for the sustained delivery of breviscapine. *International Journal of Pharmaceutics*, *301*(1-2), 15–24. doi:10.1016/j.ijpharm.2005.04.001 PMID:16023316

Chapter 3
An Innovative Approach as Self-Emulsifying Drug Delivery System for Phytoconstituents

Swati Gokul Talele
Sandip Institute of Pharmaceutical Sciences, Nasik, India

Eknath Damu Ahire
https://orcid.org/0000-0001-6542-884X
Divine College of Pharmacy, Nasik, India

Gokul Shravan Talele
Matoshri College of Pharmacy, Nasik, India

Deelip Vasantrao Derle
M.V.P. College of Pharmacy, Nasik, India

ABSTRACT

In recent years, herbal drugs have flourished as the method of rehabilitation of choice in numerous parts of the world and most of populations consider them as alternative conventional medicaments. However, most of the herbal drugs show poor solubility and bioavailability, which ultimately leads to diminished efficacy and frequency of administration. Consequently, self-emulsifying drug delivery system has been highlighted for poor water-soluble herbal medicaments. Self-emulsifying drug delivery system is an isotropic mixture of phytoconstituents, oil, surfactant, and cosurfactant, and subsequent to oral administration spontaneously endures self-emulsification and forms without emulsion as soon as it comes in contact gastric fluid. Most of the researchers and industrialists are attracted towards this novel and emerging technology as it offers various advantages. The chapter focuses on the mechanism of self-emulsifying, benefits of herbal SEDDS, factors affecting herbal SEDDS with formulation and characterisation of it.

DOI: 10.4018/978-1-7998-4453-2.ch003

1. INTRODUCTION

In India herbal medicaments are considered as safe and utilized consistently since from ancient times and believed as an ancient science of medication (Vaidya et al., 2007).To a certain extent, the term herbal medicines are well-defined in *"Ayurveda"*, (Sharma, 2003; Mukherjeeet al., 2007). *"Unani"* system of medicine. and Chinese practice(Holland, 2000; Porkert, 1974). India's Ayurvedic medicine custom is thought to be more than 5,000 years old and herbal medicines stay a vital component of life (Garodia et al., 2007). Today, still most of countries depend on herbal medicines to fulfil the essential needs of medications. Even the World Health Organization (WHO) stated that 80% of the promising world's population rely on traditional medicament for therapy and considered as prime treatment (Yadav, et .al., 2014).In current years, many of the Phyto constitutes which are strongly utilized in major diseases shows poor water solubility, low bioavailability and many other restrictions including lack of dose proportion, intrasubject and intersubject variability. (Robinson, J.R. 1996)

Major barrier in the development of formulations are low dissolution and bioavailability due to poor water solubility of these phytoconstituents. For this the various techniques are widely utilized including solid dispersion, micronization, salt formation for solubility enhancement. In micronization, due to size reduction phyto-constitutes causes poor wettability whereas salt formation may lead to aggregate formation which restricts use of these techniques.

Currently, lipid based technology widely accepted as a novel approach to increase solubility and bioavailability of water insoluble phytoconstituent's.

On the basis of literature, one of the phytoconstituent, curcumin is isolated from the rhizomes of turmeric(*Curcuma longa* Linn.) having enormous assortment of valuable pharmacological effects including antioxidant, anti-inflammatory, anticarcinogenic (Ruby et. al., 1995; Gescher et. al., 2001; Sharma et. al., 2005; Sharma et al., 2001), hypocholesterolemic (Rao et al., 1970), antibacterial(Ramaprasad et al., 1956), wound healing, antispasmodic, anticoagulant, antitumor(Ammon et al., 1991) and hepatoprotective (Subramanian et al., 1999)activities and effectively inoculated in SEDDS formulations .It shows additional benefits such as compelling free radical scavenger, having superoxide anions, singlet oxygen, hydroxyl radicals scavenging and lipid peroxidation inhibitory actions (Ukil et. al., 2005; Tonnesen et. al., 1992). Similarly phytoconstituents having hepatoprotective activity derived from Cardus Marianus (L.) Gaertn. (Family-Asteraceae).is also incorporated in SEDDS formulation due to its poor water solubility(Dixit et. al., 2007) .Numerous updated literature reports that self-emulsifying drug delivery system can be successfully utilized for hydrophobic phytoconstituent's showing improvement in dissolution and bioavailability Self emulsifying formulations rapidly diffuse in gastrointestinal fluids and leads to the formation of micro and nano emulsion containing soluble phytoconstituent with rapid absorption through lymphatic pathways.

In a nutshell this chapter furnishes an efficient compilation of ample ranging information on all the crucial vistas of the self-emulsifying formulations in herbal medicaments. Thus pave the way in the formulation and application in SEDDS for accelerated advancement into the herbal Phyto constitutes.

Definition and Bioavailability of SEDDS

SEDDS are defined as isotropic mixtures of drug/ phytoconstituents, oil, surfactant and co-surfactant that have unique ability of forming fine o/w micro-emulsion upon mild agitation followed by dilution in aqueous media, such as gastrointestinal fluid as shown in Figure 1. The self –emulsification occurs

Figure 1. Formulation Process of Phytoconstituents SEDDS

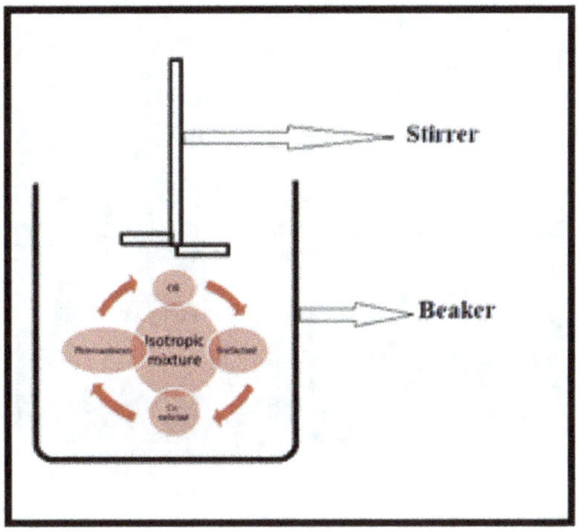

due to motility of the stomach and intestine and as shown in Figure 2 SNEDDS shows improvement in bioavailability by lymphatic transport phenomenon. (P.P. Constantin ides, 1995; Jessy Shaji et al., 2005; Swati et al., 2015).

Lipid Formulation Classification System

As shown in Figure 3 the lipid formulations are classified as Type I, II, IIIA, IIIB and IV.(Bhupendra et al. 2007) Type I, which contains only mixtures of lipid constituents, but without surfactants and co-surfactants, shows coarse particle size while all other types tend to result in globule size in the nanometer ranges. While Type I is without surfactants and co-surfactants, all of the remaining types of LFC'S contain different percentages of each of these constituents. Type I SEDDS requires digestion whereas

Figure 2. SEDDS improving bioavailability of Phytoconstituents after oral adsorption

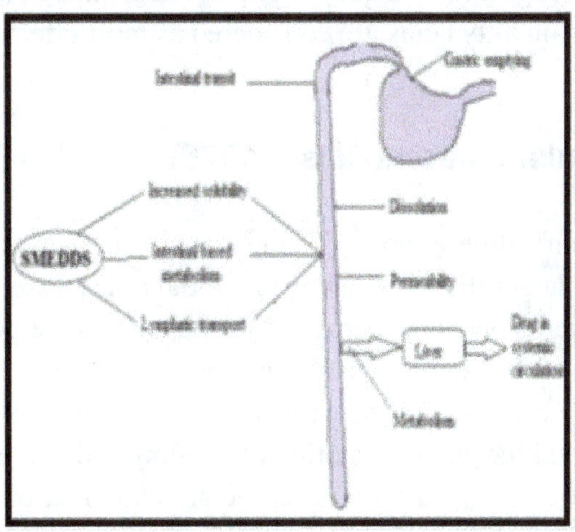

Figure 3. Lipid formulation classification system

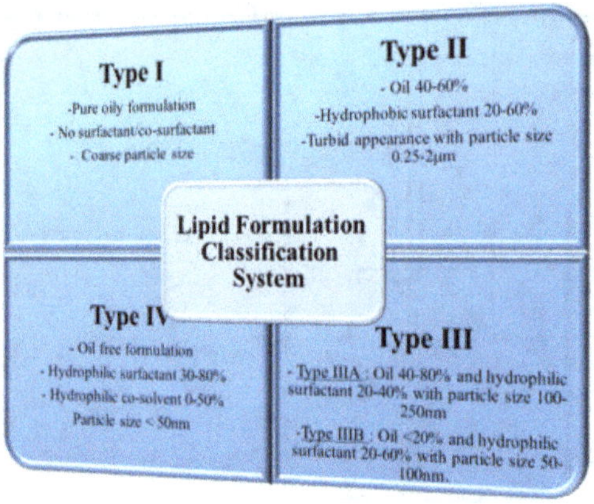

from Type II to Type IV digestion not necessary. Types II to Type IV are quite suited for formulation of various kinds of phytoconstituents.(Pouton, 2000; Pouton et al. 2008; Pouton, 1985)

Factors Affecting SEDDS Formulations (Pouton,, 1985)

As shown in Fig 4, various factors affected SEDDS formulation which give emphasizes as follows,

1) Drugs which shows log P values lower than 2 are not considered as suitable candidate. Even high dose drugs are not suitable, unless and until they show better solubility in any one component of SEDDS formulation.
2) Solubility of the drug in oily phase is essential to maintain the drug in solubilized form. If drug shows greater solubility in surfactant and cosurfactant than oil, ultimately lead to precipitation due to lowering of solvent capacity of surfactant and cosurfactant.
3) Equilibrium solubility measurement can be carried out to predict probable chances of precipitation in the GIT.
4) Lipid polarity also plays an important function in release of drug from SEDDS. Higher polarity leads to rapid release of drugs into the aqueous phase. HLB value in the range of 10-15 and mono-glycerides of medium chain fatty acids are considered as most effectual for SEDDS formulation.

Mechanism of Self-Emulsification (Reiss, 1975)

The mechanism of self emulsification is not well implicated. But as per Reiss when entropy change leads to dispersion and if it is larger than free energy essential to increase the surface area between the oil and aqueous phases of the dispersion, then only formulation undergo self-emulsification. Using light microscopy, the process of self-emulsification was observed and it was predicted that the ease of emulsification process may be related with the ease with water penetrates the oil-water interface with the development of liquid crystalline phases resulting in swelling at the interface and leads to disruption followed by droplet formation. The specificity of surfactant combination obligatory for formation of

Figure 4. Factors affecting SEDDS Formulation

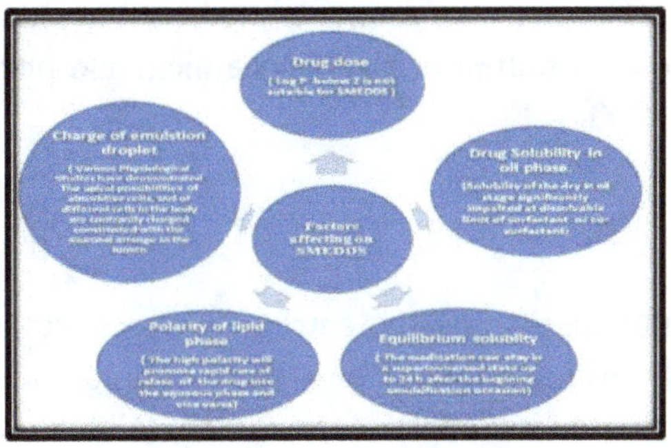

liquid crystalline phase. liquid crystalline interface plays an important role in stabilization of emulsion with barrier for coalescence.

Major Benefits of Herbal SEDDS (Bhupendra et al., 2007; Vergote et. al., 2001)

- SEDDS of herbal formulation shows better bioavailability with dose reduction.
- Oral absorption of SEDDS herbal formulation shows more consistent plasma drug profile.
- SEDDS herbal formulation leads to avoidance of first pass effect.
- SEDDS herbal formulation offers ease of manufacturing and scale up.
- SEDDS of herbal formulations offers protection from hostile environmental in GIT.
- Herbal formulation of SEDDS necessitates simple mixing with agitator during manufacturing thus avoid of complicated manufacturing process.
- SEDDS of herbal formulations administered by filling in hard or soft gelatin capsule or suitably converted into various solid dosage forms utilizing spray drying, extrusion and spherization and granulation techniques.

Key Components in Self-Emulsifying Drug Delivery System of Herbal Phytoconstituents

Phytoconstituents

Today scientist enormously highlighted that 40 to 50% new chemical entities shows low solubility with poor bioavailability and for development of SEDDS phytoconstituents aqueous solubility considered as an important issue. As per the Lipinski's rule of five.

(Lipinski et. al., 1997) which aid in determination of aqueous solubility of drug or phytoconstituents and mostly poor solubility occurs when there are more than 5 hydrogen-bond donors and greater than 10 hydrogen bond acceptors with a molecular weight > 500 and Log P>5.

A drug or phytoconstituents is considered to be highly soluble when the highest dose, strength is soluble in 250 ml or less over a pH range 1–7.5 at 37 °C. on the other side, if the drug solubility is less than 100 µg/ml or the dose to solubility ratio is greater than 250 ml then it is considered poorly soluble. Most of the phytoconstituent as curcumin with log P value four formulated with hydrophobic excipients and considered Type II and Type IIIA whereas some of the phytoconstituents shows poor aqueous solubility including vanilla and nutmeg oil with a log P value nearer to 2 formulated as Type III B and type IV using hydrophilic excipients. Hence above example, predicts that parameters to determine solubility somewhat controversy because of variation in physicochemical and physiological activities of phytoconstituents. (O'Driscoll et al., 2008)

Lipids

Lipids play a vital role in solubilization and the entry of phytoconstituents in lymphatic circulation. Various lipids, including triglycerides, diglycerides, phospholipids, fatty acids, cholesterol, natural, synthetic or semisynthetic lipids used in SEDDS formulation. (Charman SA & et. al., 1992) Amongst long and medium chain triglycerides with variation in degrees of saturations preferred in self-emulsifying formulations (Pouton et al., 2008).

As per literature survey, Mekjaruskul et al revealed that in herbal formulations of SEDDS, modified long and medium chain triglycerides utilized more as compared to other triglycerides.Even various natural oils including peanut oil, soyabean oil, castor oil, olive oil used to increase solubility of herbal extracts (Mekjaruskul et al., 2013). But solubility of curcumin in capryo 190 and in Labrafac Lipophile was 42.34± 0.27 mg/ml and 20.24 ±0.15 mg/ml, respectively as compared to corn oil as 7.58± 0.09 mg/ml. (Setthacheewakul et. al, 2010) as per study conducted by Setthacheewakul and others. Also Ramshankar et. al prepared SEDDS of curcumin (Yadav et al., 2008) using castor oil, but solubility was obtained as 0.44 ± 0.063 mg/ml. Thus the study signifies that capacity of natural oil to solubalise every herbal extract cannot efficient as compare to other triglycerides including Labrafac PG, Maisine 35-1, Labrafac, Lipophile WL 1349 and capryol 90. Quercetin, polyphenolic flavonoid extensively shows various pharmacological activity including antiviral, antidiabetic, anti-inflammatory and act as an antioxidant effectively formulated into Quarcetin-SEDDS. This formulation was prepared with medium chain monoglycerides as campul showed strong antioxidant properties as compared to pure quercetin due to enhancement in solubility and absorption of quercetin. (Jain et al., 2013)

Phospholipids

The formulation of a Gentiopicrin (obtained from gentians and especially from gentian root)-phospholipid complex in a SEDDS formulation was prepared by Gao.(Gao et al., 2009. Gentiopicrin is an active phytoconstituents exhibiting anti-inflammatory, anti-bacterial and hepatoprotective activities. The low oral bio-availability is limiting the use of the agent. To improve the bioavailability, a Gentiopicrin-phospholpid complex is manufactured and further loaded into a self-microemulsifying drug delivery system consisting of MAISINE™35-1

Gentiopicrin an active phytoconstituent which possess effective anti-inflammatory, antibacterial and hepatoprotective activity obtained from the roots of Gentians formulated by utilizing phospholipid. Gentiopicrin-phospholipid complex then loaded in SEDDS by utilizing maisine, labrasol and transcutol. In vivo study revealed that relative bioavailability of Gentiopicrin-phospholipid SEDDS formulation was observed as 703.62% in contrast to phytoconstituent Gentiopicrin.(Gao et al., 2009)

.Even morin as flavonols isolated from fruits, vegetables and medicinal plants showing anti-inflammatory, anticancer, antioxidant, antihypertensive activities with low oral bioavailability .hence phospholipid was utilized and forms a complex with morin and then this complex converted into SEDDS formulation utilizing Labrafil M 1944 CS, cremophore RH40 and transcutol in ratio of 3:5:3(w/w/w).After oral administration it shows 6.2 fold increased in bioavailability as compared to plain morin suspension (Zhang. et. al., 2011). Similarly Jeoung HeeY oo et Studied lutein(Jeoungetal.,2010), an oxygenated carotenoid obtained naturally from green vegetables shows low solubility was formulated into SEDDS. Optimum formulation containing phospholipid as Phosal 53MCT, labrasol and transcutol shows dissolution within 5 min as compared to commercial product of lutein (Eyelac®). Thus, it has been speculated that herbal Phyto constitutes shows improvement in bioavailability and absorption due to digestion of phospholipid phytoconstituent complex by action of pancreatic lipase and then converted into chylomicron and carried via lymphatic system into systemic circulation.

Fatty Acids

A traditional Chinese medicinal herb Puerarialobata containing Puerarin and Puerarialobataisoflavone used for the treatment of hypertension, senile ischemic cerebrovascular disease, and angina pectoris. To improve invitro dissolution and oral absorption, development of SEDDS of Puerarialobataisoflavone using ethyl oleate as long chain ethyl oleate,tween 80 and transcutol was performed and notably SEDDS formulation possess increase in bioavailbilityupto 2.5 fold as compared to Yufengningxin tablets (Puerarialobataisoflavone tablets) (Cu et. al., 2005).

Ginkgo biloba extract (GBE) has become extensively used herbal remedy for increasing cognitive function in elder community. The optimized formulation of SEDDS –GBE consist ethyl oleate as long chain fatty acid, Tween 80 and Cremophor EL 35, 2-propanediol. The in vitro dissolution rate and bioavailability of the active components of GBE SEDDS form were notably faster than those of the GBE tablets (Jingling et. al, 2008). From above study it was concluded that fatty acids can be used for formulation of herbal SEDDS.

Surfactants

To solubilized the hydrophobic moiety, surfactant is considered as an important factor which has undergoes self emulsification and ultimately it leads to enhancement of dissolution rate.surfactant also reduces drug precipitation .Intestinal cell membrane can be get disorder due to surfactant partition with enhancement in permeability.

Intestinal cell membrane which act as permeability barrier get disorder due to surface partition and contribute to enhancement in permeability. As per literature survey scientist elaborated opening of tight junction by utilizing surfactant labrasol offers enhancement in permeability. Nonionic surfactant widely utilized as compare to other ionic surfactant as it shows less toxicity and more bilologicalcompatibility. To achieve spontaneous emulsification HLB value greater than 12 considered as prime objective.To prevent precipitation of phytoconstituents in intestinal lumen various surfactant mainly utilized including Tween 20, 80, Cremophor EL, Labrosol and Gelucire. Literature review also focuses on the hurdle arise due to higher concentration of hydrophilic surfactant forms supersaturated system and lead to precipitation when it comes in contact with aqueous medium in gastrointestinal tract. However precitation can be prevented by incorporating polymers as polyvinyl pyrollidone (PVP) and hydroxyl propyl methylcellulose.(Jeounget. al., 2010; Jingling et. al, 2008; XiJ et al, 2009; Chen et al., 2012)

Cosurfactants

Various cosurfactants or cosolvent like propylene glycol, polyethylene glycol ethanol, transcutol, which aid in solubilization of herbal SEDDS, ultimately, enhance stability of SEDDS with deduction in interfacial tension. But it is essential to take into account that many of the volatile cosurfactant evaporating into soft and hard gelatin capsules and offers precipitation of phytoconstituents (Jeounget. al., 2010; Jingling et. al, 2008; Zhao et al., 2010).

Solubility Studies

The saturated solubility study of the herbal phytoconstituents was performed in various excipients including oils, surfactants, and co surfactants. In this study, an excess amount of the herbal phytoconstituents (approximately 5 mg) was added to each of vehicle approximately 5 ml (solid or semisolid vehicles were melted first) in glass vials and the mixture was heated to near about 60° C in water bath under continuous stirring to assist drug solubilization. The mixture was allowed to place near about at ambient temperature for 48 hours to accomplish equilibrium. The equilibrated sample was centrifuged for around 15 min at 5,000 rpm. Drug which remains in saturated form was separated by filtering with a membrane filter (0.45 µm). The concentration of soluble phytoconstituents was determined by ultraviolet spectrophotometer or by using high performance liquid chromatography. The excipients provided higher solubility for herbal phytoconstituents are selected for further exploration in formulating the SEDDS (Mekjaruskul et al, 2013; Zhang et al., 2012b).

Pseudo Ternary Phase Diagrams (Wanwenetal., 2011b; Swati et al., 2015)

Pseudo ternary phase diagrams of oil, surfactant/ co surfactant (S/CoS) and water were constructed by utilizing water titration method as shown in Fig 5 .(Zhao et al., 2010)

;Shao et al., 2010). The mixtures of oil and S/CoS at definite weight ratios were diluted with water in a drop wise manner. For construction of each phase diagram at a different ratio of S/CoS including 1:1, 2:1, 3:1, 1:2 and 1:3 wt/wt, a transparent and homogenous mixture of oil and S/CoS homogeneous blends of oil and Smix in proportion 1:9 to 9:1 w/w were produced by vortexing for 5 min. Then each prepared mix was titrated with water and observed visually for phase clarity .Weight estimation was utilized to decide the concentration of water at which turbidity-to- clearness and clearness to-turbidity transition happened. The obtained result was then used to determine the margins of the emulsion area were analogous to the preferred value of oils, as well as the S/CoS mixing ratio. **CHEMIX SOFTWARE** was utilized for preparation of phase diagram.

CHARACTERIZATION & EVALUATION of SEDDS (Swat et al., 2015; Swati et al., 2017))

The primary means of self-emulsification assessment is visual evaluation. The efficiency of self emulsification could be estimated by determining droplet size distribution, percent drug content, phase separation study, dispersibility test, Effect of drug loading on droplet size, zeta potential determination.

Figure 5. Pseudo Ternary Phase Diagram

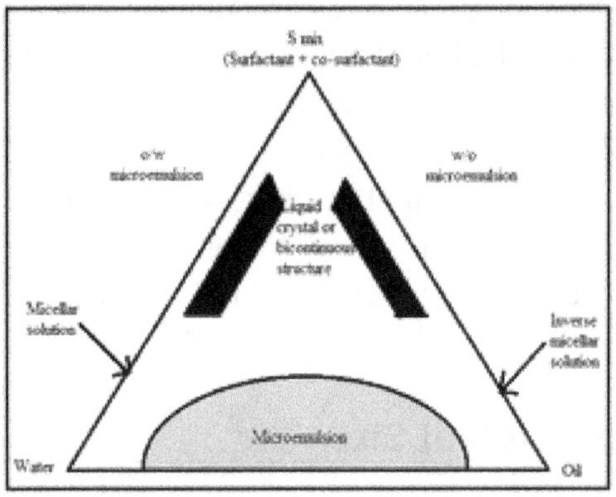

Droplet Size and Particle Size Measurement

The molecular size of the SEDDS is dictated by photon correlation spectroscopy or SEM (Scanning Electron Microscopy) which can measure sizes somewhere around 10 to 5000 nm. Particle size distribution following self emulsification is considered as an essential to evaluate an emulsion system. The smaller the particle size, more will be the drug absorption supported by greater surface area. It is notable that the when surfactant was added to SEDDS it leads to stabilization of film with condensation whereas cosurfactant leads to expansion of film. Consequently, the general extent of surfactant to co-surfactants affect the Particle size. Studies also revealed by scientist that inequality in the CH chains and the presence of double bond leads to nano-emulsion formation with lesser droplet size

Determination of Percentage Drug Content

The herbal SEDDS formulation was taken in a 100 ml volumetric flask, and added 100 ml of solvent. At that point blend was shaken for 1 hour in mechanical shaker and kept aside for 24 hour. After 24 hour, separated the arrangement through Whatman filter paper (0.45 μm) . The obtained filtrate was then investigated using an ultraviolet spectrophotometer. The percent drug content was then determined using absorbance and standard graph.

Phase Separation Study

One milliliter SEDDS was added to glass test tube containing 5 ml of 0.1 N hydrochloric acid, buffer pH 6.8 and distilled water. After altering the test tube for 3-4 times, every blend was put away for a time of 2 hour and phase separation was observed visually .

Zeta Potential Measurement

Zeta potential for micro emulsion can be determined using a suitable Zetasizer. Zeta potential or electrokinetic potential is related to stability of microemulsion and potential is measured from tightly bound surface and electroneutral surface. The zeta potential confers the degree of repulsion between adjacent, similarly charged particles in emulsion namely called colloidal dispersion. Emulsion which contains smaller particles causes more repulsion exceeds to attraction and leads to stabilization of emulsion and when emulsion shows lowest zeta potential, it shows attraction proceeds repulsion and formation of floccules will take place and proceed to breaking of emulsion.

As per study conducted by Zhang et al., zeta potential of curcumin SEDDS was considerably higher than blank SEDDS, may be due to formation of intermolecular hydrogen bonds in the midst of the hydroxyl groups in curcumin and some relative groups containing oxygen or nitrogen atoms in surfactant, co-surfactant and oil created the change in the surface electrostatic double layer of droplets .(Zhang et al., 2012b)

Effect of Drug Loading on Droplet Size

Effect of drug loading on globule size of micro-emulsion was studied using optimized composition formulation were prepared with or without drug. The resultant SEDDS preconcentrate, 0.5 mL was diluted to 100 mL with double distilled water and the mean globule size of the subsequent small scale emulsion was controlled by Motic computerized Microscope.

Thermodynamic Stability Study

The objective of thermodynamic stability is to evaluate the phase separation and effect of temperature variation on SEDDS formulation. SEDDS were diluted with aqueous medium were centrifuged at 15,000 rpm for 15 min and then observed visually for phase separation. Further formulation were subjected to freeze thaw cycles (-2^{0}C for 2 days followed by + 40^0 C for 2 days) and were observed for appearance, phase separation.

In-Vitro Release Study

Herbal SEDDS in vitro dissolution study was performed using dissolution apparatus II (Paddle Type) at 37 ± 0.5° C using the dissolution media. During the study, 5 ml of the aliquots was removed at predetermined time intervals (5, 10, 15, 25, 30, 45 and 60 min) from dissolution medium and replaced with fresh media. The amount of herbal phytoconstituents released in the dissolution medium was determined by using an ultraviolet spectrophotometer or by using high performance liquid chromatography.

Herbal SEDDS Solidification Techniques

Most of formulations available as liquid SEDDS but due to some drawbacks of hard gelatin capsule, scientist attempted to transform liquid SEDDS into solid SEDDS. Following are some techniques which convoluted conversion of liquid SEDD to solid SEDDS as shown in Fig 6.

Adsorption Technique

In this process addition of liquid SEDDS to inert adsorbent as solid carrier was accomplished in suitable blender and free flowing powder was obtained. Jeoung Hee Yoo et. al. developed solid SEDDS of lutein

Figure 6. Various solidification techniques for solid SNEDDS of herbal Phytoconstituents

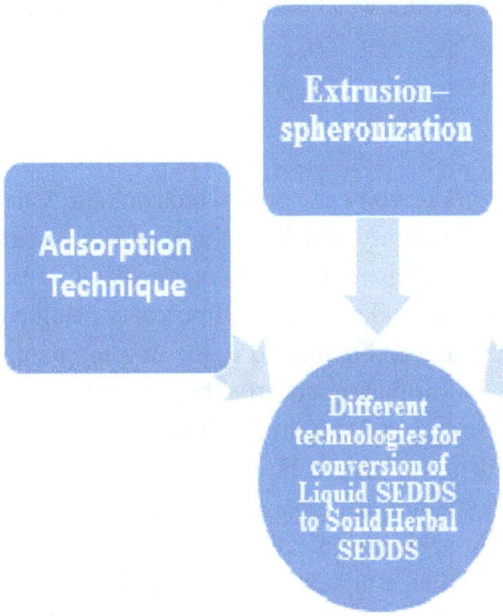

by using carrier as Aerosil 200 and observed that drug dissolution enhance enormously as compare to lutein powder.(Cui et. al., 2005)

Extrusion-Spheronization

It is the most accepted technique for producing pellets of liquid SEDDS of herbal extract. This technique involves four steps initially granulation where there is preparation of wet mass and then extrusion which involves transforming the wet mass into cylinders .Afterwards, spheronization leads to splitting of the extrudate and encompassing of the particles into spheres (Sagar et al., 2016).

Isoi et. al. developed Silymarin SEDDS by using SES (Akoline MCM), Miglyol, Tween 80, microcrystalline cellulose and lactose monohydrate and then transformed into pellets. and pharmacokinetic data showed effective improvement in vivo bioavailability with enhancement in lymphatic absorption. In another study Setthacheewakul et al. converted liquid SEDDS to curcumin pellets and shows increased bioavailability and stability. This proves extrusion and spheronization efficiently utilized as solidification technique for herbal extract (Iosi et. al., 2011).

Spray Drying

Briefly, a solid adsorbent carriers having larger surface area and adsorption capacity are selected for conversion of liquid SEDDS to solid SEDDS. In spray drying technique suspension was prepared by suspending adsorbent in suitable vehicle and then blended with liquid SEDDS . The homogenous suspension was obtained by stirring at 200-300 rpm by using magnetic stirrer at room temperature for 15 minutes. The resultant suspension was then spray dried in a laboratory spray dryer. The resultant powder was collected from the collecting chamber and cyclones. Shanmugam et al, prepared solid SEDDS containing oil as phospholipid by using colloidal silica as inert material Enhancement in bioavailability of solid SEDDS as compare to plain lutein powder was observed (Shanmugam et. al., 2011).

CONCLUSION

Most of the herbal drugs shows poor aqueous solubility with low bioavailability and eventually causes increase in dosing frequency. To enhance solubility and henceforth of herbal extract, SEDDS is an innovative approach utilized successfully for all herbal phytoconstituents. Additionally liquid herbal SEDDS can be converted into granules, pellets and as fine solid powders using adsorption, extrusion and spherization and by spray drying technique and exploited to the development of most acceptable, stable SEDDS for herbal drugs. Because of various prospective benefits, these advances will rebuild the interest of pharmaceutical industrialist in self emulsifying herbal formulations. Furthermore this approach causes noteworthy addition as avoidance of hepatic first pass effect, reduction in gastric irritation with controlled and sustained release formulation of herbal drugs. Lastly, based on present research, SEDDS of herbal drugs considered as novel approach to overcome the hurdles caused by conventional drug delivery of herbal drugs and considered as a new boon in herbal therapy. Efficiently curcumin, Gentiopicrin, lutein and quercetin, Pueraria lobata isoflavone converted into self-emulsifying formulation. Thus, this novel approach requires further exploration and research to bring out a spacious range of commercially available self-emulsifying formulations.

REFERENCES

Ammon, H. P. T., & Anazodo, M. L. (1991). Curcumin: A potent inhibitor of leukotriene B4 formation in rat peritoneal polymorphonuclear neutrophils (PMNL). *Planta Medica*, *58*, 226.

Ammon, H. P. T., Safayhi, H., Mack, T., & Sabieraj, J. (1993). Mechanism of. *Medica (Stuttgart)*, *57*, 1–7.

Charman, S. A., Charman, W. N., Rogge, M. C., Wilson, T. D., Dutko, F. J., & Pouton, C. W. (1992). Self-emulsifying drug delivery systems: Formulation and biopharmaceutic evaluation of an investigational lipophilic compound. *Pharmaceutical Research*, *9*(1), 87–93. doi:10.1023/A:1018987928936 PMID:1589415

Chen, L. J., Liu, Y., Li, L., & Gao, F. (2012). Enhanced bioavailability of total paeony glycoside by self-microemulsifying drug delivery system. *Yao Xue Xue Bao*, *47*(12), 1678–1686. PMID:23460976

Constantinides, P. P. (1995). Lipid microemulsions for improving drug dissolution and oral absorption: Physical and biopharmaceutical aspects. *Pharmaceutical Research*, *12*(11), 1561–1572. doi:10.1023/A:1016268311867 PMID:8592652

Cui, S., Zhao, C., Chen, D., & He, Z. (2005). Self-microemulsifying drug delivery systems (SMEDDS) for improving in vitro dissolution and oral absorption of Pueraria lobata isoflavone. *Drug Development and Industrial Pharmacy*, *31*(4-5), 349–356. doi:10.1081/DDC-54309 PMID:16093200

Dixit, N., Baboota, S., Kohli, K., Ahmad, S., & Ali, J. (2007). Silymarin: A review of pharmacological aspects and bioavailability enhancement approaches. *Indian Journal of Pharmacology*, *39*(4), 172. doi:10.4103/0253-7613.36534

Gao, D., Han, I., & Wang, J. (2009). Self micro emulsifying drug delivery system loaded with gentiopicrin phospholipid complex for oral delivery; preparation in vivo characterization and in vivo evaluation abstract 2009. *AAPS Annual meeting and exposition.*

Garodia, P., Ichikawa, H., Malani, N., Sethi, G., & Aggarwal, B. B. (2007). From ancient medicine to modern medicine: Ayurvedic concepts of health and their role in inflammation and cancer. *Journal of the Society for Integrative Oncology*, *5*(1), 25–37. doi:10.2310/7200.2006.029 PMID:17309811

Gescher, A. J., Sharma, R. A., & Steward, W. P. (2001). Cancer chemoprevention by dietary constituents: A tale of failure and promise. *The Lancet. Oncology*, *2*(6), 371–379. doi:10.1016/S1470-2045(00)00392-2 PMID:11905754

Holland, A. (1999). *Voices of Qi: an introductory guide to traditional Chinese medicine*. North Atlantic Books.

Iosio, T. A. M. A. R. A., Voinovich, D. A. R. I. O., Perissutti, B., Serdoz, F., Hasa, D., Grabnar, I., Acqua, S. D., Zara, G. P., Muntoni, E., & Pinto, J. F. (2011). Oral bioavailability of silymarin phytocomplex formulated as self-emulsifying pellets. *Phytomedicine*, *18*(6), 505–512. doi:10.1016/j.phymed.2010.10.012 PMID:21111585

Jain, S., Jain, A. K., Pohekar, M., & Thanki, K. (2013). Novel self-emulsifying formulation of quercetin for improved in vivo antioxidant potential: Implications for drug-induced cardiotoxicity and nephrotoxicity. *Free Radical Biology & Medicine*, *65*, 117–130. doi:10.1016/j.freeradbiomed.2013.05.041 PMID:23792276

Li, W., Yi, S., Wang, Z., Chen, S., Xin, S., Xie, J., & Zhao, C. (2011). Self-nanoemulsifying drug delivery system of persimmon leaf extract: Optimization and bioavailability studies. *International Journal of Pharmaceutics*, *420*(1), 161–171. doi:10.1016/j.ijpharm.2011.08.024 PMID:21884770

Lipinski, C. A., Lombardo, F., Dominy, B. W., & Feeney, P. J. (1997). Experimental and computational approaches to estimate solubility and permeability in drug discovery and development settings. *Advanced Drug Delivery Reviews*, *23*(1-3), 3–25. doi:10.1016/S0169-409X(96)00423-1 PMID:11259830

Mekjaruskul, C., Yang, Y. T., Leed, M. G., Sadgrove, M. P., Jay, M., & Sripanidkulchai, B. (2013). Novel formulation strategies for enhancing oral delivery of methoxyflavones in Kaempferia parviflora by SMEDDS or complexation with 2-hydroxypropyl-β-cyclodextrin. *International Journal of Pharmaceutics*, *445*(1-2), 1–11. doi:10.1016/j.ijpharm.2013.01.052 PMID:23376503

Mukheriee, P. K., & Wahile, A. (2006). Integrated approaches towards drug development from Ayurveda and other Indian system of medicines. *Journal of Ethnopharmacology*, *103*(1), 25–35. doi:10.1016/j.jep.2005.09.024 PMID:16271286

Muley, S., Nandgude, T., & Poddar, S. (2016). Extrusion–spheronization a promising pelletization technique: In-depth review. *Asian Journal of Pharmaceutical Sciences, 11*(6), 684-699.

Porkert, M. (1974). *The theoretical foundations of Chinese medicine: Systems of correspondence* (Vol. 3). MIT Press.

Pouton, C. W. (1985). Self-emulsifying drug delivery systems: Assessment of the efficiency of emulsification. *International Journal of Pharmaceutics*, *27*(2-3), 335–348. doi:10.1016/0378-5173(85)90081-X

Pouton, C. W. (2000). Lipid formulations for oral administration of drugs: Non-emulsifying, self-emulsifying and 'self-microemulsifying'drug delivery systems. *European Journal of Pharmaceutical Sciences*, *11*, S93–S98. doi:10.1016/S0928-0987(00)00167-6 PMID:11033431

Pouton, C. W., & Porter, C. J. (2008). Formulation of lipid-based delivery systems for oral administration: Materials, methods and strategies. *Advanced Drug Delivery Reviews*, *60*(6), 625–637. doi:10.1016/j.addr.2007.10.010 PMID:18068260

Prajapati, B. G., & Patel, M. M. (2007). Conventional and alternative pharmaceutical methods to improve oral bioavailability of lipophilic drugs. *Asian Journal of Pharmaceutics*, *1*(1), 1–8.

Ramaprasad, C., & Sirsi, M. (1956). Indian medicinal plants: Curcuma longa; in vitro antibacterial activity of curcumin and the essential oil. *Journal of Scientific and Industrial Research, C*, 15, 239–241.

Ramshankar, Y. V., Suresh, S., & Devi, K. (2008). Novel self-emulsifying formulation of curcumin with improved dissolution, antiangiogenic and anti-inflammatory activity. *Clinical Research and Regulatory Affairs*, *25*(4), 213–234. doi:10.1080/10601330802600893

Rao, D. S., Sekhara, N. C., Satyanarayana, M. N., & Srinivasan, M. (1970). Effect of curcumin on serum and liver cholesterol levels in the rat. *The Journal of Nutrition*, *100*(11), 1307–1315. doi:10.1093/jn/100.11.1307 PMID:5476433

Reiss, H. (1975). Entropy-induced dispersion of bulk liquids. *Journal of Colloid and Interface Science*, *53*(1), 61–70. doi:10.1016/0021-9797(75)90035-1

Robinson, J. R. (1996). Introduction: semi-solid formulations of oral drug delivery. *Bulletin Technique-Gattefosse*, 11-14.

Ruby, A. J., Kuttan, G., Babu, K. D., Rajasekharan, K. N., & Kuttan, R. (1995). Anti-tumour and antioxidant activity of natural curcuminoids. *Cancer Letters*, *94*(1), 79–83. doi:10.1016/0304-3835(95)03827-J PMID:7621448

Setthacheewakul, S., Kedjinda, W., Maneenuan, D., & Wiwattanapatapee, R. (2011). Controlled release of oral tetrahydrocurcumin from a novel self-emulsifying floating drug delivery system (SEFDDS). *AAPS PharmSciTech*, *12*(1), 152–164. doi:10.120812249-010-9568-8 PMID:21181511

Shaji, J., & Joshi, V. (2005). Self-micro emulsifying drug delivery system (SMEDDS) for improving bioavailability of hydrophobic drugs and its potential to give sustain release dosage form. *Indian Journal of Pharmaceutical Education*, *39*(3), 130.

Shanmugam, S., Baskaran, R., Balakrishnan, P., Thapa, P., Yong, C. S., & Yoo, B. K. (2011). Solid self-nanoemulsifying drug delivery system (S-SNEDDS) containing phosphatidylcholine for enhanced bioavailability of highly lipophilic bioactive carotenoid lutein. *European Journal of Pharmaceutics and Biopharmaceutics*, *79*(2), 250–257. doi:10.1016/j.ejpb.2011.04.012 PMID:21550401

Shao, B., Tang, J., Ji, H., Liu, H., Liu, Y., Zhu, D., & Wu, L. (2010). Enhanced oral bioavailability of Wurenchun (Fructus Schisandrae Chinensis extracts) by self-emulsifying drug delivery systems. *Drug Development and Industrial Pharmacy*, *36*(11), 1356–1363. doi:10.3109/03639045.2010.480975 PMID:20849350

Sharma, A. K. (2003). Panchkarma Therapy in Ayurvedic Medicine. In L. C. Mishra (Ed.), *Scientific Basis for Ayurvedic Therapies*. CRC Press. doi:10.1201/9780203498583.ch4

Sharma, R. A., Gescher, A. J., & Steward, W. P. (2005). Curcumin: The story so far. *European Journal of Cancer*, *41*(13), 1955–1968. doi:10.1016/j.ejca.2005.05.009 PMID:16081279

Sharma, R. A., McLelland, H. R., Hill, K. A., Ireson, C. R., Euden, S. A., Manson, M. M., ... Steward, W. P. (2001). Pharmacodynamic and pharmacokinetic study of oral Curcuma extract in patients with colorectal cancer. *Clinical Cancer Research*, *7*(7), 1894–1900. PMID:11448902

Talele, S. G. (2017). Response Surface Methodology as a Tool for Optimization of self-nanoemulsified Drug Delivery System of Quetiapine Fumarate. *Asian Journal of Pharmaceutics (AJP)*, *11*(4).

Talele, S. G., & Gudsoorkar, V. R. (2016). Novel approaches for solidification of SMEDDS. *Int J Pharm Biosci*, *15*, 90–101.

Tang, J., Sun, J., Cui, F., Zhang, T., Liu, X., & He, Z. (2008). Self-emulsifying drug delivery systems for improving oral absorption of ginkgo biloba extracts. *Drug Delivery*, *15*(8), 477–484. doi:10.1080/10717540802039089 PMID:18720135

Tennesen, H. H., & Greenhill, J. V. (1992). Studies on curcumin and curcuminoids. XXII: Curcumin as a reducing agent and as a radical scavenger. *International Journal of Pharmaceutics*, *87*(1-3), 79–87. doi:10.1016/0378-5173(92)90230-Y

Ukil, A., Maity, S., Karmakar, S., Datta, N., Vedasiromoni, J. R., & Das, P. K. (2003). Curcumin, the major component of food flavour turmeric, reduces mucosal injury in trinitrobenzene sulphonic acid-induced colitis. *British Journal of Pharmacology*, *139*(2), 209–218. doi:10.1038j.bjp.0705241 PMID:12770926

Vaidya, A. D. B., & Devasagayam, T. P. A. (2007). Recent advances in Indian herbal drug research guest editor: Thomas Paul Asir Devasagayam current status of herbal drugs in India: an overview. Academic Press.

Vergote, G. J., Vervaet, C., Van Driessche, I., Hoste, S., De Smedt, S., Demeester, J., Jain, R. A., Ruddy, S., & Remon, J. P. (2001). An oral controlled release matrix pellet formulation containing nanocrystalline ketoprofen. *International Journal of Pharmaceutics*, *219*(1-2), 81–87. doi:10.1016/S0378-5173(01)00628-7 PMID:11337168

Xi, J., Chang, Q., Chan, C. K., Meng, Z. Y., Wang, G. N., Sun, J. B., Wang, Y. T., Tong, H. H. Y., & Zheng, Y. (2009). Formulation development and bioavailability evaluation of a self-nanoemulsified drug delivery system of oleanolic acid. *AAPS PharmSciTech*, *10*(1), 172–182. doi:10.120812249-009-9190-9 PMID:19224372

Yadav, M., Bhatia, V. J., Doshi, G., & Shastri, K. (2014). Novel techniques in herbal drug delivery systems. *International Journal of Pharmaceutical Sciences Review and Research*, *28*(2), 83–89.

Yoo, J. H., Shanmugam, S., Thapa, P., Lee, E. S., Balakrishnan, P., Baskaran, R., Yoon, S.-K., Choi, H.-G., Yong, C. S., Yoo, B. K., & Han, K. (2010). Novel self-nanoemulsifying drug delivery system for enhanced solubility and dissolution of lutein. *Archives of Pharmacal Research*, *33*(3), 417–426. doi:10.100712272-010-0311-5 PMID:20361307

Zhang, J., Peng, Q., Shi, S., Zhang, Q., Sun, X., Gong, T., & Zhang, Z. (2011). Preparation, characterization, and in vivo evaluation of a self-nanoemulsifying drug delivery system (SNEDDS) loaded with morin-phospholipid complex. *International Journal of Nanomedicine*, *6*, 3405. PMID:22267925

Zhang, L., Zhu, W., Yang, C., Guo, H., Yu, A., Ji, J., ... Zhai, G. (2012). A novel folate-modified self-microemulsifying drug delivery system of curcumin for colon targeting. *International Journal of Nanomedicine*, *7*, 151. PMID:22275831

Zhao, Y., Wang, C., Chow, A. H., Ren, K., Gong, T., Zhang, Z., & Zheng, Y. (2010). Self-nanoemulsifying drug delivery system (SNEDDS) for oral delivery of Zedoary essential oil: Formulation and bioavailability studies. *International Journal of Pharmaceutics*, *383*(1-2), 170–177. doi:10.1016/j.ijpharm.2009.08.035 PMID:19732813

Chapter 4
Nutraceuticals:
An Effective and Safe Way From Microbes of Marine Sources

Charu Gupta
AIHRS, Amity University, Noida, India

Dhan Prakash
AIHRS, Amity University, Noida, India

ABSTRACT

Therapeutic compounds can be derived from various natural sources like plants, animals, marine organisms, and micro-organisms. Although the marine biota accounts for around 50% of the total world biodiversity, their potential as a rich source of bioactive products and their applications in both pharmaceutical and nutraceutical industries have only recently been identified through several scientific studies. Marine biotechnology is an upcoming area that involves about the study of marine microorganisms and animals including algae, sponges, and coral as a novel source of bioactive substances that can be used in the treatment of various human diseases like cancer, anaemia, diarrhea, obesity, diabetes, atopic dermatitis, Crohn's disease, etc. Very limited scientific data is available on the bioactive potential of marine microorganisms. This chapter deals with the exploitation of microbes from marine sources as potential sources for various nutraceuticals and their possibilities for applications in a variety of diseases and as functional food supplement.

1. INTRODUCTION

It is well known that more than 70% of our planet's surface is covered by oceans. Experts estimated that the biological diversity in marine environment is higher than in tropical rain forests. Marine water contains enormous amounts of biodiversity which makes it as a source of huge amounts and wide varieties of novel bioactive compounds. Many marine organisms are soft bodied and have a sedentary life style necessitating chemical means of defense. Therefore, they have evolved the ability to synthesize toxic compounds or to obtain them from marine microorganisms. These compounds help them deter preda-

DOI: 10.4018/978-1-7998-4453-2.ch004

tors, keep competitors at bay or paralyze their prey. The overwhelming biological diversity of marine microbes has so far only been explored to a very limited extent. This diversity is believed to give rise to an equally high diversity of secondary metabolites synthesized by the marine micro-fauna and micro-flora. Natural products released into the water are rapidly diluted and, therefore, need to be highly potent to have any effect. It is increasingly recognized that a huge number of natural products and novel chemical entities exist in the oceans, with biological activities that may be useful in the quest for finding drugs with greater efficacy and specificity for the treatment of many human diseases (Mayer and Lehmann, 2000; Proksch et al., 2002).

The oceans are the source of a large group of structurally unique natural products that are mainly accumulated in invertebrates such as sponges, tunicates, bryozoans, and molluscs. Macroalgae, also called seaweed, are the most popular type of algae in the nutraceutical industry as it provides a great variety of food and food ingredients especially in Asian countries like Korea, Japan and China. It is estimated that the annual production value of macro-algae is US$5 billion in 2007 (Pickering et al., 2007). About 2400 natural products have been isolated from macro-algae belonging to the classes Rhodophyceae, Phaeophyceae and Chlorophyceae (Elena, 2003). Presently seaweeds constitute commercially important marine renewable resources which are providing valuable ideas for the development of new drugs against diabetes, microbial infections and inflammations (Bhagavathy et al., 2011). Algal constituents include acids, alkaloids, amines, antibacterial, antifungal, antiviral substances, lipids, sterols, steroids, fatty acids, phenolic compounds, phytochromes, pigments, proteins, peptides, amino acids, sugar, alcohols and vitamins. *Gracilaria opuntia* belongs to the family Rhodophyceae (Red algae) and possesses various biological activities.

Marine microorganisms have received mounting attention in bio-discoveries due to their exclusive physicochemical characteristics which have been acquired as an adaptation to prevailing extreme conditions in the marine environment. It has been noticed that those unique marine microbes and their biologically active metabolites are potential sources to be used as sustainable food and pharmaceutical ingredients (Dewapriya and Kim, 2014). Most of the bioactive compounds are having numerous biological activities which are found to act as nutraceuticals for humans and animals. Marine organisms thus represent a valuable source of bioactive compounds. The biodiversity of the marine environment and the associated chemical diversity constitute practically an unlimited resource for the development of new bioactive products (Aneiros and Garateix, 2004). Marine organisms such as sponges, tunicates, bryozoans, molluscs, bacteria, microalgae, macro-algae and cyanobacteria have recently been utilized for biotechnology. Compounds produced from these organisms are effective as therapeutics for infectious and non-infectious disease, with a high specificity for target molecules, usually an enzyme.

In the nutraceutical industry marine algae are majorly used as sources of food and food ingredients (Tseng, 2001). Microalgae and macro-algae are the two main categories of algae and both have applications as nutraceuticals. Microalgae, the most primary and simply-organized members of marine plant life, are rich sources of food ingredients, such as β-carotene, Vitamins C, A, E, H, B_1, B_2, B_6 and B_{12}, astaxanthin, polysaccharides and polyunsaturated fatty acids (Grobbelaar, 2004). As such, bioactive molecules from microalgae are commercially produced, used as food additives and also incorporated into infant milk formulations and dietary supplements (Volkman, 2003). Several of these compounds (especially the tunicate metabolite ET-743) show pronounced pharmacological activities and are interesting candidates for new drugs primarily in the area of cancer treatment. Other compounds are currently being developed as an analgesic (ziconotide from the mollusc (*Conus magus*) or to treat inflammation. Numerous natural products from marine invertebrates show striking structural similarities to known metabolites of microbial origin; suggesting that microorganisms (bacteria, microalgae) are at least involved in their biosynthesis or are in fact the true sources of these respective metabolites. This assumption is corroborated by several studies on natural products from sponges that proved these compounds to be localized in symbiotic bacteria or cyanobacteria. Recently, molecular methods have successfully been applied to study the microbial diversity in marine sponges and to gain evidence for an involvement of bacteria in the biosynthesis of the bryostatins in the bryozoan *Bugula neritina* (Proksch et al., 2002).

2. MARINE MICROORGANISMS AS SOURCE OF NUTRACEUTICALS

A study reported that some unidentified prokaryotic communities such as the JS1 and DSAG groups occur widely in organic rich deep marine sediments associated with methane hydrates along the Pacific Ocean margin. These microbial communities can be stratified in deep marine sediments, and surrounding geochemical and geological settings strongly affect the community structure. It is becoming more and more evident that many classes of microorganisms exist only in the sea (Inagaki et al., 2006). Due to limited literature on the culturing techniques and media formulation for culturing marine microbes, pharmaceutical industries have not been able to fully utilize this enormous resource. The myth still prevails that marine microorganisms are difficult to culture, if not uncultivable. However, a number of reports in recent past have proven that marine microorganisms can now be cultured successfully (Okami, 1993). Most of the developed and underdeveloped countries have since shifted their focus to the marine habitat and new marine oriented programs are emerging worldwide. Major classes of microbes like bacteria and fungi are now the target of biomedical study and intriguing novel metabolites are being produced. Coastal bacterial samples grown under saline conditions yield new antibiotics, antitumor, and anti-inflammatory compounds (Trischman, 1994). In fact, the symbiotic microbial consortia also prove to be a source of bioactive compounds with pharmaceutical potential. Bacteria and fungi have been sampled from the surfaces of marine plants and the internal tissues of invertebrates and, marine fungi seem to be of increasing interest (Belofsky et al., 1998).

2.1 Marine Bacteria

Marine bacteria are prolific producers of valuable secondary metabolites as they thrive in harsh oceanic climates. The marine isolate *Pseudomonas,* Gram-negative, γ-proteo-bacteria is not well explored and only a limited number have been reported as producers of bioactive compounds. A bacterium strain KMM 3042 that is aerobic, non-pigmented, produces some bioactive substances such as pyrroles, pseudopeptide pyrrolidinedione, phloroglucinol, phenazine, benzaldehyde, quinoline, quinolone, phenanthren, phthalate, andrimid, moiramides, zafrin and bushrin (Romanenko et al., 2008a). Some of these bioactive compounds are antimicrobial agents, and dibutyl phthalate and di-(2-ethylhexyl) phthalate have been reported to be cathepsin-B inhibitors (Isnansetyo and Kamei, 2009). *Stenotrophomonas* strains isolated from sponge, sea urchin, and ophiura specimens showed remarkable antimicrobial and antifungal inhibitory activity. Although negligible activity was observed against *Candida albicans,* these strains could substantially inhibit Gram-positive microorganisms. It is noteworthy that *S. maltophilia* is an opportunistic pathogen and also possess bio-controlling capabilities (Romanenko et al., 2008b). Another study from the same group, directed against low molecular weight antimicrobial metabolites from marine ark shell *Anadara broughtoni* associated heterotrophic bacteria, revealed antimicrobial, hemolytic and surface activities in butanol extracts of cells or cell-free supernatant of six active strains (Romanenko et al., 2008c). Yet another recently discovered genus of bioactive substance producing marine bacteria is *Pseudoalteromonas*, the seawater species *P. phenolica* was reported to inhibit methicillin resistant *Staphylococcus aureus* strains due to a brominated biphenyl compound, 3,3'',5,5''-tetrabromo-2,2''-diphenyldiol (Isnansetyo and Kamei, 2003). Some strains of *P. luteoviolacea* also seem to have activity against protists (Bhatnagar & Kim, 2010).

Egan et al., 2002 reported that the yellow pigment of *Pseudoalteromonas tunicata* has anti-fungal activity which was later identified as a tambjamine (4-methoxypyrrole-containing bioactive compounds) like alkaloid and re-designated as YP1 (Franks et al., 2005). These tambjamines have been isolated from marine invertebrates and have been previously reported to possess antimicrobial, anti-tumorigenic, immunosuppressive, anti-proliferative and ichthyodeterrent activities (Bhatnagar and Kim, 2010). There are many evidences those points towards the colonizing bacteria at the surface of higher organisms as the source of these compounds (König et al., 2006). This has further been proven by Burke and colleagues by elucidation of YP1 biosynthetic pathway in *P. tunicate* (Burke et al., 2007).

2.2 Marine Fungi

Marine derived fungi have been widely studied for their bioactive metabolites and have proven to be a rich and promising source of novel anticancer, antibacterial, anti-plasmodial, anti-inflammatory and antiviral agents (Bhadury et al., 2006; Newman and Hill, 2006). Some marine fungi have unique new carbon frameworks which are exceptional in nature. Compounds produced by such fungi are of interest as new lead structures for medicine as well as for plant protection. Responding to the great demand for natural compounds from marine derived fungi, Kjer *et al.* (2010) have defined a detailed protocol for their isolation and cultivation from various marine organisms (sponges, algae and mangrove plants) in order to characterize and elucidate the structure of secondary metabolites produced by these fungi. A couple of years ago, Du *et al.* (2007) isolated a novel anthraquinone derivative with naphtha [1,2,3-de] chromene-2,7-dione skeleton, and named it aspergiolide A. It was isolated from a marine filamentous fungus, *Aspergillus glaucus* in the Fujian province of China, and was found to exhibit cytotoxicity against K562 and P388 cell lines. The same group has also worked on the antitumor activities of alkaloids isolated from a *Penicillium* sp. derived from deep ocean sediment.

They isolated two new meleagrin analogs, meleagrin D and E, and two new diketopiperazines, roquefortine H and I which showed weak cytotoxicity as compared to the previously reported meleagrin B and meleagrin that induced HL-60 cell apoptosis or arrested the cell cycle through G2/M phase, respectively. They proposed that the distinct substitutions on the imidazole ring could have a significant influence on the cytotoxicity of these alkaloids (Du et al., 2010). A number of novel compounds and metabolites with bioactive potential continue to be isolated and characterized from marine derived fungi, which are capable of producing not only antimicrobial but also antifouling compounds. In 2006, a bioassay-guided isolation and purification procedure was used to obtain a novel antifouling and antimicrobial compound from a marine-derived fungus *Ampelomyces* sp. The isolate, 3-chloro-2,5-dihydroxybenzyl alcohol effectively inhibited larval settlement of the tubeworm *Hydroides elegans* and of cyprids of the barnacle *Balanus amphitrite* and was non-toxic; suggestive of a potent anti-foulant and/or antibiotic activity (Kwong et al., 2006). Another study from the same group concerned the antibiotic and antifouling compound production by the marine derived fungus *Cladosporium sp.* F14. They reported that in nutrient enriched cultivation media, this strain produced antibiotic and antifouling compounds in the presence of glucose or xylose

(Xiong et al., 2009). In the search for novel antimitotic and antifungal substances from marine-derived fungi, a scientific study reported that low concentration of the ethanol extracts of the culture broth of a *Fusarium sp.* (strain 05JANF165) were bioactive. Their search for the basis of this bioactivity led to the identification and purification of a new antifungal antibiotic and the chemical structure was elucidated as Fusarielin E (Gai et al., 2007).

Another Korea based study resulted in the isolation of a novel antibacterial dioxopiperazine, dehydroxybisdethiobis-methylthio-gliotoxin, and the previously reported bisdethiobis-methylthiogliotoxin and gliotoxin, from the broth of a marine derived fungus of the genus *Pseudallescheria* and its structure was assigned through NMR. All three compounds exhibited potent antibacterial activity against the methicillin resistant and multidrug resistant *Staphylococcus aureus*, whereas Gliotoxin showed a significant radical scavenging activity against 1,1-diphenyl-2-picrylhydrazyl (DPPH) (Li et al., 2006). Another study from the same source, reported two novel antibacterial aspyrone derivatives viz. Chlorohydroaspyrones A and B, and the previously described aspyrone, asperlactone, and penicillic acid from the broth of a marine isolate of the fungus *Exophiala* and were found to have mild antibacterial activity against *Staphylococcus aureus* (Zhang et al., 2008). Marine fungi have also been reported to possess a nematicidal effect. Nematicidal and antimicrobial metabolites were reported previously from marine ascomycete *Lachnum papyraceum* (Karst.) Karst III and the production of novel isocoumarin derivatives were achieved under halogenated conditions (Stadler et al., 1995). Inspired by this work, Nenkep *et al.* (2010) reported the isolation of halogenated benzoquinones (bromochlorogentisylquinones A and B), with significant radical scavenging activity against DPPH, from a marine derived *Phoma* herbarum strain.

2.3 Actinomycetes

Actinomycetes from natural sources are widely recognized to produce secondary metabolites, including many antimicrobials such as streptomycin, erythromycin, and tetracycline, with original and ingenious structures and potent biological activities (Takahashi and Omura, 2003). Therefore, actinomycetes are considered to be a potent resource for new lead compounds in drug development. Many marine isolates of actinomycetes have been reported to be producers of novel antitumor (Olano, 2009), antimalarial (Prudhomme, 2008) and antimicrobial agents (El-Gendy et al., 2008; McArthur et al., 2008). In the exploration of marine derived actinomycetes as a source of antitumor compounds, Cho *et al.* (2007) isolated four new 3-methyl-4-ethylideneproline-containing peptides, Lucentamycins A-D from the fermentation broth of a marine derived actinomycete, *Nocardiopsis lucentensis* (strain CNR-712). Out of the four compounds, Lucentamycins A and B were observed to have significant *in vitro* cytotoxicity against HCT-116 human colon carcinoma Cho *et al.* (2007). In another report, five isoquinoline quinones, four new derivatives, Mansouramycin A-D, and the known 3-methyl-7- (methylamino)-5,8-isoquinolinedione were isolated from the ethyl acetate extract from the marine derived Mei37 isolate of *Streptomyces* sp. These isolated compounds, when subjected to cytotoxicity analysis against 36 tumor cell lines, indicated significant cytotoxicity with great degree of selectivity for non-small cell lung cancer, breast cancer, melanoma, and prostate cancer cells (Hawas et al., 2009) suggesting their potential as anticancer drugs.

In the same year, Perez and coworkers isolated a macrodiolide Tartrolon D from the fermentation broths of *Streptomyces* sp. MDG-04-17-069. The tartrolons are a class of compounds that have attracted a great deal of attention owing to their interesting biological properties. The isolated tartrolon in this study was found to display strong cytotoxic activity against three human tumor cell lines viz. lung (A549), colon (HT29), and breast (MDA-MB-231) (Pérez et al., 2009). Yet another study reported the secondary metabolites of a marine *Saccharomonospora* sp. that yielded a novel alkaloid Lodopyridone, which was found to be cytotoxic to HCT-116 human colon cancer cells (Maloney et al., 2009).

Marine actinomycetes are not only known for their anti-tumor and anti-cancerous potential, they are well documented as antimicrobial agents too. A California based study was successful in isolating a series of chlorinated bisindole pyrroles, Lynamicins A–E from a novel strain of a marine actinomycete, *Marinispora*. This isolate demonstrated broad-spectrum activity against both Gram-positive and Gram-negative organisms. When tested for their antimicrobial spectrum against a panel of 11 pathogens, these compounds showed activity against drug-resistant pathogens such as methicillin-resistant *Staphylococcus aureus* and vancomycin-resistant *Enterococcus faecium* (McArthur et al., 2008). Carlson *et al.* (2009) have reported the isolation of novel dienoyl tetramic acids tirandamycin C and tirandamycin D with activity against vancomycin resistant *Enterococcus faecalis*, from the marine environmental isolate *Streptomyces* sp. 307-9. These compounds were structurally similar to the previously identified compounds Tirandamycins A and B with a slight variation in the pattern of pendant oxygenation on the bicyclic ketal system.

Maskey *et al.* (2004) isolated Trioxacarcins A, B and C along with three new derivatives designated as Trioxacarcins D, E and F, from the ethyl acetate extract of *Streptomyces* sp. isolate B8652. All trioxacarcins showed high anti-bacterial activity whereas some of them showed high anti-tumor and anti-malarial activity. In another study, crude extract of a marine *Streptomyces* strain obtained from deep sea sediments, was used to isolate five structurally similar compounds which were found to have potent antifouling activity (Xu et al., 2010). On the other hand, a marine-derived *Actinomyces* strain (NPS554) isolated from Japan yielded two trialkyl-substituted aromatic acids, Lorneic acid A and B. It was observed that Lorneic acid-A had significant inhibition activity against phosphodiesterase (PDE) 5 (Iwata et al., 2009). It is worth noting here that PDE5 inhibitors are of pharmacological importance in erectile dysfunctions and pulmonary hypertension.

2.4 Microalgae

Cyanobacteria are a diverse group of Gram-negative bacteria, also known as blue-green algae that produce an array of secondary compounds with selective bioactivity against vertebrates, invertebrates, plants, microalgae, fungi, bacteria, viruses and cell lines (Lopes et al., 2010). They produce a wide variety of secondary metabolites with antifungal, antiviral, antibiotic and other activities, which make them an interesting candidate of potential pharmaceutical importance. Certain anticancer compounds, which were initially thought to be obtained from marine sources, are now known to be produced by cyanobacteria (Luesch et al., 2002). Ulithiacyclamide and Patellamide A belong to Cyanobactins, produced by cyanobacteria, which have potent antimalarial, antitumor, and multidrug reversing activities (Sivonen et al., 2010). Recently, two new bioactive marine cyanobacterial natural products, Viridamides A and B have been reported. It was observed that Viridamide A showed anti-trypanosomal and anti-leishmanial activity. The producer organism being blackish-green, mat-forming, filamentous cyanobacterium identified as *Oscillatoria nigroviridis* (Simmons et al., 2008). Green algae have also been reported as producers of antiprotozoal molecules. In a recent study, Allmendinger *et al.* (2010) screened the antiprotozoal activity of crude extracts of four green marine algae (*Cladophora rupestris, Codium fragile sp. tomentosoides, Ulva intestinalis* and *Ulva lactuca*). All algal extracts showed antiprotozoal activity against *T. brucei rhodesiense*, and leishmanicidal activity (Allmendinger et al., 2010). This study was reportedly the first study to show antiprotozoal activity of British marine algae.

In addition, Desbois et al. (2009) isolated an antibacterial polyunsaturated fatty acid, eicosapentaenoic acid (EPA) from the marine diatom, *Phaeodactylum tricornutum Bohlin*, which showed activity against a range of both Gram-positive and Gram-negative bacteria, including Methicillin Resistant *Staphylococcus aureus* (MRSA) (Desbois et al., 2009). Both micro- and macroalgae are used as nutraceuticals. Studies have shown that microalgae are rich sources of β-carotene, Vitamins C, A, E, H, B1, B2, B6 and B12, astaxanthin, polysaccharides and polyunsaturated fatty acids (Grobbelaar, 2004). As such, bioactive molecules from microalgae are commercially produced, used as food additives and also incorporated into infant milk formulations and dietary supplements (Volkman, 2003).

Macroalgae, also called seaweed, are the most popular type of algae in the nutraceutical industry as it provides a great variety of food and food ingredients especially in Asian countries like Korea, Japan and China. Agarose is one of the main products from macroalgae, however macroalgae are also sources of metabolites and natural products with unique nutritional and therapeutic properties. These metabolites and natural products include proteins, furanone, polyunsaturated fatty acids, L-α kainic acid, phenotics, pigments, phlorotannins, phycocolloids (carrageenan and agar) and minerals. Similarly, red and brown seaweeds are alternative sources of vitamins, minerals, and proteins (Plaza et al., 2008) and are good sources of essential fatty acids (Gomez-Ordonez et al., 2010). They have been used to prepare bioactive peptides and to improve protein digestibility. Recently, antihypertensive bioactive peptides have been isolated that may act as angiotensin-converting enzyme (ACE) inhibitors (Kim et al., 2011).

2.5 Symbiotic Marine Micro-Organisms

Study of symbiotic microorganisms is a rapidly growing field as some reports from the recent past suspect that a number of metabolites obtained from algae and invertebrates may be produced by their associated microorganisms. Sponge associated microbes are known for their tremendous activities covering a wide range of biological functions (Thomas et al., 2010). Recently, Baker *et al.* (2009) isolated and identified a diverse range of fungi from *Haliclona simulans*. They used variety of media for identification and determination of antimicrobial activities, if any. They isolated 19 different genotypes belonging to *Agaricomycotina, Mucoromycotina, Saccharomycotina,* and *Pezizomycotina*; some of these isolates showing antimicrobial inhibition of *Escherichia coli, Bacillus sp., Staphylococcus aureus,* and *Candida glabrata* (Baker et al., 2009). The sponge-microbial association is a potential chemical and ecological phenomenon, which provides sustainable resource for developing novel pharmaceutical leads. Keeping in view the importance of antimicrobial potential of marine sponge associated microbes, targeting sponge microsymbionts is an essential focus nowadays (Gandhimathi et al., 2008; Selvin et al., 2009). A marine derived fungal strain M-3, isolated from marine red alga *Porphyra yezoensis* was screened for its antifungal activity against *Pyricularia oryzae* by Byun *et al.* (2003). As a result, a novel Diketopiperazine was isolated from the culture extracts and its structure was also elucidated by spectroscopic methods. A study in 2004, reported hemolysis and inhibition of *Candida albicans* by employing the butanolic extracts of the algal associated species *Pseudoalteromonas issachenkonii* cultures. Further analysis of the ethyl acetate extracts revealed that the basis of this antifungal activity was isatin (indole-2,3-dione) (Byun et al., 2003).

Similarly, a red-brown hemolytic pigment was also discovered by Kalinovskaya et al., 2004. Apart from great ecological value from the habitat point of view, coral reefs are the most species-rich environments in the oceans harboring a number of microbial species proving to be a rich and unexplored source of novel bioactive compounds (Radjasa et al., 2004). Another study reported antibacterial and anti-larval compounds from marine gorgonian associated bacterium *Bacillus amyloliquefaciens* isolated from the South China Sea gorgonian, *Junceella juncea*. The broth of this strain showed strong antibacterial activity towards *Escherichia coli, Bacillus subtilis,* and *Staphyloccocus aureus* and anti-larval activity towards the larvae of bryozoan *Bugula neritina*. Certain species of marine bacteria known as colonists of marine macro-organisms have also been reported to have antimicrobial potential. In a report, 42 strains of marine bacterial isolates showed antimicrobial activity and were assigned to genera *Alteromonas, Pseudomonas, Bacillus and Flavobacterium* (Zheng et al., 2005). Certain mycoparasitic and fungicolous fungi are known to colonize other fungal physiological structures and are known to be the source of effective bioactive agents (Soman et al., 2001). A study conducted in the United States in 2002 reported five new natural products, Phomadecalins A, B, C and D, and Phomapentenone A, from cultures of *Phoma* sp., a mitosporic fungal colonist isolated from the stromata of *Hypoxylon* sp. These compounds were found to be active against Gram-positive bacteria, *Bacillus subtilis* (ATCC 6051) and *Staphylococcus aureus* (ATCC 29213) (Che et al., 2002).

3. CLASSIFICATION OF MARINE NUTRACEUTICALS ON THE BASIS OF CHEMICAL NATURE

Marine nutraceuticals can be broadly classified into Marine lipids (micro-algal origin), Polysaccharides derived from macro algae, Marine probiotics, Marine natural pigments, Chitin and other related products, Bioactive marine peptides/enzymes and Vitamins.

3.1 Lipids

Lipids derived from marine microalgae are used in larval nutrition of aquaculture especially for enrichment of live feeds. Their other biological properties are anti-inflammatory, anti-allergic, anti-viral and therapeutic. The wide spectrum of the properties is due to the presence of various components like polyunsaturated fatty acids (PUFA), highly unsaturated fatty acids (HUFA) and other substances.

Various nutraceuticals derived from marine microbes and their biological activities are given in Table 1.

3.2 Polysaccharides

Bacterial polysaccharides are a class of pharmaceutically important secondary metabolites. It has been found that exopolysaccharides (EPS) from marine bacteria contain novel formulations with a variety of properties like thickening, coagulating, adhesion, stabilizing and gelling, which makes them suitable candidates for industrial applications. Moreover, good viscosity and pseudo-plastic properties of EPS render them resistant to the extremities of temperature, pH and salinity making them more industry friendly (Satpute et al., 2007). Certain marine bacterial species are known as prolific producers of biosurfactants, bioemulsifiers and exopolysaccharides. In a study, an exopolysaccharide (EPS-2) having immunomodulatory and antiviral effects on immunocompetent cells, has been reported from *Geobacillus thermodenitrificans* obtained from a shallow marine vent of Volcano Island (Italy). Bacteria not only produce secondary metabolites against other organisms, but they also produce certain compounds which help in cleaning their environment (Arena et al., 2009).

Table 1. Major Nutraceuticals from marine microbes and their activity (Adopted from: Raposo et al., 2013; Bhatnagar and Kim, 2010)

Lipid/Fatty acid	Biological action/ Function
Microalgal Source	
Eicosapentaenoic acid (EPA)	Nutraceutical; antimicrobial and anti-inflammatory
alpha-Linolenic acid (GLA)	Integrity of tissue and delay of aging
Arachidonic acid (ARA)	Aggregative and vaso-constrictive of platelets
Docosahexaenoic acid (DHA)	Nutraceutical and brain development
Brassicasterol and stingmasterol	Hyper-cholesterolemic
Alpha-amino-butyric acid (AABA)	Neuro-transmitter, antioxidant and anti-inflammatory
Okadaic acid	Antifungal and promotion of the secretion of nerve growth factor (NGF)
Microcolin-A	Immunosuppressive
Cyanobacteria Source	
Dolastatin -10 Dolastatin- 15 Curacin A Toyocamycin	Anti-microtubule; and the synthetic analogue, TZT-1027, as antitumor Anti-microtubule; and the synthetic analogue, ILX-651, as antitumor Anti-microtubule Antifungal
Actinomycetes Source	
Resistoflavine Marinomycin A Daryamide C Violacein	Anti-cancerous and antibacterial Antitumor and antibiotic Antitumor Antiprotozoal
Bacterial Source	
Macrolactin S Pyrone I and II MC21-B	Antibacterial Antibacterial Antibacterial
Fungal source	
Meleagrin Oxaline Alternaramide	Antitumor Antitumor Antibacterial
Algal source	
Norharman Calothrixin-A Eicosapentanoic acid (EPA)	Enzyme inhibitor Antimalarial and anti-cancerous
Symbiotic microbes	
Macrolactin V DAPG BE-43472B	Antibacterial and anti-larval Antibacterial (anti-MRSA, anti-VRSA and anti-VRE) Antibacterial (anti-MRSA and anti-VRE)

Some polysaccharides are also derived from macro algae. Seaweeds contain higher amounts of the polysaccharides like agar, alginates and carrageenan. These act as food fiber and are collectively called phyco-colloids or hydrocolloids. Being rich in fiber, seaweeds exhibit health benefits like reducing the absorption of toxins, anti-carcinogenic and antioxidant properties.

Some of the important bioactive polysaccharides isolated from the macroalgae (seaweeds) that possess the potential to be used as nutraceuticals are Fucoidan, Sphinganine amide and caulerpicin (green algae), Carrageenan, Alginic acid and xylofucans, Hyperoxaluria, Sulfated polysaccharides, and Alginates. All these compounds possess wide range of biological properties such as antioxidant, antiangiogenic, antibacterial, antiviral and antitumor activities anticoagulant, immuno-modulating, hypolipidemic, and anti-inflammatory (Ande et al., 2017). In addition to the phyco-colloids, seaweeds are sources of biologically active phytochemicals like carotenoids, phycobilins, fatty acids, vitamins, sterols, tocopherol, phycocyanins and others.

Macroalgae are also rich sources of insoluble and soluble dietary fiber and are mainly composed of indigestible sulfated polysaccharides. Examples of structural and storage polysaccharides found in red and brown seaweeds include fucan, agar, laminaran, carrageenan and alginate. The alginates from brown seaweeds are utilized as hydrocolloids due to their biological activity. Food and cosmetics industries use fucans from brown seaweeds (Suleria et al., 2015). Das *et al.* (2008) studied the degradation of a model polyaromatic hydrocarbon, anthracene, an organic pollutant, by a marine *Bacillus circulans* strain. In addition, the produced biosurfactant depicted a high degree of emulsification of various hydrocarbons. It was observed that this bacterium utilized anthracene as a carbon substrate for the production of biosurfactant. This group also investigated another biosurfactant producing marine bacterium with an ability to remove metal from solutions with efficiency dependent on the concentration of the metal as well as on the biosurfactant (Das et al., 2009).

3.3 Bryostatins: Bryozoan Origin

The marine bryozoan, *Bugula neritina*, is the sole source of the bryostatins, a family of macrocyclic lactones with anticancer activity. Bryostatins are actually the bacterial products as *B. neritina* harbors the uncultivated gamma proteobacterial symbiont '*Candidatus Endobugula sertula*'. The clinical studies of bryostatins are also under going to study their potential for the treatment of leukemias, lymphomas, melanomas and solid tumors (Davidson et al., 2001). Their mode of action is that they act through protein kinase C signal transduction to alter cellular activity.

3.4 Probiotics: Marine Lactic Acid Bacteria (LAB) Origin

Microbial diversity of marine environments is very rich and can be helpful to develop safe and effective probiotics. Novel marine probiotics can be an effective alternative for fighting the antibiotic resistance. *Lactobacillus* and *Bifidobacterium* are found to possess anti-mutagenic (Chalova et al., 2008) and immunomodulatory (Forsythe and Bienenstock, 2010) activity in host animal. Different strains of marine probiotic bacteria are *Lactobacillus (L. casei, L. acidophilus, L. rhamnosus* GG (ATCC 53013), *L. johnsonii* La-1), *Bifidobacterium (B. bifidum, B. longum, B. infantis, B. breve, B. adolescentis), Leuconostoc spp. (Ln. lactis, Ln. mesenteroides subsp. cremoris, Ln. mesenteroides subsp. dextranicum)* and *Streptococcus spp. (S. salivarius subsp. thermophiles*). The problem posed during the development of new marine probiotics is the isolation and identification of potential strain. Application of biotechnological and molecular biological tactics is necessary for the development of marine probiotic strains for use of aquatic industry (Ande et al., 2017).

3.5 Pigments: Marine Algae

Besides polysaccharides and lipids, marine macro and micro algae also provide various types of the bioactive natural pigments. The natural pigments of the marine algae provide food by photosynthesis and also provide the pigmentation. In addition to these, the natural pigments are also found to exhibit health benefits which make them one of the important marine nutraceuticals. Chlorophyll-a, Lutein, zeaxanthin and canthaxanthin possess anti-mutagenic properties; pheophytin-a exhibits neuroprotective, and anti-inflammatory action; Chlorophyll-a, Pheophorbide-a, Pyropheophytin-a, Phycoerythrobilin, Lutein, Fucoxanthin, Phycocyanin, Astaxanthin, Zeaxanthin and Canthaxanthin are all good antioxidants. Alpha-Carotene is also used as a food additive (Ande et al., 2017).

3.6 Chitosan: Chitin

Chitosan is a natural polymer derived from chitin and it is the second most abundant polysaccharide after cellulose. Chitin is recovered from processing discards of shrimp, crab, lobster, and crayfish following de-proteinization and demineralization. The chitin so obtained may then be deacetylated to afford chitosan. Fungal cell walls are also rich in chitin. Chitin and chitosan are used as biomaterials in a variety of application in edible film industry, additives, for improving nutritional quality, Recovery of solid materials from food processing waste, in purification of water etc. The other biological properties of chitosan are antioxidant, hypocholesterolaemic, antimicrobial, and anti-inflammatory activities (Je and Kim, 2012).

Chitosan disrupts the barrier properties of the outer membrane of Gram-negative bacteria due to ionic interaction between the cationic groups of the chitosan molecules and the anionic groups of the microbial cell membrane, which can rupture the cell membrane. Sulfuryl chitin, phosphoryl chitin and some chitin derivatives prepared by nitrous acid deamination of DAC, inhibited bacterial growth and increased cytotoxicity of a macrophage cell line. NTM-DAC had higher bacterial inhibition activity than carboxy-methyl chitosan.

Chitosan can also function as an antifungal agent by forming gas-permeable coats, interference with fungal growth and stimulation of various defense processes like, build-up of chitinases, production of proteinase inhibitors and stimulators of callous synthesis. The antioxidant property could be attributed to the ability of chitosan to chelate metals and combine with lipids. Derivatives of chitosan, namely, N,O-carboxymethyl chitosan, N,O-carboxymethyl chitosan lactate, N,O-carboxymethyl chitosan acetate and N,O- carboxymethyl chitosan pyrrolidine carboxylate had also exhibited the antioxidant activity. Chitosan possesses special properties for use in pharmaceutical, biomedical, food industry, health, and agriculture due to its biocompatibility, biodegradability and nontoxic nature. Through encapsulation, it is being used as a vehicle for nutraceutical compounds and pharmacological compounds. Chitosan derivatives may also be produced in order to obtain more effective products for certain applications (Ande et al., 2017).

3.7 Bioactive Peptides/Enzymes: Marine Origin

Peptides refer to the specific protein fragments that exhibit a specific biological activity. Some of the peptides may exhibit multifunctional properties like opioid, immunomodulatory, antibacterial, anti-thrombotic and antihypertensive activity (Kim, 2012). Bio-functional peptides have a size range of 2 to 20 amino acid residues and are encrypted within the sequence of the parent protein and are released during processing. They can be formed either by acid or alkaline hydrolysis. The major bioactivities of peptides are antihypertensive (ACE inhibitory), antioxidant, antimicrobial, anti-hypoallergenic activity and cell immunity. Proteins isolated from bacteria such as *Dunaliella, Phaeodactylum tricornutum* and *Arthrospira platensis* possess potent antioxidant and anti-inflammatory activity which can be effectively used in aquaculture practices. Similarly, enzymes such as superoxide dismutase and carbonic anhydrase derived from *Porphyridium, Anabaena, Isochrysis galbana and Amphidinium carterae* play an important role in regulating the metabolite waste (CO_2).

3.8 Vitamins: Marine Micro-Algal Origin

Marine microalgae are also known to have good amount of alpha-carotene. Microalgae like, *Arthrospira, Isochrysis galbana, Porphyridium cruentum and Tetraselmis* are rich in vitamin C, K, A, E and alpha-carotene which possess strong antioxidant activity. Vitamins A (particularly provitamin-A, alpha-carotene) and E (particularly alpha-tocopherol) serve as excellent antioxidants and free radical scavengers that protect cells from damage by oxidants. Research has shown that vitamin E has a number of extraordinary beneficial effects as a specific antioxidant, acting together with vitamin C and alpha-carotene, in improving antioxidant defenses in the body. Fat soluble vitamin K isolated from Pavlova helps in blood clotting or coagulation. The role of antioxidant vitamins in health and disease control has been well documented (Suleria et al., 2015).

4. CLASSICAL EXAMPLES OF SOME MARINE MICROFLORA AND THEIR NUTRACEUTICAL POTENTIAL

Oceans have borne most of the biological activities on our planet. A number of biologically active compounds with varying degrees of action, such as anti-tumor, anti-cancer, anti-microtubule, anti-proliferative, cytotoxic, photo-protective, as well as antibiotic and anti-fouling properties, have been isolated to date from marine sources. The marine environment also represents a largely unexplored source for isolation of new microbes (bacteria, fungi, actinomycetes, microalgae-cyanobacteria and diatoms) that are potent producers of bioactive secondary metabolites. Extensive research has been done to unveil the bioactive potential of marine microbes (free living and symbiotic) and the results are amazingly diverse and productive. Some of these bioactive secondary metabolites of microbial origin with strong antibacterial and antifungal activities are being intensely used as antibiotics and may be effective against infectious diseases such as HIV, conditions of multiple bacterial infections (penicillin, cephalosporines, streptomycin, and vancomycin) or neuropsychiatric sequelae. Research is also being conducted on the general aspects of biophysical and biochemical properties, chemical structures and biotechnological applications of the bioactive substances derived from marine microorganisms, and their potential use as cosmeceuticals and nutraceuticals. Some of the research studies on bioactive molecules from marine sources are discussed below.

Seaweeds provide a rich source of bioactive molecules. In this study, the anti-microbial potential of Red sea weed, *Gracilaria opuntia* was investigated against clinically important microorganism such as *Escherichia coli*, *Staphylococcus aureus*, *Klebsiella pneumonia* and *Pseudomonas putida* that cause diseases in diabetic patients. Crude extracts prepared from aqueous, ethanol and methanol extraction procedures revealed that aqueous extraction procedure have a wide range of antimicrobial activity against all the test pathogens. The overall antibacterial activity assessed from the above results indicates the presence of active constituents in the extractions of seaweeds which can be explored for the production of significant molecules which could be used in pharmaceutical industry (Rayapu et al., 2017).

In a similar study on *Gracilaria edulis*, their phytochemical, antibacterial and antifungal activities of crude extracts were investigated. The methanol and aqueous extracts of *Gracilaria edulis* showed the presence of a number of metabolites such as alkaloids, saponin, phenols, terpenoids, proteins, flavonoids, glycosides, coumarins and tannins. The red algae showed the significant antibacterial activity against the clinical pathogens of *Pseudomonas aeroginosa, Staphylococcus aureus, Bacillus cereus, Bacillus subtilis, Streptococcus pyogenes, Salmonella typhi* as well as the fungus *Aspergillus niger, Aspergillus flavus, Rhizopus indicus* and *Candida albicans*. The methanol extract showed the broader spectrum of antibacterial and antifungal activity when compared with aqueous extract (Rajakumar and Allwin, 2017). In another study, the phytochemical and biological evaluation of some *Sargassum* species from Persian Gulf was also studied. These plants contain important phytochemical constituents and have various potential biological activities. The study investigated the presence of phytochemical constituents and total phenolic quantity of the seaweeds *Sargassum angustifolium, Sargassum oligocystum* and *Sargassum boveanum*. Cytotoxicity of seaweeds was tested against HT-29, HeLa and MCF-7 cell lines. Antioxidant potential of these 3 *Sargassum* species was also analyzed. *Sargassum angustifolium* had the highest content of total phenolics and showed the highest antioxidant activity. Cytotoxic results showed that all species could inhibit cell growth effectively, for *S. oligocystum, S. angustifolium* and *S. boveanum* respectively. Thus considerable phytochemicals and moderate cytotoxic activity of *S. angustifolium, S. oligocystum* and *S. boveanum* make them appropriate candidate for further studies and identification of their bioactive principles (Mehdinezhad et al., 2016).

In another study on algae, the screening of their phytochemicals from their extracts and testing on their antibacterial, antifungal and antioxidant potential was carried out. Solvent extracts of five different micro-algal strains including *Tetraselmis sp., Dunaliella sp., Chlorella sp., Synechocystis sp.,* and *Oscillatoria* sp. were screened for seven phytochemical activities. Antimicrobial activity of solvent extracts was tested against seven bacterial and three fungal strains. The antioxidant potential of solvent extracts was analyzed using the DPPH scavenging assay. Flavonoids were predominantly found in all the solvent extracts. Micro-algal strains showed better antifungal than antibacterial activity. Acetone extract of *Dunaliella* sp. showed highest percentage DPPH scavenging activity. The extracts showing highest antimicrobial and DPPH scavenging activity were subjected to GC-HRMS. The results showed the presence of Octadecanoic acid-4-hydroxy-methyl ester, benzoic acid, hexadecanoic acid and Tetradecanoic acid, confirming the bioactive compounds in the algal extracts (Rajendran et al., 2014).

5. OTHER MARINE SOURCES OF NUTRACEUTICALS

It is noteworthy that marine sources have also demonstrated tremendous abilities as producers of anticancer compounds and secondary metabolites which act against infectious diseases and inflammation. Blunt et al. (2004) listed that in marine environment sponges (37%), coelenterates (21%) and microorganisms (18%), are major sources of biomedical compounds, followed by algae (9%), echinoderms (6%), tunicates (6%), molluscs (2%) bryozoans (1%), etc. (Blunt et al., 2004).

6. CONCLUSION

From the above discussion it is quite pertinent to conclude that the marine environment harbors variety of microbial flora that have capability to produce a wide array of bioactive metabolites that can be used both in nutrition and pharmaceuticals to formulate new drugs that are effective against various drug resistant pathogens. Though the saga of marine microbial bioactive metabolites is continuing with new compounds being added day by day, our knowledge is still a miniscule of what exists deep in the oceans. Interdisciplinary research and collaborative endeavors are required amongst scientists, medical practitioners, marine microbiologists and biotechnologists, to provide innovative approaches to marine based biomedical research. It is worth giving serious consideration to the exploitation of marine microbial life and the associated secondary metabolites, aided by genomic analyses, applying metabolic approach and employing combined biomedical and biotechnological efforts, which would lead to discovery of some novel, lead compounds of a varied degree of bioactivity.

7. ACKNOWLEDGMENT

The authors are grateful to Dr. Ashok K. Chauhan, Founder President and Mr. Atul Chauhan, Chancellor, Amity University UP, Noida, India for the encouragement, research facilities and financial support.

8. ETHICAL ISSUES

There is none to be declared.

9. CONFLICT OF INTEREST

The author(s) confirm that this article content has no conflict of interest.

REFERENCES

Allmendinger, A., Spavieri, J., Kaiser, M., Casey, R., Hingley-Wilson, S., Lalvani, A., Guiry, M., Blunden, G., & Tasdemir, D. (2010). Antiprotozoal, anti-mycobacterial and cytotoxic potential of twenty-three British and Irish red algae. *Phytotherapy Research*, *24*(7), 1099–1103. doi:10.1002/ptr.3094 PMID:20077438

Ande, M.P., Syamala, K., Rao, P.S., Mohan, K.M. & Lingam, S.S. (2017). Marine Nutraceuticals. *Aquaculture Times*, *3*(2), 6-9.

Aneiros, A., & Garateix, A. (2004). Bioactive peptides from marine sources: Pharmacological properties and isolation procedures. *Journal of Chromatography. B, Analytical Technologies in the Biomedical and Life Sciences*, *803*(1), 41–53. doi:10.1016/j.jchromb.2003.11.005 PMID:15025997

Arena, A., Gugliandolo, C., Stassi, G., Pavone, B., Iannello, D., Bisignano, G., & Maugeri, T. L. (2009). An exopolysaccharide produced by *Geobacillus thermodenitrificans* strain B3-72: Antiviral activity on immunocompetent cells. *Immunology Letters, 123*(2), 132–137. doi:10.1016/j.imlet.2009.03.001 PMID:19428560

Baker, P. W., Kennedy, J., Dobson, A. D. W., & Marchesi, J. R. (2009). Phylogenetic Diversity and Antimicrobial Activities of Fungi Associated with *Haliclona simulans* Isolated from Irish Coastal Waters. *Marine Biotechnology (New York, N.Y.), 11*(4), 540–547. doi:10.100710126-008-9169-7 PMID:19083060

Belofsky, G. N., Jensen, P. R., Renner, M. K., & Fenical, W. (1998). New cytotoxic sesquiterpenoid nitrobenzoyl esters from a marine isolate of the fungus *Aspergillus versicolor. Tetrahedron, 54*(9), 1715–1724. doi:10.1016/S0040-4020(97)10396-9

Bhadury, P., Mohammad, B. T., & Wright, P. C. (2006). The current status of natural products from marine fungi and their potential as anti-infective agents. *Journal of Industrial Microbiology & Biotechnology, 33*(5), 325–337. doi:10.100710295-005-0070-3 PMID:16429315

Bhagavathy, S., Sumathi, P., & Bell, I. J. B. (2011). Green algae chlorococcumhumicola-a new source of bioactive compounds with antimicrobial activity. *Asian Pacific Journal of Tropical Biomedicine, 1*(1), S1–S7. doi:10.1016/S2221-1691(11)60111-1

Bhatnagar, I., & Kim, S.-K. (2010). Immense Essence of Excellence: Marine Microbial Bioactive Compounds. *Marine Drugs, 8*(10), 2673–2701. doi:10.3390/md8102673 PMID:21116414

Blunt, J. W., Copp, B. R., Munro, M. H. G., Northcote, P. T., & Prinsep, M. R. (2004). Marine Natural products. *Natural Product Reports, 21*(1), 1–49. doi:10.1039/b305250h PMID:15039834

Burke, C., Thomas, T., Egan, S., & Kjelleberg, S. (2007). The use of functional genomics for the identification of a gene cluster encoding for the biosynthesis of an antifungal tambjamine in the marine bacterium *Pseudoalteromonas tunicata. Environmental Microbiology, 9*(3), 814–818. doi:10.1111/j.1462-2920.2006.01177.x PMID:17298379

Byun, H. G., Zhang, H., Mochizuki, M., Adachi, K., Shizuri, Y., Lee, W. J., & Kim, S. K. (2003). Novel antifungal diketopiperazine from marine fungus. *The Journal of Antibiotics, 56*(2), 102–106. doi:10.7164/antibiotics.56.102 PMID:12715868

Carlson, J. C., Li, S., Burr, D. A., & Sherman, D. H. (2009). Isolation and Characterization of Tirandamycins from a Marine-Derived *Streptomyces* sp. *Journal of Natural Products, 72*(11), 2076–2079. doi:10.1021/np9005597 PMID:19883065

Chalova, V., Lingbeck, J., Kwon, Y., & Ricke, S. (2008). Extracellular antimutagenic activities of selected probiotic *Bifidobacterium* and *Lactobacillus spp*. as a function of growth phase. *Journal of Environmental Science and Health. Part B, Pesticides, Food Contaminants, and Agricultural Wastes, 43*(2), 193–198. doi:10.1080/03601230701795262 PMID:18246512

Che, Y., Gloer, J. B., & Wicklow, D. T. (2002). Phomadecalins, A-D Phomapentenone: A New Bioactive Metabolites from *Phoma* sp. NRRL 25697, a Fungal Colonist of *Hypoxylon Stromata. Journal of Natural Products, 65*(3), 399–402. doi:10.1021/np010519o PMID:11908990

Cho, J. Y., Williams, P. G., Kwon, H. C., Jensen, P. R., & Fenical, W. (2007). Lucentamycins A–D, cytotoxic peptides from the marine-derived actinomycete *Nocardiopsis lucentensis. Journal of Natural Products*, *70*(8), 1321–1328. doi:10.1021/np070101b PMID:17630797

Das, P., Mukherjee, S., & Sen, R. (2008). Improved bioavailability and biodegradation of a model polyaromatic hydrocarbon by a biosurfactant producing bacterium of marine origin. *Chemosphere*, *72*(9), 1229–1234. doi:10.1016/j.chemosphere.2008.05.015 PMID:18565569

Das, P., Mukherjee, S., & Sen, R. (2009). Biosurfactant of marine origin exhibiting heavy metal remediation properties. *Bioresource Technology*, *100*(20), 4887–4890. doi:10.1016/j.biortech.2009.05.028 PMID:19505818

Davidson, S. K., Allen, S. W., Lim, G. E., Anderson, C. M., & Haygood, M. G. (2001). Evidence for the Biosynthesis of Bryostatins by the Bacterial Symbiont "*Candidatus Endobugula sertula*" of the Bryozoan *Bugula neritina. Applied and Environmental Microbiology*, *67*(10), 4531–4537. doi:10.1128/AEM.67.10.4531-4537.2001 PMID:11571152

Desbois, A. P., Mearns-Spragg, A., & Smith, V. J. (2009). A fatty acid from the diatom *Phaeodactylum tricornutum* is antibacterial against diverse bacteria including multi-resistant *Staphylococcus aureus* (MRSA). *Marine Biotechnology (New York, N.Y.)*, *11*(1), 45–52. doi:10.100710126-008-9118-5 PMID:18575935

Dewapriya, P., & Kim, S. (2014). Marine microorganisms: An emerging avenue in modern nutraceuticals and functional foods. *Food Research International*, *56*, 115–125. doi:10.1016/j.foodres.2013.12.022

Du, L., Feng, T., Zhao, B., Li, D., Cai, S., Zhu, T., Wang, F., Xiao, X., & Gu, Q. (2010). Alkaloids from a deep ocean sediment-derived fungus *Penicillium* sp. and their antitumor activities. *The Journal of Antibiotics*, *63*(4), 165–170. doi:10.1038/ja.2010.11 PMID:20186171

Du, L., Zhu, T., Fang, Y., Liu, H., Gu, Q., & Zhu, W. (2007). Aspergiolide A, a novel anthraquinone derivative with naphtho(1,2,3-de)chromene-2,7-dione skeleton isolated from a marine-derived fungus *Aspergillus glaucus. Tetrahedron*, *63*, 1085–1088. doi:10.1016/j.tet.2006.11.074

Egan, S., James, S., Holmström, C., & Kjelleberg, S. (2002). Correlation between pigmentation and antifouling compounds produced by *Pseudoalteromonas tunicata. Environmental Microbiology*, *4*(8), 433–442. doi:10.1046/j.1462-2920.2002.00322.x PMID:12153584

El-Gendy, M. M., Hawas, U. W., & Jaspars, M. (2008). Novel bioactive metabolites from a marine derived bacterium *Nocardia* sp. ALAA 2000. *The Journal of Antibiotics*, *61*(6), 379–386. doi:10.1038/ja.2008.53 PMID:18667786

Elena, M. (2003). Mailiohydrin, a cytotoxic chamigrene dibromohydrin from a phillippine *Laurencia* species. *Journal of Natural Products*, *64*, 790–791.

Forsythe, P., & Bienenstock, J. (2010). Immunomodulation by commensal and probiotic bacteria. *Immunological Investigations*, *39*(4-5), 429–448. doi:10.3109/08820131003667978 PMID:20450286

Franks, A., Haywood, P., Holmström, C., Egan, S., Kjelleberg, S., & Kumar, N. (2005). Isolation and structure elucidation of a novel yellow pigment from the marine bacterium *Pseudoalteromonas tunicata*. *Molecules (Basel, Switzerland)*, *10*(10), 1286–1291. doi:10.3390/10101286 PMID:18007521

Gai, Y., Zhao, L. L., Hu, C. Q., & Zhang, H. P. (2007). Fusarielin E, a new antifungal antibiotic from *Fusarium* sp. *Chinese Chemical Letters*, *18*(8), 954–956. doi:10.1016/j.cclet.2007.05.048

Gandhimathi, R., Arunkumar, M., Selvin, J., Thangavelu, T., Sivaramakrishnan, S., Kiran, G. S., Shanmughapriya, S., & Natarajaseenivasan, K. (2008). Antimicrobial potential of sponge associated marine actinomycetes. *Journal de Mycologie Médicale*, *18*(1), 16–22. doi:10.1016/j.mycmed.2007.11.001

Gomez-Ordonez, E., Jimenez-Escrig, A., & Ruperez, P. (2010). Dietary fibre and physico-chemical properties of several edible seaweeds from the Northwestern Spanish coast. *Food Research International*, *9*(9), 2289–2294. doi:10.1016/j.foodres.2010.08.005

Grobbelaar, J. U., & Bornman, C. H. (2004). Algal biotechnology: Real opportunities for Africa. *South African Journal of Botany*, *70*(1), 140–144. doi:10.1016/S0254-6299(15)30274-X

Hawas, U. W., Shaaban, M., Shaaban, K. A., Speitling, M., Maier, A., Kelter, G., Fiebig, H. H., Meiners, M., Helmke, E., & Laatsch, H. (2009). Mansouramycins A-D, cytotoxic isoquinolinequinones from a marine streptomycete. *Journal of Natural Products*, *72*(12), 2120–2124. doi:10.1021/np900160g PMID:19921834

Inagaki, F., Nunoura, T., Nakagawa, S., Teske, A., Lever, M., Lauer, A., Suzuki, M., Takai, K., Delwiche, M., Colwell, F. S., Nealson, K. H., Horikoshi, K., D'Hondt, S., & Jorgensen, B. B. (2006). Biogeographical distribution and diversity of microbes in methane hydrate-bearing deep marine sediments on the Pacific Ocean Margin. *Proceedings of the National Academy of Sciences of the United States of America*, *103*(8), 2815–2820. doi:10.1073/pnas.0511033103 PMID:16477011

Isnansetyo, A., & Kamei, Y. (2003). MC21-A, a bactericidal antibiotic produced by a new marine bacterium, *Pseudoalteromonas phenolica* sp. nov. O-BC30T against methicillin-resistant *Staphylococcus aureus*. *Antimicrobial Agents and Chemotherapy*, *47*(2), 480–488. doi:10.1128/AAC.47.2.480-488.2003 PMID:12543647

Isnansetyo, A., & Kamei, Y. (2009). Bioactive substances produced by marine isolates of *Pseudomonas*. *Journal of Industrial Microbiology & Biotechnology*, *36*(10), 1239–1248. doi:10.100710295-009-0611-2 PMID:19582493

Iwata, F., Sato, S., Mukai, T., Yamada, S., Takeo, J., Abe, A., Okita, T., & Kawahara, H. (2009). Lorneic Acids, Trialkyl-Substituted Aromatic Acids from a Marine-Derived Actinomycete. *Journal of Natural Products*, *72*(11), 2046–2048. doi:10.1021/np900353y PMID:19856955

Je, J. Y., & Kim, S. K. (2012). Chitosan as potential marine nutraceutical. *Advances in Food and Nutrition Research*, *65*, 121–135. doi:10.1016/B978-0-12-416003-3.00007-X PMID:22361183

Kalinovskaya, N. I., Ivanova, E. P., Alexeeva, Y. V., Gorshkova, N. M., Kuznetsova, T. A., Dmitronek, A. D., & Nicolau, D. V. (2004). Low-molecular-weight, biologically active compounds from marine *Pseudoalteromonas* species. *Current Microbiology*, *48*(6), 441–446. doi:10.100700284-003-4240-0 PMID:15170241

Kim, E. Y., Kim, D. G., Kim, Y. R., Hwang, H. J., Nam, T. J., & Kong, I. S. (2011). An improved method of protein isolation and proteome analysis with *Saccharina japonica* (Laminariales) incubated under different pH conditions. *Journal of Applied Phycology*, *23*(1), 123–130. doi:10.100710811-010-9550-6

Kim, S. K. (2012). Marine Medical Foods: Implications and Applications, Animals and microbes. *Advances in Food and Nutrition Research*, 65.

Kjer, J., Debbab, A., Aly, A. H., & Proksch, P. (2010). Methods for isolation of marine-derived endophytic fungi and their bioactive secondary products. *Nature Protocols*, *5*(3), 479–490. doi:10.1038/nprot.2009.233 PMID:20203665

König, G., Kehraus, S., Seibert, S., Abdel-Lateff, A., & Müller, D. (2006). Natural products from marine organisms and their associated microbes. *ChemBioChem*, *7*(2), 229–238. doi:10.1002/cbic.200500087 PMID:16247831

Kwong, T. F., Miao, L., Li, X., & Qian, P. Y. (2006). Novel Antifouling and Antimicrobial Compound from a Marine-Derived Fungus *Ampelomyces* sp. *Marine Biotechnology (New York, N.Y.)*, *8*(6), 634–640. doi:10.100710126-005-6146-2 PMID:16924374

Li, X., Kim, S. K., Nam, K. W., Kang, J. S., Choi, H. D., & Son, B. W. (2006). A new antibacterial dioxopiperazine alkaloid related to gliotoxin from a marine isolate of the fungus *Pseudallescheria*. *The Journal of Antibiotics*, *59*(4), 248–250. doi:10.1038/ja.2006.35 PMID:16830893

Lopes, V. R., Fernández, N., Martins, R. F., & Vasconcelos, V. (2010). Primary screening of the bioactivity of brackish water cyanobacteria: Toxicity of crude extracts to *Artemia salina* larvae and *Paracentrotus lividus* embryos. *Marine Drugs*, *8*(3), 471–482. doi:10.3390/md8030471 PMID:20411110

Luesch, H., Harrigan, G. G., Goetz, G., & Horgen, F. D. (2002). The cyanobacterial origin of potent anticancer agents originally isolated from sea hares. *Current Medicinal Chemistry*, *9*(20), 1791–1806. doi:10.2174/0929867023369051 PMID:12369878

Maloney, K. N., Macmillan, J. B., Kauffman, C. A., Jensen, P. R., Dipasquale, A. G., Rheingold, A. L., & Fenical, W. (2009). Lodopyridone, a structurally unprecedented alkaloid from a marine actinomycete. *Organic Letters*, *11*(23), 5422–5424. doi:10.1021/ol901997k PMID:19883103

Maskey, R. P., Helmke, E., Kayser, O., Fiebig, H. H., Maier, A., Busche, A., & Laatsch, H. (2004). Anti-cancer and antibacterial trioxacarcins with high anti-malaria activity from a marine *Streptomycete* and their absolute stereochemistry. *The Journal of Antibiotics*, *57*(12), 771–779. doi:10.7164/antibiotics.57.771 PMID:15745111

Mayer, A. M. S., & Lehmann, V. K. B. (2000). Marine pharmacology. *The Pharmacologist*, *42*, 62–69. PMID:16901686

McArthur, K. A., Mitchell, S. S., Tsueng, G., Rheingold, A., White, D. J., Grodberg, J., Lam, K. S., & Potts, B. C. (2008). Lynamicins A-E, chlorinated bisindole pyrrole antibiotics from a novel marine actinomycete. *Journal of Natural Products*, *71*(10), 1732–1737. doi:10.1021/np800286d PMID:18842058

Mehdinezhad, N., Ghannadi, A., & Yegdaneh, A. (2016). Phytochemical and biological evaluation of some *Sargassum* species from Persian Gulf. *Research in Pharmaceutical Sciences, 11*(3), 243–249. PMID:27499794

Nenkep, V. N., Yun, K., Li, Y., Choi, H. D., Kang, J. S., & Son, B. W. (2010). New production of haloquinones, bromochlorogentisylquinones A and B, by a halide salt from a marine isolate of the fungus *Phoma herbarum. The Journal of Antibiotics, 63*(4), 199–201. doi:10.1038/ja.2010.15 PMID:20224602

Newman, D. J., & Hill, R. T. (2006). New drugs from marine microbes: The tide is turning. *Journal of Industrial Microbiology & Biotechnology, 33*(7), 539–544. doi:10.100710295-006-0115-2 PMID:16598493

Okami, Y. J. (1993). The search for bioactive metabolites form marine bacteria. *Marine Biotechnology (New York, N.Y.), 1*, 59–65.

Olano, C., Méndez, C., & Salas, J. A. (2009). Antitumor compounds from marine actinomycetes. *Marine Drugs, 7*(2), 210–248. doi:10.3390/md7020210 PMID:19597582

Pérez, M., Crespo, C., Schleissner, C., Rodríguez, P., Zúñiga, P., & Reyes, F. (2009). Tartrolon D, a cytotoxic macrodiolide from the marine-derived actinomycete *Streptomyces* sp. MDG-04-17-069. *Journal of Natural Products, 72*, 2192–2194. doi:10.1021/np9006603 PMID:19968258

Pickering, T. D., Posa, S., & Reuben, J. S. (2007). Intentional introductions of commercially harvested alien seaweeds. *Botanica Marina, 50*(5/6), 338–350. doi:10.1515/BOT.2007.039

Plaza, M., Cifuentes, A., & Ibanez, E. (2008). In the search of new functional food ingredients from algae. *Trends in Food Science & Technology, 19*(1), 31–39. doi:10.1016/j.tifs.2007.07.012

Proksch, P., Proksch, P., Edrada, R. A., & Ebel, R. (2002). Drugs from the sea – current status and microbiological implications. *Applied Microbiology and Biotechnology, 59*(2-3), 125–134. doi:10.100700253-002-1006-8 PMID:12111137

Prudhomme, J., McDaniel, E., Ponts, N., Bertani, S., Fenical, W., Jensen, P., & Le Roch, K. (2008). Marine actinomycetes: A new source of compounds against the human malaria parasite. *PLoS One, 3*(6), e2335. doi:10.1371/journal.pone.0002335 PMID:18523554

Radjasa, O. K. (2004). Marine invertebrate-associated bacteria in coral reef ecosystems as a new source of bioactive compounds. *J. Coast. Dev., 7*, 65–70.

Rajakumar, R., & Allwin Prem Singh, Y. (2017). Preliminary Phytochemical and Antimicrobial studies on the crude extract of red algae *Gracilaria edulis* against clinical isolates. *European Journal Pharmaceutical and Medical Research, 4*(07), 763–766.

Rajendran, N., Selvan, K., Sobana, P., & Logeswar, V., Kathiresan, T., & Vennison, J. (2014). Phytochemicals, Antimicrobial and Antioxidant Screening From Five Different Marine Microalgae. *Journal of Chemical and Pharmaceutical Sciences, 2*, 78–85.

Raposo, M. F. D., de Morais, R., & de Morais, A. (2013). Health applications of bioactive compounds from marine microalgae. *Life Sciences, 93*(15), 479–486. doi:10.1016/j.lfs.2013.08.002 PMID:23994664

Rayapu, L., Makkar, F., Chakraborty, K., & Valluru, L. (2017). Phytochemical Evaluation and Antimicrobial Activity of *Gracilaria Opuntia*: An Important Anti-Diabetic Red Marine Macroalgae. *International Journal of Current Pharmaceutical Research*, *9*(6), 37–41. doi:10.22159/ijcpr.2017v9i6.23426

Romanenko, L. A., Uchino, M., Kalinovskaya, N. I., & Mikhailov, V. V. (2008a). Isolation, phylogenetic analysis and screening of marine mollusc-associated bacteria for antimicrobial, hemolytic and surface activities. *Microbiological Research*, *163*(6), 633–644. doi:10.1016/j.micres.2006.10.001 PMID:19216104

Romanenko, L. A., Uchino, M., Tanaka, N., Frolova, G. M., Slinkina, N. N., & Mikhailov, V. V. (2008b). Occurrence and antagonistic potential of *Stenotrophomonas* strains isolated from deep-sea invertebrates. *Archives of Microbiology*, *189*(4), 337–344. doi:10.100700203-007-0324-8 PMID:18034228

Romanenko, L. A., Uchino, M., Tebo, B. M., Tanaka, N., Frolova, G. M., & Mikhailov, V. V. (2008c). *Pseudomonas marincola* sp. nov., isolated from marine environments. *International Journal of Systematic and Evolutionary Microbiology*, *58*(3), 706–710. doi:10.1099/ijs.0.65406-0 PMID:18319482

Satpute, S. K., Banat, I. M., Dhakephalkar, P. K., Banpurkar, A. G., & Chopade, B. A. (2007). Biosurfactants, bioemulsifiers and exopolysaccharides from marine microorganisms. *Biotechnology Advances*, *28*(4), 436–450. doi:10.1016/j.biotechadv.2010.02.006 PMID:20172021

Selvin, J., Shanmughapriya, S., Gandhimathi, S., Kiran, G. S., Ravji, T. R., Natarajaseenivasan, K., & Hema, T. A. (2009). Optimization and production of novel antimicrobial agents from sponge associated marine actinomycetes *Nocardiopsis dassonvillei* MAD08. *Applied Microbiology and Biotechnology*, *83*(3), 435–445. doi:10.100700253-009-1878-y PMID:19190903

Simmons, T. L., Engene, N., Ureña, L. D., Romero, L. I., Ortega-Barría, E., Gerwick, L., & Gerwick, W. H. (2008). Viridamides A and B, lipodepsipeptides with antiprotozoal activity from the marine cyanobacterium *Oscillatoria nigro*-Viridis. *Journal of Natural Products*, *71*(9), 1544–1550. doi:10.1021/np800110e PMID:18715036

Sivonen, K., Leikoski, N., Fewer, D. P., & Jokela, J. (2010). Cyanobactins-ribosomal cyclic peptides produced by cyanobacteria. *Applied Microbiology and Biotechnology*, *86*(5), 1213–1225. doi:10.100700253-010-2482-x PMID:20195859

Soman, A. G., Gloer, J. B., Angawi, R. F., Wicklow, D. T., & Dowd, P. F. (2001). Vertilecanins: New Phenopicolinic Acid Analogs from *Verticillium lecanii*. *Journal of Natural Products*, *64*(2), 189–192. doi:10.1021/np000094q PMID:11429997

Stadler, M., Anke, H., & Sterner, O. (1995). Metabolites with nematicidal and antimicrobial activities from the ascomycete *Lachnum papyraceum* (Karst.) Karst. III. production of novel isocoumarin derivatives, isolation and biological activities. *The Journal of Antibiotics*, *48*(3), 261–266. doi:10.7164/antibiotics.48.261 PMID:7730162

Suleria, H. A. R., Osborne, S., Masci, P., & Gobe, G. (2015). Marine-Based Nutraceuticals: An Innovative Trend in the Food and Supplement Industries. *Marine Drugs*, *13*(10), 6336–6351. doi:10.3390/md13106336 PMID:26473889

Takahashi, Y., & Omura, S. (2003). Isolation of new actinomycete strains for the screening of new bioactive compounds. *The Journal of General and Applied Microbiology*, *49*(3), 141–154. doi:10.2323/jgam.49.141 PMID:12949697

Thomas, T. R. A., Kavlekar, D. P., & LokaBharathi, P. A. (2010). Marine Drugs from Sponge-Microbe Association–A Review. *Marine Drugs*, *8*(4), 1417–1468. doi:10.3390/md8041417 PMID:20479984

Trischman, J. A., Tapiolas, D. M., Jensen, P. R., Dwight, R., McKee, T. C., Ireland, C. M., Stout, T. J., & Clardy, J. (1994). Salinamides A and B: Anti-inflammatory depsipeptides from a marine *Streptomycete*. *Journal of the American Chemical Society*, *116*(2), 757–758. doi:10.1021/ja00081a042

Tseng, C. K. (2001). Algal biotechnology industries and research activities in China. *Journal of Applied Phycology*, *13*(4), 375–380. doi:10.1023/A:1017972812576

Volkman, J. K. (2003). Sterols in microorganisms. *Applied Microbiology and Biotechnology*, *60*(5), 495–506. doi:10.100700253-002-1172-8 PMID:12536248

Xiong, H., Qi, S., Xu, Y., Li, M., & Qian, P.-Y. (2009). Antibiotic and antifouling compound production by the marine-derived fungus *Cladosporium* sp. F14. *J. Hydro-. Environmental Research*, *2*, 264–270.

Xu, Y., He, H., Schulz, S., Liu, X., Fusetani, N., Xiong, H., Xiao, X., & Qian, P. Y. (2010). Potent antifouling compounds produced by marine *Streptomyces*. *Bioresource Technology*, *101*(4), 1331–1336. doi:10.1016/j.biortech.2009.09.046 PMID:19818601

Zhang, D., Yang, X., Kang, J. S., Choi, H. D., & Son, B. W. (2008). Chlorohydroaspyrones A and B, antibacterial aspyrone derivatives from the marine-derived fungus *Exophiala* sp. *Journal of Natural Products*, *71*(8), 1458–1460. doi:10.1021/np800107c PMID:18661951

Zheng, L., Han, X., Chen, H., Lin, W., & Yan, X. (2005). Marine bacteria associated with marine macroorganisms: The potential antimicrobial resources. *Annals of Microbiology*, *55*, 119–124.

Chapter 5
Effect of NDDS on Polyherbal Formulation

Sandeep Onkar Waghulde
https://orcid.org/0000-0001-5855-9606
Konkan Gyanpeeth Rahul Dharkar College of Pharmacy and Research Institute, Raigad, India

Nilofar A. Khan
Konkan Gyanpeeth Rahul Dharkar College of Pharmacy and Research Institute, Raigad, India

Nilesh Gorde
Konkan Gyanpeeth Rahul Dharkar College of Pharmacy and Research Institute, Raigad, India

ABSTRACT

In India, in ancient times, people used plant materials to make drug polyherbal formulations. Herbal drugs have enormous therapeutic potential which can be explored through various beneficial drug delivery systems and novel drug delivery systems. Great advancement has been made in the uses of plant therapeutics on the development of novel herbal formulations like polymeric nanoparticles, nanocapsules, liposomes, phytosomes, nanoemulsions, microsphere, transferosomes, and ethosomes. These formulations have reported having various advantages over the traditional formulations such as improved solubility and bioavailability, reduced toxicity, controlled drug delivery, protections of plant actives from degradation. Also, having the drug targeting properties with improved selectivity, drug delivery, and effectiveness with dose reduction not only increases the safety but also patient compliance.

1. INTRODUCTION

From time immemorial it has been the endeavour of the physician and the apothecary to provide patients with the best possible forms of medicines so that recovery from disease is faster and complete. The drugs are delivered in a suitable formulation keeping in view the safety, efficacy and acceptability among other factors, and the formulation is usually known as dosage form or drug delivery system. With the progress in all spheres of science and technology, the dosage forms have evolved from simple mixtures and pills

DOI: 10.4018/978-1-7998-4453-2.ch005

to highly sophisticated technology intensive drug delivery systems, which are known as Novel Drug Delivery Systems (NDDS). (Mandal & Mandal, 2010) In the past few decades, considerable attention has been focused on the development of novel drug delivery system for herbal drugs. (Saraf, 2010) Herbal drugs are becoming more popular in the modern world for their application to cure variety of diseases with less toxic effects and better therapeutic effects. However, some limitations of herbal extracts/ plant actives like instability in highly acidic pH, liver metabolism etc. has led to drug levels below therapeutic concentration in the blood resulting in less or no therapeutic effect. Incorporation of novel drug delivery technology to herbal or plant actives minimizes the drug degradation or pre systemic metabolism and serious side effects by accumulation of drugs to the non targeted areas and improves the ease of administration in the paediatric and geriatric patients. (Goyal, et al., 2011) Conventional dosage forms including prolonged-release dosage forms are unable to meet the ideal prerequisites of novel carriers like ability to deliver the drug at a rate directed by the need of the body and to channel the active entity of herbal drug to the site of action.

For good bioavailability, natural products must have a good balance between hydrophilicity (for dissolving into the gastrointestinal fluids) and lipophilicity (to cross lipidic biomembranes). Many phytoconstituents like polyphenolics have good water solubility, but are, nevertheless, poorly absorbed (Manach, et al., 2004) either due to their multiple-ring large size molecules which cannot be absorbed by simple diffusion, or due to their poor miscibility with oil and other lipids, severely limiting their ability to pass across the lipid –rich outer membranes of the enterocytes of the small intestine. (Chauhan, et al., 2009)

Novel herbal drug carriers cure particular disease by targeting exactly the affected zone inside a patient's body and transporting the drug to that area. Novel drug delivery system is advantageous in delivering the herbal drug at predetermined rate and delivery of drug at the site of action which minimizes the toxic effects with increase in bioavailability of drugs. In novel drug delivery technology, control of the distribution of drug is achieved by incorporating the drug in carrier system or in changing the structure of the drug at molecular level. Incorporation of herbal drugs in the delivery system also aids to increase in solubility, enhanced stability, protection from toxicity, enhanced pharmacological activity, improved tissue macrophage distribution, sustained delivery and protection from physical and chemical degradation. For example, liposomes act as potential vehicles to carry anti cancer agents by increasing amount of drug in tumour area and decrease the exposure or accumulation of drug in normal cells/tissues thereby preventing tissue toxicity effects. The phytosomal carriers have been studied for effective delivery of herbal extracts of ginseng (Ginkgo biloba) etc. In the present chapter, an attempt has been made to touch upon various aspects and applications related to novel herbal drug formulations and its Effect of NDDS on Polyherbal formulation (Dhiman & Nanda et al., 2012).

In the past, almost all the medicines were from the plants; the plant being man's only chemist for ages. Herbs are staging a comeback, herbal 'renaissance' is happening all over the globe and more and more people are taking note of herbal therapies to treat various kinds of ailments in place of mainstream medicine. (Sharma & Verma, 2016)

Knowledge and use of plants as herbal medicines has occurred in various populations throughout human evolution (Yadav & Bhatia, 2014). World Health Organization (WHO) has defined herbal medicines as finished, labeled medicinal products that contain active ingredients, aerial or underground parts of the plant or other plant material or combinations. WHO estimates that 80% of the world populations presently use herbal medicine for primary health care (Devi, et al., 2010). However, during the second half of the twentieth century, especially in the Western world, herbal medicines were gradually replaced by allopathic medicines. Allopathic treatments are currently more widely used than traditional medicines, especially in developed countries. However, most developing countries continue to use these natural medicines, most likely because obtaining a synthetic drug is expensive (Bonifacio, et al., 2014). The therapeutic and phytochemical importance of herbal medicine has been built for the improvement of human health, but its broader application is restricted due to the low bioavailability, the problems come with poor lipid-soluble compounds due to limited membrane permeability. Many herbal products demonstrated low therapeutic action due to their solubility problems which finally resulted in low bio-availability despite their extraordinary potential.(Seema, 2014)

During past decades, lot of attention has been given on the improvement of novel drug delivery systems for herbal drugs. Novel herbal drug carriers help in cure of particular disease by targeting the affected area inside a patient's body and transporting the drug to that area. Novel drug delivery system is advantageous in delivering the herbal drug at optimum rate and delivery of drug at the site of action which minimizes the toxicity and enhances bioavailability of the drugs. In novel drug delivery technology, control of the distribution of drug is achieved by incorporating the drug in carrier system or in changing the structure of the drug at molecular level (Mandal & Mandal. 2010). Herbal drugs are becoming more popular in the modern world for their application to cure variety of diseases with less toxic effects and better therapeutic effects (Saraf, 2010). However some limitations of herbal extracts/ plant actives like instability in highly acidic pH, liver metabolism etc. led to drug levels below therapeutic concentration in the blood resulting in less or no therapeutic effect (Goyal, et al., 2011). Incorporation of novel drug delivery technology to herbal or plant actives minimizes the drug degradation or pre systemic metabolism, and serious side effects by accumulation of drugs to the non-targeted areas and improves the ease of administration in the paediatric and geriatric patients. Various novel drug delivery systems such as liposomes, niosomes, microspheres and phytosomes have been reported for the delivery of herbal drugs. Incorporation of herbal drugs in the delivery system also aids to increase in solubility, enhanced stability, protection from toxicity, enhanced pharmacological activity, improved tissue macrophage distribution, sustained delivery and protection from physical and chemical degradation. For example, liposomes act as potential vehicles to carry anti-cancer agents by increasing amount of drug in tumour area and decrease the exposure or accumulation of drug in normal cells/tissues thereby preventing tissue toxicity effects (Manach, et al., 2004).

It is apparent, for any variety of chemical approach, that dependence on the present-day pattern of information exchange in logic fundamentals or memory devices will entail defect-tolerant computer architectures with suitable, intellectual software. (Waghulde, Sandeep, Naik, Pravin. 2017) On the other hand, it may be promising to develop other routes which require more complex architectures and unlike principles of information exchange where the problems associated with idleness, current density, recital speed, and especially contact confrontation and charge redistribution at the lead-to-molecule interface are less relevant (Schmid, 2011).

Also there is increasing evidence that many current drug therapies simply suppress symptoms and ignore the underlying disease processes. In contrast, many natural products appear to address the cause of many diseases and yield superior clinical results. Unfortunately, most physicians and patients are not aware that these natural alternatives exist. But research in this field is a never ending process. (Smith, 2009) The method by which a drug is delivered can have a significant effect on its efficacy. Some drugs have an optimum concentration range within which maximum benefit is derived, and concentrations above or below this range can be toxic or produce no therapeutic benefit at all. On the other hand, the very slow progress in the efficacy of the treatment of severe diseases has suggested a growing need for a multidisciplinary approach to the delivery of therapeutics to targets in tissues. From this, new ideas on controlling the pharmacokinetics, pharmacodynamics, non-specific toxicity, immunogenicity, biorecognition and efficacy of drugs were generated. These new strategies, often called drug delivery systems (DDS), are based on interdisciplinary approaches that combine polymer science, pharmaceutics, bioconjugate chemistry and molecular biology. (Charman, et al., 1999)

Novel drug delivery system is a novel approach to drug delivery that addresses the limitations of the traditional drug delivery systems. Modern medicine cures a particular disease by targeting exactly the affected zone inside a patient's body and transporting the drug to that area. Drug delivery system is the method by which an optimum amount of the concerned drug is administered to the patient in such a way that it reaches exactly the 'site of action' and starts working then and there. Novel drug delivery system attempts to eliminate all the disadvantages associated with conventional drug delivery systems. There are various approaches by which novel drug delivery can be achieved. (Musthaba, et al., 2009)

In one of the Novel drug delivery i.e. Transdermal which is the non-invasive delivery of medications from the surface of skin-the largest and most accessible organ of human body- through its layers, to the circulatory system. TDDS offers many advantages over conventional injection and oral methods. It reduces the load that the oral route commonly places on the digestive tract and liver. It enhances patient compliance and minimizes harmful side effects of a drug caused from temporary overdose. Another advantage is convenience, especially notable in patches that require only once weekly application. Such a simple dosing regimen can aid in patient adherence to drug therapy. In combination of Herbal it may possibly enhance the therapeutic effects with less side effects (Waghulde, et al., 2013). The present article was aimed to provide insight of different types of drug delivery systems incorporating active ingredients and potential advantages of such systems.

2. NOVEL DRUG DELIVERY APPROACHES

Various drug delivery and drug targeting systems are currently under development to minimize drug degradation and loss, to prevent harmful side-effects and to increase drug bioavailability and the fraction of the drug accumulated in the required zone. Among drug carriers one can name soluble polymers, microparticles made of insoluble or biodegradable natural and synthetic polymers, microcapsules, cells, cell ghosts, lipoproteins, liposomes and micelles. The carriers can be made slowly degradable, stimulireactive (e.g. pH- or temperature-sensitive) and even targeted (e.g. by conjugating them with specific antibodies against certain characteristic components of the area of interest). Targeting is the ability to direct the drug-loaded system to the site of interest. Two major mechanisms can be distinguished for addressing the desired sites for drug release: (i) passive and (ii) active targeting. An example of passive targeting is the preferential accumulation of chemotherapeutic agents in solid tumors as a result of the enhanced vascular permeability of tumor tissues compared with healthy tissue. A strategy that could allow active targeting involves the surface functionalization of drug carriers with ligands that are selectively recognized by receptors on the surface of the cells of interest. Since ligand-receptor interactions can be highly selective, this could allow a more precise targeting of the site of interest. Controlled drug release and subsequent biodegradation are important for developing successful formulations. Potential release mechanisms involve: (i) desorption of surface-bound / adsorbed drugs; (ii) diffusion through the carrier matrix; (iii) diffusion (in the case of nanocapsules) through the carrier wall; (iv) carrier matrix erosion and (v) a combined erosion / diffusion process. The mode of delivery can be the difference between a drug's success and failure, as the choice of a drug is often influenced by the way the medicine is administered. (Graham & Neil, 1990) Sustained (or continuous) release of a drug involves polymers that release the drug at a controlled rate due to diffusion out of the polymer or by degradation of the polymer over time. Pulsatile release is often the preferred method of drug delivery, as it closely mimics the way by which the body naturally produces hormones such as insulin. It is achieved by using drug-carrying respond to specific stimuli (e.g. exposure to light, changes in pH or temperature). (Sungthongjeen, et al., 2004) For over 20 years, researchers have appreciated the potential benefits of nanotechnology in providing vast improvements in drug delivery and drug targeting. Improving delivery techniques that minimize toxicity and improve efficacy offers great potential benefits to patients, and opens up new markets for pharmaceutical and drug delivery companies. Other approaches to drug delivery are focused on crossing particular physical barriers, such as the blood–brain barrier, in order to better target the drug and improve its effectiveness; or on finding alternative and acceptable routes for the delivery of protein drugs other than via the gastrointestinal tract, where degradation can occur (Sahoo & Labhasetwar, 2003). Presently novel drug delivery systems have been widely utilized only for allopathic drugs, but they have their own limitations hence, turning to safe, effective and time-tested Ayurvedic herbal drug formulation would be a preferable option.

The novel carriers should ideally fulfill two prerequisites. Firstly, it should deliver the drug at a rate directed by the needs of the body, over the period of treatment. Secondly, it should channel the active entity of herbal drug to the site of action. Conventional dosage forms including prolonged-release dosage forms are unable to meet none of these. In phyto-formulation research, developing nano dosage forms (polymeric nanoparticles and nanocapsules, liposomes, solid lipid nanoparticles, phytosomes and nanoemulsion etc.) have a number of advantages for herbal drugs, including enhancement of solubility and bioavailability, protection from toxicity, enhancement of pharmacological activity, enhancement of stability, improving tissue macrophages distribution, sustained delivery, protection from physical and chemical degradation etc. Thus the nano sized novel drug delivery systems of herbal drugs have a potential future for enhancing the activity and overcoming problems associated with plant medicines. The strength of drug delivery systems is their ability to alter the pharmacokinetics and biodistribution of the drug. Nanoparticles have unusual properties that can be used to improve drug delivery. Where larger particles would have been cleared from the body, cells take up these nanoparticles because of their size. Complex drug delivery mechanisms are being developed, including the ability to get drugs through cell walls and into cells.

Efficiency is important because many diseases depend upon processes within the cell and can only be impeded by drugs that make their way into the cell. Triggered response is one way for drug molecules to be used more efficiently. (Devi et al., 2010; Drexler 1992; Nishizawa et al., 1995; Kulkarni et al., 2010) Liposomes, which are biodegradable and essentially non-toxic vehicles, can encapsulate both hydrophilic and hydrophobic materials (Medina et al., 2004). Liposome based drug delivery systems offer the potential to enhance the therapeutic index of anti-cancer agents, either by increasing the drug concentration in tumor cells and/or by decreasing the exposure in normal tissues exploiting enhanced permeability and retention effect phenomenon and by utilizing targeting strategies (Sharma et al., 2006). The main advantages of using liposomes include: i) the high biocompatibility, ii) the easiness of preparation, iii) the chemical versatility that allows the loading of hydrophilic, amphiphilic, and lipophilic compounds, and iv) the simple modulation of their pharmacokinetic properties by changing the chemical composition of the bilayer components (Terreno et al., 2008). Delivery of agents to the reticuloendothelial system (RES) is easily achieved, since most conventional liposomes are trapped by the RES. The application of novel approaches can also improve the efficacy of herbal cosmetic formulations on the human body

(Chanchal & Swarnlata, 2008). Similarly the other vesicular systems like nanoemulsion, ethosomes and transferosomes are highly useful assemblies and find various advantages in the delivery of herbal medicines; some of them are summarized in present article. The phytosome process has also been applied to many popular herbal extracts including Ginkgo biloba, grape seed, hawthorn, milk thistle (Barzaghi, 1990), green tea, and ginseng. The flavonoid and terpenoid components of these herbal extracts lend themselves quite well for the direct binding to phosphatidyl choline. Phytosome is produced by binding individual components of herbal extracts to phosphatidyl choline, resulting in a dosage form that is better absorbed and thus, produces better results than the conventional herbal extracts. The results indicate that the absorption of silybin from silybin phytosome is approximately seven times greater compared to the absorption of silybin from regular milk thistle extract. Drugs can be embedded or dissolved in nanoparticles and can also be adsorbed or coupled on the surface (Yuan & Yi, 2003). Encapsulating drugs within NPs can improve the solubility and pharmacokinetics of drugs, and, in some cases, enable further clinical development of new chemical entities that have stalled because of poor pharmacokinetic properties (Alexis et al., 2008).

The major carrier materials of nanoparticles are synthetic biodegradable high molecular polymer and natural polymer. The former usually includes poly-α-cyanoacrylate alkyl esters, polyvinyl alcohol, polylactic acid, and polylacticcoglycolic acid, etc. The latter is usually divided into two classes: proteins (albumin, gelatin and vegetable protein) and polysaccharides (cellulose, starch and its derivatives, alginate, chitin and chitosan, etc.) (Xiao & Li, 2002; Ajazuddin & Saraf, 2010).

3. IMPORTANCE OF NOVEL DRUG DELIVERY FOR HERBAL DRUGS

Our country has a vast knowledge base of Ayurveda whose potential is only being realized in the recent years. However, the drug delivery system used for administering the medicine to the patient is traditional and out-of-date, resulting in reduced efficacy of the drug. In case of herbal extracts, there is a great possibility that many compounds will be destroyed in the highly acidic pH of the stomach. Other components might be metabolized by the liver before reaching the blood. As a result, the required amount of the drug may not reach the blood. If the drug does not reach the blood at a minimum level, which is known as 'minimum effective level' then there will be no therapeutic effect (Devi et al., 2010).

Phytopharmaceuticals are pharmaceuticals using traditional compounds derived from botanicals instead of chemicals. Natural ingredients are more easily and more readily metabolized by the body. Therefore they produce fewer, if any, side effects and provide increased absorption in the bloodstream resulting in more thorough and effective treatments. Pharmaceuticals made from chemical compounds are prone to adverse side effects. The human body will have a tendency to reject certain chemical compounds which do not occur naturally. These rejections occur in the form of side effects; some as mild as minor headaches, and others as severe as to be potentially lethal. It is important to note while phytopharmaceuticals produce fewer to no side effects, chemical interactions with other prescription drugs can occur. Furthermore, as they are single and purified compounds, they can be easily standardized making it easier to incorporate them in modern drug delivery systems compared to herbs (Norman, 2001).

Lipid-based drug delivery systems have been investigated in various studies and have shown their potential in controlled and targeted drug delivery. Pharmacosomes are amphophilic phospholipid complexes of drugs bearing active hydrogen that bind to phospholipids. They impart better biopharmaceutical properties to the drug, resulting in improved bioavailability. Phytosomes are novel compounds comprising of lipophilic complexes of components of plant origin like Silybum Marianum, Ginkgo Biloba, ginseng and so on, with phospholipid. (Semalty et al., 2009) They are also called as phytolipids delivery system. They have high lipophilicity and improved bioavailability and therapeutic properties. These are advanced form of herbal extract that have improved pharmacokinetic and pharmacological parameter, whose result can advantageously be used in treatment of acute liver diseases, either metabolic or infective origin. Phytosomes are produced by a patent process in which individual component of herbal extract like flavonolignans and terpenoids are bound on a molecular level to the phospholipids like phosphatidyl choline through a polar end. Phytosomes are used as a medicament and have wide scope in cosmetology. Many areas of phytosomes are to be revealed in future in the prospect of pharmaceutical application. Phytosomes forms a bridge between the convectional delivery system and novel delivery system (Joshi et al., 2008).

Incorporation of novel drug delivery technology to herbal or plant actives minimizes the drug degradation or presystemic metabolism, and serious side effects by accumulation of drugs to the non targeted areas and improves the ease of administration in the paediatric and geriatric patients. Various novel drug delivery systems such as liposomes, niosomes, microspheres and phytosomes have been reported for the delivery of herbal drugs. Incorporation of herbal drugs in the delivery system also aids to increase in solubility, enhanced stability, protection from toxicity, enhanced pharmacological activity, improved tissue macrophage distribution, sustained delivery and protection from physical and chemical degradation. For example, liposomes act as potential vehicles to carry anti cancer agents by increasing amount of drug in tumour area and decrease the exposure or accumulation of drug in normal cells/tissues thereby preventing tissue toxicity effects (Uhumwangho & Okor, 2005). The phytosomal carriers have been studied for effective delivery of herbal extracts of ginseng, ginkgo biloba etc. Direct binding of phosphatidyl choline to herbal extract components led to better absorption characteristics as compared to conventional delivery of herbal extracts. Other vesicular assemblies like microspheres, nanoemulsions, polymeric nanoparticles etc. have been proved beneficial to carry herbal components. The present review article was aimed to provide an overview of different types of drug delivery systems incorporating active ingredients and potential advantages of such systems. (Goyal et al., 2011) If the herbs themselves or the purified phytopharmaceuticals or phytosomes are incorporated in novel drug delivery systems, we can get the benefits of both. Thus it is important to incorporate the novel drug delivery system in Indian Ayurvedic medicines to combat serious diseases.

4. HERBAL NOVEL DRUG DELIVERY APPROACHES

As herbal novel drug delivery systems have lot of potential, several researchers are working towards developing novel drug delivery systems like mouth dissolving tablets, sustained and extended release formulations, mucoadhesive systems, transdermal dosage forms, microparticles, microcapsules, nanoparticles, implants etc. of herbs. Some of them are at the laboratory stage and some have reached to the marked. Some of the research work done in this area is summarized below.

Asoka Life science Limited launched Res-Q, the world's first poly-herbal mouth dissolving tablet, fast mouth dissolving drug. It has a novel drug delivery system that imparts increased efficacy. In Ayurvedic medicine segment, this is the first attempt to make medicines more effective in managing chronic ailments. Res-Q is a poly-herbal medicine highly effective for lung problems and other respiratory ailments like asthma. This unique mouth dissolving drug delivery system ensures that the drug reaches the blood directly and the first pass metabolism is bypassed. It dissolves in mouth by mixing with the saliva and get absorbed. This Res-Q provides relief from respiratory distress within fifteen minutes. This way, this drug resembles the efficacy of Sorbitrate, a revolutionary mouth dissolving drug used in cardiac distress (Parakh & Gothoskar, 2003).

A patent describes an orally administrable formulation for the controlled release or stable storage of a granulated herb, comprising a granulated herb and a carrier, the formulation release of 75% of the active ingredients between 4 and 18 h after administration. The active ingredients are selected from the group consisting of hypericin, hyperforin and echinacosides. The invention seeks to provide improved herbal preparations, whose preparations offer a convenient oral dosage form of herbs for supplying optimum plasma concentrations of the biologically active compounds that facilitates user compliance. The oral-controlled and stable release dosage form of granulated herb is in either matrix formulations such as matrix tablets or in multi-particulate formulations like microcapsules put into two piece capsules that are done in order to obtain a drug delivery system, which will ensure a steady supply of the active components for a sustained period (Blatt et al., 1999).

Another US patent invention is a new stable herbal drug formulation in the form of sustained-release microgranules containing Gingko Biloba extract as well as the process for preparing it. Plant extracts have poor flowability and compressibility properties. Thus, formulation of such extracts in the form of sustained release tablets is difficult, as it requires homogeneous mixtures of extracts with pharmaceutical excipients during all compression steps. Microgranules can be manufactured by a number of different processes, for example extrusion-spheronization, fluid air bed process or a coating-pan method. Extrusion-spheronization is suitable for pellets with high content of active substance, but need more equipment. For the manufacture of the granules of the invention, the coating-pan method is preferred, as it requires only simple equipment and operation (Marechal et al., 2006).

A study on palatal mucoadhesive tablet containing a herbal formulation showed the sustained release abilities of buccal adhesive tablets comprising of mucoadhesive polymers. The ingredients of the herbal formulation i.e. sage, Echinacea, Lavender and Mastic gum have previously demonstrated antimicrobial activity. In the study, the herbal formulation comprised of these four herbal medicinals was incorporated into a slow dissolving mucoadhesive tablet, designed to fit the palate. Results indicated that the adhesive tablet containing the herbal formulation is effective in reducing oral malodor and VSC levels (Sterer et al., 2008). An investigation aimed to formulate transdermal films incorporating herbal drug components such as Boswellic acid (Boswellia serrata) and curcumin (Curcuma longa) is one of the first few attempts to utilize ayurvedic drugs through transdermal drug delivery system (TDDS), which utilizes skin as a site for continuous drug administration into the systemic circulation. Thus this delivery system avoids the first pass metabolism of the drug without the pain associated with injection; moreover, the system provides a sustained drug delivery with infrequent dosing via zero-order kinetics and the therapy can be easily terminated at any time. Use of turmeric in TDDS for the local action of the drug at the site of administration can also be considered as a new version of ayurvedic turmeric poultice or lepa (Verma et al., 2007).

A patent describes the herbal-based oral composition for periodic retention within the buccal cavity of a human, comprising of a mixture of herbs like Radix Polygoni Multiflori, Rhizoma Drynariae, Rhizoma Ligustici Chuanxiong, Calculus Bovis, Indigo Naturalis, Herba Ecliptae, Pericarpium Trichosanthis, Radix Sophorae Flavescentis, Spina Gleditsiae, Radix Angelicae Sinensis, Fructus Mori and Halitum. The formulations selected for oral retention were from the group consisting of gels, pastes and chewing gums. The herbal ingredients are selected and prepared to provide a composition that is effective at causing human scalp and facial hair to darken, to reduce loss of scalp hair and to promote hair growth after a period of repeated usage (Chung et al., 2001).

In a study by Ma and colleagues, the effect and mechanism of Shuanghua aerosol (SHA) was investigated on upper respiratory tract infections in children aged from 3 to 14 years. Shuanghua aerosol consists of Flos Chrysanthemum Indicum, Flos Lonicera, Herba Houttuynia, Radix Bupleurum and methane. The control treatment was Shuanghuanglian aerosol (SHLA), which consists of Flos Lonicera, Fructus Forsythia and Radix Scutellaria. The authors conclude that SHA has obvious anti-inflammatory and antiviral effects and has a good curative effect in treating infantile upper respiratory tract infections (Ma et al., 2000).

ArthriBlend-SR is a marketed formulation containing herbal extracts and nutrients to support healthy joints and connective tissues in the body. It is a proprietary clinically validated blend of natural actives for joint care applications. The composition has the added advantage of sustained release technology, which benefits the continuous management of symptoms of arthritis. The blend contains Glucosamine sulfate, Boswellin (Boswellia serrata extract) and Curcumin C3 Complex (Curcuminoids from Curcuma longa), ingredients that work synergistically to support the management of inflammatory conditions such as arthritis. It will provide a slow release profile of 80–90% active ingredient release, in an 8hR period. The benefits of a sustained release formulation are particularly relevant to the bioavailability of glucosamine (Arthri, 2009).

Nowadays, people are opting for herbal medicines for their better therapeutic values and lesser adverse effects, so there is a need to develop a novel drug delivery system and a targeting system for herbal drugs. (Ansari et al., 2012) Novel drug delivery system, not only provides a safe and effective delivery, enabling people to regain faith over herbal drug delivery systems but also increases the market for herbal drugs. Several other novel drug delivery systems can be used for enhancing the efficacy of drugs.(Pinto, 2010; Vyas & Khar, 2002; Deepa et al., 2012) Sublingual delivery of phytoconstituents, for rapid action of the drug as it bypasses the first pass metabolism which is the main problem of herbal drugs, Muco adhesive Drug delivery can also be used for targeted delivery of drugs which increases the bioavailability of drug locally. Floating Drug delivery of drugs which are stable at gastric pH for their absorption in upper GI tract and Niosomes can also be used in place of liposomes and are less toxic than liposomes since they have non–ionic carrier system. Unlike liposomes, they don't undergo any free radical oxidation.

5. HERBAL NOVEL DRUG DELIVERY SYSTEMS

5.1 Phytosome

The term, Phyto " means plant while", some "means cell-like". Phytosomes is vesicular drug delivery system in which phyto constituents of herb extract surround and bound by lipid (one phyto-constituent molecule linked with at least one phospholipid molecule). Phytosome protect valuable component of herbal extract from destruction by digestive secretion and gut bacteria and because of which they show better absorption which produces better bioavailability and improved pharmacological and pharmacokinetic parameters than conventional herbal extract (Pawar & Bhangale, 2015) and the difference between phytosomes and liposome shown in fig.1.

Figure 1. Schematic representation of the structure of phytosome (A) and major difference between liposome and phytosome (B) (Jing et al., 2014)

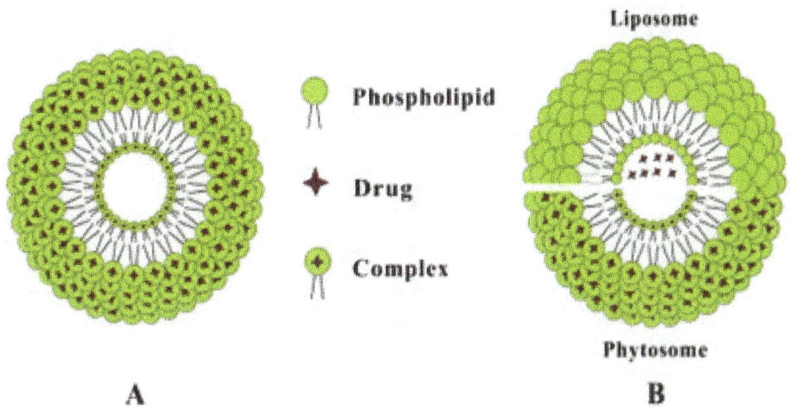

5.1.1 Advantages of Phytosomes (Dhandapani, et al., 2014)

1. Increased bioavailability due to phospholipid complex.
2. Improved absorption in GIT.
3. Increased bioavailability causes improved therapeutic effect.
4. Less dose requirement due to high bioavailability.
5. Higher stability.
6. High lipophilicity causes high penetrability, hence forth used in cosmetics over liposomes
7. Greater clinical benefits.
8. Phosphatidyl choline acts as liver protective other than a carrier

5.1.2 Method for preparation for Phytosomes

5.2 Liposome

Liposomes are concentric bilayered vesicle in which an aqueous volume is entirely enclosed by a membranous lipid bilayer mainly composed of natural or synthetic phospholipids. The name liposome is derived from two Greek words: "Lipos" meaning fat and "Soma" meaning body. A liposome can be formed at a variety of sizes as uni-lamellar or multi-lamellar construction, and its name relates to its structural building blocks, phospholipids, and not to its size. A liposome does not necessarily have lipophobic contents, such as water, although it usually does. Liposomes are artificially prepared vesicles made of lipid bilayer. Liposomes can be filled with drugs, and used to deliver drugs for cancer and other diseases. Liposomes can be prepared by disrupting biological membranes, for example by sonication. Liposomes are micro particulate or colloidal carriers, usually 0.05- 5.0 μm in diameter which form spontaneously when certain lipids are hydrated in aqueous media. Liposomes are composed of relatively biocompatible and biodegradable material, and they consist of an aqueous volume entrapped by one or more bilayer of natural and/or synthetic lipids. Drug with widely varying lipophilicity can be encapsulated in liposomes,

Figure 2. Method for preparation for Phytosomes (Patela et al., 2009)

Phospholipids

↓

Dissolved in organic solvents containing Drug/ Extract

↓

Solution of Phospholipids in organic solvent

↓

Solvent with drug/extract

↓

Drying

↓

Formation of thin film

↓

Hydration

↓

Formation of Phytosomal suspension

either in the phospholipids bilayer, in the entrapped aqueous volume or at the bilayer interface (Mansoori et al., 2012) the drug encapsulated in liposomes shown in fig 3.

5.2.1 Liposome Classification Based on Structural Features (Kulkarni et al., 2011)

1. MLV - Multilamellar large vesicles

Figure 3. Drug encapsulation in Liposomes (63)

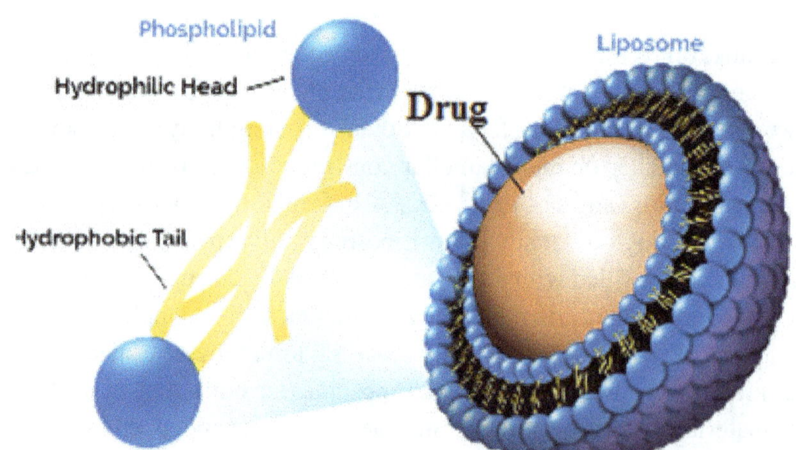

2. OLV - Oligolamellar vesicles
3. UV - Unilamellar vesicles
4. SUV- Small unilamellar vesicles
5. MUV - sized unilamellar vesicles
6. LUV - Large unilamellar vesicles
7. GUV - Giant unilamellar vesicles
8. MVV -Multivesicular vesicles

5.2.2 Liposome Classification Based on Method of Liposome Preparation

1. REV -Single or oligolamellar vesicle made by reverse phase evaporation method.
2. MLV / REV -Multilamellar vesicles made by reverse phase evaporation method.
3. SPLV -Stable plurilamellar vesicles.
4. FAT-MLV Frozen and thawed MLV
5. VET- Vesicles prepared by extrusion method.
6. FUV-Vesicles prepared by fusion
7. FPV -Vesicles prepared by French press
8. DRV- Dehydration rehydration vesicles
9. BSV- Bubblesomes

5.2.3 Advantages of Liposome (Dua et al., 2012)

1. Provides selective passive targeting to tumor tissues (Liposomal doxorubicin).
2. Increased efficacy and therapeutic index.
3. Increased stability via encapsulation.
4. Reduction in toxicity of the encapsulated agents.
5. Site avoidance effect.
6. Improved pharmacokinetic effects (reduced elimination, increased circulation life times).
7. Flexibility to couple with site specific ligand to achieve active targeting
8. Biodegradable and flexible
9. Can incorporate micro and macro molecules
10. Can carry both water and lipid soluble drugs

5.2.4 General Method of Liposomes Preparation and Drug Loading

5.3 Niosomes

Niosomes are microscopic lamellar structures formed on admixture of a nonionic surfactant, cholesterol and a charge inducing agent with subsequent hydration in aqueous media. Niosomes possess an infra-structure consisting of hydrophobic and hydrophilic moieties together and as a result can accommodate drug molecules with a wide range of solubility's. Niosomes have been evaluated in many pharmaceutical applications. In such therapeutic applications, important advantages of using niosomes include their ability to reduce systemic toxicity by encapsulation of treatment agents and minimize clearance of such

Figure 4. Liposomes preparation (Thapa et al., 2013)

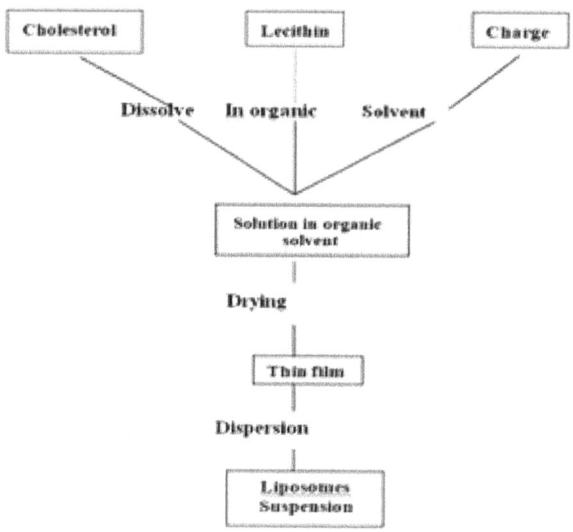

agents from the body by slow drug release (Mohamed et al., 2012) and the structure of niosome shown in the figure 3.

5.3.1 Types of Niosomes (Rahimpour & Hamishehkar, 2012)

Niosomes are classified based on number of bilayer, size and method of preparation.

1. Mulitlamellar- 0.5µm to 10µm in diameter.
2. Larger unilamellar- 0.1µm to 1µm in diameter.
3. Small unilamellar – 25-500nm in diameter.

5.3.2 Advantages of Niosome (Rahimpour Y. And Hamishehkar H, 2012)

1. Niosomes are biodegradable, biocompatible, non-toxic and non-immunogenic.
2. Niosomes are able to encapsulate large amount of materials in a small volume of vesicles.
3. Niosomes have better patient adherence and satisfaction and also better effectiveness than conventional oily formulations.
4. Niosomes can entrap wide range of chemicals (hydrophilic, lipophilic and amphiphilic drugs) due to its unique structure.
5. The characteristics of niosome such as shape, fluidity and size can be easily controlled by changing in structural composition and method of production.
6. Niosomes can be prescribed via different administration routes such as oral, Parenteral and topical, etc. with different dosage forms such as semisolids, powders, suspensions.
7. Due to chemical stability of structural composition, the storage of the niosome is easy.

Figure 5. Structure of Niosome (Sharma et al., 2018)

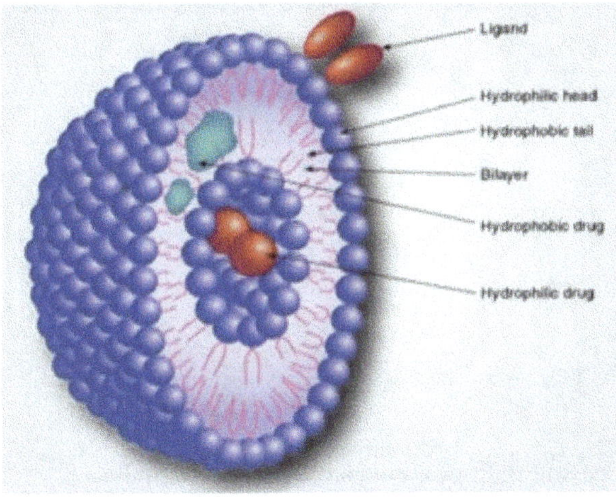

5.4 Transfersomes

The term and concept of Transfersome were introduced in 1991 by Gregor Cevc. The name means "carrying body", and is derived from the Latin word "transferre", meaning to carry across, and the Greek word "soma", fora "body". A Transfersome carrier is an artificial vesicle which resembles the natural cell vesicle. Thus it is suitable for targeted and controlled drug delivery. Transfersome is a highly adaptable and stress-responsive, complex aggregate. It is an ultra-deformable vesicle which possesses an aqueous core surrounded by the complex lipid bilayer. Interdependency of local composition and shape of the bilayer makes the vesicle both self-regulating and self-optimizing. This enables the Transfersome to cross various transport barriers efficiently, and then act as a drug carrier for non-invasive targeted drug delivery and sustained release of therapeutic agents. These self-optimized aggregates, with the ultra-flexible membrane, are able to deliver the drug reproducibly either into or through the skin, depending on the choice of administration or application, with high efficiency these vesicular transfersome are several orders of magnitudes more elastic than the standard liposome and thus well suited for the skin penetration. Transfersomes overcome the skin penetration difficulty by squeezing themselves along the intracellular sealing lipid of the stratum corneum. Flexibility of transfersome membrane is achieved by mixing suitable surface-active components in the proper ratios (Pawar et al., 2015)

5.4.1 Advantages of Transfersomes (Sachan R., Parashar T., et al, 2013)

1. Transfersomes can deform and pass through narrow constriction (from 5 to 10 times less than their own diameter) without measurable loss.
2. They have high entrapment efficiency, in case of lipophilic drug near to 90%.
3. This high deformability gives better penetration of intact vesicles.
4. They can act as a carrier for low as well as high molecular weight drugs e.g. analgesic, anesthetic, corticosteroids, sex hormone, anticancer, insulin, gap junction protein, and albumin.
5. Transfersomes possess an infrastructure consisting of hydrophobic and hydrophilic moieties together and as a result can accommodate drug molecules with wide range of solubility.

Figure 6. Undeformable Vesicle (Transfersome) (Walve et al., 2011)

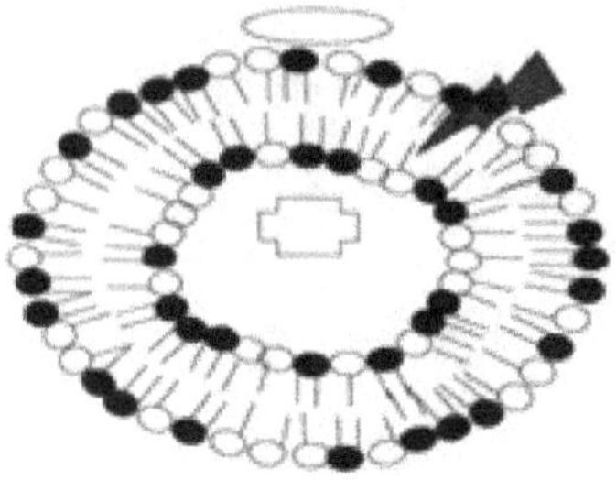

6. They act as depot, releasing their contents slowly and gradually.
7. They can be used for both systemic as well as topical delivery of drug.
8. They are biocompatible and biodegradable as they are made from natural phospholipids similar to liposomes.
9. They protect the encapsulated drug from metabolic degradation.
10. Easy to scale up, as procedure is simple, do not involve lengthy procedure and unnecessary use or pharmaceutically unacceptable additives.

5.5 Dendrimers

Dendrimers are spheroid or globular nanostructures of polymeric materials. They are highly branched, monodisperse nanoparticles that bind the drug at the surface or entrap within their inner cores. There is a unique property of branching around the inner space that has huge effect on physical and chemical properties. Preparations of these particles are either by divergent or convergent methods. The size grows linearly while the number of surface groups put in. They have very low poly disparity index and ranging dimension increment by stepwise from 1-10 nm. The performance and individual properties of dendrimers can be at variance deeply from their linear complements. Due to very low polydispersity of Dendrimers, they contribute to their efficacy as drug delivery strategy (Yadav D., Suri S. et al. 2011)

5.5.1 Advantages of Dendrimer (Mishra Ina, 2011)

1. Medication to the affected part inside a patient's body directly.
2. Target drug delivery: Dendrimers are suitable for targeting solid tumors due to increased permeability, limited drainage in tumour vasculature which will lead to accumulation of macromolecules in tumor (enhanced permeation rate). There is also reduction in amount of drug used via targeted delivery (attaching site specific ligand at surface or magnetic guidance) and thus reduction in systemic toxicity.
3. Controlled and sustained release of drugs can also be obtained.
4. Drugs can be easily made to remain within layers of skin and not penetrate in systemic circulation.
5. Bypassing the gastric medium and hence the eschewing the variation due to effect of gastric secretions.

Figure 7. Structure of a Dendrimer (Zeng, F.; Zimmerman, 1997)

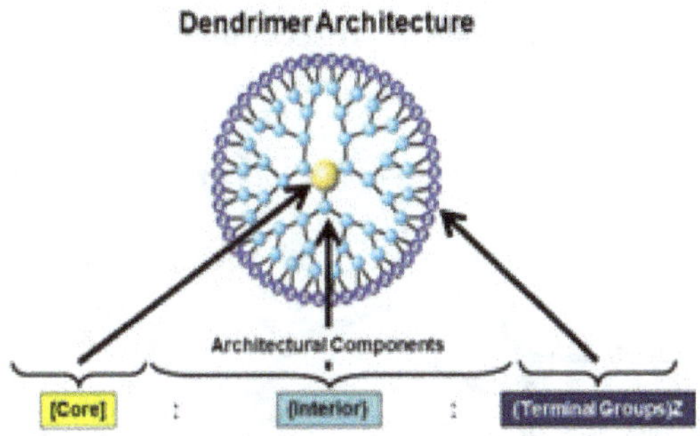

6. Increase in therapeutic efficacy, decrease in side effects: decreased clearance of drug via altered distribution of drug in organs at site of localization and transportation due to controlled and sustained release of the drug.
7. Relatively high drug loading.
8. Preservation of drug activity: as drugs can be incorporated into the systems without any chemical reaction.

5.5.2 Currently, There are Three Methods for Using Dendrimers in Drug Delivery (Kushwaha K.S., Rastogi A., et al, 2012 and Zhang L., Pornpattananangkul D., et al, 2010)

1. The drug is attached to the periphery of the dendrimer to form dendrimer prodrugs,
2. The drug is coordinated to the outer functional groups via ionic interactions, or
3. The dendrimer acts as a unimolecular micelle by encapsulating a pharmaceutical through the formation of a dendrimer drug (i.e., host–guest) supramolecular assembly. The latter approach is of interest for multiple reasons and provides an opportunity to encapsulate pharmacologically active compounds and to study the supramolecular assemblies formed in these systems.
4. Dendrimers possess several unique properties that make them a good nanoparticle platform for antimicrobial drug delivery.

5.5.3 Mechanism of Drug Delivery Through Dendrimers

The well defined 3D structure and many functional surface groups, drug molecules can be loaded both in the interior of the dendrimers as well as attached to the surface groups (as shown in the figure). Dendrimers can function as drug carriers either by encapsulating drugs within the dendritic structure, or by inter-acting with drugs at their terminal functional groups via electrostatic or covalent bonds (prodrug).

5.5.4 There are Broadly Two Mechanisms for Drug Delivery

A) First, is by in vivo degradation of drug dendrimer conjugate (covalent bonding of drug to dendrimer), which depends on presence of suitable enzymes or an environment capable of degrading bonds.

B) The second one is by releasing the drug due to changes in physical environment such as pH, temperature. This approach is independent of the external factors and takes place in cavities of the core (endo-receptor) or outer shell of receptor (exo-receptor)

Figure 8. A Dendrimer molecule with drug molecules loaded at terminal surface of Branches

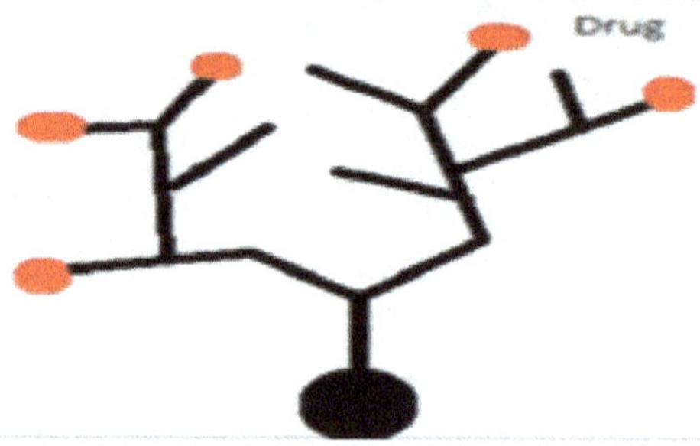

There are two types of delivery, one is to a specific type of cell and other as a controlled release from a depot (which may be present in circulation or imbedded in some suitable tissue) 1. Psividas biosilicon allows drug molecules to be held in Nano-sized particles that release a tiny pulse of drug as the biosilicon dissolves. Biosilicon shows resistance to degradation in acid environment. A dendrimer of higher generations consists of shell. A shell consists of a central core and alternating two layers of monomers around it. Amines constitute the central core which may sometimes be replaced by sugar. All core molecules have multiple and identical reaction site. Amine is the simplest core molecule present with three functional sites. The surface of all full generations consists of multiple amines, while the surface of the half generations consists of multiple acids. These two kinds of surfaces provide the means of attachment of multiple different functional components

5.6 Ethosomes

Ethosomes are the slight modification of well established drug carrier liposome. Ethosomes are lipid vesicles containing phospholipids, alcohol (ethanol and isopropyl alcohol) in relatively high concentration and water. Ethosomes are soft vesicles made of phospholipids and ethanol (in higher quantity) and water. The size range of ethosomes may vary from tens of nanometers (nm) to microns (μ) ethosomes permeate through the skin layers more rapidly and possess significantly higher transdermal flux. (Nikalje A. P., Tiwari S., 2012)

5.6.1 Advantages of Ethosomes (P.Tarun, Soniya, et al, 2013)

1. Delivery of large molecules (peptides, protein molecules) is possible.
2. It contains non-toxic raw material in formulation.
3. Enhanced permeation of drug through skin for transdermal drug delivery.
4. Ethosomal drug delivery system can be applied widely in Pharmaceutical, Veterinary, Cosmetic fields.

Figure 9. Structure of Ethosomes (Nikalje & Tiwari, 2012)

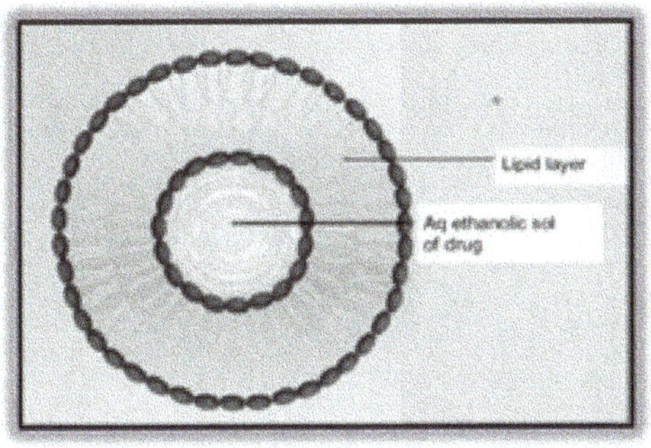

5. High patient compliance: The ethosomal drug is administrated in semisolid form (gel or cream) hence producing high patient compliance.
6. Simple method for drug delivery in comparison to Iontophoresis and Phonophoresis and other complicated methods
7. The Ethosomal system is passive, non-invasive and is available for immediate commercialization.

5.6.2 Preparation Methods for Ethosomes

5.7 Transdermal Delivery Of Drugs (Selvam RP, Singh AK, et al, 2010)

Transdermal drug delivery systems (TDDS) are defined as self-contained, discrete dosage forms which, when applied to intact skin, deliver the drug(s), through the skin, at a controlled rate to systemic. Transdermal delivery system provides the advantage of controlled drug delivery, enhanced bioavailability, reduction in side effects and easy application[20]. This patch is a medicated adhesive pad that is design to release the active ingredient at a constant rate over a constant period of several hours to days after

Figure 10. Hot method for the preparation of Ethosomes

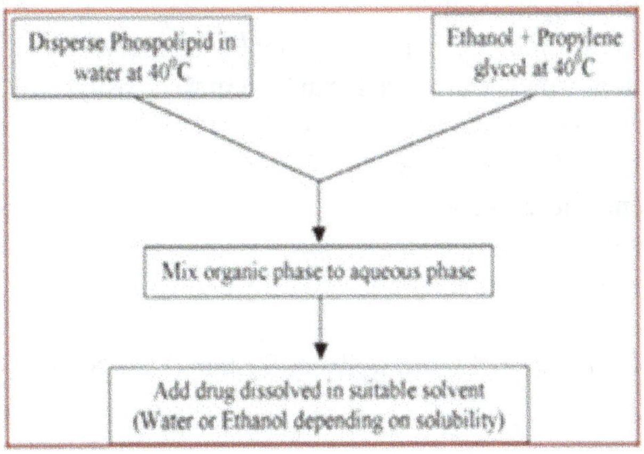

Figure 11. Cold method for the preparation of Ethosomes

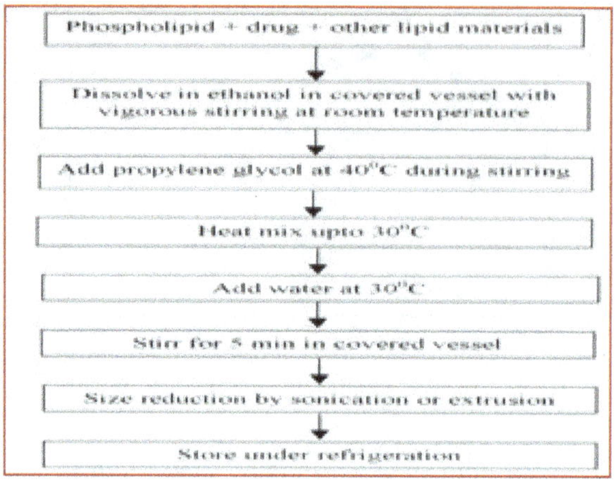

application to the skin. The drug present in transdermal patch permeates into systemic circulation by diffusion through various layer of skin which lead further to effected organ. This system provides drug delivery at control rate, high bio availability, easy application, sustainable action.

5.7.1 Advantages of Transdermal Drug Delivery (Latheeshjlal L, Phanitejaswini P, et al, 2011, Chien YW, 1992, Banker GS, Rhodes CT. 1990, Guy RH. 1996, Benson HAE. 2005 and Guy RH, Hadgraft J, et al, 1987)

1. TDDS is a drug delivery system in which a device usually known as patch is adhered on the skin surface to deliver the drug into the systemic circulation through the skin at predefined concentration for therapeutic effects, which avoids additional limitations due to other dosage forms.
2. It offers constant permeation of drugs through the skin giving constant serum drug level, the goal of therapy.
3. It can be used as an alternate to oral drug delivery system for those patients, who find difficulty in taking drugs through oral route.
4. It can be used as an alternative for nauseated or unconscious patients.
5. Patients having gastrointestinal problems can be given drugs through TDDS as there will be no direct contact between drug and stomach.
7. Like intravenous infusion, it also gives constant plasma level.
8. If toxicity develops from TDDS, patch can be removed easily.
9. It is very convenience as application of drug is very easy.
10. It eliminates first pass mechanism.
11. It reduces systemic drug interactions.
12. It offers long duration of action.
13. Self administration can be done.

5.7.2 Disadvantages of Transdermal Drug Delivery System (Dass S, Dey SK. 2013)

1. Many hydrophilic drugs cannot pass or very slowly permeates the skin. This will affect the therapeutic efficacy of the drug.
2. Many problems like itching, edema, erythema etc. may be seen due to patches.
3. The barrier function of the skin may change from person to person, or with ages or with different sites on same person.
4. There may be some possibility of irritation at the site of drug administration.
5. Uneconomic system of drug delivery.
6. It is not use in acute condition, only used in chronic conditions
7. TDDS is not compatible with ionic drugs.
8. Dumping of dose may occur.
9. Drugs having affinity for both lipophilic and hydrophilic phases are used.
10. High drug level in blood cannot be attained.

5.7.3 Main Ingredients Used For the Preparation of Transdermal Drug Delivery System (Kumar KPS, Bhowmik D, et al, 2010 and Patil PM, Chaudhari PD, et al, 2012)

Liners- It provides the protection of patches during storage and the liner should be removed previous to use.

Adhesive- It served to adhere the components of the patch together along with adhering the patch to skin.

Membrane- Its controls the drug releases from the multi-layer patches. It's also known as the permeation enhancer.

Drug- Drug reservoir is direct contact with release liner.

Backing- protects the patches from outer environment

5.7.4 Method of Preparing Transdermal Patches (Shrivastava D. 2012, Sharma A. 2012 and Ghinaiya M. 2013)

Method of preparation of TDDS was summarized by modifying the earlier reported methods. The patches were prepared by solvent casting method. The polymer (for example PVP/HPMC) was taken in a beaker with a minimum quantity of the solvent. Then 2/3rd of the solvent was mixed with the other polymers (for example PVA) and was added firstly with stirring at lower rpm and later at a higher speed. The plasticizer was added and homogeneously mixed and the drug was included with enduring agitation and the volume was made up. The films were cast onto a suitably designed and fabricated glass mould and then dried in oven at 40°C. The films were removed by using sharp blade by inserting along the edges of the film. The dried films were wrapped in butter paper and stored in a closed container away from light and in cool place.

Transdermal Patches

Figure 12. Method of Preparing

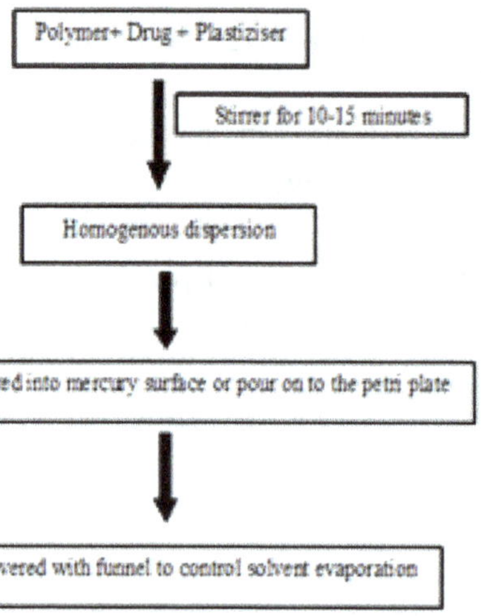

5.7.5 Mechanism of Action of Transdermal Patches (Rasheed SH, Haribabu R, et al. 2011)

The function of the transdermal patch and the flow of the active drug ingredient from the patch to the circulatory system via skin transpire through different methods. For a systemically active drug to reach

Figure 13. Transdermal Drug delivery (94)

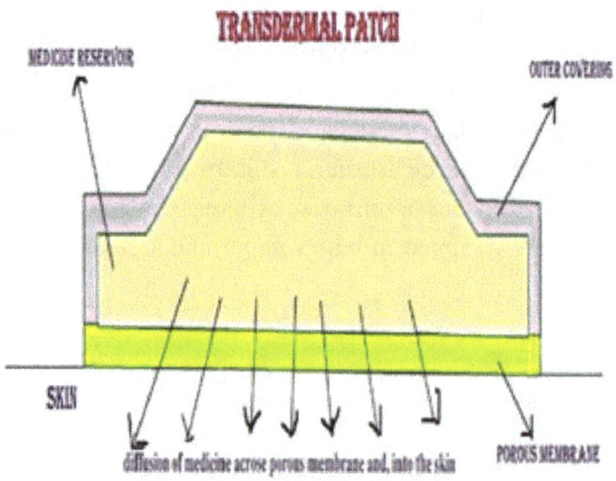

a target tissue, it has to take some physicochemical properties which make easy the sorption of the drug through the skin and enter the microcirculation.

5.8 Nanoparticles

Nanoparticles are nano- or sub–nano-sized structures composed of synthetic or semi-synthetic polymers. In recent times, nanoparticles of herbal medicines have attracted much attention. Nanoparticles are colloidal systems with particles varying in size from 10 nm to 1000 nm. It is an effective system as the formulation is encapsulated in it easily and can easily reach the effective site. The nano-spheres are the solid-core spherical particulates which are nano metric in size (Chaturvedi M, Kumar M, et al, 2011). The nano-spheres have a matrix type structure in which the active ingredient is dispersed throughout (the particles), whereas the nanocapsules have a polymeric membrane and an active ingredient core. Nanonization possesses many advantages, such as increasing compound solubility, reducing medicinal doses, and improving the absorbency of herbal medicines compared with the respective crude drugs preparations (Ajazuddin, Saraf S. 2010)

5.8.1 Advantages of Herbal Nanoparticles Delivery System (Yadav M, Bhatia VJ, Doshi G, et al. 2014, Sharma M. 2014, Mohnaraj VJ, Chen Y. 2016 and Atram S. 2014)

1. Nanoparticles are the choice of formulation, to promote the drugs through the biological barriers and increase the bioavailability of drugs.
2. Particles size and surface is easily manipulated for both active and passive targeting for parenterals.
3. Traditional medicines have advantage of low risk of side effects, widespread availability, low cost and efficacious for lifestyle diseases for prolonged period of time.
4. Controlled and sustained release of the drug during transportation and at site of localization, altering organ distribution of the drug.
5. Nanoparticle improves the absorbency of the herbal formulation and reduces the dose of formulation. Because of this, its solubility is increased and the drug can reach the target site, as compared to other systems.
6. When drug is encapsulated within nanoparticles, it results in improvement of the solubility and pharmacokinetics of drugs.
7. Quantity of component becomes less with improving quality of dug effect.
8. Fewer raw materials are required to achieve the desired effect and control drug delivery to provide exact specification regarding dug dose form.
9. Carry maximum amount of drug to the site of action by passing all barriers. Such as the acidic PH of stomach increase prolong circulation of drug into blood due to small particles size.

5.9 Nanoparticle Synthesis (Geckeler KE. J. 1993, Wang W. 2008, Schwarz, James A. 2004, Iwaki T, Kakihara Y, et al, 2003, Sohn BH, Cohen RE, 1991and Boris I Kharisov, et al, 2014)

5.9.1 Polymer Nanoparticle

Polymer Nanoparticles are defined as solid, colloidal particles in the range of 10-1000 nm. Polymer Nanoparticle is known as nanosphere and nanocapsules. These can be prepared either from preformed polymers or by direct polymerization of monomers. Different methods like solvent evaporation, salting out, dialysis, supercritical fluid evaporation and rapid expansion of supercritical solution are being used. The choice of preparation method is made on the basis of a number of factors such as the type of polymeric system, area of application, size requirement etc. The polymeric nanoparticles which are synthesized by any of these techniques are proved for efficient therapeutic activity

5.9.2 Metallic Nanoparticles

Metal nanoparticle is used to describe nanosized metals with dimension (length, width and thickness) range between 1-100 nm. There are various liquid phase methods for preparing metallic nanoparticles, such as chemical reduction, sol gel, and reversed micelle. Nobel metal Nanoparticles with spherical shaped and size, were produced continuously by the chemical reduction methods.

Metal nanoparticles are widely used due to their characteristic features such as large surface enriches, provides specific electronic structure between molecular and metallic states and process a large number of low coordination sites. These are used in magnetic separation of labelled cells and other biological entities, therapeutic drug, gene and radionuclide delivery, radio frequency methods for the catabolism of tumours via hyperthermia, and contrast enhancement agents for magnetic resonance imaging.

5.9.3 Magnetic Nanoparticles

Magnetic Nanoparticles have been synthesized with number of different compositions and phases including pure metals like CO, Fe and Ni, metal alloys such as FePt, CoPt . Using magnetic nanoparticles particle size of approximately 3 nm can be obtained. The size of particles will be hundreds of atoms which enable us to make recording media of up to 1 Tb/in2 in recording density which can be achieved by correctly organizing the particles. Various methods are been reported few among them are coprecipitation, sonochemistry, colloidal method, solvothermal, combustion synthesis, hydrothermal method, microemulsion and thermal decomposition methods. The key applications of MNPs are in Bio separation where the conjugation of the target biomolecules and MNPs which are functionalized with specific receptors, forms complexes and can be easily attracted by the applied magnetic field and extracted from the pristine mixture, thus providing a convenient and time-saving approach for bioseparation as compared to conventional method like centrifugation and filteration. This technology is also used in biosensing, drug delivery, magnetic resonance imaging and hyperthermia.

Figure 14. Schematic representation for preparation of metallic Nanoparticles

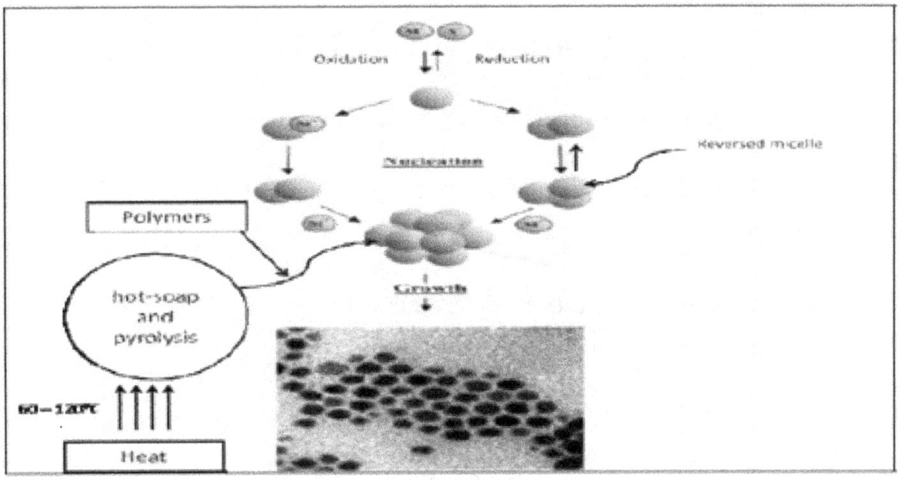

5.10 Microsphere (Mukherjee PK, Harwansh RK, et al, 2015)

Microsphere comprises of small spherical particles, with diameters in the micrometer range, typically 1 μm to 1000 μm (1 mm). Microspheres are sometimes referred to as micro-particles. Microspheres can be manufactured from various natural and synthetic materials. Glass microspheres, polymer microspheres and ceramic microspheres are commercially available. Microspheres are classified as biodegradable or non-biodegradable. Biodegradable microspheres include albumin microspheres, modified starch microspheres, gelatin microspheres, polypropylene dextran microspheres, polylactic acid microspheres, etc. According to the current literature reports on non-biodegradable microspheres, polylactic acid is the only polymer approved to be used by people, and it is used as a controlled-release agent. Solid and hollow microspheres vary widely in density and therefore are used for different applications. Hollow microspheres are typically used as additives to lower the density of a material. In addition, reports on immune microsphere and magnetic microsphere are also common in recent years. Immune microsphere possesses the immune competence as a result of the antibody and antigen being coated or adsorbed on the polymer microspheres.

5.10.1 Advantage of Microsphere formulation (Chaturvedi M, Kumar M, et al, 2011)

1. Administration of medication via micro-particulate system is advantageous because microspheres can be ingested or injected, and they can be tailored for desired release profiles and used for site-specific delivery of drugs and in some cases can even provide organtargeted release.
2. Drug can be easily released from the formulation.
3. It can protect the specific function of drugs, and can release the drugs into an outer phase for a long period.

5.10.2 Application of Microspheres in Pharmaceutical Industry (Mathur M. 2013)

1. For Taste and odor masking.
2. To delay the volatilization.
3. For Separation of incompatible substances.
4. For Improvement of flow properties of powders.
5. To Increase the stability of the drug against the external conditions.
6. For Safe handling of toxic substances.
7. To improve the solubility of water insoluble substances by incorporating dispersion of such material in aqueous media

5.10.3 Application of Novel Drug Delivery System in Enhancing the Therapeutic Potential of Phytoconstituents

In modern drug discovery era, various chemically synthesized new molecules are approved by FDA and are coming on the market, having wide therapeutic efficacy, but the adverse effects are associated with this therapy causes serious adverse effects which could be life threatening. Conventional therapy provides non-targetability in tissues and organs due to peak and valley fluctuations, and a frequent dose of administration can produce troublesome for allopathic medicines lead to poor patient compliance. (Jing J, Sklar EG, et al, 2008) The controlled release drug delivery system provides drug release at a controlled rate and maintains the overall therapeutic concentration of the drug in the body. In ancient times, herbal remedies and natural extract are consumed by people to cure various diseases. These herbal remedies contain hundreds of phytoconstituents present, which is working simultaneously against the disease. In recent times, the interest of people in phytopharmaceuticals has been increasing day-by-day among physicians and patients, and it is evident from the global market of herbal medicine and phytopharmaceuticals that has increased from $18 billion from 2005 and $26 from 2011. (Solecki RS, Shanidar IV.1975, Salanki A, Kutty SK. 2007 and Park K. 2014) Various dietary products and supplements are also derived from the natural origin are also gaining more interest in the industry and the global market for phytopharmaceuticals. Some phytoconstituents derived from the natural origin are having a poor solubility and low bioavailability resulting in a narrow therapeutic index, which hinders his novel efficiency, so formulation scientist is working on targeting and controlled drug release of phytoconstituents to provide better therapeutic effect and increased patient compliance.(Hoffman AS. 2008 and Srikanth P, Raju N, et al, 2013) The three main goals of novel drug delivery system (NDDS) is by providing sustained drug release, selected targeting to the site of action and increased patient compliance (Figure 15).

NDDS not only reduce the frequency of administration but also reduce the Peak and valley fluctuations which lead to enhanced bioavailability. The applications of NDDS in phytopharmaceuticals have been widely investigated, and various commercial formulations of phytoconstituents are available in the global market which people will consume and take benefit from it. In Phytoformulation research, various drug delivery vehicles, such as liposomes, polymeric

nanoparticles, microemulsion, microspheres, solid lipid nanoparticles (SLNs), are used in which phytoconstituent is solubilized and release the drug in a sustained manner. (Huang X, Brazel CS. 2001, Jha SK, Dey S, et al, 2011, Vasir JK, Tambwekar K, et al, 2003, Müller RH, Mäder K, et al, 2000, Brannon-Peppas L. 1995 and Musthaba SM, Baboota S, et al, 2009) The list of drug delivery vehicles used in illustrated in (Figure 16).

Figure 15. Goals of novel drug delivery system

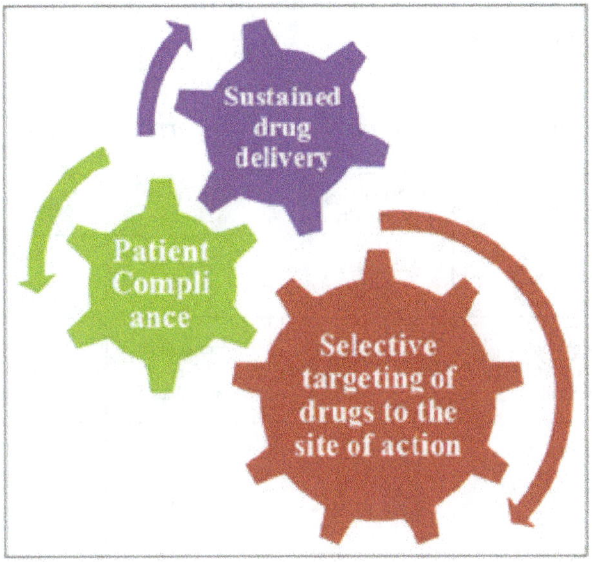

5.11 LIPOSOMES

Liposomes are discovered in 1970 as drug delivery vehicles for targeting at the active site into desired concentration. These are concentric bilayer vesicles in which the aqueous volume is entirely closed by lipid bilayer mainly composed of phospholipids. Liposomes are biocompatible, non-toxic, and biodegradable in nature; hence, it is widely used in enhancing the therapeutic efficacy of various phytoconstituents.

Figure 16. Novel drug delivery carriers in herbal formulations

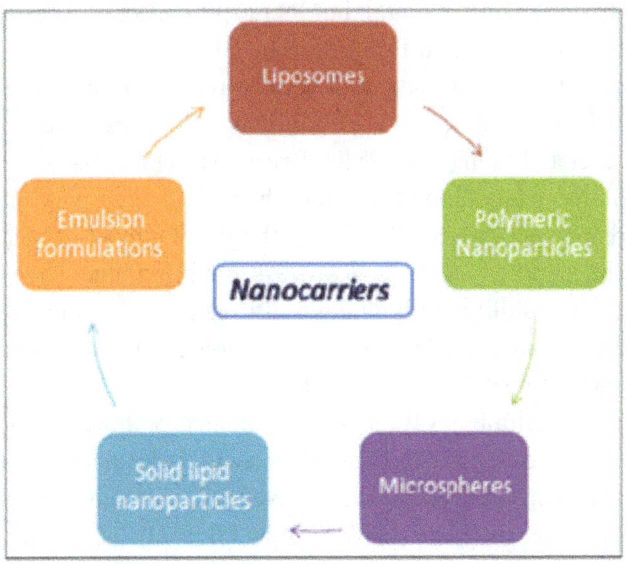

The advantages of liposomes in herbal formulations are given below. (Allen TM, Cullis PR. 2013, Xu X, Burgess DJ. 2011 and Flaten GE, Chang TT, et al, 2013) The potential applications of liposomes in phytoconstituents are given in Table 1.

Table 1. Studies reporting enhanced bioavailability after incorporation into liposomes

Phyto constituent	Chemical nature and source	Pharmacological activity	Method of delivering	Clinical significance	References
Quercetin	Pentahydroxyflavone, obtained from *Sophora japonica* L.	Antioxidant and antineoplastic	Elastic liposomes	Encapsulation efficiency was increased by 97%	Priprem A, Sutthiparinyanont S, et al, 2015
Curcumin	Diarylheptanoid, obtained from *Curcuma longa*	Anticancer, Anti-inflammatory, wound healing properties	Transdermal delivery of liposomes	Improved bioavailability and clinical efficacy	Li L, Braiteh FS, Kurzrock R. 2005
Vincristine	Bisindole alkaloid, obtained from *Catharanthus roseus*	Broad spectrum anticancer activity against lung and prostate cancer	Intravenous liposome delivery	Overcome Neurotoxicity problems and other side effects	Zhigaltsev IV, Maurer N, et al. 2005
Paclitaxel	Taxol nucleus, obtained from *Taxus bacatta* and *Taxus bevifolia*	Broad anticancer activity against almost all types of cancer	Injectable liposomal delivery	Improved antitumor activity by selective targeting in cancerous cells	Yang T, Cui FD, et al. 2007
Colchicine	Benzofuran compound, obtained from *Colchicum autumnale*	Anti-gout	Delivering liposome through film dispersion	Optimum encapsulation efficiency and stability	K. Chakraborty, A. Shivakumar, et al, 2018

5.12 Nanoparticles

Nanoparticle can be used to target the herbal medicines to individual organ which improves the selectivity, solubility, drug delivery, safety, effectiveness and reduces the frequent dose. The nanoparticle size drug delivery enhances the entire surface area of the drugs therefore allocating quicker dissolution in the blood. Reduction in toxicity while maintaining therapeutic effects. The enhanced permeation and retention of nanoparticles can cross Blood Brain Barrier (BBB).

Nanoparticles can enter the human body in several ways, via Lungs where a rapid translocation through the blood stream to the vital organs is possible including the Blood Brain Barrier (BBB) and absorption by Intestinal tract and Skin (Hoet PMH, Brnske HI, et al, 2004).

Nanosized herbal medicines can potentially enhance the biological activity and overcome the problems associated with pure herbal drugs. New challenges in the development of nanotechnology based drug delivery system include the feasibility of scale up process that bring innovative therapeutic echniques to the market quickly, and the possibility of obtaining multifunctional systems to fulfil several biological and therapeutic requirements. Nanoparticles may exert toxicological effect; nanotoxicology has emerged as a new branch of toxicology for studying undesirable effect of

Nanoparticle. In the past, health innovations were evaluated on their efficacy and improved patient quality of life. Currently, health care costs must also be considered. Nanotherapeutic prod cts, which are more complex in structure and more expensive than conventional alternatives, are designed to provide an overall reduction in health care costs (Leonard K, Ahmmad B, et al, 2011). This reduction in health care

Figure 17. Release of drug molecules to the targeted site+ (Wang W. 2008)

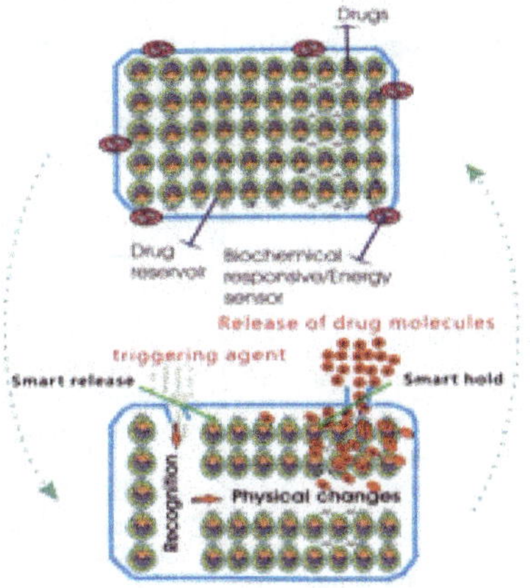

costs is likely to be obtained by increasing the nanotherapeutic efficacy, reducing the length of in-patient stay, reducing personal health care costs, and the effective treatment of expensive major diseases. The nanomedicine-related drug market is directly affected by the pharmaceutical regulatory environment, health care policies, demographics, and the wider economic environment.

5.13 Emulsion Based Formulations

Emulsions are thermodynamically unstable formulations of oil and water phase, stabilized by a suitable emulsifying agent. Microemulsions are thermodynamically stable and are isotropic mixtures of oil, water, and surfactant with a droplet size of 100-200 nm. Microemulsion is widely used drug delivery formulations to improve the solubility of poorly soluble drugs. Microemulsions possess various advantages

Table 2. Studies reporting enhanced bioavailability after incorporation into polymeric nanoparticles

Phyto constituent	Chemical nature and source	Pharmacological activity	Clinical significance	References
Hypericin	Napthodianthrone, obtained from *Hypericum perforatum*	Photosensitizer used in radiotherapy	Improved lipophilicity in physiologically active media and improved their Diagnostic applications	Tian Q, Wang W, et al. 2009
Ginseng	Steroidal compound, obtained from *Panax ginseng,Panax quinquefolius*	Antioxidant activity	Enhanced stability, therapeutic action, and drug release	Zeisser-Labouebe M, Lange N, et al, 2006
Glycyrrhizic acid	Steroidal saponin, obtained from *Glycyrrihiza glabra*	Antihypertensive, useful in hepatitis	Improved drug release and encapsulation efficiency	Khemani M, Sharon M, et al, 2012
Berberine	Isoquinoline compound, obtained from Berberis aquifolium	Anticancer	Sustain the delivery of phytoconstituent lead to enhanced duration of action	Chang CH, Huang WY, et al. 2011 and Kumar R, Kumar MS, et al, 2012

Table 3. Studies reporting enhanced clinical significance of Emulsion Based Formulations

Phyto constituent	Chemical nature and source	Pharmacological activity	Clinical significance	References
Curcumin	Diarylheptanoid, obtained from *Curcuma longa*	Anticancer activity, anti-inflammatory activity	Improved permeation and enhancement ratio via transdermal delivery	Chen L, Zhao X, et al. 2013
Triptolide	Diterpenoid triepoxide,obtained from Chinese herb, *Tripterygium wilfordii*	Useful in autoimmune disorders, antineoplastic	provides improved percutaneous permeability and better-sustained release profile	Yin YM, Cui FD, et al. 2009
Docetaxel	Taxol comound, obtained from taxus species (*Taxus bacatta, Taxus brevifolia*)	Broad spectrum antimitotic compound	Docetaxel microemulsion provides improved apical to basolateral transport across Caco-2 cells	Chaturvedi M, Kumar M, et al, 2011

such as good thermodynamic stability, ease of manufacturing, fewer chances of drug degradation, and improved stability (Mujaffar F, Singh UK, et al, 2013 and Sintov AC. 2015).

Microspheres are widely used as drug delivery carrier for targeting of various agents that cause dose-dependent adverse effects. In recent times, microspheres are widely used to enhance the therapeutic potential of various poorly soluble phytoconstituets. Various techniques such as gastroretentive bloating microspheres, microencapsulation, emulsification, and calcium alginate based beads are used widely for herbal drug delivery.

Table 5. Studies reporting enhanced bioavailability upon incorporating herbal drug into phytosomes

Phyto constituent	Chemical nature and source	Pharmacological activity	Clinical significance	References
Ginkgo biloba	Kew tree or maiden hair tree,obtained as dried leaves belong to family Gingkoaceae	Cardioprotective, antioxidant	Increased antioxidant activity as compare to commercial formulation	Naik SR, Pilgaonkar VW, et al, 2006
Curcumin	Diarylheptanoid, obtained from *Curcuma longa*	Anti-inflammatory, anticancer	Chitosan microspheres provide improved drug targeting and bioavailability	Zhang J, Tang Q, et al, 2013
Quercetin	Pentahydroxyflavone, obtained from *Sophora japonica* L.	Antineoplastic	Better encapsulation efficacy and drug release	Rasaie S, Ghanbarzadeh S, et al, 2014
Epigallocatechins	Catechin nucleus, obtained from various species of Terminalia plant	Anticancer and antioxidant	Catechins in phytosomes have better antioxidant activity as compared to commercial formulation	Kidd PM. 2009

Table 6. Shows the studies enhancing the therapeutic potential of phytoconstituents upon incorporation into microspheres

Phyto constituent	Chemical nature and source	Pharmacological activity	Clinical significance	References
Rutin	Flavonoid glycoside, obtained from *Carpobrotus edulis*	Antioxidant	Microspheres shows sustained release behavior for the drug within 20 hr, and still maintain existed within 180 hr	Jiang HL, Cui YL, et al, 2013
Camptothecin	Quinoline alkaloid, obtained from *Camptothecin acuminata*	Antineoplastic	CPT encapsulated in PLGA microspheres should retain its antitumor potency for longer period of time	Tong W, Wang L, et al, 2003
Quercetin	Pentahydroxyflavone, obtained from *Sophora japonica* L.	Antioxidant and anti-inflammatory	Controlled drug delivery for effective management of arthritis	Natarajan V, Krithica N, et al, 2011
Ginsenosides	Steroidal glycoside, obtained from Panax species (*Panax ginseng, Panax notofolium)*	Anticancer, Immunomodulator	PLA microspheres shows improved drug release behavior and encapsulation efficiency	Zhang D, Guan LI, et al, 2008

5.14 Topical Drug Delivery Approaches

Delivery of phytoconstituents via skin is widely investigated for enhancing permeation and therapeutic efficacy. The topical delivery possesses major advantages such as avoidance of first pass metabolism, decrease adverse effects associated with oral and intravenous (IV) doses, effective maintenance of cars, and improved therapeutic efficacy. Various strategies are used to enhance the transdermal permeation including transdermal patches, ethosomes, transferosomes, and SLNs. (Prausnitz MR, Langer R. 2008 and Benson HE, Watkinson AC. 2011)

The transdermal patch utilizing rate controlling membrane to sustain the delivery of the drug via the skin into the blood stream. (Pastore MN, Kalia YN, et al, 2015 and Dhiman S, Thakur GS, et al, 2011) The main limitation in transdermal patch approach that it causes skin irritation or skin infection due to the high frequency applied through iontophoresis, which will overcome by the novel vesicular carriers such as transferosomes and ethosomes, which supplies essential nutrients results in maintain the integrity of the skin.

Ethosomes are phospholipid based vesicles contains a high Ethosomes content of ethanol (20-50%) which itself act as a permeation enhancer in transdermal delivery. Compare to other carriers, ethosomes have the capability to permeate the drug more deeply and more efficiently into the systemic circulation. (Verma P, Pathak K. 2010 and Akiladevi D, Sachinandan D. 2010) On the other hand, transferosomes are also used as potential carriers for topical delivery. Transferosomes utilizing the osmotic pressure and hydration to increase permeation. These topical approaches would prove as an effective drug delivery of phytoconstituents as compared to oral and IV.

Table 7. shows various studies which increase permeation of phytoconstituents through topical drug delivery strategies

Phyto constituent	Pharmacological activity	Formulation strategy	Clinical significance	References
Khellin	Anti-acne, used in psoriasis	Transdermal patch using iontophoresis	Transdermal gel containing khellin was able to permeate more deeply and provide more effective treatment of psoriasis	Marconi B, Mancini F, et al. 1999
Caffeine from the extract of *Paullinia cupana*	CNS stimulant	Transdermal patch	Transdermal patch was effective releasing all components simultaneously as compare to commercial formulation	Heard CM, Johnson S, et al, 2006
Curcumin	Anticancer, antioxidant and anti inflammatory	Transferosomes	Formulation shows higher entrapment efficiency and higher permeation of drug from transfersomal ge	Patel R, Singh SK, et al, 2009
Capsaicin	Analgesic and antirheumatic	Transferosomes	Better analgesic activity via topical delivery as compare to commercially available oral formulation	Xiao-Ying L, Luo JB, et al, 2006
Triptolide	Used in auto-immune disease	SLNs	The anti-inflammatory activity is higher in SLN dispersion for rheumatoid arthritis	Mei Z, Chen H, et al, 2003 and Mei Z, Li X, et al, 2005

5.15 Controlled Release Devices

6. CONCLUSION

Herbal medicine is globally accepted as an alternative system of therapy in the pharmaceuticals. But the drug delivery system for herbal drugs is quite traditional and out of date. Herbal drugs/plant actives possess a lot of therapeutic potential that should be explored via application of novel drug delivery technology. Large molecular size, lipid solubility, degradation in acidic stomach are certain problems which limit the therapeutic activity of these extracts in vivo though these possess excellent bioactivity in vitro. An extensive research is going on in the area of novel drug delivery and targeting for plant actives and extracts. However, research in this area is still at the exploratory stage. A number of plant constituents like flavonoids, tannins, terpenoids etc. showed enhanced therapeutic effect at similar or less dose when incorporated into novel drug delivery vesicles as compared to conventional plant extracts. Hence, there is a great potential in development of novel drug delivery system for valuable herbal drugs as it provides

Table 8. Shows various studies which increase

Active Constituent	Pharmacological activity	Application of ethosomal formulations	References
Sophora Alopecuroides	Anti-endotoxic, anti-cancer and anti-inflammatory	Ethosome enhances delivery of drugs through the stratum corneum barrier into the deep layer of the skin.	Zhaowu Z, Xiaoli W, et al, 2009
Matrine	Antibacterial, anti-inflammatory, anti-rheumatism and anti-tumour	Increase the per cutaneous permeation and improve anti-inflammatory effect	Brown K, Scott BM. 2014

efficient and economical drug delivery. Also, the trend of incorporating NDDS for herbal drugs has also been adopted at industrial scale.

Table 9. Recent patents on novel drug delivery system of phytoconstituents

Patient number	Inventor	Publishing date	Description	References
US 20140141108 A1	Kenneth Brown, Brandi M Scott	2014-05-22	This present invention relates to an herbal composition (red quebracho extract) that treats various diseases, including bloating, constipation and there of.	Pushpangadan P, Rao C, et al, 2007
US 20070042062 A1	Palpu Pushpangadan, Chandana Rao, Ajay Rawat, Dadala Kumar	2007-02-27	This present invention relates to novel herbal formulation contain *Curcuma longa* and *Zingiber officinale* Linn. rhizomes extract for the treatment of diabetes mellitus	Kurzrock R, Li L, et al, 2011
US 7968115 B2	Razelle Kurzrock, Lan Li, Kapil Mehta, Bharat Bhushan Agarawal	2011-06-28	This present invention relates to the novel liposomal formulation of curcumin for the treatment of pancreatic, breast, and melanoma cancer	Kim JH. 2010
US 20100104646 A1	Ji Hwal Kim	2010-04-29	This present invention deals with nanoparticle composition comprises mixture of *Zanthoxylum piperitum, Cnidium officinale* encapsulated It using lecithin and chitosan to produce lecithin-capsuled nanoparticles	Ji Hwal Kim. 2006
EP 2437725 A1	Manu Chaudhary, Vijay Naithani	2012-04-11	This present invention deals with topical microemulsion composition comprises various ratio of oil, water, and surfactant and herbal phytoconstituent includes *Piper nigrum, Zingiber officinale, Piper longum, Cinnamomum zeylanicum, Cinnamomum tamala, Vitex negundo, Boswellia serrate* that will used for the treatment of rheumatoid arthritis	Chaudhary Manu, Naithani Vijay. 2012

REFERENCES

Ajazuddin, S. S., & Saraf, S. (2010). Applications of novel drug delivery system for herbal formulations. *Fitoterapia*, *81*(7), 680–689. doi:10.1016/j.fitote.2010.05.001 PMID:20471457

Akiladevi, D., & Sachinandan, D. (2010). Ethosomes: A noninvasive approach for transdermal drug delivery. *International Journal of Current Pharmaceutical Research*, *2*, 1–4.

Alexis, F., Basto, P., Levy-Nissenbaum, E., Radovic-Moreno, A. F., Zhang, L., Pridgen, E., & Farokhzad, O. C. (2008). HER-2-targeted nanoparticle-affibody bioconjugates for cancer therapy. *ChemMedChem*, *3*(12), 1839–1843. doi:10.1002/cmdc.200800122 PMID:19012296

Allen, T. M., & Cullis, P. R. (2013). Liposomal drug delivery systems: From concept to clinical applications. *Advanced Drug Delivery Reviews*, *65*(1), 36–48. doi:10.1016/j.addr.2012.09.037 PMID:23036225

Amit, J., Sunil, C., Vimal, K., & Anupam, P. (2008). The pharma review. New Delhi: Kongposh Publications Pvt, Ltd.

Anju, D., & Arun, N. (2012). Novel Herbal Drug Delivery System (NHDDS): The need of Hour, 2012, International Conference on Environment. *Chemistry and Biology IPCBEE*, *49*, 34. doi:10.7763/IPCBEE

Ansari, S. H., Islam, F., & Sameem, M. (2012, July). Influence of nanotechnology on herbal drugs: A Review. *Journal of Advanced Pharmaceutical Technology & Research*, *3*(3), 142–146. doi:10.4103/2231-4040.101006 PMID:23057000

Arthri Blend, S. R. (2009). A formulation containing herbal extracts and nutrients to support healthy joints and connective tissues in the body. *Nutraceuticals World*. Retrieved from http://findarticles.com/particles/mi_hb223/is_6_7/ai_n29102045/

Ashwani, G., & Kumar, S. (2011). Potential of novel drug delivery systems for herbal drugs. *Indian Journal of Pharmaceutical Education and Research*, *45*(3), 225–235.

Atram, S. (2014). Recent development of herbal formulation. A novel drug delivery system. InternationalAyurveda. *Medical Journal*, *2*(6), 952–958.

Banker, G. S., & Rhodes, C. T. (1990). *Modern pharmaceutics* (3rd ed.). Marcel Dekkar, Inc.

Barzaghi, N., Crema, F., Gatti, G., Pifferi, G., & Perucca, E. (1990). Pharmacokinetic studies on IdB 1016, a silybin- phosphatidylcholine complex, in healthy human subjects. *European Journal of Drug Metabolism and Pharmacokinetics*, *15*(4), 333–338. doi:10.1007/BF03190223 PMID:2088770

Benson, H. A. E. (2005). Transdermal drug delivery: Penetration enhancement techniques. *Current Drug Delivery*, *2*(1), 23–33. doi:10.2174/1567201052772915 PMID:16305405

Benson, H. E., & Watkinson, A. C. (2011). *Topical and transdermal drug delivery: Principles and practice*. Wiley Online Library. doi:10.1002/9781118140505

Blatt, Y., & Kimmelman, E. (1999). *Microencapsulated and controlled-release herbal formulations*. United States Patent 6340478.

Bonifácio, B. V., Silva, P. B., Ramos, M. A., Negri, K. M., Bauab, T. M., & Chorilli, M. (2014). Nanotechnology-based drug delivery systems and herbal medicines: A review. *International Journal of Nanomedicine*, *9*(1), 1–15. doi:10.2147/IJN.S52634 PMID:24363556

Brannon-Peppas, L. (1995). Recent advances on the use of biodegradable microparticles and nanoparticles in controlled drug delivery. *International Journal of Pharmaceutics*, *116*(1), 1–9. doi:10.1016/0378-5173(94)00324-X

Brown, K., & Scott, B. M. (2014). *Herbal supplements and methods of use thereof.* US Patent (US 20140141108 A1).

Chakraborty, K., & Shivakumar, A. (2018). Nano-technology in herbal medicines. *RE:view*. Advance online publication. doi:10.13140/RG.2.2.32261.24808

Chanchal, D., & Swarnlata, S. (2008). Novel approaches in herbal cosmetics. *Journal of Cosmetic Dermatology*, *7*(2), 89–95. doi:10.1111/j.1473-2165.2008.00369.x PMID:18482010

Chang, C. H., Huang, W. Y., Lai, C. H., Hsu, Y. M., Yao, Y. H., Chen, T. Y., Wu, J.-Y., Peng, S.-F., & Lin, Y. H. (2011). Development of novel nanoparticles shelled with heparin for berberine delivery to treat Helicobacter pylori. *Acta Biomaterialia*, *7*(2), 593–603. doi:10.1016/j.actbio.2010.08.028 PMID:20813208

Charman, W. N., Chan, H. K., Finnin, B. C., & Charman, S. A. (1999). Drug delivery: A key factor in realising the full therapeutic potential of drugs. *Drug Development Research*, *46*(3–4), 316–327. doi:10.1002/(SICI)1098-2299(199903/04)46:3/4<316::AID-DDR18>3.0.CO;2-E

Chaturvedi, M., Sinhal, A., Kumar, M., & Saifi, A. (2011). Recent developments in novel drug delivery systems of herbal drugs. *International Journal of Green Pharmacy*, *5*(2), 87–94. doi:10.4103/0973-8258.85155

Chauhan, N. S., Rajan, G., & Gopalakrishna, B. (2009). Phytosomes: A potential phyto-phospholipid carriers for herbal drug delivery. *Journal of Pharmacy Research*, *2*(7), 1267–1270.

Chen, L., Zhao, X., Cai, J., Guan, Y., Wang, S., Liu, H., & Li, J. (2013). Triptolide-loaded microemulsion-based hydrogels: Physical properties and percutaneous permeability. *Acta Pharmaceutica Sinica. B*, *3*(3), 185–192. doi:10.1016/j.apsb.2013.05.001

Chien, Y. W. (1992). *Novel drug delivery systems, drugs and the Pharmaceutical sciences, 50.* Marcel Dekkar.

Chung, H., & Burk, H. (2001). *Herbal-based oral composition and process for producing the same.* European Patent EP0862446.

Cornell, B. A., Braach-Maksvytis, V. L., King, L. G., Osman, P. D., Raguse, B., Wieczorek, L., & Pace, R. J. (1997). A biosensor that uses ion-channel switches. *Nature*, *387*(6633), 580–583. doi:10.1038/42432 PMID:9177344

Dass, S., & Dey, S. K. (2013). A novel approach towards transdermal drug delivery system: A precise review. *Indo American Journal of Pharmaceutical Research*, *3*(6), 4680–4696.

Devi, V. K., Jain, N., & Valli, K. S. (2010). Importance of novel drug delivery systems in herbal medicines. *Pharmacognosy Reviews*, *4*(7), 27–31. doi:10.4103/0973-7847.65322 PMID:22228938

Devi, V. K., Jain, N., & Valli, K. S. (2010). Importance of novel drug delivery systems in herbal medicines. *Pharmacognosy Reviews*, *4*(7), 27–31. doi:10.4103/0973-7847.65322

Dhandapani, N. V., & Sumanraj, K. S. (2014). Phytosomes-A review. *International Journal of Pharma Sciences*, *4*(4), 622–625.

Dhiman, S., & Thakur, G. S. (2011). Transdermal patches: A recent approch to new drug delivery system. *International Journal of Pharmacy and Pharmaceutical Sciences*, *3*, 26–34.

Drexler, K. E. (1992). *Nanosystems: Molecular machinery, manufacturing, and computation*. John Wiley & Sons.

Dua, J. S., & Rana, A. C. (2012). Liposome: Methods Of Preparation And Applications. *IJPSR*, *3*(2), 14–20.

Fatima Grace, X., & Rahul Raj, S. (2014). Herbal ethosomes—A Novel Approach in Herbal Drug Technology. *American Journal of Ethnomedicine*, *1*(4), 226–230.

Flaten, G. E., Chang, T. T., Phillips, W. T., Brandl, M., Bao, A., & Goins, B. (2013). Liposomal formulations of poorly soluble camptothecin: Drug retention and biodistribution. *Journal of Liposome Research*, *23*(1), 70–81. doi:10.3109/08982104.2012.742537 PMID:23210622

Freiberg, S., & Zhu, X. X. (2004). Polymer microspheres for controlled drug release. *International Journal of Pharmaceutics*, *282*(1–2), 1–18. doi:10.1016/j.ijpharm.2004.04.013 PMID:15336378

Geckeler, K. E. J., & Stirn, J. (1993). Stirn Polyreaktionen Mechanismen,Systematik, Relevanz. *Naturwissenschaften*, *80*(11), 487–500. doi:10.1007/BF01140804 PMID:8264805

Ghinaiya, M. (2013). Formulation and evaluation of transdermal patch of an antihypertensive drug. *International Journal of Pharma Sciences*, *4*, 3664–3682.

Goyal, A., & Kumar, S. (2011). Potential of novel drug delivery system for herbal drugs. *Indian Journal of Pharmaceutical Education and Research*, *45*, 225–235.

Graham, S., & Neil, B. (1990). Controlled drug delivery systems. *La Chimica e l'Industria*, *6*, 25–38.

Guy, R. H. (1996). Current status and future prospects of transdermal drug delivery. *Pharmaceutical Research*, *13*(12), 1765–1769. doi:10.1023/A:1016060403438 PMID:8987069

Guy, R. H., Hadgraft, J., & Bucks, D. A. W. (1987). Transdermal drug delivery and cutaneous metabolism. *Xonobiotica*, *7*(3), 325–343. doi:10.3109/00498258709043943 PMID:3107225

Heard, C. M., Johnson, S., Moss, G., & Thomas, C. P. (2006). In vitro transdermal delivery of caffeine, theobromine, theophylline and catechin from extract of Guarana, Paullinia cupana. *International Journal of Pharmaceutics*, *317*(1), 26–31. doi:10.1016/j.ijpharm.2006.02.042 PMID:16600539

Hirai, S., Kim, Y. I., Goto, T., Kang, M. S., Yoshimura, M., Obata, A., & Kawada, T. (2007). Inhibitory effect of naringenin chalcone on inflammatory changes in the interaction between adipocytes and macrophages. *Life Sciences*, *81*(16), 1272–1279. doi:10.1016/j.lfs.2007.09.001 PMID:17915259

Hoet, P. H., Brüske-Hohlfeld, I., Salata, O. V., & Brnske, H. I. (2004). Nano particles known and unknown health risk. *J. Nanobiotecnol*, *2*(1), 12. doi:10.1186/1477-3155-2-12 PMID:15588280

Hoffman, A. S. (2008). The origin and evolution of controlled drug delivery systems. *Journal of Controlled Release*, *132*(3), 153–163. doi:10.1016/j.jconrel.2008.08.012 PMID:18817820

Huang, X., & Brazel, C. S. (2001). On the importance and mechanisms of burst release in matrix-controlled drug delivery systems. *Journal of Controlled Release*, *73*(2–3), 121–136. doi:10.1016/S0168-3659(01)00248-6 PMID:11516493

Ina, M. (2011). Dendrimer: A novel drug delivery system. *Journal of Drug Delivery and Therapeutics*, *1*(2), 70–74.

Iwaki, T., Kakihara, Y., Toda, T., Abdullah, M., & Okuyama, K. (2003). Preparation of high coercivity magnetic fe Pt nanoparticles by liquid process. *Journal of Applied Physics*, *94*(10), 6807–6811. doi:10.1063/1.1619577

Iwaki, T., Kakihara, Y., Toda, T., Abdullah, M., & Okuyama, K. (2003). Preparation of High coercivity magnetic FePt nanoparticles by liquid process. *Journal of Applied Physics*, *94*(10), 6807–6811. doi:10.1063/1.1619577

Jha, S. K., & Dey, S. (2011). Microemulsions-potential carrier for improved drug delivery. *Asian J. Biomed PharmSci*, *1*, 5–9.

Jiang, H. L., Cui, Y. L., & Qi, Y. (2013). Microencapsulation of rutin in chitosan-coated alginate microspheres through internal gelation technique. *Advanced Materials Research*, *716*, 433–458. doi:10.4028/www.scientific.net/AMR.716.455

Jin, J., Sklar, G. E., Min Sen Oh, V., & Chuen Li, S. (2008). Factors affecting therapeutic compliance: A review from the patient"s perspective. *Therapeutics and Clinical Risk Management*, *4*(1), 269–286. doi:10.2147/TCRM.S1458 PMID:18728716

Kharisov, B. I., Dias, H. V. R., Kharissova, O. V., Vázquez, A., Peña, Y., & Gómez, I. (2014). Solubilization, dispersion and stabilization of magnetic Nanoparticles in water and non aqueous solvent: Recent trends. *RSC Advances*, *4*(85), 45354–45381. doi:10.1039/C4RA06902A

Khemani, M., Sharon, M., & Sharon, M. (2012). Encapsulation of berberine in nano-sized PLGA synthesized by emulsification method. *ISRN Nanotechnol.*, *34*, 12–21. doi:10.5402/2012/187354

Kidd, P. M. (2009). Bioavailability and activity of phytosome complexes from botanical polyphenols: The silymarin, curcumin, green tea, and grape seed extracts. *Alternative Medicine Review*, *14*(3), 226–246. PMID:19803548

Kim, J. H. (2010). *Nanoparticle composition for prevention of hair loss and promotion of hair growth.* US patent (US 20100104646 A1).

Kim, J. H. (2006). *Nanoparticle composition for prevention of hair loss and promotion of hair growth.* (US20100104646A1).

Kulkarni, P. R., & Yadav, J. D. (2011). Liposomes: A novel drug delivery system. *International Journal of Current Pharmaceutical Research, 3*(2), 10–18.

Kulkarni, V., & Waghulde, S. (2010). Nanomedicine: The newer generation fusion molecular nanotechnology. *RJPBCS, 1*(3), 551–557.

Kumar, K. P. S., & Bhowmik, D. (2010). Transdermal drug delivery system-A novel drug delivery system and its market scope and opportunities. *International Journal of Pharmacy and Biological Sciences, 1*, 1–21.

Kumar, R., & Kumar, M. S. (2012). Multiple emulsions: A review. *International Journal of Advances in Pharmaceutical Research, 2*, 9–19.

Kurzrock, R., & Li, L. (2011). *Liposomal formulation of curcumin for the treatment of cancer.* US patent (US 20070042062 A1).

Kushwaha, K. S., & Rastogi, A. (2012). Novel drug delivery system for anticancer drug: A review. *International Journal of Pharm Tech Research, 4*(2), 542–553.

Latheeshjlal, L., & Phanitejaswini, P. (2011). Transdermal drug delivery systems: An overview. *International Journal of Pharm Tech Research, 3*(4), 2140–2148.

Leonard, K., Ahmmad, B., Okamura, H., & Kurawaki, J. (2011). In situ green synthesis of biocompatible ginseng capped gold nanoparticles with remarkable stability. *Colloids and Surfaces. B, Biointerfaces, 82*(2), 391–396. doi:10.1016/j.colsurfb.2010.09.020 PMID:20980131

Li, J., Wang, X., & Zhang, T. (2014). phytosome-A-and-major-difference-between phytosome and liposome. *Asian Journal of Pharmaceutical Sciences, 10*(2). Advance online publication. doi:10.1016/j.ajps.2014.09.004

Li, L., Braiteh, F. S., & Kurzrock, R. (2005). Liposome-encapsulated curcumin: In vitro and in vivo effects on proliferation, apoptosis, signaling, and angiogenesis. *Cancer, 104*(6), 1322–1331. doi:10.1002/cncr.21300 PMID:16092118

Ma, B., Duan, X., & Wang, Z. (2000). Clinical and experimental study on Shuanghua aerosol in treating infantile upper respiratory tract infection. *Chinese Journal of Integrated Traditional and Western Medicine, 20*(9), 653–655. PMID:11789167

Manach, C., Scalbert, A., Morand, C., Rémésy, C., & Jiménez, L. (2004). Polyphenols: Foodsources and bioavailability. *The American Journal of Clinical Nutrition, 79*(5), 727–747. doi:10.1093/ajcn/79.5.727 PMID:15113710

Manach, C., Scalbert, A., Morand, C., Rémésy, C., & Jiménez, L. (2004). Polyphenols: Foodsources and bioavailability. *The American Journal of Clinical Nutrition, 79*(5), 727–747. doi:10.1093/ajcn/79.5.727 PMID:15113710

Mandal, S. C., & Mandal, M. (2010). Current status and future prospects of new drug delivery system. *Pharmacy Times*, *42*(4), 13–16.

Mansoori, M. A., & Agrawal, S. (2012). A review on liposome. *IJARPB*, *2*(4), 453–464.

Manu, C., & Vijay, N. (2012). *Topical micro-emulsions for the treatment of rheumatic disorders*. (EP 2437725 A1)

Marconi, B., Mancini, F., Colombo, P., Allegra, F., Giordano, F., Gazzaniga, A., Orecchia, G., & Santi, P. (1999). Distribution of khellin in excised human skin following iontophoresis and passive dermal transport. *Journal of Controlled Release*, *60*(2–3), 261–268. doi:10.1016/S0168-3659(99)00080-2 PMID:10425331

Marechal, D., & Wg, Y. (2006). *Sustained-release microgranules containing gingko biloba extract and the process for manufacturing these*. United States Patent 7569236.

Mathur, M. (2013). Approaches for improving the pharmacological and pharmacokinetic properties of herbal drugs. *Int. Res. J Pharm. App. Sci.*, *3*(4), 40–50.

Medina, O. P., Zhu, Y., & Kairemo, K. (2004). Targeted liposomal drug delivery in cancer. *Current Pharmaceutical Design*, *10*(24), 2981–2989. doi:10.2174/1381612043383467 PMID:15379663

Mei, Z., Chen, H., Weng, T., Yang, Y., & Yang, X. (2003). Solid lipid nanoparticle and microemulsion for topical delivery of triptolide. *European Journal of Pharmaceutics and Biopharmaceutics*, *56*(2), 189–196. doi:10.1016/S0939-6411(03)00067-5 PMID:12957632

Mei, Z., Li, X., Wu, Q., Hu, S., & Yang, X. (2005). The research on the anti-inflammatory activity and hepatotoxicity of triptolide-loaded solid lipid nanoparticle. *Pharmacological Research*, *51*(4), 345–351. doi:10.1016/j.phrs.2004.10.007 PMID:15683748

Mishra, D., & Panda, G. (2012). Novel drug delivery system for herbal formulation in cancer treatment. *World Journal of Pharmaceutical Research*, *6*(15), 341–353.

Mohamed, S., & El-Ridy, A. (2012). Niosomes as A novel pharmaceutical formulation encapsulating the hepatoprotective drug silymarin. *International Journal of Pharmacy and Pharmaceutical Sciences*, *4*(1), 549–559.

Mohnaraj, V. J., & Chen, Y. (2016). Nanoparticles-A review. *Tropical Journal of Pharmaceutical Research*, *5*(1), 561–573.

Mujaffar, F., & Singh, U. K. (2013). Review of microemulsion as futuristic drug delivery. *International Journal of Pharmacy and Pharmaceutical Sciences*, *5*, 39–51.

Mukherjee, P. K., & Harwansh, R. K. (2015). *Bioavailability of herbal products: Approach toward improved pharmacokinetics. Evidence-based validation of Herbal Medicine*. Elsevier, Inc. doi:10.1016/B978-0-12-800874-4.00010-6

Müller, R. H., Mäder, K., & Gohla, S. (2000). Solid lipid nanoparticles (SLN) for controlled drug delivery—A review of the state of the art. *European Journal of Pharmaceutics and Biopharmaceutics*, *50*(1), 161–177. doi:10.1016/S0939-6411(00)00087-4 PMID:10840199

Musthaba, S. M., Baboota, S., Ahmed, S., Ahuja, A., & Ali, J. (2009). Status of novel drug delivery technology for phytotherapeutics. *Expert Opinion on Drug Delivery*, *6*(6), 625–637. doi:10.1517/17425240902980154 PMID:19505192

Naik, S. R., Pilgaonkar, V. W., & Panda, V. S. (2006). Evaluation of antioxidant activity of Ginkgo biloba phytosomes in rat brain. *Phytotherapy Research*, *20*(11), 1013–1016. doi:10.1002/ptr.1976 PMID:16909446

Natarajan, V., Krithica, N., Madhan, B., & Sehgal, P. K. (2011). Formulation and evaluation of quercetin polycaprolactone microspheres for the treatment of rheumatoid arthritis. *Journal of Pharmaceutical Sciences*, *100*(1), 195–205. doi:10.1002/jps.22266 PMID:20607810

Nikalje, A. P., & Tiwari, S. (2012). Ethosomes: A Novel Tool for Transdermal Drug Delivery. *IJRPS*, *2*(1), 1–20.

Nishizawa, M., Menon, V. P., & Martin, C. R. (1995). Metal nanotubule membranes with electrochemically switchable ion-transport selectivity. *Science*, *268*(5211), 700–702. doi:10.1126cience.268.5211.700 PMID:17832383

Norman, G. B. (2001). A handbook for practice on a scientific basis (2nd ed). Stuttgart: Medpharm Scientific Publishers and CRC Press.

Parakh, S. R., & Gothoskar, A. V. (2003). Review of mouth dissolving tablet technologies. Pharmaceutical Technology. Duluth, MN: Advanstar Communications, ETATS-UNIS.

Park, K. (2014). Controlled drug delivery systems: Past forward and future back. *Journal of Controlled Release*, *190*, 3–8. doi:10.1016/j.jconrel.2014.03.054 PMID:24794901

Parth, S., & Surajpal, V. (2016). Global need for novel herbal drug formulations. *International Journal of Pharmacognosy and Phytochemical Research*, *8*(9), 1535–1544.

Pastore, M. N., Kalia, Y. N., Horstmann, M., & Roberts, M. S. (2015). Transdermal patches: History, development and pharmacology. *British Journal of Pharmacology*, *172*(9), 2179–2209. doi:10.1111/bph.13059 PMID:25560046

Patel, R., & Singh, S. K. (2009). Development and characterization of curcumin loaded transferosomes for transdermal delivery. *Journal of Pharmaceutical Sciences*, *1*, 71–80.

Patela, J., & Patelb, R. (2009). An overview of phytosomes as an advanced herbal drug delivery system. *Asian Journal of Pharmaceutical Sciences*, *4*(6), 363–371.

Patil, P. M., & Chaudhari, P. D. (2012). Recent trend in challenges and opportunities of transdermal drug delivery system. *International Journal of Drug Development and Research*, *4*, 39–50.

Pawar, H. A., & Bhangale, B. D. (2015). Phytosome as a Novel Biomedicine: A Microencapsulated. *Drug Delivery System*, *7*(1), 6–12.

Pawar, P., & Kalamkar, R. (2015). Ethosomes: A novel tool for herbal drug delivery. *Ijppr. Human*, *3*(4), 191–202.

Pinto, J. F. (2010). Site specific drug delivery systems within gastro intestinal tract: From the mouth to the colon. *International Journal of Pharmaceutics*, *395*(1-2), 44–52. doi:10.1016/j.ijpharm.2010.05.003 PMID:20546856

Prausnitz, M. R., & Langer, R. (2008). Transdermal drug delivery. *Nature Biotechnology*, *26*(11), 1261–1268. doi:10.1038/nbt.1504 PMID:18997767

Prausnitz, M. R., Mitragotri, S., & Langer, R. (2004). Current status and future potential of transdermal drug delivery. *Nature Reviews. Drug Discovery*, *3*(2), 115–124. doi:10.1038/nrd1304 PMID:15040576

Priprem, A., Sutthiparinyanont, S., Na, H.-K., Surh, Y.-J., & Chulasiri, M. (2015). Effect of formulations of nanosized quercetin liposomes on COX-2 and NF-kB in MCF-10A cells. *Pharmaceutical Nanotechnology*, *1*(1), 26–34. doi:10.2174/2211738511301010026

Pushpangadan, P., & Rao, C. (2007). *Novel antidiabetic herbal formulation*. US Patent (US 20070042062 A1).

Rahimpour, Y., & Hamishehkar, H. (2012). Niosomes as Carrier in Dermal Drug Delivery. In Recent advances in novel drug carrier systems (pp. 141–164). doi:10.5772/51729

Rasaie, S., & Ghanbarzadeh, S. (2014). Nano phytosomes of quercetin: A promising formulation for fortification of food products with antioxidants. *Pharmaceutical Sciences*, *20*, 96–101.

Rasheed, S. H., & Haribabu, R. (2011). Transdermal drug delivery system. Simplified medication regimen- A review. *Research Journal of Pharmaceutical, Biological and Chemical Sciences*, *2*, 223–238.

Sachan, R., & Parashar, T. (2013). Drug carrier Transfersomes: A novel tool for transdermal drug delivery system. *Int. J. Res. Dev. Pharm. Lex et Scientia*, *2*(2), 309–316.

Sahoo, S. K., & Labhasetwar, V. (2003). Nanotech approaches to drug delivery and imaging. *Drug Discovery Today*, *8*(24), 1112–1120. doi:10.1016/S1359-6446(03)02903-9 PMID:14678737

Saklani, A., & Kutty, S. K. (2008). Plant derived compounds in clinical trials. *Drug Discovery Today*, *13*(3–4), 161–171. doi:10.1016/j.drudis.2007.10.010 PMID:18275914

Schmid, G. (2011). *Nanoparticles: From theory to application*. John Wiley & Sons.

Schwarz, J. A. (2004). *Dekker encyclopedia of Nanoscienceand nanotechnology*. Marcel Dekker.

Seema, A. (2014). Recent development of herbal formulation- a novel drug. *Int. Ayur Med J.*, *2*(6), 952–958.

Selvam, R. P., & Singh, A. K. (2010). Transdermal drugdelivery systems for antihypertensive drugs-A review. *International Journal of Pharmaceutical and Biomedical Research*, *1*(1), 1–8.

Semalty, A., Semalty, M., Rawat, B. S., Singh, D., & Rawat, M. S. (2009). Pharmacosomes: The lipid-based new drug delivery system. *Expert Opinion on Drug Delivery*, *6*(6), 599–612. doi:10.1517/17425240902967607 PMID:19519287

Sharma, A. (2012). Transdermal approach of antidiabetic drug glibenclamide: A review. *Int. J. Pharm. Res. Dev.*, *3*, 25–32.

Sharma, D., Ali, A. A. E., & Aate, J. R. (2018). Niosomes as novel drug delivery system: Review article. *Pharmatutor*, *6*(3), 58–65. doi:10.29161/PT.v6.i3.2018.58

Sharma, G., Anabousi, S., Ehrhardt, C., & Ravi Kumar, M. N. (2006). Liposomes as targeted drug delivery systems in the treatment of breast cancer. *Journal of Drug Targeting*, *14*(5), 301–310. doi:10.1080/10611860600809112 PMID:16882550

Sharma, M. (2014). Application of nanotechnology based dosage form for delivery of herbal drugs. *Research and Reviews: Journal of Pharmaceutics and Nanotechnology*, *2*(1), 23–30.

Shrivastava, D. (2012). Transdermal approach of antidiabetic drug glibenclamide: A review. *World Journal of Pharmacy and Pharmaceutical Sciences*, *1*, 532–544.

Sintov, A. C. (2015). Transdermal delivery of curcumin via microemulsion. *International Journal of Pharmaceutics*, *481*(1–2), 97–103. doi:10.1016/j.ijpharm.2015.02.005

Smith, A. (2009). *The benefits of natural medicine*. Retrieved from http://ezinearticles.com/?expert=Alden_Smith

Sohn, B. H., & Cohen, R. E. (1991). *Chem Mater. Processible optically transparent block copolymer films containing super paramagnetic iron oxide nano preparation*. Academic Press.

Solecki, R. S., & Shanidar, I. V. (1975). A neanderrhal flower burial in northern Iraq. *Science*, *190*, 880–881.

Srikanth, P., & Raju, N. (2013). A review on oral controlled drug delivery. *Int. J. Adv. Pharm.*, *3*, 51–58.

Sterer, N., Nuas, S., Mizrahi, B., Goldenberg, C., Weiss, E. I., Domb, A., & Davidi, M. P. (2008). Oral malodor reduction by a palatal mucoadhesive tablet containing herbal formulation. *Journal of Dentistry*, *36*(7), 535–539. doi:10.1016/j.jdent.2008.04.001

Sungthongjeen, S., Puttipipatkhachorn, S., Paeratakul, O., Dashevsky, A., & Bodmeier, R. (2004). Development of pulsatile release tablets with swelling and rupturable layers. *Journal of Controlled Release*, *95*(2), 147–159. doi:10.1016/j.jconrel.2003.10.023

Tarun, P., & Soniya. (2013). Ethosomes: A recent vesicle of transdermal drug delivery system. *International Journal of Research and Development in Pharmacy and Life Sciences*, *2*(2), 285–292.

Terreno, E., Delli Castelli, D. D., Cabella, C., Dastrù, W., Sanino, A., Stancanello, J., ... Aime, S. (2008). Paramagnetic liposomes as innovative contrast agents for magnetic resonance (MR) molecular imaging applications. *Chemistry & Biodiversity*, *5*(10), 1901–1912. doi:10.1002/cbdv.200890178

Thapa, R. K., & Khan, G. M. (2013). Herbal Medicine Incorporated nanoparticles: Advancements in herbal treatment. *Asian Journal of Biomedical and Pharmaceutical Sciences*, *3*(24), 7–14.

Tian, Q., Wang, W., He, X., Zhu, X., Huang, W., Zhang, C., & Chen, X. (2009). Glycyrrhetinic acid-modified nanoparticles for drug delivery: Preparation and characterization. *Chinese Science Bulletin*, *54*(18), 3121–3126. doi:10.100711434-009-0249-5

Tong, W., Wang, L., & D'Souza, M. J. (2003). Evaluation of PLGA microspheres as delivery system for antitumor agentcamptothecin. *Drug Development and Industrial Pharmacy*, *29*(7), 745–756. doi:10.1081/ddc-120021774

Uhumwangho, M. U., & Okor, R. S. (2005). Current trends in the production and biomedical applications of liposomes: A review. *Journal of Medicine and Biomedical Research*, *4*(1), 9–21. doi:10.4314/jmbr.v4i1.10663

Varde, N. K., & Pack, D. W. (2004). Microspheres for controlled release drug delivery. *Expert Opinion on Biological Therapy*, *4*(1), 35–51. doi:10.1517/14712598.4.1.35

Vasir, J. K., Tambwekar, K., & Garg, S. (2003). Bioadhesive microspheres as a controlled drug delivery system. *International Journal of Pharmaceutics*, *255*(1–2), 13–32. doi:10.10160378-5173(03)00087-5

Verma, H., & Prasad, S. B. (2013). Herbal drug delivery system: A modern era prospective. *International Journal of Current Pharmaceutical Review and Research*, *4*, 88–101.

Verma, M., & Gupta, P. K. (2007). Development of transdermal drug dosage formulation for the anti-rheumatic ayurvedic medicinal plants. *Ancient Science of Life*, *11*, 66–69.

Verma, P., & Pathak, K. (2010). Therapeutic and cosmeceutical potential of ethosomes: An overview. *Journal of Advanced Pharmaceutical Technology & Research*, *1*(3), 274–282. doi:10.4103/0110-5558.72415

Vyas, S. P., & Khar, R. K. (2002). *Targeted and controlled drug delivery novel carrier systems* (1st ed.). CBS Publishers.

Waghulde, S., & Naik, P. (2013). Development, recent inventions and evaluation techniques of transdermal drug delivery system—A review. *International Journal of Pharmaceutical and Phytopharmacological Research*, *3*(2), 152–160.

Waghulde, S., & Naik, P. (2017). An overview of therapeutic applications. *Advances in Medical Technologies and Clinical Practice*, •••, 1–25. doi:10.4018/978-1-5225-0751-2.ch001

Walve, J. R., & Bakliwal, S. R. (2011). Transfersomes: A surrogated carrier for transdermal drug delivery system. *International Journal of Applied Biology and Pharmaceutical Technology*, 2(1), 204–213.

Wang, W. (2008). *Why is a novel drug delivery system important for herbal or ayurvedic medicines*. Retrieved from http://www.articlealley.com/article_673669_17.html

Xiao, Y. L., & Li, B. (2002). Chine. *Trad. Herb. Drugs*, *33*, 385–388.

Xiao-Ying, L., Luo, J. B., Yan, Z. H., Rong, H. S., & Huang, W. M. (2006). Preparation and in vitro and in vivo evaluations of topically applied capsaicin transfersomes. *Yao Xue Xue Bao*, *41*(5), 461–466.

Xu, X., & Burgess, D. J. (2011). Liposomes as carriers for controlled drug delivery. *Advances in Delivery Science and Technology*, *3*, 195–220.

Yadav, D., & Suri, S. (2011). Novel Approach: Herbal Remedies And Natural Products In Pharmaceutical Science As Nano Drug Delivery Systems. *IJPT*, *3*(3), 3092–3116.

Yadav, M., Bhatia, V. J., & Doshi, G. (2014). Novel techniques in herbal drug delivery systems. *International Journal of Pharmaceutical Sciences Review and Research, 28*(2), 83–89.

Yang, T., Cui, F. D., Choi, M. K., Lin, H., Chung, S. J., Shim, C. K., & Kim, D. D. (2007). Liposome formulation of paclitaxel with enhanced solubility and stability. *Drug Delivery, 14*(5), 301–308. doi:10.1080/10717540601098799

Yin, Y. M., Cui, F. D., Mu, C. F., Choi, M. K., Kim, J. S., Chung, S. J., ... Kim, D. D. (2009). Docetaxel microemulsion for enhanced oral bioavailability: Preparation and in vitro and in vivo evaluation. *Journal of Controlled Release, 140*(2), 86–94. doi:10.1016/j.jconrel.2009.08.015

Yuan, D. F., & Yi, Y. M. (2003). Her. *El Medico, 22*, 113–114.

Zeisser-Labouèbe, M., Lange, N., Gurny, R., & Delie, F. (2006). Hypericin-loaded nanoparticles for the photodynamic treatment of ovarian cancer. *International Journal of Pharmaceutics, 326*(1–2), 174–181. doi:10.1016/j.ijpharm.2006.07.012

Zeng, F., & Zimmerman, S. C. (1997). Dendrimers in Supramolecular Chemistry: From Molecular Recognition to Self-Assembly. *Chemical Reviews, 97*(5), 1681–1712. doi:10.1021/cr9603892

Zhang, D., & Guan, L. I. (2008). *Preparation and characterization of biodegradable polylactide (PLA) microspheres encapsulating ginsenoside Rg3, 24*. Chem Res. Chin. University.

Zhang, J., Tang, Q., Xu, X., & Li, N. (2013). Development and evaluation of a novel phytosome-loaded chitosan microsphere system for curcumin delivery. *International Journal of Pharmaceutics, 448*(1), 168–174. doi:10.1016/j.ijpharm.2013.03.021

Zhang, L., Pornpattananangku, D., Hu, C. M., & Huang, C. M. (2010). Development of nanoparticles for antimicrobial drug delivery. *Current Medicinal Chemistry, 17*(6), 585–594. doi:10.2174/092986710790416290

Zhaowu, Z., Xiaoli, W., Yangde, Z., & Nianfeng, L. (2009). Preparation of matrine ethosome, its percutaneous permeation in vitro and anti-inflammatory activity in vivo in rats. *Journal of Liposome Research, 19*(2), 155–162. doi:10.1080/08982100902722381

Zhigaltsev, I. V., Maurer, N., Akhong, Q. F., Leone, R., Leng, E., Wang, J., ... Cullis, P. R. (2005). Liposome-encapsulated vincristine, vinblastine and vinorelbine: A comparative study of drug loading and retention. *Journal of Controlled Release, 104*(1), 103–111. doi:10.1016/j.jconrel.2005.01.010

Chapter 6
Nanoparticles for the Enhancement of the Therapeutic Efficacy of Herbal Formulations

Mohammad Irfan Ali
Suresh Gyan Vihar University, Jaipur, India

Jyotsna Dayma
Suresh Gyan Vihar University, Jaipur, India

Sarmad Moin
https://orcid.org/0000-0003-2521-2731
Suresh Gyan Vihar University, Jaipur, India

ABSTRACT

Nano dosage forms the drug delivery method of herbal formulation used for improving the efficacy and overwhelming the problems related to plant medicines. Therefore, incorporation of the nano-sized carrier in conventional plant-derived medicine is essential to cure more chronic and lifestyle diseases. Several nano dosage forms like polymeric nanoparticles, liposomes, lipid nanoparticles, nano-emulsion, proliposomes, etc. has great advantages for herbal medicine including bioavailability, enhancement of solubility, improvement of pharmacological activity, protection from toxicity, stability enhancement, sustained delivery, improving the distribution of macrophages, protection from chemical, and physical degradation. The chapter focused on the advantages of nano herbal formulations over traditional herbal formulations.

DOI: 10.4018/978-1-7998-4453-2.ch006

1. INTRODUCTION

Nanotechnology is a domain of science that amalgamates different streams of science and technology. The most peculiarity about nanotechnology is, it conducted at the scale, which is nearby 1 to 100nm, hence the name "Nanotechnology". Nanotechnology is a multifaceted discipline that covers technology and research from the fields of physics, biology, and chemistry. The incredible growth in this emerging field has unlocked new limits for the synthesis, exploration, and utilization of nanoparticles.

The nanoparticles are commonly found in nature because of various events like photochemical and volcanic activities, combustion process, cooking of food, automobile exhausts, and creation of reactive oxygen species (ROS) is of prime importance. Metals like gold, silver, platinum, copper, palladium, iron and zinc are used for the fabrication of nanoparticles (Haleemkhan *et al.*, 2015). These nanoparticles have applications in particles in diverse fields. Even though nanoparticles can be produced by using many physicochemical methods, their production using non-toxic and environmentally benevolent biological methods are attractive, especially for application in medicine (Shah *et al.*, 2015). Plants have this uniqueness to reduce the metal ions on their surface and far-flung from the site of ion penetration. Lower organisms like algae, actinomycetes, bacteria, and fungi also possess the potential to produce nanoparticles. A nanoparticle from biological sources reduces environmental impact compared with some of the physicochemical production approaches and be able to use to fabricate enormous amounts of nanoparticles that are devoid of impurity and have a well-defined dimension and morphology (Makarov *et al.*, 2014).

Synthesis of nanoparticles can be achieved mainly by following two approaches either a "top-down" approach or a "bottom-up" approach (Sepeur *et al.*, 2013). In the top-down approach, reduction in dimension from appropriate starting material is accomplished by numerous physical and chemical treatments (Meyers *et al.*, 2006). Irregularities in the outer surface structure and surface chemistry of the nanoparticles is the main drawback of this approach. The dependency of various physical features of nanoparticles on the outer surface structure again imparts limitations on this approach (Thakkar *et al.*, 2010).

On the contrary, the bottom-up approach involves the fabrication of nanoparticles from smaller entities like atoms, molecules, and smaller particles and mostly relies on biological and chemical methods (Mukherjee *et al.*, 2001). In this approach first, the building blocks of the nanoparticles are formed which is then followed by assembling the nano-structure to produce the final particle (Thakkar *et al.*, 2010).

1.1 Nanoparticles in Herbal Formulation

Since primordial times, the herbal formulation has been extensively used globally for their superior therapeutic values and scarcer antagonistic effects as compared to contemporary therapeutics (Arulanandraj et al., 2018, Kesharwani et al., 2019). For a long period, the herbal formulation was not exploited for the fabrication of novel medicine due to the deficiency of processing difficulties and scientific justification. However, nowadays, the modern research can fulfil the scientific needs of the herbal drug for development of nano-drug delivery systems like microspheres, lipid nanoparticles, nanoparticles, liposomes and other carrier system (Figure 1). The foremost benefit of nano-drug delivery systems for directed drug delivery increases the solubility, reduces dosage frequency absorption and reduce elimination (Yadev *et al.*, 2011) that depicted in figure 2.

Berberine is an isoquinoline alkaloid naturally occurring in *Berberis vulgaris* L. have the anti-tumor properties against esophageal cancer, brain tumor, colon cancer, and human leukemic cell lines; (Reichard

Figure 1. Various type of nanocarrier used in Herbal drug delivery

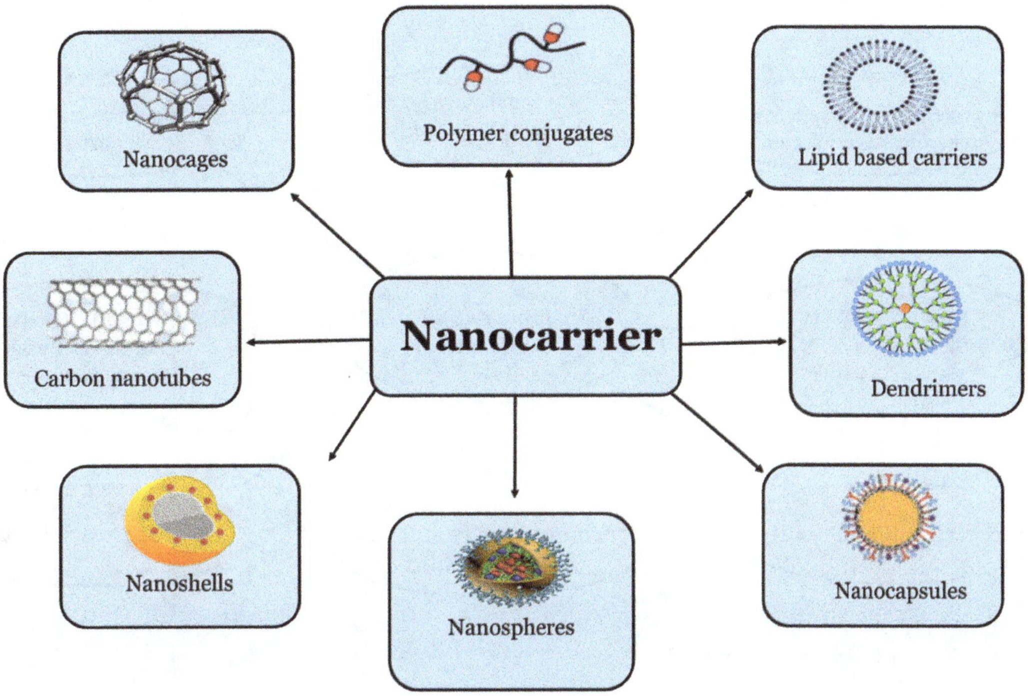

et al., 2007). Berberine loaded nanoparticles are efficaciously synthesized using single emulsion, ionic gelation, multiple emulsion methods used for sustained release of the drug (Arulanandraj *et al.*, 2018).

The fabrication of nanoparticles from *Centella asiatica* extract to protect from moisture entrapped in Chitosan- alginate nanoparticles by ionic gelation technique (Okonogai *et al.*, 2008). However, because of its undersized half-life, rapid metabolism, deprived water solubility, fast elimination, poor bioavailability its applications were limited (Anand *et al.*, 2007). Nanoparticles of curcumin synthesized by wet milling technique overcome these problems and improving the efficacy of herbal formulation (Bisht *et al.*, 2007).

Dehydrated roots of *Salvia miltiorrhiza* L. Danshen, are extensively used for improving blood stasis, promoting circulation, cerebrovascular diseases coronary heart disease, and hyperlipidemia (Zhou *et al.*, 2006). Nano formulation of Salvia miltiorrhiza reveals the higher antioxidant potential and the discharge pattern than the conventional formulation (Liu *et al.*, 2008). Loaded nanoparticles of *Salvia miltiorrhiza* with phospholipids complex also enhanced bioavailability orally (Peng *et al.*, 2008).

Cuscuta chinensis used as anti-aging, anti-cancer and immune-modulatory effects and Nanoparticles of *Cuscuta chinensis* produced by nano-precipitation exhibits higher antioxidant activities as well as hepatoprotective at lower concentration method activity (Yen *et al.*, 2008). Paclitaxel is an anticancer drug extracted from the *Taxus brevifolia* Nutt bark. Integration of paclitaxel into nanoparticles to enhance its anti-tumoral activity, improve bioavailability, drug stability, sustained release of the drug (Breuning *et al.*, 2008). Quercetin is a chemically flavonoid isolated from *Spohora japonica* L. used as antioxidant, anticancer, and antiviral agent. The nano-encapsulation of Quercetin with poly-D, L-lactide prepared

Figure 2. Various advantages of Herbal nanocarrier

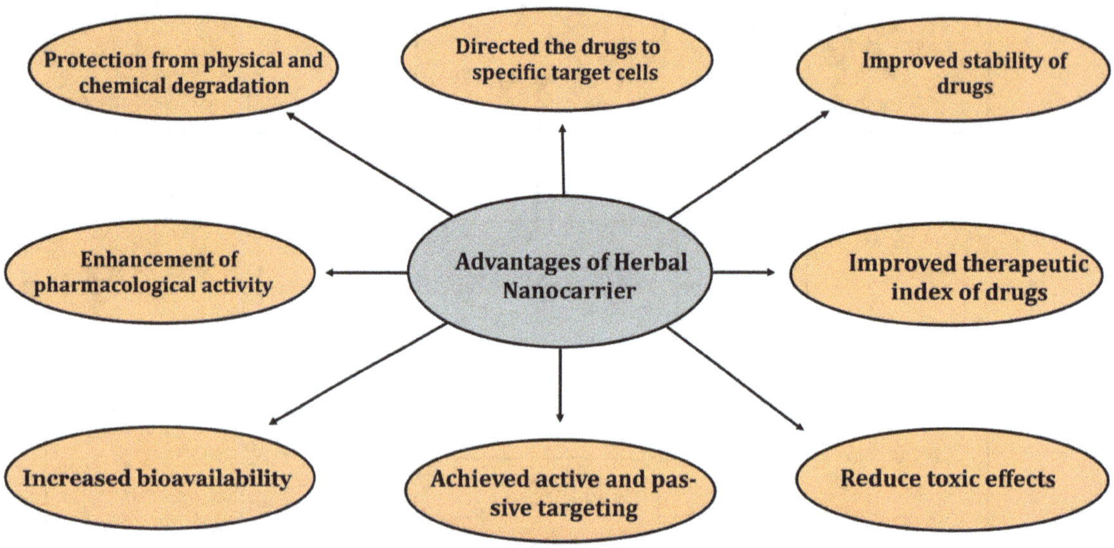

by solvent evaporation technique enhances the therapeutic effectiveness and bioavailability (Kumar *et al.*, 2010).

Kaempferia parviflora (KP) is used for male sexual function and enhancement of physical fitness. Little absorption by the oral route of the main bioactive component, methoxy flavones occur in the traditional method. Nanosuspensions produced by the spray drying method has relatively high stability, high intestinal absorption and fast dissolution rate (Mekjaruskul and Sripanidkulchai 2020).

An herbal formulation of kaempferol (KA) containing flavonoid with antiangiogenic potential used in eye diseases, corneal neovascularization for the inhibited formation of the vessel. Encapsulation of kaempferol (KA), with gelatin nanoparticles (GNP) used for corneal neovascularization treatment by topical distribution, have better therapeutic effects, greater bioavailability and sluggish discharge of the constituents (Chuang *et al.*, 2019).

Herbal extract used to stimulating hair growth exhibits anti-inflammatory activities however, its efficacy has been limited due to little ability to penetration into follicles of hair. The prepared hydrogels by poly(γ-glutamic acid) (PGA) containing herbal extract mixtures into chitosan (CS). Hydrogel nanoparticle formulation is as a potential efficacy for enhancing hair growth by the accumulation of hair growth stimulating compounds into hair follicles (Kim *et al.*, 2019). Nanoparticles used in herbal formulation mentioned in Table 1.

Table 1. Nanoparticles in herbal formulation

S. N.	Nano-formulation	Carrier/Method	Application	References
1.	Curcumin-loaded nanoformulation	Poly(2-propyl-2-oxazine) (A-pPrOzi-A)	Anti-metastatic potential	Lübtow *et al.*, 2019
2.	*Leucas aspera* nanoparticles	Precipitation method.	Anticancerous activity in prostate cancer.	Mohan *et al.*, 2017
3.	*Artemissia annua* Nanoparticle	Encapsulation	Antimalarial action	Sathyavathi *et al.*, 2010
4.	Berberine loaded nanoparticles	Single or multiple emulsion, and ionic gelation approaches	Anti-tumor properties	Reichard *et al.*, 2007
5.	*Centella asiatica* nanoparticles	Chitosan- alginate nanoparticles by ionic gelation technique	Treatment of leprosy, cancer, allergy and syphilis	Okonogai *et al.*, 2008
6.	Curcumin nanoparticles	wet milling technique	Anticancer	Bisht *et al.*, 2007
7.	Nano-coated *Salvia miltiorrhiza*	Dry method	Antioxidant property	Liu *et al.*, 2008
8.	Nanocoated *Cuscutta chinensis*	Nano-precipitation method	Heptoprotective and antioxidant activities	Yen *et al.*, 2008
9.	Genistein nanoparticles	Nano-precipitation method	Osteoporosis, breast and uterine cancer, cardiovascular diseases,	Tang *et al.*, 2011
10.	Paclitaxel nanoparticles	lipid based nanoparticles	Anticancer	Dong *et al.*, 2009
11.	Quercetin nanoparticles	PLA (poly-D, L-lactide) by solvent evaporation technique	Antioxidant activity	Kumar *et al.*, 2010

1.2 Plant Mediated Synthesis of Nano-Formulation

Nanoparticles synthesized from plant extract provides advancement over other methods because of its simplicity, cost-effective, environment-friendly and relatively reproducible and readily scalable properties (Iravani, 2011). The plant may act as both, reducing agents as well as stabilizing components in the fabrication of nanoparticles (Kumar and Yadav, 2011). A wide category of nanoparticles can be synthesized from plant extract as different plant extracts have diverse amalgamations of organic reducing components (Mukunthan and Balaji, 2012). Production of nanoparticles by using medicinal plant extracts involves the mixing of a plant extract with a metal salt solution at room temperature. Nanoparticles of gold, silver and many other novel metals have been synthesized in this way (Li *et al.*, 2011).

In medicine, silver nanoparticles from plant extract are used in the treatment of various ailments, even cancer. Silver nanoparticles synthesized from geraniol and *Melia azedarach* showed inhibitory effect on fibrosarcoma "Wehi 164 cancer cell line" (Safaepour *et al.*, 2009) and cancer cell line of HeLa cervical (Sukirtha *et al.*, 2011) respectively. Similarly, the superior hypoglycaemic potential of silver nanoparticles over the extract of *Cassia fistula* bark alone was revealed by Daisy and Saipriya in 2012. This finding could be proved very beneficial in the management of diabetes mellitus.

Silver nanoparticles have been proved to be a very effective antimicrobial agent. High antimicrobial activity against both Gram-negative (*E. coli*) and Gram-positive (*Streptococcus aureus*) microorganisms were shown by silver nanoparticles synthesized using *Ocimum sanctum* leaf extracts (Singhal *et al.*, 2011). Silver nanoparticles obtained from the aromatic swath of screw pine inflorescence were found more genotoxic but fewer cytotoxicity as compared to Ag+ ion (Panda *et al.*, 2011). Baskaralingam *et al.*, (2012) used an extract of *Calotropis gigantea* leaf to synthesize silver nanoparticles. These nanoparticles had antibacterial potential against *Vibrio alginolyticus*. Similarly, the extract of *Cinnamomum camphora* leaf which is endowed with a plethora of secondary metabolites like phenolics, terpenoids, polysaccharides, and flavones was employed for the synthesis of gold and silver nanoparticles and proved to be bactericidal at a concentration of 45 μg/mL (Huang *et al.*, 2007). Gold and silver nanoparticles of different shapes from the extract of *Dioscorea bulbifera* tuber were produced by Ghosh *et al.*, 2011. They found that these nanoparticles in blend with antibiotics have a synergistic effect against Pseudomonas aeruginosa, *Escherichia coli* and *Acinetobacter baumannii* (Ghosh *et al.*, 2012).

Silver nanoparticles produced from *Syzygium cumin* have a greater antioxidant potential comparison with the antioxidant potential of seeds *in vitro* (Banerjee and Narendhirakannan, 2011). Plant-derived nanoparticles varied in different shapes and sizes depending upon various factors. Silver nanoparticles produced from decoction of *Citrus sinensis* peel at 60 °C with average size around 10 nm have a broad spectrum antibacterial potential (Kaviya *et al.*, 2011b) as compared to nanoparticles synthesized at reduces temperature up to 25 °C this is because at low-temperature average size of the particles is increased up to 35 nm hence, show reduced activity. Prathna *et al.*, (2011a) stated the fabrication of silver nanoparticles by using an extract of *Azadirachta indica* leaves and concluded that by enhancing the reaction time as of 30 min to 4 h, the particle size progressively increases as of around 10 nm to around 35 nm. Prathna *et al.*, (2011b) reported the production of spherical 50 nm silver nanoparticles using extracts of *Citrus limon*. The citric acid found in the extracts was the main reducing agent. One-step fabrication of silver nanoparticles by using *Papaver somniferum* and *Trachyspermum ammi* extracts was worked out by Vijayaraghavan *et al.*, (2012). The aqueous decoction of *Trachyspermum ammi* created nanoparticles of size range 87–998 nm of different triangular shapes and the aqueous decoction of *Papaver somniferum* produced spherical shaped microparticles of size range 3–8 μm. An exceptionally stable silver nanoparticle (16–40 nm) from the secondary metabolites obtained from the extract of Datura leaf was produced by Kesharwani *et al.*, (2009). Kasthuri *et al.*, (2009) synthesized triangular and hexagonal gold nanoparticles from HAuCl4 by using the dilute extract of *Phyllanthus amarus* containing phyllanthin. Decreasing the dilution of the extract produced by spherical nanoparticles.

Narayanan and Sakthivel (2008) synthesized gold nanoparticles by using a decoction of *Coriandrum sativum* leaf of size from 7 to 58 nm with different shapes such as spherical, decahedral, triangular). Production of spherical and triangular gold and silver nanoparticles by using a decoction of *Tanacetum vulgare* fruit (Dubey *et al.*, 2010). An FTIR study discovered the carbonyl groups act as a reducing agent. Liu *et al.*, (2012) developed an assay based on nanoparticle for quantifying antioxidant properties of tea. Palladium nanoparticles having a size of 15 nm were produced by using the extract of Glycine max soybean leaf (Kumar *et al.*, 2012) whereas Lee *et al.*, (2011) employed copper for synthesizing nanoparticles (40–100 nm) using magnolia leaf extract.

The nanoparticles synthesized by using the decoction of *Syzygium cumini* (L.) seed have stronger antioxidant potential as compared to the crude extract (Banerjee and Narendhirakannan, 2011). The gold nanoparticles from seed aqueous extract of *Abelmoschus esculentu* reported antifungal potential against *Puccinia graminis* tritci, *Aspergillus flavus*, *Aspergillus niger* and *Candida albicans* (Jayaseelan *et al.*, 2013) The production of gold nanoparticles by chloroauric acid ($HAuCl_4$) by using plant extracts of *Angelica*, *Hamamelis*, *Hypericum*, exploited in medical and biological applications (Pasca *et al.*, 2014). A number of nanoparticles synthesized from plants listed in Table 2.

1.3 Algae and Cyanobacteria Mediated Nano-Formulation

Cyanobacteria produce a number of chemically diverse and bioactive compounds like cyclic peptides, fatty acid amides, lipopeptides, and alkaloids. Many marine cyanobacteria are used for the fabrication of herbal formulation and extraction of the bioactive compound, which remains effective against cancer by inducing apoptosis. The current scenario not even 10% of bioactive components extracted from microalgae have commercialized attributable to complications related to its solubility. Nano-formulations overcome these problems and produced an extensive variety of nanoparticles and their polymerized forms may perhaps be an emergent approach for the progress of new cancer drugs (Bajpai *et al.,* 2018). Phycocyanin is a natural anti-inflammatory extracted from cyanobacteria and its nano-formulation with propylene glycol inclosing vesicles used to improve the delivery of phycocyanin to the deep skin layers. Algae are the ridiculous source of biologically active substances therefore used in intra- or extracellular biosynthesis of nanoparticles. Among various algae, microalgae are regarded as cell factories for biological synthesis of nanoparticles, because of their high biomass productivity and growth rate. Furthermore, they have been proved as a potential microorganism for detoxification of heavy metal through bioremediation and production of various metabolites that are exploiting commercially. They not only collect metals by chemical transformation and chelation, but are also produce bio-mineral structures and metal nanoparticles (Jenaa *et al.,* 2013 and Jena *et al.,* 2014). The fabrication of nanoparticles of metal from algae is made by collecting, washing, drying and grinding of algal biomass. Later on grinded algal biomass is dissolved in solution containing the metal precursors, an organic or inorganic salt (e.g. $HAuCl_4$, $AgNO_3$, Lead acetate, etc.) in distinct experimental situations to react with redox agents like oxygen and energy sources like oven and microwave for a definite time until the existence of nanoparticles is noticed (Merin *et al.,* 2010, Arockiya, *et al.,* 2012).

Gold nanoparticles produced by using *Turbinaria conoides* (marine brown algae) and antibacterial activity shows maximum inhibition against *Streptococcus* sp. and moderate inhibition counters to *Bacillus subtilis* and *Klebsiella pneumonia* (Mittal *et al.,* 2013). A novel biological synthetic approach was reported as rapid, simple and green for the fabrication of silver nanoparticle by using *Kappaphycus alverazii* and blend of algal culture of *Chaetoceros calcitrans, Chlorella salina, Isochrysis galbana* and *Tetraselmis gracilis* (Ganesan *et al.,* 2013 and Sharma *et al.,* 2014). Seaweeds were also used as reducing and capping agents in the fabrication of the novel metal nanoparticles. The silver nanoparticles show good antibacterial activity hence may be used in medicine as sterile clothing and wound dressing in hospitals (Shiny, *et al.,* 2013). Abboud *et al.,* in 2014, revealed that the water-soluble compounds diterpenoids are found in the extract of *Bifurcaria Bifurcata* responsible for the reduction and stabilization of CuO nanoparticles and concluded that these synthesized CuO nanoparticles had antibacterial potential against Gram-negative and Gram-positive bacteria. Cyanobacteria or Blue-green algae are photosynthetic bacteria that have the capacity to synthesize different metal nanoparticles like Copper, Silver, Gold, and Palladium. For example, Silver nanoparticles produced by aqueous extract and live biomass of *Spirulina platensis* (Tsibakhashvili *et al.,* 2011 and Mahdieha *et al.,* 2012). Cyanobacteria can synthesize nanoparticles in both intracellular and extracellular environments. *Synechocystis* sp. (Focsan *et al.,* 2011) and *Plectonema boryanum* (Lengke *et al.,* 2006) both were reported for the fabrication of gold nanoparticle intracellularly. The interaction of *P. boryanum* biomass with aqueous palladium (II) chloride ($PdCl_2$) at 25-100 °C for 28 days reported for the fabrication of palladium nanoparticles (Fleet *et al.,* 2007 and Lengke *et al.,* 2007). Cyanobacteria, *P. boryanum* accumulate gold from aqueous gold (III)-chloride and also encourage the precipitation of amorphous gold (I) sulphide at their cell walls (Lengke *et al.,*

Table 2. Nanoparticles synthesized by Plants

Plants	Plant part used	Nanoparticle	Size	Reference
Aloe vera	Leaves	In_2O_3NPs	5-50 nm	Maensiria *et al.*, 2008
Aloe vera	Leaves	ZnONPs	25-40 nm	Gunalana *et al.*, 2012
Aloe indica	Leaves	AgNPs	29-36 nm	Natarajan *et al.*, 2012
Aloe vera	Leaves	AuNPs	-	Chandran *et al.*, 2006
Acalypha indica	Leaves	CuO NPs	26-30 nm	Sivaraj *et al.*, 2014
Amaranthus polygonoides	Leaves	AgNPs	40-50 nm	Firdhouse and Lalitha, 2013
Ananas comosus	Fruits	AuNPs	-	Basavegowda *et al.*, 2013
Avena sativa	Leaves	AuNPs	-	Armendariz *et al.*, 2004
Azadirachta indica	Leaves	AgNPs, AuNPs	50–100 nm	Shankar *et al.*, 2004
Boswellia ovalifoliolata, Shorea tumbuggaia, Svensonia hyderobadensis Thespesia populnea and Vinca rosea	Leaves	AgNPs	-	Savithramma *et al.*, 2012
Brassica juncea, Festuca rubra and Medicago sativa.	In vivo synthesis	AgNPs	-	Marchiol *et al.*, 2014
Calotropis Gigantea	Leaves	ZnONPs	30-35 nm	Vidya *et al.*, 2013
Calotropis procera	Latex	ZnONPs	5-40 nm	Singh *et al.*, 2011
Calotropis procera	Latex	Cu NPs	15 ± 1.7 nm	Harne *et al.*, 2012
Camellia sinensis	Leaves	Fe_2O_3NPs	60 nm	Ahmmad *et al.*, 2013
Capsicum annuum	Leaves	AgNPs	10-12	Li *et al.*, 2007
Carica papaya	Leaves	AgNPs	2-5 nm	Komal and Arya, 2013
Chrysanthemum morifolium	Flowers	AgNPs	20-50 nm	He *et al.*, 2013
Cinnamommum camphora	Leaves	AgNPs	55–80 nm	Huang *et al.*, 2007
Cinnamon zeylanicum	Bark	AgNPs	31-40 nm	Sathishkumar *et al.*, 2009
Coriandrum sativum	Leaves	AgNPs	26 nm	Sathyavathi *et al.*, 2010
Cycas	Leaves	AgNPs	3.29	Jha and Prasad, 2010
Diopyros kaki	Leaves	PtNPs	2 - 12 nm	Song *et al.*, 2010
Emblica officinalis	Leaves	AgNPs, AuNPs	10–20 nm, 15–25 nm	Ankamwar *et al.*, 2005
Eucalyptus camaldulensis	Leaves	AuNPs	6–20 nm	Haratifar *et al.*, 2009
Gliricidia sepium	Leaves	AgNPs	27 nm	Rajesh *et al.*, 2009
Jatropha curcas	Seeds	AgNPs	15 - 50 nm	Bar *et al.*, 2009
Leucas martinicensis	Leaves	AgNPs	20-25 nm	Ashokkumar *et al.*, 2014
Medicago sativa	Leaves	AuNPs	15–200 nm	Singh *et al.*, 2006
Medicago sativa	Leaves	AuNPs	4–10 nm	Gardea-Torresdey *et al.*, 2002
Momordica charantia	fruit peel extract	AuNPs	10-100 nm	Pandey *et al.*, 2012
Moringa oleifera	Leaves	AgNPs	57 nm	Prasad *et al.*, 2011
Murraya koenigii	Leaves	AgNPs	20 nm	Philip 2011 and Philip *et al.*, 2011
Olax scandens	Leaves	AgNPs	20-60 nm	Mukherjee *et al.*, 2014
Olea Europaea	Leaves	AgNPs	20-25 nm	Khalil *et al.*, 2013
Passiflora tripartite	Fruits	Fe_3O_4 NPs	22.3±3 nm	Kumar *et al.*, 2014
Piper nigrum	Leaves and Stem	AgNPs	7–50nm and 9–30 nm respectively	Paulkumar *et al.*, 2014
Portulaca oleracea	Leaves	AgNPs	60 nm	Firdhouse and Lalitha, 2013
Sesbania	Leaves	AuNPs	6–20 nm	Sharma *et al.*, 2007
Solanum tricobatum, Syzygium cumini, Centella asiatica and Citrus sinensis	Plant Powder	AgNPs	53, 41, 52 and 42 nm respectively	Logeswari *et al.*, 2013
Tamarindus indica	Leaves	AuNPs	-	Ankamwar *et al.*, 2005
Trianthema decandra	Root extract	AuNPs, AgNPs	33–65 nm, 36–74 nm	Geethalakshmi and Sarada, 2012
Triticum aestivum	Leaves	AuNPs	10–30 nm	Armendariz *et al.*, 2002
Vitis vinifera	Raisin	SeNPs	3-18 nm	Sharma *et al.*, 2014
Glycyrrhiza glabra	Aquous extract	AgNPs	9nm	Osvelia *et al.*, 2016
Zea mays	Aquous extract	AgNPs	-	Patra and Baek, 2017

2006) and to destabilize gold (I) thiosulfate complex to zero-valent gold sulfate-reducing bacteria was used (Fleet *et al.,* 2006). *P. boryanum* related to gold (I) thiosulphate improved the accumulation of nanoparticles of size ranging ≤10 nm in membrane vesicles. However, in the existence of $AuCl_4$– 1–10 µm size octahedral gold platelets were observed (Kannan *et al.,* 2010).

In the case of extracellular synthesis of nanoparticles, copper oxide nanoparticles from *Phormidium* cyanobacterium were observed on the hydrolysis of cationic copper by chelating protein or reductase enzyme secreted by bacteria. The SDS-PAGE analysis of chelating proteins or reductase enzymes revealed their importance in the reduction and stabilization of copper nanoparticles (Rahman *et al.,* 2009). Sulfated polysaccharides have also been proved as reducing and stabilizing agents in the synthesis of iron oxide nanoparticles (Fe3O4-NPs) by aqueous extract of *Sargassum muticum* (Mahdavi *et al.,* 2013). The extracellular fabrication of silver nanoparticles from aqueous extracts of *Spirulina platensis* was achieved by challenging the extract with the silver nitrate solution. Formation of dark brown solution established the silver ion reduction to silver nanoparticles. This biotransformation occurs at the beginning of the reaction and UV visible spectra indicated the presence of silver nanoparticles (Sharma *et al.,* 2015). Nanoparticle synthesized by algae and cyanobacteria listed in Table 3.

Table 3. Nanoparticles synthesized by algae and cyanobacteria

Algae	Nanoparticle	Size	Reference
Bifurcaria bifurcate	CuONPs	Average size 20.66 nm	Abboud *et al.,* 2014
Caulerpa peltata, Hypnea Valencia and Sargassum myriocystum	ZnONPs	36 nm	Nagarajan and Kuppusamy, 2013
Chaetoceros calcitrans, Chlorella salina, Isochrysis galbana and *Tetraselmis gracilis*	AgNPs	53.1-71.9 nm	Merin *et al.,* 2010
Chlorococcum humicola	AgNPs	430 nm	Jenaa *et al.,* 2013
Kappaphycus alverazii	AgNPs	50-60 nm	Ganesan *et al.,* 2013
Oscillatoria willei	AgNPs	100-200 nm	Ali *et al.,* 2011
Padina gymnospora	AgNPs	25-40 nm	Shiny *et al.,* 2013
Phormidium cyanobacterium	CuONPs	10-40 nm	Rahman *et al.,* 2009
Sargassum muticum	Fe_3O_4 NPs	18 ± 4 nm	Mahdavi *et al.,* 2013
Sargassum wightii	AuNPs	30-100nm	Oza *et al.,* 2012
Scenedesmus sp.	AgNPs	15-20 nm	Jena *et al.,* 2014
Spirulina Platensis	AuNPs	20-30 nm	Kalabegishvili *et al.,* 2012
Spirulina platensis	AgNPs	11.6 nm	Mahdieha *et al.,* 2012
Spirulina platensis	AgNPs	75-235 nm	Tarafdar *et al.,* 2013
Turbinaria conoides	AgNPs	96 nm	Rajeshkumar *et al.,* 2012

1.4 Fungi Mediated Production of Nanoparticles

Fungi are eukaryotic organisms that usually function as decomposers. Their worth mentioning abilities include discharging of enzymes to hydrolyze complex substances to digesting extracellular food, which are exploited as an energy source. Therefore, the exploration of fungi in nano-biotechnology is considered very important. In this respect, fungi have been engrossed more consideration on biogenic synthesis of metallic nanoparticles due to their metal bioaccumulation capability.

Fungi have the colossal number of secretory components, which bring about the capping and reduction of nanoparticles. Production of nanoparticles by using fungi has numerous benefits as they have tolerance with a high concentration of metal in the medium, easily scaled up for mass production of nanoparticles, good mono-dispersion of nanoparticles, much higher protein expressions and reduced cost (Vahabi *et al.,* 2011). For example, green fabrication of nanoparticles of copper oxide by using *Penicillium aurantiogriseum, P. waksmanii P. citrinum* and was successfully carried out by Sanghi and Verma, 2008. Bio-reduction of aqueous chloroaurate (AuCl4) ions was bringing out using fungus *Verticillium* sp (Mukherjee *et al.,* 2001), *Fusarium oxysporum* (Mukherjee *et al.,* 2002), *Aspergillus flavus* (Vigneshwaran *et al.,* 2007) used for the formation of gold nanoparticle with quite well-defined shape and size. In this reaction, the chloroaurate ions adsorbed on the surface of fungal cells by electrostatic interaction between positively charged groups of enzymes found in the mycelial cell wall. *Aspergillus fumigates* (Bhainsa *et al.,* 2006) *Trichoderma reesei* (Vahabi *et al.,* 2011), *A. flavus* (Moharrer *et al.,* 2012 and Ninganagouda *et al.,* 2013) and A. niger (Vivekanandan *et al.,* 2012) fungus resulted in the rapid fabrication of silver nanoparticles.

Mostly, fungi are considered as the most favored organisms for the fabrication of extracellular nanoparticles. The extracellular fabrication of silver nanoparticles by using the seed media supernatant of *Schizophyllum radiatum* was reported by Metuku *et al.,* 2013. Nitrate dependent reductase enzyme may be accountable for the metal ion reduction in some microorganisms. This enzyme is conjugated along with an electron donor like quinine and reduces the metal ion into elemental form. Bansal *et al.,* in 2004 and 2005 found that proteins have been involved in the production of zirconia nanoparticles and it was also revealed that the secreted proteins were capable of hydrolyzing silica, titania, and zirconium ions extracellularly. Extracellular fabrication of nanoparticles in size range 47 nm was obtained from fungus *Aspergillus terreus* (Zare et al., 2013).

Although extracellular fabrication of nanoparticles has advantages like low cost, simpler extraction and purification process (Das *et al.,* 2014), intracellular production is also very important in the case of bioremediation which involves heavy metals removal like Cu and Pt from the contaminated environment. Also, the removal of this fungi and its accumulated metal contaminant from the contaminated sample is very easy. A remarkable study on white-rot fungus *Coriolus versicolor* conducted by Sanghi *et al.,* for the production and accumulation of intracellular silver nanoparticles (Sanghi and Verma, 2009).

Mycosynthesized nanoparticles along with antimicrobial activity also show antitumor potential under optimum conditions. For example, Magdi *et al.,* 2014 reported the antitumor activity of mycosynthesised nanoparticles against human colon carcinoma, human breast cancer, and human hepatocellular carcinoma cells. Xue *et al.,* 2016 had identified *Arthroderma fulvum* fungal strain used for synthesizing silver nanoparticles. Biofabricated silver nanoparticles exhibit considerable antifungal potential against the *Candida* spp., *Fusarium* spp., *Aspergillus* spp. Various nanoparticles synthesized by fungus mentioned in Table 4.

Table 4. Nanoparticles synthesized by Fungi

Fungi	Nanoparticle	Size	Reference
Aspergillus flavus	AgNPs	7 nm	Moharrer *et al.*, 2012
A. tubingensis	TiO_2 NPs	<100 nm	Tarafdar *et al.*, 2013
Alternaria alternate	AgNPs	20-60 nm	Gajbhiye *et al.*, 2009
Coriolus versicolor	AgNPs	10-75nm	Sanghi *et al.*, 2008
Fusarium oxysporum	AgNPs	1-100 nm	Ishida *et al.*, 2013
F. semitectum	AgNPs	10-60nm	Basavaraja *et al.*, 2007
Ganoderma lucidum	AgNPs	10-70 nm	Karwa *et al.*, 2011
Geotrichum Candidum	AuNPs	65-70 nm	Joerger *et al.*, 2000
Penicillium citrinum	CuONPs	91-295 nm	Honarya *et al.*, 2012
P. waksmanii	CuONPs	80-179 nm	Honarya *et al.*, 2012
P.citrinum	AgNPs	340-450 nm	Goswami *et al.*, 2013
P. aurantiogriseum	CuONPs	89-250 nm	Honarya *et al.*, 2012
Streptomyces glaucus	AgNPs	4-25 nm	Tsibakhashvili *et al.*, 2011
Schizophyllum radiatum	AgNPs	10-40 nm	Metuku *et al.*, 2013
Streptomyces sp.	MnSNPs, ZnSNPs	10-20 nm	Waghmare *et al.*, 2011
Streptomyces sp.	AgNPs	68.13 nm	Chauhan *et al.*, 2013
Macrophomina phaseolina	AgNPs	-	Chowdhury *et al* 2014
Aspergillus flavus	TiO2	12–15 nm	Raliya *et al.*, 2015
Arthroderma fulvum	AgNPs	15.5- 17.5 nm	Xue *et al.*, 2016

2. CONCLUSION

Enhancement of the therapeutic efficacy of herbal formulation has been getting attention due to the surging of chronic and acute diseases. However, many problems associated with herbal medicines like low oral absorption, poor solubility, poor bioavailability, unpredictable toxicity, and instability limit their exploitation. In order to eradicate such problems, "Nanotechnology" has recognized the attractive remedies that will encounter the problem related to the herbal formulation. It has been projected that the effective and valuable importance of the herbal remedies being exploited with the nanoparticles will improve the efficacy of present drug delivery systems.

REFERENCES

Abboud, Y., Saffaj, T., Chagraoui, A., El Bouari, A., Brouzi, K., Tanane, O., & Ihssane, B. (2014). Biosynthesis, characterization and antimicrobial activity of copper oxide nanoparticles (CONPs) produced using brown alga extract (*Bifurcaria bifurcata*). *Applied Nanoscience*, *4*(5), 571–576. doi:10.100713204-013-0233-x

Ahmmad, B., Leonard, K., Islam, M. S., Kurawaki, J., Muruganandham, M., Ohkubo, T., & Kuroda, Y. (2013). Green synthesis of mesoporous hematite (a-Fe2O3) nanoparticles and their photocatalytic activity. *Advanced Powder Technology*, *24*(1), 160–167. doi:10.1016/j.apt.2012.04.005

Ali, D. M., Sasikala, M., Gunasekaran, M., & Thajuddin, N. (2011). Biosynthesis and characterization of silver nanoparticles using marine cyanobacterium, *Oscillatoria willei*. *Digest Journal of Nanomaterials and Biostructures*, *6*, 385–390.

Anand, P., Kunnumakkara, A. B., Newman, R. A., & Aggarwal, B. B. (2007). Bioavailability of Curcumin: Problems and Promises. *Molecular Pharmaceutics*, *4*(6), 807–818. doi:10.1021/mp700113r PMID:17999464

Ankamwar, B., Daml, C., Ahmad, A., & Sastry, M. (2005). Biosynthesis of Gold and Silver Nanoparticles Using *Emblica Officinalis* Fruit Extract, Their Phase Transfer and Trans metallationinan Organic Solution. *Journal of Nanoscience and Nanotechnology*, *5*(10), 1665–1671. doi:10.1166/jnn.2005.184 PMID:16245525

Armendariz, V., Gardea-Torresdey, J. L., Jose-Yacaman, M., Gonzalez, J., Herrera, I., & Parsons, J. G. (2002). Gold nanoparticles formation by oat and wheat biomasses. *Proceedings –Waste Research Technology Conference at the Kansas City*.

Armendariz, V., Herrera, I., Peralta-videa, J. R., Jose-yacaman, M., Troiani, H., Santiago, P., & Gardea-Torresdey, J. L. (2004). Size controlled gold nanoparticle formation by *Avena sativa* biomass: Use of plants in nanobiotechnology. *Journal of Nano Research*, *6*(4), 377–382. doi:10.100711051-004-0741-4

Arockiya, F., Parthiban, C., Ganesh-Kumar, V., & Anantharaman, P. (2012). Biosynthesis of antibacterial gold nanoparticles using brown alga, *Stoechospermum marginatum* (kützing). *Spectrochimica Acta. Part A: Molecular and Biomolecular Spectroscopy*, *99*, 166–173. doi:10.1016/j.saa.2012.08.081 PMID:23063860

Arulanandraj, N., Dhivya, S., & Gopal, V. (2018). A review on Herbal Nanoparticles. *PharmaTutor.*, *6*(5), 32–37. doi:10.29161/PT.v6.i5.2018.32

Ashokkumar, S., Ravi, S., Kathiravan, V., & Velmurugan, S. (2014). Rapid biological synthesis of silver nanoparticles using *Leucas martinicensis* leaf extract for catalytic and antibacterial activity. *Environmental Science and Pollution Research International*, *21*(19), 11439–11446. doi:10.100711356-014-3012-7 PMID:24906826

Bajpai, V. K., Shukla, S., Kang, S. M., Hwang, S. K., Song, X., Huh, Y. S., & Han, Y. K. (2018). Developments of Cyanobacteria for Nano-Marine Drugs: Relevance of Nano-formulation s in Cancer Therapies. *Marine Drugs*, *16*(6), E179. doi:10.3390/md16060179 PMID:29882898

Banerjee, J., & Narendhirakannan, R. (2011). Biosynthesis of silver nanoparticles from *Syzygium cumini* (L.) seed extract and evaluation of their in vitro antioxidant activities. *Digest Journal of Nanomaterials and Biostructures*, *6*, 961–968.

Bansal, V., Rautray, D., Ahamd, A., & Sastry, M. (2004). Biosynthesis of zirconia nanoparticles using the fungus *Fusarium oxysporum*. *Journal of Materials Chemistry*, *14*(22), 3303–3305. doi:10.1039/b407904c

Bansal, V., Rautray, D., Bharde, A., Ahire, K., Sanyal, A., Ahmad, A., & Sastry, M. (2005). Fungus-mediated biosynthesis of silica and titania particles. *Journal of Materials Chemistry*, *15*(26), 2583–2589. doi:10.1039/b503008k

Bar, H., Bhui, D. K., Sahoo, G. P., Sarkar, P., Pyne, S., & Misra, A. (2009). Green synthesis of silver nanoparticles using seed extract of *Jatropha curcas. Colloids and Surfaces. A, Physicochemical and Engineering Aspects*, *348*(1-3), 212–216. doi:10.1016/j.colsurfa.2009.07.021

Basavaraja, S., Balaji, S. D., Lagashetty, A., Rajasab, A. H., & Venkataraman, A. (2007). Extracellular biosynthesis of silver nanoparticles using the fungus *Fusarium semitectum. Materials Research Bulletin*, *43*(5), 1164–1170. doi:10.1016/j.materresbull.2007.06.020

Basavegowda, N., Sobczak-Kupiec, A., Malina, D., Yathirajan, H. S., Keerthi, V. R., Chandrashekar, N., Dinkar, S., & Liny, P. (2013). Plant mediated synthesis of gold nanoparticles using fruit extracts of *ananas comosus* (L.) (pineapple) and evaluation of biological activities. *Advanced Materials Letters*, *4*(5), 332–337. doi:10.5185/amlett.2012.9423

Baskaralingam, V., Sargunar, C. G., Lin, Y. C., & Chen, J. C. (2012). Green synthesis of silver nanoparticles through *Calotropis gigantea* leaf extracts and evaluation of antibacterial activity against *Vibrio alginolyticus. Nanotech Dev.*, *2*(1), e3. doi:10.4081/nd.2012.e3

Bhainsa, K. C., & D'Souza, S. F. (2006). Extracellular biosynthesis of silver nanoparticles using the fungus *Aspergillus fumigates. Colloids and Surfaces. B, Biointerfaces*, *47*(2), 160–164. doi:10.1016/j.colsurfb.2005.11.026 PMID:16420977

Bisht, S., Feldmann, G., Soni, S., Ravi, R., Karikar, C., Maitra, A., & Maitra, A. (2007). Polymeric nanoparticles-encapsulated curcumin (nanocurcumin): A novel strategy for human cancer therapy. *Journal of Nanobiotechnology*, *5*(3), 2–18. doi:10.1186/1477-3155-5-3 PMID:17439648

Breuning, M., Bauer, S., & Goepferich, A. (2008). Polymers and Nanoparticles: Intelligent tools for intracellular targeting. *European Journal of Pharmaceutics and Biopharmaceutics*, *68*(1), 112–128. doi:10.1016/j.ejpb.2007.06.010 PMID:17804211

Chandran, P., Chaudhary, M., Pasricha, R., Ahmad, A., & Sastry, M. (2006). Synthesis of Gold Nanotriangles and Silver Nanoparticles using *Aloe vera* Plant Extract. *Biotechnology Progress*, *22*(2), 577–583. doi:10.1021/bp0501423 PMID:16599579

Chauhan, R., Kumar, A., & Abraham, J. (2013). A Biological Approach to the Synthesis of Silver Nanoparticles with *Streptomyces* sp JAR1 and its Antimicrobial Activity. *Scientia Pharmaceutica*, *81*(2), 607–621. doi:10.3797cipharm.1302-02 PMID:23833724

Chowdhury, S., Basu, A., & Kundu, S. (2014). Green synthesis of protein capped silver nanoparticles from phytopathogenic fungus *Macrophomina phaseolina* (Tassi) Goid with antimicrobial properties against multidrug-resistant bacteria. *Nanoscale Research Letters*, *9*(1), 365. doi:10.1186/1556-276X-9-365 PMID:25114655

Chuang, Y. L., Fang, H. W., Ajitsaria, A., Chen, K. H., Su, C. Y., Liu, G. S., & Tseng, C. L. (2019). Development of Kaempferol-Loaded Gelatin Nanoparticles for the Treatment of Corneal Neovascularization in Mice. *Pharmaceutics*, *11*(12), E635. doi:10.3390/pharmaceutics11120635 PMID:31795237

Daisy, P., & Saipriya, K. (2012). Biochemical analysis of Cassia fistula aqueous extracts and phytochemically synthesized gold nanoparticles as hypoglycemic treatment for diabetes mellitus. *International Journal of Nanomedicine*, *7*, 1189–1202. doi:10.2147/IJN.S26650 PMID:22419867

Das, V., Thomas, R., Varghese, R., Soniya, E. V., Mathew, J. & Radhakrishnan, E. K. (2014). Extracellular synthesis of silver nanoparticles by the Bacillus strain CS 11 isolated from industrialized area. *Biotech, 4*, 121-126.

Dong, X., Mattingly, C. A., Tseng, M., Cho, M., Adams, V. R., & Mumper, R. J. (2009, May). Development of new lipid based paclitaxel nanoparticles using sequential simplex optimization. *European Journal of Pharmaceutics and Biopharmaceutics*, *72*(1), 9–17. doi:10.1016/j.ejpb.2008.11.012 PMID:19111929

Dubey, S. P., Lahtinen, M., & Sillanpaa, M. (2010). Green synthesis and characterizations of silver and gold nanoparticles using leaf extract of Rosa rugosa. *Colloids and Surfaces. A, Physicochemical and Engineering Aspects*, *364*(1-3), 34–41. doi:10.1016/j.colsurfa.2010.04.023

Firdhouse, M. J., & Lalitha, P. (2013). Biomimetic synthesis of silver nanoparticles using aqueous extract of *amaranthus polygonoides. International Journal of Pharma and Bio Sciences*, *4*, 588–595.

Fleet, M. F., & Southam, G. (2006). Morphology of Gold Nanoparticles Synthesized by Filamentous Cyanobacteria from Gold(I)-Thiosulfate and Gold(III)-Chloride Complexes. *Langmuir*, *22*(6), 2780–2787. doi:10.1021/la052652c PMID:16519482

Fleet, M. F., & Southam, G. (2007). Synthesis of palladium nanoparticles by reaction of filamentous cyanobacterial biomass with a palladium (II) chloride complex. *Langmuir*, *23*(17), 8982–8987. doi:10.1021/la7012446 PMID:17658865

Focsan, M., Ardelean, I. I., Craciun, C., & Astilean, S. (2011). Interplay between gold nanoparticle biosynthesis and metabolic activity of cyanobacterium *Synechocystis* sp. PCC 680. *Nanotechnology*, *22*(48), 485101–485109. doi:10.1088/0957-4484/22/48/485101 PMID:22072064

Gajbhiye, M., Kesharwani, J., Ingle, A., Gade, A., & Rai, M. (2009). Fungus-mediated synthesis of silver nanoparticles and their activity against pathogenic fungi in combination with fluconazole. *Nanotechnology. Biology and Medicine (Aligarh)*, *5*, 382–386. PMID:19616127

Ganesan, V., Devi, J. A., Astalakshmi, A., Nima, P., & Thangaraja, A. (2013). Eco- Friendly Synthesis of Silver Nanoparticles using a Sea Weed, *Kappaphycus Alvarezii* (Doty) Doty ex P.C.Silva. *International Journal of Engineering and Advanced Technology*, *2*(5).

Gardea-Torresdey, J. L., Parsons, J. G., Gomez, E., Peralta-Videa, J., Troiani, H. E., & Santiago, P. (2002). Formation and growth of Au nanoparticles inside live alfalfa plants. American Chemical Society, 2, 397–401. doi:10.1021/nl015673+

Geethalakshmi, R., & Sarada, D. V. L. (2012). Gold and silver nanoparticles from *Trianthema decandra*: Synthesis, characterization, and antimicrobial properties. *International Journal of Nanomedicine*, *7*, 5375–5384. doi:10.2147/IJN.S36516 PMID:23091381

Ghosh, S., Patil, S., Ahire, M., Kitture, R., Jabgunde, A., Kale, S., Pardesi, K. Bellare, J., Dhavale, D.D. & Chopade, B.A. (2011). Synthesis of gold nano-anisotrops using *Dioscorea bulbifera* tuber extract. *Journal of Nanomaterial.*

Ghosh, S., Patil, S., Ahire, M., Kitture, R., Kale, S., Pardesi, K., Cameotra, S. S., Bellare, J., Dhavale, D. D., & Chopade, B. A. (2012). Synthesis of silver nanoparticles using Dioscorea bulbifera tuber extract and evaluation of its synergistic potential in combination with antimicrobial agents. *International Journal of Nanomedicine*, *7*, 483–496. PMID:22334779

Goswami, A. M., Sarkar, T. S., & Ghosh, S. (2013). An Ecofriendly synthesis of silver nano-bioconjugates by *Penicillium citrinum* (MTCC9999) and its antimicrobial effect. *AMB Express*, *3*(1), 16. doi:10.1186/2191-0855-3-16 PMID:23433075

Gunalana, S., Sivaraja, R., & Rajendran, V. (2012). Green synthesized ZnO nanoparticles against bacterial and fungal pathogens. *Progress in Natural Science*, *22*(6), 693–700. doi:10.1016/j.pnsc.2012.11.015

Haleemkhan, A.A., Naseem, & Vardhini, B. V. (2015). Synthesis of nanoparticles from Plant Extract. *International Journal of Modern Chemistry and Applied Sciences, 2*(3), 195-203.

Haratifar, E., Shahverdi, H. R., Shakibaie, M., Moghaddam, K. M., Amini, M., Montazeri, H., & Shahv, A. R. (2009). Semi-Biosynthesis of Magnetite-Gold Composite Nanoparticles Using an Ethanol Extract of *Eucalyptus camaldulensis* and Study of the Surface Chemistry. *Journal of Nanomaterials*, *5*, 962021.

Harne, S., Sharma, A., Dhaygude, M., Joglekar, S., Kodam, K., & Hudlikar, M. (2012). Novel route for rapid biosynthesis of copper nanoparticles using aqueous extract of Calotropis procera L. latex and their cytotoxicity on tumor cells. *Colloids and Surfaces. B, Biointerfaces*, *95*, 284–288. doi:10.1016/j.colsurfb.2012.03.005 PMID:22483347

He, Y., Du, Z., Lv, H., Jia, Q., Tang, Z., Zheng, X., Zhang, K., & Zhao, F. (2013). Green synthesis of silver nanoparticles by *Chrysanthemum morifolium* Ramat extract and their application in clinical ultrasound gel. *International Journal of Nanomedicine*, *8*, 1809–1815. doi:10.2147/IJN.S43289 PMID:23687447

Honarya, S., Barabadi, H., Gharaeifathaba, D. E., & Naghibi, F. (2012). Green synthesis of copper oxide nanoparticles using *Penicillium aurantiogriseum, Penicillium citrinum* and *Penicillium waksmanii. Digest Journal of Nanomaterials and Biostructures*, *7*, 999–1005.

Huang, J. L., Li, Q. B., Sun, D. H., Lu, Y. H., Su, Y. B., Yang, X., Wang, H., Wang, Y., Shao, W., He, N., Hong, J., & Chen, C. (2007). Biosynthesis of silver and gold nanoparticles by novel sundried Cinnamomum camphora leaf. *Nanotechnology*, *18*(10), 105104. doi:10.1088/0957-4484/18/10/105104

Iravani, S. (2011). Green synthesis of metal nanoparticles using plants. *Green Chemistry*, *13*(10), 2638–2650. doi:10.1039/c1gc15386b

Ishida, K., Cipriano, T. F., Rocha, G. M., Weissmuller, G., Gomes, F., Miranda, K., & Rozental, S. (2013). Silver nanoparticle production by the fungus *Fusarium oxysporum*: Nanoparticle characterisation and analysis of antifungal activity against pathogenic yeasts. *Memorias do Instituto Oswaldo Cruz*, *109*(2), 1–9. doi:10.1590/0074-0276130269 PMID:24714966

Jayaseelan, C., Ramkumar, R., Rahuman, A. A., & Perumal, P. (2013). Green synthesis of gold nanoparticles using seed aqueous extract of *Abelmoschus esculentus* and its antifungal activity. *Industrial Crops and Products*, *45*, 423–429. doi:10.1016/j.indcrop.2012.12.019

Jena, J., Pradhan, N., Nayak, R. R., Dash, B. P., Sukla, L. B., Panda, P. K., & Mishra, B. K. (2014). Microalga *Scenedesmus* sp.: A Potential Low-Cost Green Machine for Silver Nanoparticle Synthesis. *Journal of Microbiology and Biotechnology*, *24*(4), 522–533. doi:10.4014/jmb.1306.06014 PMID:24394192

Jenaa, J., Pradhana, N., Dashb, B. P., Suklaa, L. B., & Pandaa, P. K. (2013). Biosynthesis and characterization of silver nanoparticles using microalga *Chlorococcum humicola* and its antibacterial activity. *International Journal of Nanomaterials and Biostructures.*, *3*, 1–8.

Jha, A. K., & Prasad, K. (2010). Green synthesis of silver nanoparticles using Cycas leaf. *International Journal of Green Nanotechnology: Physical Chemistry*, *1*, 110–117.

Joerger, R., Klaus, T., & Granqvist, C. G. (2000). Biologically Produced Silver-Carbon Composite Materials for Optically Functional Thin-Film Coatings. *Advanced Materials*, *12*(6), 407–409. doi:10.1002/(SICI)1521-4095(200003)12:6<407::AID-ADMA407>3.0.CO;2-O

Kalabegishvili, T., Kirkesali, E., Frontasyeva, M. V., & Pavlov, S. S. (2012). Synthesis of Gold Nanoparticles by Blue-Green Algae *Spirulina Platensis. Proceedings of the international conference nanomaterials: applications and properties.*

Kannan, B., & Narayanan, N. S. (2010). Biological synthesis of metal nanoparticles by microbes. *Advances in Colloid and Interface Science*, *156*(1-2), 1–13. doi:10.1016/j.cis.2010.02.001 PMID:20181326

Karwa, A., Gaikwad, S., & Rai, M. (2011). Mycosynthesis of Silver Nanoparticles Using Lingzhi or Reishi Medicinal Mushroom, *Ganoderma lucidum* (W. Curt.:Fr.) P. Karst. and their Role as Antimicrobials and Antibiotic Activity Enhancers. *International Journal of Medicinal Mushrooms*, *13*(5), 483–491. doi:10.1615/IntJMedMushr.v13.i5.80 PMID:22324414

Kasthuri, J., Kathiravan, K., & Rajendiran, N. (2009). Phyllanthin-assisted biosynthesis of silver and gold nanoparticles: A novel biological approach. *Journal of Nanoparticle Research*, *11*(5), 1075–1085. doi:10.100711051-008-9494-9

Kaviya, S., Santhanalakshmi, J., Viswanathan, B., Muthumary, J., & Srinivasan, K. (2011b). Biosynthesis of silver nanoparticles using Citrus sinensis peel extract and its antibacterial activity. *Spectrochimica Acta. Part A: Molecular and Biomolecular Spectroscopy*, *79*(3), 594–598. doi:10.1016/j.saa.2011.03.040 PMID:21536485

Kesharwani, J., Yoon, K. Y., Hwang, J., & Rai, M. (2009). Phytofabrication of silver nanoparticles by leaf extract of Datura metel: Hypothetical mechanism involved in synthesis. *Journal of Bionanoscience.*, *3*(1), 39–44. doi:10.1166/jbns.2009.1008

Kesharwani, R. K., Misra, K., & Singh, D. B. (2019). Perspectives and challenges of tropical medicinal herbs and modern drug discovery in the current scenario. *Asian Pacific Journal of Tropical Medicine*, *12*(1), 1–7. doi:10.4103/1995-7645.250337

Khalil, M. M. H., Ismail, E. H., El-Baghdady, K. Z., & Mohamed, D. (2013). Green synthesis of silver nanoparticles using olive leaf extract and its antibacterial activity. *Arabian Journal of Chemistry*, *7*(6), 1131–1139. doi:10.1016/j.arabjc.2013.04.007

Kim, H. S., Kwon, H. K., Lee, D. H., Le, T. N., Park, H. J., & Kim, M. I. (2019). Poly(γ-Glutamic Acid)/Chitosan Hydrogel Nanoparticles For Effective Preservation And Delivery Of Fermented Herbal Extract For Enlarging Hair Bulb And Enhancing Hair Growth. *International Journal of Nanomedicine*, *14*, 8409–8419. doi:10.2147/IJN.S227514 PMID:31695374

Komal, R., & Arya, V. (2013). Biosynthesis and characterization of silver nanoparticles from aqueous leaf extracts of *Carica papaya* and its antibacterial activity. *International Journal of Nanomaterials and Biostructures.*, *3*, 17–20.

Kumar, A., Yadev, S. K., Pakade, Y. B., Singh, B., & Yadev, S. C. (2010). Development of biodegradable nanoparticles for delivery of quercetin. *Colloids and Surfaces. B, Biointerfaces*, *15*(2), 184–192. doi:10.1016/j.colsurfb.2010.06.002 PMID:20598513

Kumar, B., Smita, K., Cumbal, L., & Debut, A. (2014). Biogenic synthesis of iron oxide nanoparticles for 2-arylbenzimidazole fabrication. *Journal of Saudi Chemical Society*, *18*(4), 364–369. doi:10.1016/j.jscs.2014.01.003

Kumar, P. R., Vivekanandhan, S., Misra, M., Mohanty, A., & Satyanarayana, N. (2012). Soybean (*Glycine max*) leaf extract based green synthesis of palladium nanoparticles. *Journal of Biomaterials and Nanobiotechnology*, *3*(01), 14–19. doi:10.4236/jbnb.2012.31003

Kumar, V., & Yadav, S. K. (2011). Synthesis of Stable, Polyshaped Silver and Gold Nanoparticles Using Leaf Extract of *Lonicera japonica* (L.). *International Journal of Green Nanotechnology.*, *3*(4), 281–291. doi:10.1080/19430892.2011.633474

Lee, H. J., Lee, G., Jang, N. R., Yun, J. H., Song, J. Y., & Kim, B. S. (2011). Biological synthesis of copper nanoparticles using plant extract. *Nanotechnology*, *1*, 371–374.

Lengke, M., Ravel, B., Fleet, M. E., Wanger, G., Gordon, R. A., & Southam, G. (2006). Mechanisms of gold bioaccumulation by filamentous cyanobacteria from gold(III)-chloride complex. *Environmental Science & Technology*, *40*(20), 6304–6309. doi:10.1021/es061040r PMID:17120557

Lengke, M. F., Fleet, M. E., & Southam, G. (2007). Synthesis of palladium nanoparticles by reaction of filamentous cyanobacterial biomass with a palladium(II) chloride complex. *Langmuir*, *23*(17), 8982–8987. doi:10.1021/la7012446 PMID:17658865

Li, S. K., Shen, Y. H., Xie, A. J., Yu, X. R., Zhang, X. Z., Yang, L. B., & Li, C. H. (2007). Rapid, room-temperature synthesis of amorphous selenium/protein composites using *Capsicum annuum* L. extract. *Nanotechnology*, *18*(40), 405101–405109. doi:10.1088/0957-4484/18/40/405101

Li, X., Xu, H., Chen, Z. S., & Chen, G. (2011). Biosynthesis of nanoparticles by microorganisms and their applications. *Journal of Nanomaterials*, *2011*, 16. doi:10.1155/2011/270974

Liu, J. R., Chen, G. F., Shih, H. N., & Kuo, P. C. (2008). Enhanced antioxidant bioactivity of Salvia miltiorrhiza (Danshen) products prepared using nanotechnology. *Phytomedicine, 15*(1-2), 23–30. doi:10.1016/j.phymed.2007.11.012 PMID:18077145

Liu, Q., Liu, H., Yuan, Z., Wei, D., & Ye, Y. (2012). Evaluation of antioxidant activity of chrysanthemum extracts and tea beverages by gold nanoparticles-based assay. *Colloids and Surfaces. B, Biointerfaces, 92*, 348–352. doi:10.1016/j.colsurfb.2011.12.007 PMID:22221458

Logeswari, P., Silambarasan, S., & Abraham, J. (2013). Ecofriendly synthesis of silver nanoparticles from commercially available plant powders and their antibacterial properties. *Scientia Iranica F., 20*, 1049–1054.

Lübtow, M. M., Nelke, L. C., Seifert, J., Kühnemundt, J., Sahay, G., Dandekar, G., Nietzer, S. L., & Luxenhofer, R. (2019). Drug induced micellization into ultra-high capacity and stable curcumin nanoformulations: Physico-chemical characterization and evaluation in 2D and 3D in vitro models. *Journal of Controlled Release, 303*, 162–180. doi:10.1016/j.jconrel.2019.04.014 PMID:30981815

Maensiria, S., Laokula, P., Klinkaewnaronga, J., Phokhaa, S., Promarakc, V., & Seraphin, S. (2008). Indium oxide (In2O3) nanoparticles using*Aloe vera*plant extract: Synthesis and optical properties. *Journal of Optoelectronics and Advanced Materials, 10*, 161–165.

Magdi, H. M., Mourad, M. H., Abd, E., & El-Aziz, M. M. (2014). Biosynthesis of silver nanoparticles using fungi and biological evaluation of mycosynthesized silver nanoparticles. *Egyptian Journal of Experimental Biology. (Bot.), 10*(1), 1–12.

Mahdavi, M., Namvar, F., Ahmad, M. B., & Mohamad, R. (2013). Green Biosynthesis and Characterization of Magnetic Iron Oxide (Fe_3O_4) Nanoparticles Using Seaweed (*Sargassum muticum*) Aqueous Extract. *Molecules (Basel, Switzerland), 18*(5), 5954–5964. doi:10.3390/molecules18055954 PMID:23698048

Mahdieha, M., Zolanvari, A., Azimeea, A. S., & Mahdiehc, M. (2012). Green biosynthesis of silver nanoparticles by *Spirulina platensis. Scientia Iranica F., 19*(3), 926–929. doi:10.1016/j.scient.2012.01.010

Makarov, V. V., Love, A. J., Sinitsyna, O. V., Makarova, S. S., Yaminsky, I. V., Taliansky, M. E., & Kalinina, N. O. (2014). Green. *Nanotechnologies: Synthesis of Metal Nanoparticles Using Plants. Acta Naturae., 6*(1), 35–44. PMID:24772325

Marchiol, L., Mattiello, A., Poscic, F., Giordano, C., & Musetti, R. (2014). In vivo synthesis of nanomaterials in plants: Location of silver nanoparticles and plant metabolism. *Nanoscale Research Letters, 9*(1), 101. doi:10.1186/1556-276X-9-101 PMID:24581279

Mekjaruskul, C., & Sripanidkulchai, B. (2020). Kaempferia parviflora Nanosuspension Formulation for Scalability and Improvement of Dissolution Profiles and Intestinal Absorption. *AAPS PharmSciTech, 21*(2), 52. doi:10.120812249-019-1588-4 PMID:31900735

Merin, D. D., Prakash, S., & Bhimba, B. V. (2010). Antibacterial screening of silver nanoparticles synthesized by marine micro algae. *Asian Pacific Journal of Tropical Medicine, 3*(10), 797–799. doi:10.1016/S1995-7645(10)60191-5

Metuku, R. P., Pabba, S., Burra, S., Bindu, S. V., Gudikandula, K., & Charya, M. A. S. (2013). Biosynthesis of silver nanoparticles from *Schizophyllum radiatum* HE 863742.1: Their characterization and antimicrobial activity. *Biotechnology.*, 3. PMID:28324427

Meyers, M. A., Mishra, A., & Benson, D. J. (2006). Mechanical properties of nanocrystalline materials. *Progress in Materials Science, 51*(4), 427–556. doi:10.1016/j.pmatsci.2005.08.003

Mittal, A. K., Chisti, Y., & Banerjee, U. C. (2013). Synthesis of metallic nanoparticles using plant extracts. *Journal of Biotechnology Advances, 31*(2), 346–356. doi:10.1016/j.biotechadv.2013.01.003 PMID:23318667

Mohan, A., Nair, S. V., & Lakshmanan, V. K. (2017). Leucas aspera nanomedicine shows superior toxicity and cell migration retarded in prostate cancer cells. *Applied Biochemistry and Biotechnology, 181*(4), 1388–1400. doi:10.100712010-016-2291-5 PMID:27812900

Moharrer, S., Mohammadi, B., Gharamohammadi, R. A., & Yargoli, M. (2012). Biological synthesis of silver nanoparticles by *Aspergillus flavus*, isolated from soil of Ahar copper mine. *Indian Journal of Science and Technology, 5*(3), 2443–2444. doi:10.17485/ijst/2012/v5i3.41

Mukherjee, P., Ahmad, A., Mandal, D., Senapati, S., Sainkar, S. R., Khan, M. I., Parishcha, R., Ajaykumar, P. V., Alam, M., Kumar, R., & Sastry, M. (2001). Fungus mediated synthesis of silver nanoparticles and their immobilization in the mycelia matrix: A novel biological approach to nanoparticle synthesis. *Nano Letters, 1*(10), 515–519. doi:10.1021/nl0155274

Mukherjee, P., Ahmad, A., Mandal, D., Senapati, S., Sainkar, S. R., Khan, M. I., Ramani, R., Parischa, R., Ajayakumar, P. V., Alam, M., Sastry, M., & Kumar, R. (2001). Bioreduction of AuCl4 - ions by the fungus, *Verticillium* sp. and surface trapping of the gold nanoparticles formed. *Angewandte Chemie International Edition, 40*(19), 3585–3588. doi:10.1002/1521-3773(20011001)40:19<3585::AID-ANIE3585>3.0.CO;2-K PMID:11592189

Mukherjee, P., Senapati, S., Mandal, D., Ahmad, A., Khan, M. I., Kumar, R., & Sastry, M. (2002). Extracellular synthesis of gold nanoparticles by the fungus *Fusarium oxysporum. ChemBioChem, 3*(5), 461–463. doi:10.1002/1439-7633(20020503)3:5<461::AID-CBIC461>3.0.CO;2-X PMID:12007181

Mukherjee, S., Chowdhury, D., Kotcherlakota, R., Patra, S., & Vinothkumar, B. (2014). Potential Theranostics Application of Bio-Synthesized Silver Nanoparticles (4-in-1 System). *Theranostics, 4*(3), 316–335. doi:10.7150/thno.7819 PMID:24505239

Mukunthan, K., & Balaji, S. (2012). Cashew apple juice (Anacardium occidentale L.) speeds up the synthesis of silver nanoparticles. *International Journal of Green Nanotechnology., 4*(2), 71–79. doi:10.1080/19430892.2012.676900

Nagarajan, S., & Kuppusamy, K. A. (2013). Extracellular synthesis of zinc oxide nanoparticle using seaweeds of gulf of Mannar, India. *Journal of Nanobiotechnology, 11*(1), 39. doi:10.1186/1477-3155-11-39 PMID:24298944

Narayanan, K. B., & Sakthivel, N. (2008). Coriander leaf mediated biosynthesis of gold nanoparticles. *Materials Letters, 62*(30), 4588–4590. doi:10.1016/j.matlet.2008.08.044

Natarajan, E., Purushothaman, B., Palanisamy, P., Somasundaram, D., & And Subathra, S. (2012). Studies on morphological characterization and antimicrobial activity of silver nanoparticles synthesized by bio and chemoreductive methods. *International Journal of Pharma and Bio Sciences, 3*, 264–273.

Ninganagouda, S., Rathod, V., Jyoti, H., Singh, D., & Prema, K. & Manzoor-Ul-Haq. (2013). Extracellular biosynthesis of silver nanoparticles using *Aspergillus flavus* and their antimicrobial activity against gram negative mdr strains. *International Journal of Pharma and Bio Sciences, 4*, 222–229.

Okonogai, S., Sirithunyalang, J., & Chen, U. (2008). Nanoencapsulation of Centella asiatica bioactive extract. *XVIth International Conference on Bioencapsulation, 4*(6), 1-4.

Osvelia, E. R., Rene, H. D., Rosa, I. S., Gabriel, A. M., Nereyda, N., María del Carmen, S. N., Facundo, R., & Claudio, C. R. (2016). Green Synthesis of Silver Nanoparticles and Their Bactericidal and Antimycotic Activities against Oral Microbes. *Journal of Nanomaterials*.

Oza, G., Pandey, S., Shah, R., & Sharon, M. (2012). A Mechanistic Approach for Biological Fabrication of Crystalline Gold Nanoparticles Using Marine Algae, *Sargassum wightii. European Journal of Experimental Biology, 2*, 505–512.

Panda, K. K., Achary, V. M. M., Krishnaveni, R., Padhi, B. K., Sarangi, S. N., Sahu, S. N., & Panda, B. B. (2011). *In vitro* biosynthesis and genotoxicity bioassay of silver nanoparticles using plants. *Toxicology In Vitro, 25*(5), 1097–1105. doi:10.1016/j.tiv.2011.03.008 PMID:21419840

Pandey, S., Oza, G., Mewada, A., & Sharon, M. (2012). Green Synthesis of Highly Stable Gold Nanoparticles using *Momordica charantia* as Nano fabricator. *Archives of Applied Science Research, 4*, 1135–1141.

Pasca, R. D., Mocanu, A., Cobzac, S. C., Petean, I., Horovitz, O., & Tomoaia-Cotisel, M. (2014). Biogenic syntheses of gold nanoparticles using plant extracts. *Particulate Science and Technology: An International Journal., 32*(2), 131–137. doi:10.1080/02726351.2013.839589

Patra, J. K., & Beak, K. H. (2017). Antibacterial Activity and Synergistic Antibacterial Potential of Biosynthesized Silver Nanoparticles against Foodborne Pathogenic Bacteria along with its Anticandidal and Antioxidant Effects. *Frontiers in Microbiology, 8*. Advance online publication. doi:10.3389/fmicb.2017.00167 PMID:28261161

Paulkumar, K., Gnanajobitha, G., Vanaja, M., & Rajeshkumar, S. (2014). *Piper nigrum*. Leaf and Stem Assisted Green Synthesis of Silver Nanoparticles and Evaluation of Its Antibacterial Activity Against Agricultural Plant Pathogens. Scientific World Journal.

Peng, Q., Tao, G., Jiao, Z., Jie, L., Dong, Z., & Zhirong, Z. (2008). Enhanced the oral bioavailability of savianolic acid B by phospholipid complex loaded nanoparticles. *Die Pharmazie, 63*, 661–666. PMID:18819519

Philip, D. (2011). *Mangifera Indica* leaf-assisted biosynthesis of well-dispersed silver nanoparticles. *Spectrochimica Acta Part A., 78*(1), 327–331. doi:10.1016/j.saa.2010.10.015 PMID:21030295

Philip, D., Unnib, S., & Aswathy, A. V. K. (2011). *Murraya Koenigii* leaf-assisted rapid green synthesis of silver and gold nanoparticles. *Spectrochimica Acta Part A., 78*(2), 899–904. doi:10.1016/j.saa.2010.12.060 PMID:21215687

Prasad, T. N. V. K. V., & Elumalai, E. K. (2011). Biofabrication of Ag nanoparticles using *Moringa oleifera* leaf extract and their antimicrobial activity. *Asian Pacific Journal of Tropical Biomedicine*, *1*(6), 439–442. doi:10.1016/S2221-1691(11)60096-8 PMID:23569809

Prathna, T. C., Chandrasekaran, N., Raichur, A. M., & Mukherjee, A. (2011a). Kinetic evolution studies of silver nanoparticles in a bio-based green synthesis process. *Colloids and Surfaces. A, Physicochemical and Engineering Aspects*, *377*(1-3), 212–216. doi:10.1016/j.colsurfa.2010.12.047

Prathna, T. C., Raichur, A. M., Chandrasekaran, N., & Mukherjee, A. (2011b). Biomimetic synthesis of silver nanoparticles by Citrus limon (lemon) aqueous extract and theoretical prediction of particle size. *Colloids and Surfaces. B, Biointerfaces*, *82*(1), 152–159. doi:10.1016/j.colsurfb.2010.08.036 PMID:20833002

Rahman, A., Ismail, A., Jumbianti, D., Magdalena, S., & Sudrajat, H. (2009). Synthesis of copper oxide nano particles by using *Phormidium* cyanobacterium. *Indonesian Journal of Chemistry.*, *9*(3), 355–360. doi:10.22146/ijc.21498

Rajesh, W. R., Jaya, R. J., Niranjan, S. K., Vijay, D. M., & Sahebrao, K. B. (2009). Phytosynthesis of Silver Nanoparticle Using *Gliricidia sepium* (Jacq.). *Current Nanoscience*, *5*(1), 117–122. doi:10.2174/157341309787314674

Rajeshkumar, S., Kannan, C., & Annadurai, G. (2012). Green synthesis of silver nanoparticles using marine brown algae *Turbinaria conoides* and its antibacterial activity. *International Journal of Pharma and Bio Sciences*, *3*, 502–510.

Raliya, R., Biswas, P., & Tarafdar, J. C. (2015). TiO_2 nanoparticle biosynthesis and its physiological effect on mung bean (Vigna radiata L.). *Biotechnology Reports (Amsterdam, Netherlands)*, *5*, 22–26. doi:10.1016/j.btre.2014.10.009 PMID:28626678

Reichard, P., Nielsen, O. S., Bauer, S., Hartmann, J. T., Schoffski, P., & Christensen, T. B. (2007). Exatecan in pretreated adult patients with advanced soft tissue sarcoma: Result of a phase-II. A study of EORTC soft tissue and bone sarcoma group. *Euro J Cnacer.*, *43*(6), 1017–1022. doi:10.1016/j.ejca.2007.01.014

Safaepour, M., Shahverdi, A. R., Shahverdi, H. R., Khorramizadeh, M. R., & Gohari, A. R. (2009). Green synthesis of small silver nanoparticles using geraniol and its cytotoxicity against Fibrosarcoma–Wehi 164. *Avicenna Journal of Medical Biotechnology*, *1*, 111–115. PMID:23407598

Sanghi, R., & Verma, P. (2008). Biomimetic synthesis and characterization of protein capped silver nanoparticles. *Bioresource Technology*, *100*(1), 501–504. doi:10.1016/j.biortech.2008.05.048 PMID:18625550

Sanghi, R., & Verma, P. (2009). Biomimetic synthesis and characterisation of protein capped silver nanoparticles. *Bioresource Technology*, *100*(1), 501–504. doi:10.1016/j.biortech.2008.05.048 PMID:18625550

Sathishkumar, M., Sneha, K., Won, W. S., Cho, C. W., Kim, S., & Yun, Y. S. (2009). *Cynamon zeylanicum* bark extract and powder mediated green synthesis of nanocrystallinesilver particles and its bactericidal activity. *Colloids and Surfaces. B, Biointerfaces*, *73*(2), 332–338. doi:10.1016/j.colsurfb.2009.06.005 PMID:19576733

Sathyavathi, R., Balamurali, K. M., Venugopal, R. S., Saritha, R., & Narayana, R. D. (2010). Biosynthesis of Silver Nanoparticles Using *Coriandrum Sativum* Leaf Extract and Their Application in Nonlinear Optics. *Advanced Science Letters*, *3*(2), 1–6. doi:10.1166/asl.2010.1099

Savithramma, N., Linga, R. M., Ankanna, S., & Venkateswarlu, P. (2012). Screening of medicinal plants for effective biogenesis of silver nano particles and efficient anti-microbial activity. *International Journal of Pharmaceutical Sciences and Research*, *3*, 1141–1148.

Sepeur, S., Laryea, N., Goedicke, S., & Groß, F. (2013). Nanotechnology: technical basics and applications. Hannover: Vincentz. 168. doi:10.1515/9783748602347

Shah, M., Fawcett, D., Sharma, S., Tripathy, S. K., & Poinern, G. E. J. (2015). Green synthesis of metallic nanoparticles via biological entities. *Material.*, *8*(11), 7278–7308. doi:10.3390/ma8115377 PMID:28793638

Shankar, S. S., Rai, S. A., Ahmad, A., & Sastry, M. (2004). Rapid synthesis of Au, Ag,and bimetallic Au core–Ag shell nanoparticles using Neem (*Azadirachta indica*) leaf broth. *Journal of Colloid and Interface Science*, *275*(2), 496–502. doi:10.1016/j.jcis.2004.03.003 PMID:15178278

Sharma, G., Jasuja, N. D., Ali, M. I., & Joshi, S. C. (2014). A Review on Nanomedicinal and Nanosensing Potential of Nanoparticles. *International Journal of Biological Chemistry.*, *8*(2), 58–54. doi:10.3923/ijbc.2014.58.84

Sharma, G., Sharma, A. R., Bhavesh, R., Park, J., Ganbold, B., Nam, J.-S., & Lee, S.-S. (2014). Biomolecule-Mediated Synthesis of Selenium Nanoparticles using Dried *Vitis vinifera* (Raisin) Extract. *Molecules (Basel, Switzerland)*, *19*(3), 2761–2770. doi:10.3390/molecules19032761 PMID:24583881

Sharma, K., Agrawal, S. S., & Gupta, M. (2015). Development and validation of uv spectrophotometric method for the estimation of curcumin in bulk drug and pharmaceutical dosage forms. *International Journal of Drug Development and Research.*, *4*(2), 375–380.

Sharma, N. C., Sahi, S. V., Nath, S., Parsons, J. G., Gardea-Torresdey, J. L., & Pal, T. (2007). Synthesis of plant-mediated gold nanoparticles and catalytic role of biomatrix-embedded nanomaterials. *Environmental Science & Technology*, *41*(14), 5137–5142. doi:10.1021/es062929a PMID:17711235

Shiny, P. J., Mukherjee, A., & Chandrasekaran, N. (2013). Marine algae mediated synthesis of the silver nanoparticles and its antibacterial efficiency. *International Journal of Pharmacy and Pharmaceutical Sciences*, *5*, 239–241.

Singh, A., Chaudhary, M., & Sastry, M. (2006). Construction of conductive multilayer films of biogenic triangular gold nanoparticles and their application in chemical vapour sensing. *Nanotechnology*, *17*(9), 2399–2405. doi:10.1088/0957-4484/17/9/055

Singh, R. P., Shukla, V. K., Yadav, R. S., Sharma, P. K., Singh, P. K., & Pandey, A. C. (2011). Biological approach of zinc oxide nanoparticles formation and its characterization. *Advanced Materials Letters*, *2*(4), 313–317. doi:10.5185/amlett.indias.204

Singhal, G., Bhavesh, R., Kasariya, K., Sharma, A. R., & Singh, R. P. (2011). Biosynthesis of silver nanoparticles using Ocimum sanctum (Tulsi) leaf extract and screening its antimicrobial activity. *Journal of Nanoparticle Research, 13*(7), 2981–2988. doi:10.100711051-010-0193-y

Sivaraj, R., Rahman, P. K., Rajiv, P., Narendhran, S., & Venckatesh, R. (2014). Biosynthesis and characterization of Acalypha indica mediated copper oxide nanoparticles and evaluation of its antimicrobial and anticancer activity. *Spectrochimica Acta. Part A: Molecular and Biomolecular Spectroscopy, 129*, 255–258. doi:10.1016/j.saa.2014.03.027 PMID:24747845

Song, J. Y., Kwon, E. Y., & Kim, B. S. (2010). Biological synthesis of platinum nanoparticles using *Diopyros kaki* leaf extract. *Bioprocess and Biosystems Engineering, 33*(1), 159–164. doi:10.100700449-009-0373-2 PMID:19701776

Sukirtha, R., Priyanka, K. M., Antony, J. J., Kamalakkannan, S., Ramar, T., & Palani, G. (2011). Cytotoxic effect of green synthesized silver nanoparticles using Meliaazedarach against in vitro HeLa cell lines and lymphoma mice model. *Process Biochemistry, 47*(2), 273–279. doi:10.1016/j.procbio.2011.11.003

Tang, J., Xu, N., Ji, H., Liu, H., Wang, Z., & Wu, L. (2011). Eudragit Nanoparticles containing genistein: Formulation, development and bioavailability assessment. *International Journal of Nanomedicine, 6*, 2429–2435. PMID:22072878

Tarafdar, A., Raliya, R., Wang, W. N., Biswas, P., & Tarafdar, J. C. (2013). Green synthesis of TiO2 Nanoparticle using *Aspergillus tubingensis. Advanced Science, Engineering and Medicine*, *5*(9), 1–7. doi:10.1166/asem.2013.1376

Thakkar, K. N., Mhatre, S. S., & Parikh, R. Y. (2010). Biological synthesis of metallic nanoparticles. *Nanomedicine; Nanotechnology, Biology, andMedicine, 6*(2), 257–262. doi:10.1016/j.nano.2009.07.002 PMID:19616126

Tsibakhashvili, N. Y., Kirkesali, E. I., Dodo, T., Pataraya, D. T., & Gurielidze, M. A. (2011). Microbial synthesis of silver nanoparticles by Streptomyces glaucus and Spirulina platensis. *Nanomaterials: Applications and Properties, 2*, 306–310.

Vahabi, K., Mansoori, G. A., & Karimi, S. (2011). Biosynthesis of Silver Nanoparticles by Fungus *Trichoderma Reesei. Insciences Journal, 1*, 65–79. doi:10.5640/insc.010165

Vidya, C., Hirematha, S., Chandraprabhab, M. N., Antonyraja, M. A. L. & Gopala, I. V. (2013). Green synthesis of ZnO nanoparticles by *Calotropis Gigantea. International Journal of Current Engineering and Technology*, 1.

Vigneshwaran, N., Ashtaputre, N. M., Varadarajan, P. V., Nachane, R. P., Paralikarand, K. M., & Balasubramanya, R. H. (2007). Biological synthesis of silver nanoparticles using the fungus *Aspergillus flavus. Materials Letters, 61*(6), 1413–1418. doi:10.1016/j.matlet.2006.07.042

Vijayaraghavan, K., Nalini, S., Prakash, N. U., & Madhankumar, D. (2012). One step green synthesis of silver nano/microparticles using extracts of Trachyspermum ammi and Papaver somniferum. *Colloids and Surfaces. B, Biointerfaces, 94*, 114–117. doi:10.1016/j.colsurfb.2012.01.026 PMID:22348989

Vivekanandan, K. E., Rajb, K. G., Kumaresana, S., & Pandib, M. (2012). Biosynthesis of silver nanoparticle activity against bacterial strain, cephalexin antibiotic synergistic activity. *International Journal of Current Science*, *4*, 1–7.

Waghmare, S. S., Deshmukh, A. M., Kulkarni, S. W., & Oswaldo, L. A. (2011). Biosynthesis and Characterization of Manganese and Zinc Nanoparticles. *Universal Journal of Environmental Research and Technology*, *1*, 64–69.

Xue, B., He, D., Gao, S., Wang, D., Yokoyama, K., & Wang, L. (2016). Biosynthesis of silver nanoparticles by the fungus Arthroderma fulvum and its antifungal activity against genera of Candida, Aspergillus and Fusarium. *International Journal of Nanomedicine*, *11*, 1899–1906. PMID:27217752

Yadev, D., Suri, S., Choudhary, A. A., & Sikender, M., & Heman, B. M. N. (2011). Novel approach, herbal remedies and natural products in pharmaceutical science as nano drug delivery systems. *International Journal of Pharm Tech Research*, *3*(3), 3092–3116.

Yen, F. L., Wu, T. H., Lin, L., Cham, T. M., & Lin, C. C. (2008). Nanoparticles formulation of *Cuscutta chinensis* prevents acetaminophen-induced hepatotoxicity in rats. *Food and Chemical Toxicology*, *46*(5), 1771–1777. doi:10.1016/j.fct.2008.01.021 PMID:18308443

Zare, B., Babaie, S., Setayesh, N., & Shahverdi, A. R. (2013). Isolation and characterization of a fungus for extracellular synthesis of small selenium nanoparticles. *Nanomedicine Journal*, *1*, 13–19.

Zhou, L., Chow, M., & Zhou, Z. (2006). Improved quality control method for Danshen products – consideration of both hydrophilic and lipophilic active componenets. *Journal of Pharmaceutical and Biomedical Analysis*, *41*(3), 744–750. doi:10.1016/j.jpba.2005.12.032 PMID:16458472

Chapter 7
Nanoparticulate Drug Delivery System:
An Emphasis on Herbal Medicines

Akshada Bakliwal
Sandip Institute of Pharmaceutical Science, Nasik, India

Swati Gokul Talele
Sandip Institute of Pharmaceutical Science, Nasik, India

Shweta Shaileshkumar Gedam
Sandip Institute of Pharmaceutical Science, Nasik, India

Vijay Sharadkumar Chudiwal
Sun Pharma, Mumbai, India

Swapnil Sharadkumar Jain
Philips Healthcare, Mumbai, India

ABSTRACT

The herbal medicines have been extensively used worldwide since ancient times and have been accepted by physicians and patients for their improved therapeutic value as they have less adverse effects in contrast with modern medicines. Phytotherapeutics requires a scientific approach to carry the components in a sustained manner to increase patient compliance and to reduce the frequency of administration. This can be accomplished by designing novel drug delivery systems (NDDS) for herbal constituents. NDDSs not only reduce the frequency of drug administration to improve patient compliance but also help to enhance the therapeutic value by dropping toxicity and enhancing the drug bioavailability. A nanotechnology is a new approach in which nano-sized drug delivery systems of herbal drugs have a prospective future for enhancing the therapeutic activity and conquer problems associated with plant medicines. Hence, the addition of the nanotechnology as an NDDS in traditional medication is essential for the treatment of more chronic diseases like cancer, diabetes, asthma, and others.

DOI: 10.4018/978-1-7998-4453-2.ch007

1. INTRODUCTION

Currently, there is a revolution from synthetic medicines to herbal or natural medicines throughout the world i.e. worldwide the peoples reverting back to herbal medications. The active molecule present in herbal or plant species provides synergistic action and also enriches its therapeutic effects and efficiency. (Kalia 2005). The effectiveness of many species of medicinal plants depends on the supply of active compounds. Most of the active molecules are hydrophobic in nature which results in enhanced systemic clearance and diminish bioavailability. (Inamdar et al., 2008). As compared to synthetic medicines, herbal medicines have enhanced therapeutic efficacy and lesser side effects. Herbal medicines are not used in the nanoparticulate drug delivery system owing to a lack of scientific explanation and processing. But nowadays, the phytopharmaceutical research solves this problem and develops a nanoparticulate drug delivery system using herbal medicaments because nanostructured systems might be able to potentiate the action of plant extracts. Most of the conventional dosage form leads to a decrease in therapeutic effect as it undergoes systemic circulation throughout the body due to their physicochemical properties. The key benefit of novel drug delivery systems (NDDS) contain targeted drug delivery, which enhances the solubility thereby increases the absorption, lessens dosage frequency whereas reduces elimination. The potency of active component can be enhanced by novel drug delivery system also other constituents which were discarded during formulation can be reintroduced into it.(Mainardes et al., 2006; Alexis et al., 2008). Before launching the new product into the market or to use it therapeutically, the nanoparticulate drug delivery system has the ability to enhance the specificity and efficacy, reduces the side effects and to release the drug in a controlled manner. (Grill et al., 2009; Venugopal et al., 2009; Yen et al., 2008; Tedesco et al., 2004).

1.1 Reasons for Selection of Nanoparticulate Drug Delivery System

The nanoparticulate drug delivery system has many advantages over traditional drug delivery systems. Many industries are working on nanoparticulate based herbal product and trying to protect their invention through patents.

More particularly, the U.S. Application No. 20110262499 discloses nano-emulsion based topical synergistic herbal formulations which are effective against acne and other skin disorder, and process for the preparation of the same in pharmaceutical acceptable dosage forms. (Chaudhary et al., 2009).

The selection of nanoparticulate drug delivery system based on the following reasons:

- Due to high loading capacity and nano-sized, delivery of the drug in higher concentration at the targeted site.
- Due to the nano-sized, faster dissolution of the drug into the blood.
- Reduces the dose of the drug formulation.
- Decreases the side effects.

1.2 Green Synthesis of Nanoparticulate Drug Delivery System

The term 'Green' refers to the nanoparticle synthesis from the metal salt which reduces the biologically active compound's property. The biologically active compounds consist of herbal extracts (leaf, root, flower, fruit, latex, whole body, aerial part, etc), microorganisms and animal extracts. The herbal extract is a better choice which is commonly used as a biologically active compound in nanoparticulate drug delivery system.

The activity of herbal drugs is based on the active constituent present in it. The active component of herbal extract provides synergistic action and increases the therapeutic efficiency. Every active moiety present in herbal extract plays an important role. (Castot et al., 1997). Moreover, the majority of the herbal drugs have low lipid solubility which reduces the bioavailability and increases the systemic clearance at the time of dose administration. The discovery of nanotechnology is considered a milestone in the medicine world. (Yadav et al., 2011; Singh et al., 2011). Nowadays to conquer various problems in case of herbals, nanotechnology becomes a great therapy. In research and development of herbal formulation, nanoparticulate dosage forms have a number of benefits for herbal drugs, including avoidance of toxicity, enhancement of the solubility and bioavailability, improvement of stability, better biological activity, controlled delivery, protection from physical and chemical degradation, and changes, improving tissue macrophages distribution. (Sungthongjeen et al., 1999; Sharma et al., 2011). Most of the active moiety of the herbal medicaments are soluble in acetone, petroleum ether, methanol and, chloroform. (Patwardhan et al.,2004). Nanotechnology will be the useful tool as many marketed herbal formulations have several side effects and lack target specificity in various chronic diseases (Currier et al., 2000).

1.3 The Necessity of Nanoparticulate Drug Delivery System for Herbal Medicaments

- Nanoparticulate drug delivery system enhances the selectivity, efficacy, safety of herbal medicament by targeting to the individual organ.
- It also reduces dosing frequency and thereby enhances patient compliance.
- It also helps to enhance the solubility and bioavailability of herbal medicaments.
- Due to high loading capacity and nano-sizes, nanotechnology delivered the drug at the site of action in high amount.

This chapter focuses on different types of nanocarriers which are formulated using herbal extracts to increase the solubility, bioavailability, efficacy and minimizes the dosing frequency and side effects.

2. NANOCARRIERS

A nanocarrier is a type of nanomaterial mainly used as a transporter for the drug molecule. Nanocarrier includes polymeric nanoparticles, polymer conjugates, lipid-based carriers, carbon nanotubes, dendrimers, and gold nanoparticles. Liposomes and micelles are the lipid-based carriers while the gold nanocages and nanoshells are examples of gold nanoparticles. Nanocarriers delivered the drug molecule either hydrophobic or hydrophilic throughout the body. Nanocarriers are made up of different types of nanomaterials. One of the disadvantages of nanocarriers is the toxicity of nanomaterial certainly used. Nanocarriers entangled herbal drug and carry an optimum quantity of it at the targeted site of action. Due to small size, drug nanoparticles circulate into the blood for a prolonged duration of time.

Nanocarriers are used in drug delivery, especially in chemotherapy. Since nanocarriers can be used to reduce the toxicity of lots of chemotherapeutic drugs also they can specifically target the small pores and higher temperatures of tumors. Also, approximately 75% of newly synthesized anticancer drugs are

Figure 1. Different types of nanocarriers

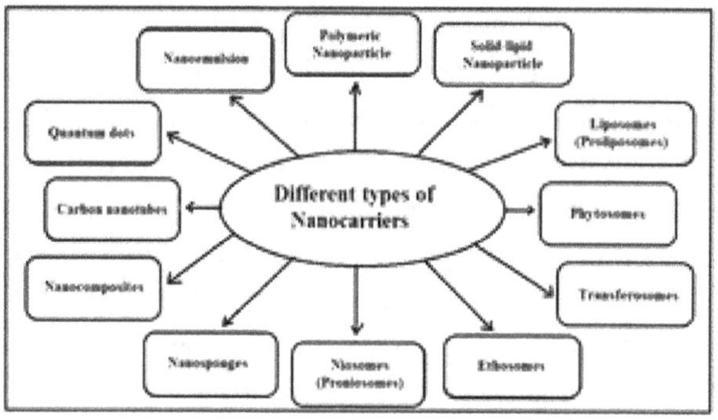

hydrophobic in nature and therefore exhibit difficulty in delivery of drug inside human cells, for such type of drug the use of micelles to effectively mask and stabilize the drug offer new possibilities.

2.1 Types of Nanocarriers

2.1.1 Nanoparticles

Nanoparticles are colloidal structures comprises of a natural or synthetic polymer having a size range from 1-1000nm. In this, the drug is dissolved, encapsulated, attached or entrapped into a nanoparticulate matrix. Nanoparticles can be either nanospheres or nanocapsules depend upon the method of preparation. The drug is uniformly distributed in nanospheres while in nanocapsules drug is enclosed with a polymer membrane. Method of preparation of nanoparticles includes solvent diffusion method, sonication method, micro-emulsion formation method, etc.

Nanoparticles have various benefits as follows:

a. Enhance solubility and bioavailability
b. Improve the shelf life of product
c. Minimize the side effects associated with dose
d. Both hydrophobic and lipophilic drugs can be incorporated (Chang et al., 2011).

2.1.2 Polymeric Nanoparticles

Polymeric nanoparticles refer to colloidal systems with the range of particle size from 10 to 1000 nm. The examples of herbal medicine used in polymeric nanoparticles include curcumin as an anti-cancer drug, after introduction into an alkaline environment, the antioxidant activity of catechin was decreased dramatically and chitosan nanoparticles for the extract of Ziziphus mauritiana and checked the effect on its immunomodulatory activity.

Table 1. Some of the Nanoparticle formulation consisting herbal medicaments

S.N.	Active constituent of plant	Biological activity	Reason of nanoparticle formulation
1	Camptothecin	Anti-cancer	To prolong circulation around tumor containing area
2	Hypocrellins	Anti-viral	To improve efficacy and stability
3	Ginkgo biloba	Brain activator	To improve metabolism an dcerebral blood flow
4	Silibinin	Hepatoprotective	To improve entrapment and stability
5	Ginseng	Anti-oxidant	To improve pharmacological response and stability

2.1.3 Ceramic Nanoparticles

Ceramic nanoparticles are inorganic systems with porous nature which newly appeared as a drug carrier. In cancer therapy, the biocompatible ceramic nanoparticles such as titania, alumina, and silica can be used. However, one of the major apprehension is that they can accumulate in the body and thus causes undesirable effects as they are non-biodegradable in nature.

2.1.4 Metallic Nanoparticles

Iron oxide nanoparticles (15–60 nm) which are metallic particles usually contain super paramagnetic agents that can be coated with phospholipids, dextran or other compounds to reduce aggregation and improve stability. Iron oxide nanoparticles are used as passive or active targeting agents. One of the novel categories of the spherical nanoparticle is a gold shell nanoparticle, comprising of a dielectric core enclosed by a thin gold shell. These particles own extremely favorable chemical and optical properties for therapeutic applications and biomedical imaging. Topical creams and ointments including silver nanoparticles are used to prevent infections of open wounds and burns.

2.1.5 Solid Lipid Nanoparticles

In the early 1990s, one of the colloidal carrier systems developed i.e. solid lipid Nanoparticles (SLNs) which combine the advantages of other colloidal systems (such as liposomes, emulsions, and polymeric nanoparticles) for drug delivery, though lessening, or, avoiding some of their disadvantages. SLNs com-

Table 2. Polymeric nanoparticle herbal formulations

S.N.	Active constituent of plant	Biological activity	Reason of polymeric nanoparticle formulation
1	Triptolide	Anti-neoplastic	To enhance solubility and reduce toxicity
2	Curcumin	Antitumor, antiamylodin, antioxidant, anti-inflammatory, and antiplatelet aggregation	To increase solubility and bioavailability
3	*Ziziphusmauritiana* plant extract	Immunomodulatory activity	To Enhance immunomodulatory activity of extract
4	Catechins	Chemopreventive, antioxidative, anticarcinogenic, anti-obesity, anti-inflammatory, antiviral	To Increase the stability of catechins

Table 3. Herbal formulations of solid lipid nanoparticle

S.N.	Active constituent of plant	Biological activity	Reason of solid-lipid nanoparticle formulation
1	Curcuminoi-ds	Antitumor, antiamylodinantioxidant,antiplatelet aggregation, and anti-inflammatory	To enhance stability of curcuminoids
2	Cryptotanshinone	Anti-bacterial, cytotoxic, Anti-inflammatory, anti-angiogenic, anti-parasitic	To enhance bioavailability

promises better protection against degradation of labile drugs, have higher physicochemical stability, and can also be produced on a large scale. SLNs composed mainly of lipids containing highly purified triglycerides, that are further stabilized by surfactants and solid at room temperature and.it can shield drug moiety against chemical degradation as the lipid particle matrix is solid. However, when the system is produced, results in lesser drug release and encapsulation efficiency as crystallization occurs. SLNs may be used in the pharmaceutical field for various routes of administration, such as parenteral, oral, and percutaneous owing to their biocompatibility and small size (50–1,000 nm). SLNs can be prepared by addition of a liquid lipid (oil) to an oil/water emulsion containing a solid lipid. They can be prepared by different methods such as warm micro-emulsion, homogenization, ultrasonication, solvent-diffusion and high-speed stirring method.

2.3 Liposomes

Liposomes are defined as the phospholipids having spherical, colloidal bilayered vesicular systems. They are bipolar amphipathic moieties with a characteristic spherical shape. The phospholipid contains to region i.e. polar head orient itself towards the aqueous media while the hydrophobic tails constitute the inner region of the membrane. They can entrap both hydrophobic as well as a hydrophilic drug within it. Hydrophilic drug occupies the aqueous domain i.e. aqueous core while lipophilic drug occupies the lipoidal domain within the bilayered membrane. The average size of liposome range from 0.05μ-5.0μ. Among various advantages associated with liposomes the noteworthy are:

a. Solubility enhancement
b. Enhancement of bioavailability
c. Programmed targeting
d. Prolongation of the duration of action
e. Stability associated problems can also be solved
f. Absorption and disposition of the constituents can also be tailored. (Wen et al., 2010).

Already enormous research has been done in this meadow but still, their stunning applications encourage researchers to ripe more benefits from this drug delivery system.

2.4 Proliposomes

Although liposomes own numerous advantages for the delivery of the drug, they still have some disadvantages of physicochemical instability (sedimentation, aggregation, fusion, phospholipid hydrolysis,

Table 4. Some of the Liposome formulation consisting herbal medicaments

S.N.	Active constituent of plant	Biological activity	Reason of liposomes formulation
1	Curcumin	Anti-cancer	To improve entrapment efficiency
2	Garlicin	Lungs	To enhanced therapeutic outcomes
3	Nux vomica	Anti-neoplastic, anti-inflammatory	To improve stability
4	Quercitin	Anti-anxiety	To improve bioavailability and reduce side effects
5	Usnic acid	Anti-mycobacterial	To enhance solubility and prolong action

sterilization and oxidation in large scale production). In order to overcome these problems a novel method for liposome production has been reported, namely Proliposomes. Proliposomes instantly form liposomal suspension when coming in contact with water as they are free-flowing particles. Stability problems of liposomes can be resolved due to its solid properties.

2.5 Phytosomes

Phytosomes is defined as the bilayered systems in which binding of drug molecules to phospholipids for the formation of lipid complexes. (Maiti et al., 2007). Phytosomes are more stable and helps to increase the bioavailability in contrast to liposomes where these constituents are only entrapment in the aqueous domain. Like liposome generated both lipophilic as well as hydrophilic domains because of which they can entrap lipophilic as well as hydrophilic drugs.(Pathan et al., 2011). To make the therapy more efficient effort have been done to prepare phytosomes of herbal drug such as, silybin, oxymatrin, embelin, etc.

2.6 Transferosomes and Ethosomes

Transferosomes and Ethosomes are phospholipid vesicles intended to administer the drug via transdermal route. Both have a common rationale of enhancing the penetration through stratum corneum barrier but the mode of action is different.(Zhaowu et al., 2009). They utilize the hydration and osmotic pressure of the skin while ethosomes have high content of ethanol (20-45%). Transferosomes are used to deliver the herbal constituents in the upper layers of skin while for deeper layer and systemic delivery twosomes are the better alternative. Usually they are give in the form of cream or gel, being non invasive they have better patient compliance.(Yan et al., 2010; Patel et al., 2009).

There are enormous examples where efficacy of herbal constituent mediate treatment is increased by adopting these delivery systems E.g. colchicine, curcumin, matrine, triptolide, etc.

2.7 Niosomes

Niosomes are multilamellar vesicles formed from non-ionic surfactants of the alkyl or dialkylpolyglycerol ether class and cholesterol. Niosomes have properties as potential drug carriers similar to liposomes. (Tangri et al., 2011). Niosomes have some advantages over the liposomes such as they are less costly, stability of phospholipids ingredients and easy to handle. (Gupta et al., 2011).

Table 5. Some of the Phytosomes formulation consisting herbal medicaments

S.N.	Active constituent of plant	Biological activity	Reason of phytosomes formulation
1	Curcumin	Anti-cancer, Anti-oxidant	To improve bioavailability
2	Embelin	Anti-fertility, Anti-bacterial	To enhance solubility
3	Ginsenosides	Immunomodulators, neutraceuticals	To enhance absorption
4	Hawthorn	Cardio-protective, anti-hypertensive	To improve efficacy and absorption
5	Marsupium	Anti-viral	To enhance bioavailability

Table 6. Some of the transferosomes formulation consisting herbal medicaments

S.N.	Active constituent of plant	Biological activity	Reason of Transferosomes formulation
1	Colchicin	Anti-gout	To reduce GIT associated side effects
2	Curcumin	Anti-cancer	To enhance permeation

2.8 Proniosomes

Proniosome gel system is step forward to niosome, which can be utilized for various applications in delivery of actives at desired site (Shukla, Tiwari 2011).. In-situ hydration of proniosomal gels formulation gets converted into the niosomes by when reacts with water from the skin(Goyal et al., 2011).The water soluble carrier particles of proniosomes are coated with surfactant which then hydrated to form niosomes before used in hot aqueous media.(Raja et al., 2011).

Some of the herbal medicaments used in proniosome formulation such as Levonorgestrel acts as a contraceptive agent, Indomethacin, piroxicam, tenoxicam acts as a NSAID, Exemestane acts as anticancer agent, captopril as an anti-hypertensive and vinpocetine as a cardiovascular and cerebral degenerative. (Yasam et al., 2014).

2.9 Nanosponges

Nanosponges are a novel class of nanoparticles with nanostructured hyper branched polymers and few nanometers wide cavities, in which a large variety of substances can be encapsulated. They have spherical nature. Nanosponges can solubilize poorly water soluble drug and provide prolonged drug release as well as improved drugs bioavailability. (Bakliwal, Talele 2018).

Table 7. Some of the Ethosomes formulation consisting herbal medicaments

S.N.	Active constituent of plant	Biological activity	Reason of Ethosomes formulation
1	Matrine	Anti-rheumatism	To improve efficacy and enhance permeation
2	Triptolide	Anti-inflammatory	To enhance bioavailability

Advantages of Nanosponges Drug Delivery System

- Nanospongesenraps wide variety of ingredients and also minimises the side effects. (Talele, Gudsoorkar).
- This technology enhances stability and flexibility of the formulation. (Patel, Oswal 2012).
- This technology offers release of drug in controlled manner for more than 12 hours.
- It also offers compatibility for the patients. (Khopade et al., 1996).
- This technology is cost effective and highly compatible with most of the ingredients.

The some of the example of herbal drugs which are encapsulated in the nanosponge formulation are camptothecin and curcumin. Camptothecin acts as an antineoplastic agent which is used to increase the solubility and bioavailability and also to reduce the side effects while curcumin is a tumor targeting agent which is also used to increase the solubility and also it minimizes the dose of drug by targeting at specific site.

2.10 Nanaocomposite

A nanocomposite is a composite material, in which one of the components has a dimension that is nanoscopic in size that is around 10^{-9} m. A nanocomposite material is made up of matrix which consists of filler and resin and they are cost effective. Nanocomposites are divided into two types viz., polymer and non-polymer based. This is one of the solubility enhancement method.

Advantages of nanocomposite drug delivery system

- To enhance the solubility
- To minimize the dosing frequency
- Targeted drug delivery

The chitosan solution and extracts of *Achyranthes aspera* and *Senna auriculata* together form a nanocomposite which is an antibacterial medical textile. Also the nanocomposites containing herbal extract of Smilax china is used in wound healing because of its antimicrobial activity.

2.11 Carbon Nanotubes

Carbon nanotubes (CNTs) are also known as a allotropes of carbon. They are made up of graphite and cylindrical in shape. In the field of nanotechnology, carbon nanotubes is one of the most commonly used additives to various structural materials. During the transport in the body, carbon nanotubes penetrate into the cells directly by keeping the drug intact without its metabolism, hence it is one of the better vehicle for the delivery of the drug. Nanotubes and fullerences are comes under the carbon nanomaterials. Carbon nanotubes have vast scope for delivery of herbal medication.

2.12 Quantum Dots

Quantum dots are one of the types of nanoparticles. It is made up of semiconductor materials having fluorescent properties. Quantum dots are key component for most of the biological applications. When comes under Ultraviolet light, they glow very quantum dots spark very luminously.

2.13 Nanoemulsion

Nanoemulsions are the optically isotropic containing system of oil and water. It offers various benefits such as enhancing the solubility and bioavailability of lipophilic drugs, easy to prepare, thermodynamically stable and having low viscosity.

The example of herbal nanoemulsions includes curcumin. In this, anti-inflammatory activity of curcumin is enhanced by formulation of nanoemulsion. Other examples of nanoemulsions include Zedoary essential oil, poly-herbal ointment, etc.

3. TOXICITY OF NANOPARTICLES

Nanotechnology is one of the growing field now-a-days. The nanotechnology is used in medical sciences to achieve the personalized medicines. Due to the small size, low dose and large surface area nanoparticles becomes most useful, but this may leads to toxicity in biological system. Because due to the small size, they have more surface area per unit mass which makes them more reactive in cellular environment. (Tanwar et al., 2006).

4. FUTURE PROSPECTS OF NANO HERBAL MEDICINES

As per future prospects, nano-pharmaceutical may alter the human body on nanoscale. So, it is important to consider both benefits and side effects of nano-pharmaceuticals. (Borodina et al., 2008; Shen et al., 2008).

5. CONCLUSION

Nanotechnology is one of the leading technologies used worldwide. In this, various types of nanomaterials and nanocarriers are used. The nanoparticulate drug delivery is most commonly used due to its safety, efficacy and targeted drug delivery. It also enhances the solubility and bioavailability, increases the therapeutic value and reduces the dosing frequency. Now-a-days, researchers focus on development of drug delivery system using herbal medicaments using a scientific justification. But there are many challenges for this like conduction of clinical research, pharmacological and toxicological evaluation, etc. Still the herbal medicines are more preferred over the conventional medicines due to its fewer side effects. This chapter focuses on different herbal drugs which are encapsulated in different formulation of nanocarriers. (Zhao et al., 2002; Arthri 2009; Devi et al., 2010; Pinto, 2010).

REFERENCES

Alexis, F., Pridgen, E., Molnar, L. K., & Farokhzad, O. C. (2008). Factors affecting the clearance and bio distribution of polymeric nanoparticles. *Molecular Pharmaceutics*, *5*(4), 505–515. doi:10.1021/mp800051m PMID:18672949

Arthri, B. S. (n.d.). A formulation containing herbal extracts and nutrients to support healthy joints and connective tissues in the body. *Nutraceuticals World*. Available from: http://findparticles.com/particles/mi_hb223/is_6_7/ai_n29102045/

Bakliwal A. A., & Talele S. G. (2018). Formulation and evaluation of nateglinide nanosponges. *Indian Drugs, 55*(2), 27-35.

Bisht, S., Feldmann, G., Soni, S., Ravi, R., Karikar, C., & Maitra, A. (n.d.). Polymeric nanoparticle-encapsulate curcumin ("nanocurcumin"): A novel strategy for human cancer therapy. *J Nanobiotechnol, 5*, 1-18.

Borodina, T. N., Rumsh, L. D., Kunizhev, S. M., Sukhorukov, G. B., Vorozhtsov, G. N., & Feldman, B. M. (2008). Entrapment of herbal extracts into biodegradable microcapsules. *Biochemistry (Moscow) Supplement Series B. Biomedical Chemistry*, *2*, 176–182.

Castot, A., Djezzar, S., Deleau, N., Guillot, B., & Efthymiou, M. L. (1997). Pharmacovigilance off the beaten track: Herbal surveillance or pharmacovigilance of medicinal plants. *Therapie*, *52*, 97–103. PMID:9231502

Chang, C. H., Huang, W. Y., Lai, C. H., Hsu, Y. M., Yao, Y. H., & Chen, T. Y. (2011). Development of novel Nanoparticles shelled with heparin for Berberine delivery to treat *Helicobacter pylori*. *Acta Biomaterialia*, *7*, 593–603.

Currier, S. J., Johnston, P. D., & Gorelick, K. J. (2000). Complementary and alternative medicine-herbal medicines. *Science & Medicine*, *7*, 40–43.

Devi, V. K., Jain, N., & Valli, K. S. (2010). Importance of novel drug delivery systems in herbal medicines. *Pharmacognosy Reviews*, *4*, 27–31.

Goyal, C., Ahuja, M., & Sharma, S. K. (2011). Preparation and evaluation of anti-inflammatory activity of gugulipid-loaded proniosomal gel. *Acta Pol Pharm Drug Res*, *68*, 147–150.

Grill, A. E., Johnston, N. W., Sadhukha, T., & Panyam, J. (2009). A review of select recent patents on novel nanocarriers. *Recent Patents on Drug Delivery & Formulation*, *3*(2), 137–142. doi:10.2174/187221109788452276 PMID:19519573

Gupta, S., Singh, R. P., Lokwani, P., Yadav, S., & Gupta, S. K. (2011). Vesicular system as targeted drug delivery system: An overview. *Int J Pharm Technol*, *3*, 987–1021.

Inamdar, N. S., Edalat, V. B., Kotwal, V. B., & Pawar, S. S. (2008). Herbal drugs in milieu of modern drugs. *Int J Green Pharm*, *2*(1), 2–8. doi:10.4103/0973-8258.39154

Kalia, A. N. (2005). *Text Book of Industrial Pharmacognosy*. Oscar Publication.

Khopade, A.J., Jain, S., & Jain, N.K. (1996). The Microsponge. *Eastern Pharmacist*, 49-53.

Mainardes, R. M., Gremião, M. P., & Evangelista, R. C. (2006). Thermoanalytical study of praziquatel-loaded PLGA nanoparticles. *Brazilian Journal of Pharmaceutical Sciences*, *42*, 523–530.

Maiti, K., Mukherjee, K., Gantait, A., Saha, B. P., & Mukherjee, P. K. (2007). Curcumin-phospholipid complex: Preparation, therapeutic evaluation and pharmacokinetic study in rats. *International Journal of Pharmaceutics*, *330*, 155–163.

Patel, E. K., & Oswal, R. J. (2012). Nanosponge and Microsponges: A Novel Drug Delivery System. *IJRP2*.

Patel, R., Singh, S. K., Singh, S., Sheth, N. R., & Gendle, R. (2009). Development and characterization of curcumin loaded transferosomes for transdermal delivery. *Journal of Pharmaceutical Sciences*, *1*, 71–80.

Pathan, R., & Bhandari, U. (2011). Preparation and characterization of embelin- phospholipid complex as effective drug delivery tool. *Journal of Inclusion Phenomena and Macrocyclic Chemistry*, *9*, 139–147.

Patwardhan, B., Vaidya, A. D., & Chorghade, M. (2004). Ayurveda and natural products drug discovery. *Current Science*, *86*, 789.

Pinto, J. F. (2010). Site-specific drug delivery systems within the gastro-intestinal tract: From the mouth to the colon. *International Journal of Pharmaceutics*, *395*, 44–52.

Raja, K., Ukken, J. P., Athul, P. V., Tamizharasi, S., & Sivakumar, T. (2011). Formulation and evaluation of maltodextrin based proniosomal drug delivery system containing anti-diabetic (glipizide) drug. *International Journal of Pharm Tech Research*, *3*, 471–477.

Sharma, A. T., Mitkare, S. S., & Moon, R. S. (2011). Multicomponent herbal therapy: A review. *International Journal of Pharmaceutical Sciences Review and Research*, *6*, 185–187.

Shen, Y. J., Zhang, Z. W., Luo, X. G., Wang, X. F., & Wang, H. L. (2008). Nanoparticles of traditional Chinese herbs inhibit thrombosis *in vivo*. *Haematologica*, *93*, 1457.

Shukla, N. D., & Tiwari, M. (2011). Proniosomal drug delivery systems – Clinical applications. *International Journal of Research in Pharmaceutical and Biomedical Sciences*, *2*, 880–887.

Singh, R. P., Singh, S. G., Naik, H., Jain, D., & Bisla, S. (2011). Herbal excipients in novel drug delivery system. *Int J ComprPharm*, *2*, 1–7.

Sungthongjeen, S., Pitaksuteepong, T., Somsiri, A., & Sriamornsak, P. (1999). Studies on pectins as potential hydrogelmatrices for controlled-release drug delivery. *Drug Development and Industrial Pharmacy*, *25*(12), 1271–1276. doi:10.1081/DDC-100102298 PMID:10612023

Talele & Gudsoorkar. (n.d.). Novel approaches for solidification of SEDDS. *Int. J Pharm and Bio.*, *4*(15), 90-101.

Tangri, P., & Khurana, S. (2011). Niosomes: Formulation and evaluation. *Int J Biopharm*, *2*, 47–53.

Tanwar, Y. S., Gupta, G. D., & Ramawa, K. G. (2006). *Development and evaluation of microparticles of Gugulipid. The PharmaReview*. Kongposh Publications Pvt., Ltd.

Tedesco, D., Steidler, S., Galletti, S., Tameni, M., Sonzogni, O., & Ravarotto, L. (2004). Efficacy of silymarin-phospholipid complex in reducing the toxicity of aflatoxin B1 in broiler chicks. *Poultry Science, 83*(11), 1839–1843. doi:10.1093/ps/83.11.1839 PMID:15554059

Venugopal, J., Prabhakaran, M. P., Low, S., Choon, A. T., Deepika, G., & Dev, V. R. (2009). Continuous nanostructures for the controlled release of drugs. *Current Pharmaceutical Design, 15*(15), 1799–1808. doi:10.2174/138161209788186344 PMID:19442191

Wen, Z., Liu, B., Zheng, Z., You, X., Pu, Y., & Li, Q. (2010). Preparation of Liposomes entrapping essential oil from AtractylodesmacrocephalaKoidz by modified RESS technique. *Chemical Engineering Research & Design, 88*, 1102–1107.

Yadav, D., Suri, S., Choudhary, A. A., Sikender, M., Hemant, K., & Beg, N. M. (2011). Novel approach: Herbal remedies and natural products in pharmaceutical science as nano drug delivery systems. *Int J Pharmtech, 3*, 3092–3116.

Yan, Z., Yuhui, W., Huanxiang, L., Guoqiang, Z., & Xinan, W. (2010). Preparation and In vitro Evaluation of EthosomalTotal Alkaloids of Sophoraalopecuroides loaded by Transmembrane pH-Gradient Method. *AAPS PharmSciTech, 1*, 1–9.

Yasam, V. R., Jakki, S. L., Natarajan, J., & Kuppusamy, G. (2014). A review on novel vesicular drug delivery. *Proniosomes. Drug Deliv, 21*, 243–249.

Yen, F. L., Wu, T. H., Lin, L. T., Cham, T. M., & Lin, C. C. (2008). Nanoparticles formulation of *Cuscutachinensis*preventsacetaminophen-induced hepatotoxicity in rats. *Food and Chemical Toxicology, 46*(5), 1771–1777. doi:10.1016/j.fct.2008.01.021 PMID:18308443

Zhao, H. R., Wang, K., Zhao, Y., & Pan, L. Q. (2002). Novel sustained-release implant of herb extract using chitosan. *Biomaterials, 23*, 4459–4462.

Zhaowu, Z., Xiaoli, W., Yangde, Z., & Nianfeng, L. (2009). Preparation of matrine ethosome, its percutaneous permeation in vitro and anti-inflammatory activity in vivo in rats. *Journal of Liposome Research, 19*, 155–162.

Chapter 8
Herbal Medicine and Its Bioactive Compounds for Treatment of Hepatitis B

Bui Thanh Tung
VNU University of Medicine and Pharmacy, Vietnam National University, Hanoi, Vietnam

Nguyen Hong Nhung
VNU University of Medicine and Pharmacy, Vietnam National University, Hanoi, Vietnam

Ta Thi Thu Hang
VNU University of Medicine and Pharmacy, Vietnam National University, Hanoi, Vietnam

Vu Khanh Linh
VNU University of Medicine and Pharmacy, Vietnam National University, Hanoi, Vietnam

ABSTRACT

Hepatitis B is an infectious disease caused by the hepatitis B virus (HBV) which is one of the most serious public health problems in the world. Some common approved drugs bring about dose-dependent adverse effects or drug resistance. Therefore, safe and useful new HBV therapeutics are essential. Medicinal plants have particular benefits to treat HBV-infected patients. Traditional medicines have many bioactive compounds that are effective as antiviral candidates including esculetin, helioxanthin, oxymatrine, epigallocatechin-3-gallate, wogonin, alkaloids, polysaccharides, etc. In this chapter, the authors summarize the pathogenesis and protein targets for the treatment of hepatitis B disease. They also indicate several medicinal plants and isolated compounds which are used for preventing and reduce symptoms of this disease.

DOI: 10.4018/978-1-7998-4453-2.ch008

1. INTRODUCTION

As stated by WHO, in 2015, the global has over 257 million cases of hepatitis B transmission (Organization, 2017). HBV causes chronic hepatitis, which can progress to cirrhosis, HBV chronic is one of the causes of hepatocellular carcinoma (HCC) (Y. Y. Zhang & Hu, 2015). In Western countries, lingering HBV infection is fairly rare and acquired mainly in a grown-up, whereas in most of Africa and Asia, most infections through blood, from child to child touch in household surroundings, from mother to child (Singh et al., 2017). HBV is considered a neglected tropical diseases (NTDs). Because, first, NTDs mainly influence populations living in subtropical and tropical areas. Second, NTDs cause stigma and discrimination due to disproportionately influence populations living in dearth. Third, by operating public health strategies, NTDs are instantaneously amenable to extensive control, elimination, or extermination. The last, NTDs are moderately neglected by study, resource distribution is not reasonable with the significance of the problem (Lemoine, Eholié, & Lacombe, 2015; O'Hara et al., 2017).

HBV infection for the first time may be asymptomatic, sickness for several days or weeks, or getting sick very quickly. Symptoms may appear after 6 months such as fatigue, loss of appetite, mild fever, nausea, vomiting, joint, muscle aches, dark urine, and yellow skin. Over time, people with chronic HBV can develop symptoms of cirrhosis and liver cancer in 15% - 40% (Harris, 2019).

The pathogenesis of HBV is considered by two factors: the first, the cause of liver hurt is elevated levels of HBV reproduction and infected hepatocytes accumulate viral products. The second, HBV infection may be either straight cytopathic, noncytopathic, or a blend of both in a private patient hang on accumulating viral products (Y. Y. Zhang & Hu, 2015).

Jesse Summers suggested that HBV reproduction in tainted cells had better be controlled due to continued amassing of viral production would lead to injury to the tainted cells. Control of cccDNA (covalently closed circular DNA) amplification is a significant aspect necessary for the possibility of hepadnaviruses to continuously infected cells, devoid of cytopathic effects. He raised the issue that HBV tenacious infection of hepatocytes hangs upon the possibility of virus-related genes to be upheld devoid of cytopathic consequence to the poisoned cells (Summers, Smith, & Horwich, 1990; Summers, Smith, Huang, & Yu, 1991). He showed that the lofty level of viral reproduction and cccDNA duplicate numbers make cytopathic alterations in both the hepatocytes and cell culture of infected animals (Lenhoff & Summers, 1994a, 1994b). HBV reproduction may also distract intracellular organelles, causing ER strain (B. Li et al., 2007) and modification of mitochondrial function (J. Chen & Siddiqui, 2007; Rahmani, Huh, Lasher, & Siddiqui, 2000; Waris, Huh, & Siddiqui, 2001), and raised reproduction may lead to exhaustion of cellular molecular sources like phospholipids which are needed for the creation of cellular coverage, lipoproteins, HBV fraught and subviral particles (Gavilanes, Gonzalez-Ros, & Peterson, 1982; Mohamadkhani et al., 2010; Norton, Gong, Mehta, Lu, & Block, 2003; Peterson, 1981).

Liver damage is also caused by the amassing of viral proteins, without HBV reproduction in hepatocytes. Chisari's group showed that (1) amassing of the viral consequence in infected cells can happen if the consequence of the viral consequences is beyond the excretion capacity of the master cell or the excretion efficiency is limited by the cellular factors, (2) the amassing of viral consequence can cause a range of main hepatocytic hurt (Chisari et al., 1987), which is similar to the histopathological modifications described in hepatitis B.

Master cells can limit viral reproduction by adjusting entrance to cellular factors and structure demanded reproduction or throughout cellular factors that are naturally opposed to stairs in the HBV lifecycle. As a result, when assessing HBV-mediated cytopathic influence, the effect of cellular limit on

HBV reproduction should also be inspected. It is supposed that HBV infection can lead to either straight cytopathic or non-cytopathic effects hang on modifications of the intracellular limit on viral replication (Y. Y. Zhang & Hu, 2015).

Clinically, HBV reproduction efficiency differences extremely from individual to individual, indicating the presence of different limits on HBV reproduction. In a few patients, HBV reproduction is allowed to touch significantly high levels, leading to liver damage. Other patients can limit the amassing of viral consequences (possibly throughout efficient virus excretion) to a not high level that wouldn't happen liver hurt. For example, immunotolerant patients with elevated HBsAg levels and serum DNA of HBV, normally do not show biochemical confirmation of liver damage (C.-J. Chu, Hussain, & Lok, 2002; Zacharakis et al., 2005). Besides distinct levels of HBV reproduction among distinct individuals, the master's limit of HBV reproduction can also be modified during the progression of HBV infection. As a result, distinct outcomes since varied efficiency of virus reproduction are most likely structured by a dynamic relation between the poisoned hepatocyte and the virus or by the HBV infection progression, not a segregated behavior of HBV itself.

HBV is a tiny DNA virus that transmits the liver. Its genome includes: the C gene encodes for the protein, which is the forerunner of the underground e antigen (HBeAg); the S gene encodes for the viral cover proteins - surface antigens (HBsAg); the P gene encodes for the virus's DNA polymerase, and the X gene encodes for an adjusting protein (Tian, Chen, & Ou, 2011). The presence of anti-IFN antibodies happened before HBV-DNA loss or HBV-DNA loss together (Porres, Carreño, Ruíz, Marrón, & Bartolomé, 1989). Therefore, IFN inhibits HBV-DNA replication. Tenofovir is a selective suppression of HBV DNA polymerase–contrary transcriptase in vitro (Lai et al., 2007). Therefore, medicines to treat chronic HBV infection, including oral nucleotide (Adefovir, Tenofovir) or nucleoside (Lamivudine, Telbivudine, Entecavir) viral inhibitors, which inhibit HBV-DNA replication.

Some medicines to treat chronic HBV infection, including oral nucleotide (Adefovir, Tenofovir) or nucleoside (Lamivudine, Telbivudine, Entecavir) viral inhibitors, and subcutaneous interferon or peginterferon (Alberti & Caporaso, 2011). However, oral nucleotide or nucleoside viral inhibitors are often resistant. Interferon or peginterferon has side effects such as fatigue, headache, high fever (Hadziyannis et al., 1990). Therefore, the search for natural compounds affecting HBV plays an important role in the treatment of HBV.

2. MEDICINAL PLANTS USING FOR TREATMENT OF HEPATITIS B VIRUS

Medicinal plants have been shown effective to inhibit hepatitis B virus activities with increased liver function. Many studies presented the effect of total medicinal plant extracts on HBV and to isolate and find out the bioactive compounds as potential drug candidates (F. Qi et al., 2013). There are so many compounds found including chrysophanol 8-O-beta-D-glucoside, wogonin, oxymatrine, artemisinin, artesunate, astragaloside IV from Radix Astragali that showed various pharmacology activities such as strong antibacterial, antifungal, and especially anti-HBV infection (Y Chen & Zhu, 2013; Cui, Wang, Kokudo, Fang, & Tang, 2010). They were isolated from medicinal plants such as *Sophora flavescens, Phyllanthus species, Astragalus, Scutellaria balcalensis, Rheum palmatum* (L. Zhang et al., 2010) Below we summarize some medicinal plants and bioactive compounds are used for the treatment hepatitis B virus infection.

2.1 Phyllanthus

The genus of *Phyllanthus* is spread over the tropical and subtropical countries with approximately 1000 species and many of them are used as herbal medicine to treat chronic liver disease (Sarin, Verma, Martín, & Mohanty, 2014). The most anti-viral herbs of *Phyllanthus* species that have been reported are *P.amarus, P.niruri, P.urninaria* (B. E. Wang, 2000). Several compounds were identified including alkaloids, flavonoids, terpenes, lignans, phenols, tannins, lactones, flavonoids. These extractions of plant *Phyllanthus* inhibit hepatitis B virus action (Dhiman & Chawla, 2005). Phyllanthus have been evaluated in preclinical and clinical and presented promising anti-viral candidates (J.-p. Liu, Lin, & McIntosh, 2001). Each of *Phyllanthus* genus has different mechanism of suppression of HBV infection. While The *P. amarus* interfere with HBV mRNA transcription invitro, *P.niruri* inhibits endogenous DNA polymerase and binds to the HbsAg of hepatitis B virus in-vitro and nontoxic to mice as well as antiviral in woodchuck (Ott, Thyagarajan, & Gupta, 1997; Venkateswaran, Millman, & Blumberg, 1987). However, Chiara Baiguea et al., investigated in the clinical trial of *P.niruri* in two years with 50 chronic HBV participants and not received an evident response to the treatment (Baiguera et al., 2018). In a recent investigation, *P. niruri* can reduce the oxidative destruction in hepatitis rats by active compound (-) – epicatechin (Shanmugam et al., 2017). Besides, niranthin isolated from *P.niruri* has an anti-HBV effect *in vitro* and *in vivo* experiments (S. Liu et al., 2014). As the result, clinical studies about these herbs should have in the future to identify exactly the role of hepatitis infection treatment. Meanwhile, *P. amarus* was indicated that it has an extraordinary outcome for HBV infection in recovery injured liver and suppression the replication of HBV, especially the rates of ALT, A/G, and SB in the treatment group was higher than in the interferon treatment group with number 73.3%, 80.0%, and 78.2%, respectively ($p<0.05$) (Baiguera et al., 2018). The previous review showed that *P.urinaria* strongly affects HBV including mechanisms such as intracellular HbsAg formation inhibition, suppressing HbsAg and HbcAg secretion, decreasing HBV DNA levels, and demonstrated practically in patient and the same result also showed in study of Ying Wu and et al (Y. Wu et al., 2015). A flavonoid was isolated from *P. urinaria*, ellagic acid, blocked HbeAg secretion in HepG2 2.2.15 cells with IC_{50} values of 0.07 µg/ml. This compound is a promising candidate therapeutic chronic HBV-infected (G. Du et al., 2018).

2.2 Scutellaria Balcalensis

Scutellaria balcalensis is the flowering plant of the genus Lamiaceae and the main application of this plant is the dried root (Q. Zhao, Chen, & Martin, 2016). The main active ingredients of these herbs are flavones including baicalin, wogonin, baicalein with a wide range of pharmacological functions. These flavones have the benefit on the nervous system, immune system, live function, anti-cancer, anti-bacterial, anti-viral, antioxidant…(T. Zhao et al., 2019). The aqueous extraction of *Scutellaria* Radix represses HBV expression in both normal and resistance of lamivudine virus in the human liver cell (Tseng, Wu, Leu, Yeh, & Chou, 2010). Especially, the recent research indicated that wogonin can repress HBV surface antigen production in-vitro ($p< 0.001$) and no adverse information (R.-L. Huang et al., 2000). The study of Qinglong and et al showed that wogonin is a potential component anti- HBV activity both in vitro and in vivo. In vitro, it reduced HBV DNA level in HepG2.2.15 live cell line as well as HBV- infected of duck, IC_{50}= 4 µg/ml at 9 days and IC_{50} values of 0.57 µg/ml at 10 days, respectively. *In vivo*, with a dose of 7-28 mg/kg for 10 days, HBsAg levels in hepatitis and plasma decreased dependently of dose treatment (Guo et al., 2007). Recently, baicalin, a flavonoid isolated from *S. balcalensis* dried root, reduced inflammation in the normal live cell stimulated by lipopolysaccharide via upregulating TUG1(Y. Huang et al., 2019). Nevertheless, this substance has anti-hepatitis A virus benefit in duck and so need more investigations about inhibitory hepatitis viral of this compound (Yun Chen et al., 2019).

2.3 Rheum Palmatum

Rheum palmatum is an herbaceous perennial in the knotweed family Polygonaceae. The active components that are isolated in ethanol extract are anthraquinones including emodin, rhein, physcion, chrysophanol, aloe-emodin, chrysophanol 8-O-β-D -glucoside. Rheum palmatum L. has various pharmacological effects such as anti-viral, liver failure, anti-metastatic, hepatitis and renal failure, antioxidant activity, anti- SARS coronavirus,… (Miraj, 2016). Anthraquinones have antibacterial, antifungal, anticancer, antiviral… (Y. Li & Jiang, 2018). *Rheum palmatum* ethanol extract and anthraquinones can inhibit HBV-DNA production and HbsAg expression in HepG2 2.2.15 cell line as well as HepAD38 cells (Z. Li, Li, Sun, & Li, 2007; Sun, Li, Li, & Li, 2007). Chrysophanol 8-O-β-D -glucoside is the most effective of inhibiting HBV DNA production and HbsAg expression with value IC_{50} values of 36.98 ± 2.28 μg/ml (Z. Li et al., 2007). In short, both in vivo and in vitro researches showed *Rheum palmatum* extract can anti-HBV activity and chrysophanol 8-O-β-D –glucoside is a potential candidate in the treatment of chronic HBV-infected.

2.4 Sophora Flavescens

Sophora flavescens belong to the genus of fabaceae family and its root has been used as traditional medicine for a long time. This herbal possess various benefits including antitumor, antimicrobial, antipyretic, antinociceptive, and anti-inflammatory pharmacological abilities (He, Fang, Huang, Wang, & Huang, 2015). The main active compounds of *Sophora flavescens* root that were identified by chromatography were matrin-type alkaloids (X. Chen, Yi, Yang, & Wang, 2004). It contains matrine, sophoridine, sophocarpine, lehmannine, sophoramine, oxymartine, oxysophocarpine, cytosine and aloperine (X. Chen et al., 2004). The aqueous extracts of *Sophora flavescens* can repress the hepatitis B virus activity of duck and major compounds consisted of oxymatrine, sophoranol and matrine that were useful substances anti-HBV production (Ye et al., 2007). The recent research determined particularly five potential compounds (flavesines G, flavesines J, alopecurine B, oxymatrine, sophoridine) that isolated from the dried root plant and played an important role to inhibit HBsAg secretion. Invitro, these alkaloids inhibition percents were more than matrin and lamivudine in HepG2.2.15 cells line (Y.-B. Zhang et al., 2018). In other studies, the researcher indicated that the compounds are potential candidates including (+) –oxysophocarpine, (-)-sophocarpine, (+)-lehmannine, (-)-13,14-dehydrosophoridine. All of them can inhibit HBsAg secretion at 48.3–79.3% and that against HBeAg secretion at 24.6–34.6%, in vitro (Ding, Liao, Huang, Zhou, & Chen, 2006). Dimmer matrin – alkaloids type isolated from this plant's root are potential to inhibit HBV production in HepG2.2.15 and all compounds were identified by spectroscopic, X-ray crystallographic and chemical methods (Y.-B. Zhang et al., 2016). Additionally, *Sophora flavescens* polysaccharides were demonstrated to protect hepatocytes by reducing hepatocytes apoptosis, prevent neutrophils and macrophages into live and improved IFN- γ and IL-6 of splenocytes in ConA-induced hepatitis mice, against HBsAg and HbeAg excretion in HepG2.2.25 cells (Yang et al., 2018). In a clinical trial, kurorione, isolated from *Sophora flavescens*, was compared with interferon- alpha2a and received no different response (C. Chen, Guo, & Liu, 2000). As the result, kurorione possess positive result in chronic HBV-infected patients (C. Chen et al., 2000). In conclusion, *Sophora flavescens* has numerious components which are the potential anti-HBV candidates including matrin- type alkaloids, Sophora flavescens polysaccharides, kurorione, (+) –oxysophocarpine, (-)-sophocarpine, (+)-lehmannine and (-)-13,14-dehydrosophoridine.

2.5 Astragalus L

Astragalus L is the genus of the legume family Fabaceae and the subfamily Faboideae and is distributed in template regions of the world with over 2,000 species. Some of them were used to protect the liver, antioxidative, immunostimulant and antiviral effects. The chemical groups of extraction are polysaccharides, saponins and phenolics that have numerous pharmacological benefits (Rios & Waterman, 1997). *Astragalus- polygonum* was more remarkable compared with *Jinshuibao capsule* in curing cirrhosis hepatitis of chronic hepatitis B (H. Chen & Weng, 2000). *In vivo, Astragalus* polysaccharide plus emodin have weak effects to inhibit HBV activity but they may use as an additional substance in treating HBV-infected patients (Dang et al., 2009). Besides, *Astragalus* polysaccharide has functions to enhance the immune responses and adjuvant of HBV DNA vaccine in mice (X. Du et al., 2012). *Astragalus L* needs more particular investigations to discover exactly anti-HBV benefits and its active compounds.

2.6 Artemisia Capillaris

Artemisia capillaris belongs to the Artemisia family with approximately 500 species (Bora & Sharma, 2011). Its leaf has a wide range of benefits including antimalarial, antihepatotoxic, antibacterial, antifungal, antioxidant and particularly anti-viral hepatitis (Yarnell & Abascal, 2010). The extracts of *Artemisia capillaris* have promising therapeutic in some hepatitis injuries like HBV-infected, liver cancer, hepatitis fibrosis (Jang, Kim, Lee, Inn, & Lee, 2015). Pumilaside A isolated from the 90% ethanol extract of *Artemisia capillaris* was the strongest inhibitory to the HBsAg(IC_{50}= 15.02 μM, SI=111.3) and HbeAg (IC_{50}= 9.00 μM, SI=185.9) secretion and the replication of HBV DNA (IC_{50}= 12.01 μM, SI= 139.2) (Y. Zhao, Geng, Sun, et al., 2014). In other research, among various substances of the 90% ethanol *A. capillaris* extract, nine chlorogenic acis analogues were the major ingredients to suppress HBV activity (Y. Zhao, Geng, Ma, et al., 2014). Additionally, the associated sources of *p*-hydroxyacetophenone and substituted cinnamic acids improved the activity inhibition of HBV DNA production with IC_{50} range from 5.8 to 74.4 μM (Y. Zhao et al., 2015). Besides, enynes in *Artemisia capillaris* was investigated the anti-HBV activity and its hydroxyl, glycosyl groups are significant for keeping activity (Geng et al., 2018).

2.7 Salvia Miltiorrhiza

Salvia miltiorrhiza is the genus of Labiatae family, it has numerous pharmacological effects including antioxidant activity, anti-microbial, anti-viral, anti-tumor, anti-inflammatory,… (B.-Q. Wang, 2010). For a long time, it has been conjugated with other drugs to effectively cure chronic HBV infection such as bufotoxin, *Polyporus umbellatus* polysaccharide (Xiong, 1993; Zhiguo, Yanpei, & Peizheng, 1999). Protocatechuic aldehyde was isolated from *Salvia miltiorrhiza* prevented usefully HBV replication both in vitro (in HepG2 2.2.15 cell line, concentrations range from 24-48 μg/mL) and in vivo (in duck with dose 25,50 or 100mg/kg/twice daily) experiments (Zhou et al., 2007). *Salvia miltiorrhiza* and this plant's active ingredients are necessary for deeper preclinical and clinical studies.

2.8 Polygonum Cuspidatum

Polygonum cuspidatum is one of the members of Polygonaceae. This herbal's dried root has been well known about a lot of good health effects such as treating cough, leucorrhea, snake bites, antiviral, antimicrobial, and so on (Huan Zhang, Li, Kwok, Zhang, & Chan, 2013). *P. cuspidatum* was indicated that it was one of the top five traditional medicines to be used for clinical HBV-infected treatment in China (L. Zhang et al., 2010). The ethanol extract of *P. cuspidatum*, as well as the water extract, suppressed HBV replication dose-dependently but the expression of HBsAg was enhanced (Chang et al., 2005). The identified components of this plant consist of quinones, stilbenes, flavonoids, coumarins, and ligan (Peng, Qin, Li, & Zhou, 2013). Polydatin isolated from *P.cuspidatum* can protect hepatocytes induced by CCl_4 (Hong Zhang et al., 2012). In short, the bioactive compounds of this plant are necessary to exact research about its anti-HBV mechanism.

2.9 Curcuma Longa

Turmeric is derived from the rhizomes of *Curcuma longa* which is the genus of the ginger family, Zingiberaceae. The mainly effective compounds are the curcuminoids that make the turmeric yellow color. Curcumin is the most important ingredient of curcuminoids and has a wide range of pharmacological effects including anti-inflammatory, anticarcinogenic, antimicrobial, cardiovascular and gastrointestinal etc. (Upadhyaya, Kesharwani & Misra, 2009; Singh et al., 2013; Akram et al., 2010; Kesharwani et al., 2015). In vitro, the water extract of Curcuma longa inhibited the hepatitis B virus production by increasing the level of p53 protein (H. J. Kim et al., 2009). In vivo, Curcuma longa reduced the expression of HBx and developed p21 and cyclin D1 in HBx- transgenic livers of mice, as the result this plant can prevent early hepatocarcinogenesis caused by HBV infection (J. Kim et al., 2011). Also in the transgenic mouse model, phytosomal formulation of curcumin has many benefits of hepatocellular carcinoma associated HBV such as inhibitory of HCC formation, enhancing of liver histopathology, reduction of lipid accumulation, the volume of a tumour, infiltration of leukocyte (Teng et al., 2019). Curcumin, a phenolic substance, suppresses HBV gene expression, and replication through reducing PGC-1 alpha regulation that enhanced the transcription of the hepatitis B virus (Rechtman et al., 2010). Curcumin can inhibit NK-kB regulation in liver cells by activating PPAR-γ, repressing ERK, increasing the cellular GSH content, and inhibits toll-like receptor-4 gene expression. It turns out that curcumin is a potential inhibitory effect of HBV (Hesari et al., 2018; Mishra et al., 2018; Kesharwani, Misra & Singh 2019). In another study, the author presented that curcumin decreased both HBsAg and HbeAg expression and also reduced HBV- DNA replication and HBV cccDNA with a dose of 20 μmol/L curcumin for 2 days in HepG2.2.15 cells. This research also indicated that the potential target of Curcumin was cccDNA which bound to protein histone and be prevented acetylation progress and in a result inhibited HBV-DNA production (Wei et al., 2017). In short, curcumin is the strongly effective of anti-HBV candidates and need deeper studies in clinical and preclinical.

Figure 1. Structure of Esculetin

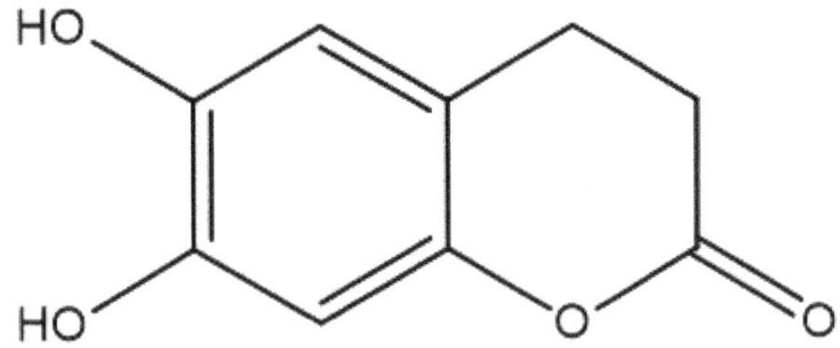

3. BIOACTIVE COMPOUNDS FROM THE MEDICINAL PLANT FOR TREATMENT OF HBV

3.1 Esculetin

Esculetin is a derivative of coumarin, was isolated from Microsorium fortunei (Moore) Ching. Esculetin has antioxidant activity and inhibitory effects on sucrose. Esculetin inhibits HBV replication *in vitro* and *in vivo* quite effectively. Besides, esculetin can significantly decrease the expression of Hepatitis B virus X (HBx) protein. Esculetin also has a potent inhibitory effect; inhibiting HBV DNA is dose-dependent, but not time-dependent. This has been demonstrated in liver samples treated with different esculetin doses, showing different levels of improvement in hepatocyte degeneration, infiltration, and necrosis (S.-X. Huang et al., 2019). The recent study showed that esculetin has low toxicity to HL-7702 cells in the chosen concentration range and the levels of DNA DHBV, HBsAg, HBeAg, alanine aminotransferase (ALT) and aspartate aminotransferase (AST) in the infected ducklings with duck hepatitis B virus (DHBV) was significantly reduced after treatment with esculetin (S.-X. Huang et al., 2019).

3.2 Helioxanthin

Helioxanthin (HE-145) is a substance belonging to the lignans group, found in Taiwania cryptomerioides Hayata, which can prevent the expression and replication of HBV in HCC cells. To clarify Helioxanthin's anti-HBV activity, the effects of helioxanthin on HBV promoter activities were examined by the luciferase reporter assay (Y.-H. Wu, 2016). The results showed that HE-145 selectively inhibits the surface antigen promoter II (SPII) and core promoter (CP) and is liver-specific because no inhibitory effect of HE-145 was found to cells other than hepatocytes such as HeLa or 293T. Additionally, HE-145 does not affect the X gene promoter (Xp) or the surface antigen I (SPI) promoter. Using EMSA analysis, the results showed that HE-145 decreased the DNA binding activity of HepA2 cell nuclear extract to cis factors on core promoter, including alpha-fetoprotein transcription factor (FTF), peroxisome proliferator-activated receptors (PPARs), PPARs binding site (PPRE), and Sp1. Unusual expression of PPAR-γ or HNF4-α reversed partially the HE-145-mediated HBV RNA suppression (Y.-H. Wu, 2016).

Figure 2. Structure of Helioxanthin

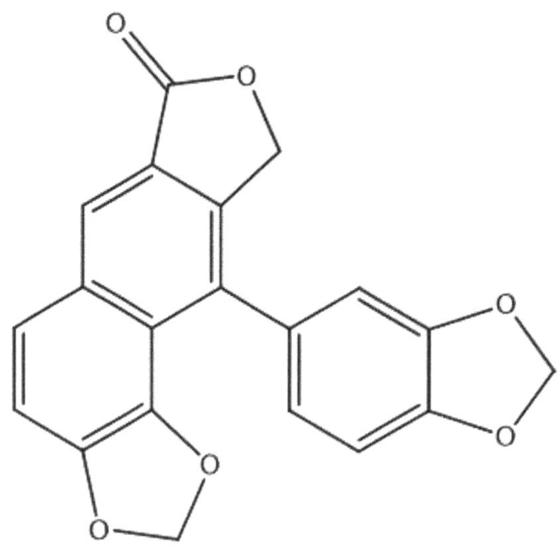

3.3 Oxymatrine

Oxymatrine is one of the quinolizidine alkaloid compounds, extracted from the Sophora japonica. Oxymatrine has a variety of effects such as protection against apoptosis, tumor and fibrotic tissue development, and inflammation. Furthermore, oxymatrine also works to improve heart failure, arrhythmia, reduce perfusion, and myocardial injury. Oxymatrine inhibits the hepatitis B virus (HBV) by downregulating the expression of heat-stress cognate 70 (Hsc70), a host protein required for HBV DNA replication to reduce resistance (Y.-P. Wang et al., 2011). Oxymatrine monotherapy (oral, 12 months) reduced blood HBV DNA by 96% and HBeAg by 70% in the chronic hepatitis B (CHB) patients resistant to lamivudine

Figure 3. Structure of Oxymatrine

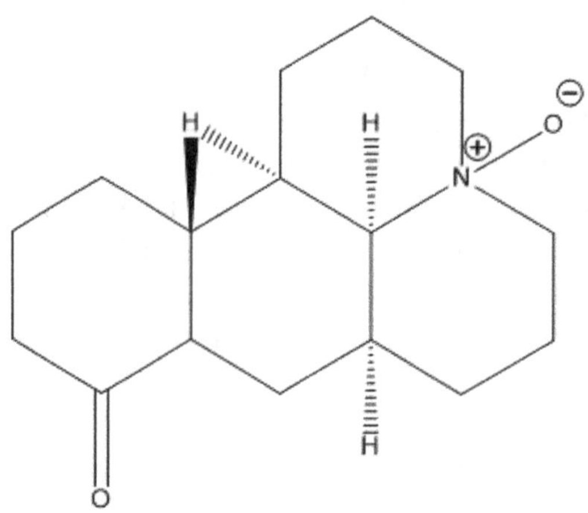

Figure 4. Structure of Epigallocatechin-3-gallate

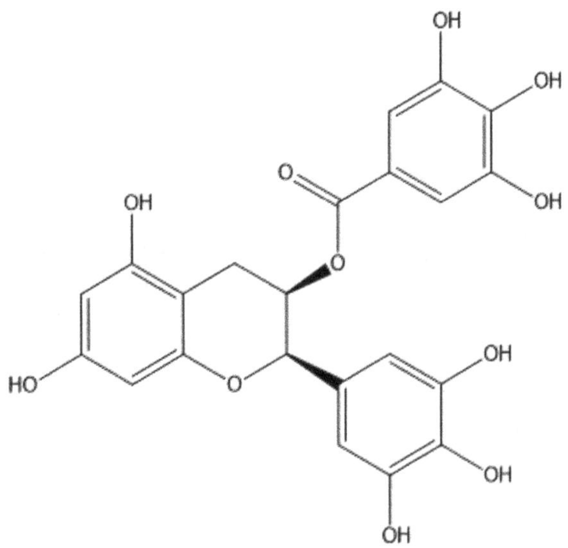

(n = 17) (Y.-P. Wang et al., 2011). The study results showed that oxymatrine treatment reduced Hcs70 mRNA and decreased intracellular HBV DNA, then inhibited replication and exhibited anti-HBV effects. Moreover, oxymatrine has an antiviral effect in the treatment of chronic hepatitis B (CHB) by reducing the expression of PD-1 on the hepatitis B virus (HBV) specific cytotoxic T lymphocyte (CTL) surface in peripheral blood in CHB patients and increase HBV-specific CTL level (Gu et al., 2012).

3.4 Epigallocatechin-3-Gallate

Epigallocatechin-3-gallate (EGCG) is a flavonoid catechin, found in the green tea plant (*Camellia sinensis*). Epigallocatechin-3-gallate is a substance that has a variety of effects such as anti-cancer, antioxidant, anti-inflammatory, anti-fibrosis (C. Chu, Deng, Man, & Qu, 2017). EGCG prevented HBV from entering immortal human primary hepatocytes at a concentration of 50 µmol/L more than 80% (Huang et al., 2014). EGCG inhibited the HBeAg and HBsAg excretion in HepG2 2.2.15 cells in a dose and time-dependent manner (Y.-H. Wu, 2016). During HBV culture, EGCG suppressed viral infection in both HA-NTCP-expressing Huh7 cells and DMSO differentiated HuS E/2 cells. In particular, EGCG induces the clathrin-dependent intracellular degradation of NTCP from the plasma membrane followed by protein breakdown. Furthermore, EGCG suppressed the clathrin-mediated endocytosis of transferrin. Finally, EGCG's ability to inhibit HBV penetration was determined using four different genotypes, from A to D (Huang et al., 2014). In another study, EGCG inhibits HBV replication because EGCG can counteract HBV-induced incomplete autoimmune through enhanced lysosome acidification (Zhong, Hu, Shu, Gao, & Xiong, 2015). According to research, HBV can induce autophagosome formation, which is needed to replicate itself. EGCG prevents HBV replication, but it is not inhibited, autophagosome creation in hepatoma cells. The autophagic procedure induced by EGCG is different from that by HBV, which is not conducive to HBV replication.

Figure 5. Structure of Wogonin

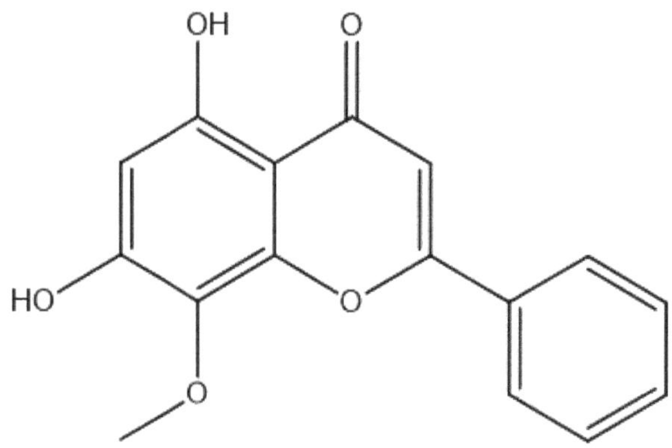

3.5 Wogonin

Wogonin is a highly biologically active flavonoid, isolated from *Scutellaria* radix. Wogonin has a variety of effects such as anti-inflammatory, anti-infection, anti-cancer, and liver disease treatment. According to research, wogonin can inhibit production (HBsAg) in cell culture without causing toxicity (R. L. Huang et al., 2000). In HepG2.2.15 cell, wogonin effectually suppressed HBV antigen secretion against both HBsAg and HBeAg with an IC_{50} of 4 μg/mL. Besides, wogonin decreased HBV DNA level in a dose-dependent manner (Guo et al., 2007). When at high concentrations, wogonin showed higher inhibition but the AST value was outside the allowable range of lower than 25 I.U./L, thus causing cytotoxicity. However, HBeAg excretion in these cells was not affected (R. L. Huang et al., 2000). Furthermore, when treated with wogonin, the linear and the relaxed circular forms of HBV DNA were greatly reduced. When treated with wogonin in infected ducks with DHBV, DHBV DNA levels were significantly reduced, showing a marked improvement. In human HBV transgenic mice, wogonin also reduced plasma HBsAg levels. In addition, wogonin has antiviral effects associated with a reduction in the initial infectious process by disrupting virus metabolism and destruction (Tai, Tsang, Chang, & Xue, 2005).

3.6 Ellagic Acid

Ellagic acid is a natural antioxidant, found in Phyllanthus niruri. Ellagic acid is resistant to HBV by blocking HBeAg secretion in HepG2 2.2.15 cells without inhibiting HBV replication, HBV polymerase activity, or blocking HBsAg secretion as a mechanism of some other substances (Shin, Kang, & Lee, 2005). After determining the effects of ellagic acid on intracellular and extracellular HBeAg and HBsAg, the results showed that intracellular HBeAg, extra- and intracellular HBsAg were unchanged while extracellular HBeAg decreased. According to the toxicity determination study, the concentration of non-toxic ellagic acid on cells was used (Shin et al., 2005). Furthermore, ellagic acid was able to effectively suppress HBeAg-induced immune tolerance in HBeAg transgenic mice (F. H. Qi et al., 2013). In this study, the author used transgenic mice producing HBeAg (HBeAg-Tg) and mouse strain C57ML/6, under the control of a metal ion-inducing promoter. The effect on the immune tolerability of HBeAg-

Figure 6. Structure of Ellagic Acid

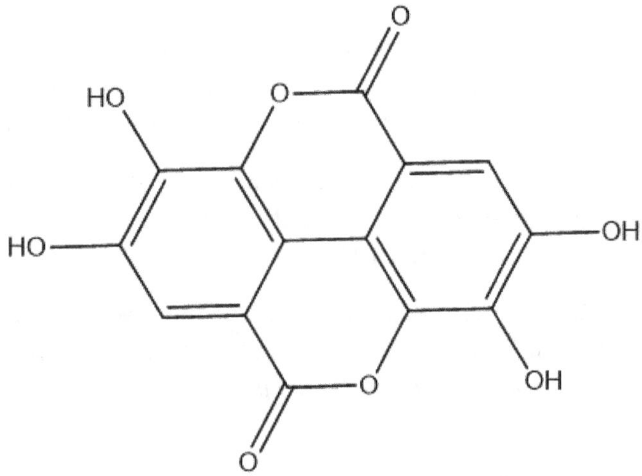

Tg and the immune tolerated release by the HBeAg secretion inhibitor, ellagic acid, was tested using T/B cell propagation, cytotoxic T-lymphocyte (CTL), HBeAg/HBeAb production, and cytokine assays. HBeAg-Tg-producing HbeAg mice based on C57ML/6 tolerated HBeAg at the T and B cell level, did not produce antibodies to HbeAg *in vivo* and *in vitro*, producing minimal levels of cytokines and reduced CTL response, while feeding mice ellagic acid (5mg/ kg body weight) suppressed HBeAg-induced immune tolerance (Kang et al., 2006).

4. CONCLUSION

Currently, the use of herbs in the treatment of HBV is a potential and effective method with fewer side-effects than the treatment with interferon-alpha or chemically synthesized drugs. The source of herbs, as well as herbal compounds, is extremely abundant, so further research is necessary to develop a treatment for HBV.

REFERENCES

Akram, M., Shahab-Uddin, A. A., Usmanghani, K., Hannan, A., Mohiuddin, E., & Asif, M. (2010). Curcuma longa and curcumin: A review article. *Rom J Biol Plant Biol*, *55*(2), 65–70.

Alberti, A., & Caporaso, N. (2011). HBV therapy: Guidelines and open issues. *Digestive and Liver Disease*, *43*, S57–S63. doi:10.1016/S1590-8658(10)60693-7 PMID:21195373

Baiguera, C., Boschetti, A., Raffetti, E., Zanini, B., Puoti, M., & Donato, F. (2018). Phyllanthus niruri versus Placebo for Chronic Hepatitis B Virus Infection: A Randomized Controlled Trial. *Complementary Medicine Research*, *25*(6), 376–382. doi:10.1159/000484927 PMID:30372693

Bora, K. S., & Sharma, A. (2011). The genus Artemisia: A comprehensive review. *Pharmaceutical Biology*, *49*(1), 101–109. doi:10.3109/13880209.2010.497815 PMID:20681755

Chang, J.-S., Liu, H.-W., Wang, K.-C., Chen, M.-C., Chiang, L.-C., Hua, Y.-C., & Lin, C.-C. (2005). Ethanol extract of Polygonum cuspidatum inhibits hepatitis B virus in a stable HBV-producing cell line. *Antiviral Research*, *66*(1), 29–34. doi:10.1016/j.antiviral.2004.12.006 PMID:15781129

Chen, C., Guo, S., & Liu, B. (2000). A randomized controlled trial of kurorinone versus interferon-alpha2a treatment in patients with chronic hepatitis B. *Journal of Viral Hepatitis*, *7*(3), 225–229. doi:10.1046/j.1365-2893.2000.00216.x PMID:10849265

Chen, H., & Weng, L. (2000). Comparison on efficacy in treating liver fibrosis of chronic hepatitis B between Astragalus Polygonum anti-fibrosis decoction and jinshuibao capsule. *Zhongguo Zhong xi yi jie he za zhi Zhongguo Zhongxiyi jiehe zazhi= Chinese journal of integrated traditional and Western medicine, 20*(4), 255.

Chen, J., & Siddiqui, A. (2007). Hepatitis B virus X protein stimulates the mitochondrial translocation of Raf-1 via oxidative stress. *Journal of Virology*, *81*(12), 6757–6760. doi:10.1128/JVI.00172-07 PMID:17428866

Chen, X., Yi, C., Yang, X., & Wang, X. (2004). Liquid chromatography of active principles in Sophora flavescens root. *Journal of Chromatography. B, Analytical Technologies in the Biomedical and Life Sciences*, *812*(1-2), 149–163. doi:10.1016/S1570-0232(04)00679-8 PMID:15556494

Chen, Y., Yao, F., Ming, K., Shi, J., Zeng, L., Wang, D., Wu, Y., Hu, Y., & Liu, J. (2019). Assessment of the Effect of Baicalin on Duck Virus Hepatitis. *Current Molecular Medicine*, *19*(5), 376–386. doi:10.2174/1566524019666190405095301 PMID:30950349

Chen, Y., & Zhu, J. (2013). Anti-HBV effect of individual traditional C hinese herbal medicine in vitro and in vivo: An analytic review. *Journal of Viral Hepatitis*, *20*(7), 445–452. doi:10.1111/jvh.12112 PMID:23730837

Chisari, F. V., Filippi, P., Buras, J., McLachlan, A., Popper, H., Pinkert, C. A., Palmiter, R. D., & Brinster, R. L. (1987). Structural and pathological effects of synthesis of hepatitis B virus large envelope polypeptide in transgenic mice. *Proceedings of the National Academy of Sciences of the United States of America*, *84*(19), 6909–6913. doi:10.1073/pnas.84.19.6909 PMID:3477814

Chu, C., Deng, J., Man, Y., & Qu, Y. (2017). Green tea extracts epigallocatechin-3-gallate for different treatments. *BioMed Research International*, *2017*, 2017. doi:10.1155/2017/5615647 PMID:28884125

Chu, C.-J., Hussain, M., & Lok, A. S. (2002). Quantitative serum HBV DNA levels during different stages of chronic hepatitis B infection. *Hepatology (Baltimore, Md.)*, *36*(6), 1408–1415. doi:10.1002/hep.1840360617 PMID:12447866

Cui, X., Wang, Y., Kokudo, N., Fang, D., & Tang, W. (2010). Traditional Chinese medicine and related active compounds against hepatitis B virus infection. *Bioscience Trends*, *4*(2). PMID:20448340

Dang, S.-S., Jia, X.-L., Song, P., Cheng, Y.-A., Zhang, X., Sun, M.-Z., & Liu, E.-Q. (2009). Inhibitory effect of emodin and Astragalus polysaccharide on the replication of HBV. *World journal of gastroenterology. WJG, 15*(45), 5669. doi:10.3748/wjg.15.5669 PMID:19960563

Dhiman, R. K., & Chawla, Y. K. (2005). Herbal medicines for liver diseases. *Digestive Diseases and Sciences, 50*(10), 1807–1812. doi:10.100710620-005-2942-9 PMID:16187178

Ding, P.-L., Liao, Z.-X., Huang, H., Zhou, P., & Chen, D.-F. (2006). (+)-12α-Hydroxysophocarpine, a new quinolizidine alkaloid and related anti-HBV alkaloids from Sophora flavescens. *Bioorganic & Medicinal Chemistry Letters, 16*(5), 1231–1235. doi:10.1016/j.bmcl.2005.11.073 PMID:16364643

Du, G., Xiao, M., Yu, S., Wang, M., Xie, Y., & Sang, S. (2018). Phyllanthus urinaria: A potential phytopharmacological source of natural medicine. *International Journal of Clinical and Experimental Medicine, 11*(7), 6509–6520.

Du, X., Zhao, B., Li, J., Cao, X., Diao, M., Feng, H., Chen, X., Chen, Z., & Zeng, X. (2012). Astragalus polysaccharides enhance immune responses of HBV DNA vaccination via promoting the dendritic cell maturation and suppressing Treg frequency in mice. *International Immunopharmacology, 14*(4), 463–470. doi:10.1016/j.intimp.2012.09.006 PMID:23006659

Gavilanes, F., Gonzalez-Ros, J. M., & Peterson, D. L. (1982). Structure of hepatitis B surface antigen. Characterization of the lipid components and their association with the viral proteins. *The Journal of Biological Chemistry, 257*(13), 7770–7777. PMID:7085648

Geng, C.-A., Yang, T.-H., Huang, X.-Y., Yang, J., Ma, Y.-B., Li, T.-Z., Zhang, X.-M., & Chen, J.-J. (2018). Anti-hepatitis B virus effects of the traditional Chinese herb Artemisia capillaris and its active enynes. *Journal of Ethnopharmacology, 224*, 283–289. doi:10.1016/j.jep.2018.06.005 PMID:29890315

Gu, X. B., Yang, X. J., Hua, Z., Lu, Z. H., Zhang, B., Zhu, Y. F., ... Pei, H. (2012). Effect of oxymatrine on specific cytotoxic T lymphocyte surface programmed death receptor-1 expression in patients with chronic hepatitis B. *Chinese Medical Journal, 125*(8), 1434–1438. PMID:22613649

Guo, Q., Zhao, L., You, Q., Yang, Y., Gu, H., Song, G., Lu, N., & Xin, J. (2007). Anti-hepatitis B virus activity of wogonin in vitro and in vivo. *Antiviral Research, 74*(1), 16–24. doi:10.1016/j.antiviral.2007.01.002 PMID:17280723

Hadziyannis, S., Bramou, T., Makris, A., Moussoulis, G., Zignego, L., & Papaioannou, C. (1990). Interferon alfa-2b treatment of HBeAg negative/serum HBV DNA positive chronic active hepatitis type B. *Journal of Hepatology, 11*, S133–S136. doi:10.1016/0168-8278(90)90180-Y PMID:2079571

Harris, A. M. (2019). Hepatitis B. *Travelers'. Health.*

He, X., Fang, J., Huang, L., Wang, J., & Huang, X. (2015). Sophora flavescens Ait.: Traditional usage, phytochemistry and pharmacology of an important traditional Chinese medicine. *Journal of Ethnopharmacology, 172*, 10–29. doi:10.1016/j.jep.2015.06.010 PMID:26087234

Hesari, A., Ghasemi, F., Salarinia, R., Biglari, H., Tabar Molla Hassan, A., Abdoli, V., & Mirzaei, H. (2018). Effects of curcumin on NF-κB, AP-1, and Wnt/β-catenin signaling pathway in hepatitis B virus infection. *Journal of Cellular Biochemistry, 119*(10), 7898–7904. doi:10.1002/jcb.26829 PMID:29923222

Huang, H.-C., Tao, M.-H., Hung, T.-M., Chen, J.-C., Lin, Z.-J., & Huang, C. (2014). (−)-Epigallocatechin-3-gallate inhibits entry of hepatitis B virus into hepatocytes. *Antiviral Research, 111*, 100–111. doi:10.1016/j.antiviral.2014.09.009 PMID:25260897

Huang, R.-L., Chen, C.-C., Huang, H.-L., Chang, C.-G., Chen, C.-F., Chang, C., & Hsieh, M.-T. (2000). Anti-hepatitis B virus effects of wogonin isolated from Scutellaria baicalensis. *Planta Medica, 66*(08), 694–698. doi:10.1055-2000-9775 PMID:11199123

Huang, R. L., Chen, C. C., Huang, H. L., Chang, C. G., Chen, C. F., Chang, C., & Hsieh, M. T. (2000). Anti-hepatitis B virus effects of wogonin isolated from Scutellaria baicalensis. *Planta Medica, 66*(8), 694–698. doi:10.1055-2000-9775 PMID:11199123

Huang, S.-X., Mou, J.-F., Luo, Q., Mo, Q.-H., Zhou, X.-L., Huang, X., Xu, Q., Tan, X.-D., Chen, X., & Liang, C.-Q. (2019). Anti-Hepatitis B Virus Activity of Esculetin from Microsorium fortunei In Vitro and In Vivo. *Molecules (Basel, Switzerland), 24*(19), 3475. doi:10.3390/molecules24193475 PMID:31557836

Huang, Y., Sun, M., Yang, X., Ma, A., Ma, Y., & Zhao, A. (2019). Baicalin relieves inflammation stimulated by lipopolysaccharide via upregulating TUG1 in liver cells. *Journal of Physiology and Biochemistry, 75*(4), 463–473. doi:10.100713105-019-00698-0 PMID:31396818

Jang, E., Kim, B.-J., Lee, K.-T., Inn, K.-S., & Lee, J.-H. (2015). A survey of therapeutic effects of Artemisia capillaris in liver diseases. *Evidence-Based Complementary and Alternative Medicine*. PMID:26366183

Kang, E. H., Kown, T. Y., Oh, G. T., Park, W. F., Park, S. I., Park, S. K., & Lee, Y. I. (2006). The flavonoid ellagic acid from a medicinal herb inhibits host immune tolerance induced by the hepatitis B virus-e antigen. *Antiviral Research, 72*(2), 100–106. doi:10.1016/j.antiviral.2006.04.006 PMID:16720052

Kesharwani, R., Misra, K., & Singh, D. (2019). Perspectives and challenges of tropical medicinal herbs and modern drug discovery in the current scenario. *Asian Pacific Journal of Tropical Medicine, 12*(1), 1–7. doi:10.4103/1995-7645.250337

Kesharwani, R. K., & Misra, K. (2011). Prediction of binding site for curcuminoids at human topoisomerase II α protein; an in silico approach. *Current Science*, 1060–1065.

Kesharwani, R. K., Srivastava, V., Singh, P., Rizvi, S. I., Adeppa, K., & Misra, K. (2015). A novel approach for overcoming drug resistance in breast cancer chemotherapy by targeting new synthetic curcumin analogues against aldehyde dehydrogenase 1 (ALDH1A1) and glycogen synthase kinase-3 β (GSK-3β). *Biotechnology and Applied Biochemistry, 176*(7), 1996–2017. doi:10.100712010-015-1696-x PMID:26113217

Kim, H. J., Yoo, H. S., Kim, J. C., Park, C. S., Choi, M. S., Kim, M., ... Yoon, S. W. (2009). Antiviral effect of Curcuma longa Linn extract against hepatitis B virus replication. *Journal of Ethnopharmacology, 124*(2), 189–196. doi:10.1016/j.jep.2009.04.046 PMID:19409970

Kim, J., Ha, H.-L., Moon, H.-B., Lee, Y.-W., Cho, C.-K., Yoo, H.-S., & Yu, D.-Y. (2011). Chemopreventive effect of Curcuma longa Linn on liver pathology in HBx transgenic mice. *Integrative Cancer Therapies, 10*(2), 168–177. doi:10.1177/1534735410380613 PMID:21190953

Lai, C.-L., Gane, E., Liaw, Y.-F., Hsu, C.-W., Thongsawat, S., Wang, Y., ... Bzowej, N. (2007). Telbivudine versus lamivudine in patients with chronic hepatitis B. *The New England Journal of Medicine*, *357*(25), 2576–2588. doi:10.1056/NEJMoa066422 PMID:18094378

Lemoine, M., Eholié, S., & Lacombe, K. (2015). Reducing the neglected burden of viral hepatitis in Africa: Strategies for a global approach. *Journal of Hepatology*, *62*(2), 469–476. doi:10.1016/j.jhep.2014.10.008 PMID:25457207

Lenhoff, R. J., & Summers, J. (1994a). Construction of avian hepadnavirus variants with enhanced replication and cytopathicity in primary hepatocytes. *Journal of Virology*, *68*(9), 5706–5713. doi:10.1128/JVI.68.9.5706-5713.1994 PMID:8057452

Lenhoff, R. J., & Summers, J. (1994b). Coordinate regulation of replication and virus assembly by the large envelope protein of an avian hepadnavirus. *Journal of Virology*, *68*(7), 4565–4571. doi:10.1128/JVI.68.7.4565-4571.1994 PMID:8207830

Li, B., Gao, B., Ye, L., Han, X., Wang, W., Kong, L., ... Li, S. (2007). Hepatitis B virus X protein (HBx) activates ATF6 and IRE1-XBP1 pathways of unfolded protein response. *Virus Research*, *124*(1-2), 44–49. doi:10.1016/j.virusres.2006.09.011 PMID:17092596

Li, Y., & Jiang, J.-G. (2018). Health functions and structure–activity relationships of natural anthraquinones from plants. *Food & Function*, *9*(12), 6063–6080. doi:10.1039/C8FO01569D PMID:30484455

Li, Z., Li, L., Sun, Y., & Li, J. (2007). Identification of natural compounds with anti-hepatitis B virus activity from Rheum palmatum L. ethanol extract. *Chemotherapy*, *53*(5), 320–326. doi:10.1159/000107690 PMID:17785969

Liu, J., Lin, H., & McIntosh, H. (2001). Genus Phyllanthus for chronic hepatitis B virus infection: A systematic review. *Journal of Viral Hepatitis*, *8*(5), 358–366. doi:10.1046/j.1365-2893.2001.00307.x PMID:11555193

Liu, S., Wei, W., Shi, K., Cao, X., Zhou, M., & Liu, Z. (2014). In vitro and in vivo anti-hepatitis B virus activities of the lignan niranthin isolated from Phyllanthus niruri L. *Journal of Ethnopharmacology*, *155*(2), 1061–1067. doi:10.1016/j.jep.2014.05.064 PMID:25009077

Miraj, S. (2016). Therapeutic effects of Rheum palmatum L.(Dahuang): A systematic review. *Der Pharma Chemica*, *8*(13), 50–54.

Mishra, H., Kesharwani, R., Singh, D., Tripathi, S., Dubey, S., & Misra, K. (2018). Computational study of curcumin, retinoic acid and its conjugates against GSK-3 beta. *Network Modeling and Analysis in Health Informatics and Bioinformatics*, *8*, 3. doi:10.100713721-018-0177-x

Mohamadkhani, A., Sayemiri, K., Ghanbari, R., Elahi, E., Poustchi, H., & Montazeri, G. (2010). The inverse association of serum HBV DNA level with HDL and adiponectin in chronic hepatitis B infection. *Virology Journal*, *7*(1), 228. doi:10.1186/1743-422X-7-228 PMID:20840785

Norton, P. A., Gong, Q., Mehta, A. S., Lu, X., & Block, T. M. (2003). Hepatitis B virus-mediated changes of apolipoprotein mRNA abundance in cultured hepatoma cells. *Journal of Virology*, *77*(9), 5503–5506. doi:10.1128/JVI.77.9.5503-5506.2003 PMID:12692252

O'Hara, G. A., McNaughton, A. L., Maponga, T., Jooste, P., Ocama, P., Chilengi, R., ... Gikungi, D. M. (2017). Hepatitis B virus infection as a neglected tropical disease. *PLoS Neglected Tropical Diseases*, *11*(10), e0005842. doi:10.1371/journal.pntd.0005842 PMID:28981505

Organization, W. H. (2017). *Global hepatitis report 2017*. World Health Organization.

Ott, M., Thyagarajan, S., & Gupta, S. (1997). Phyllanthus amarus suppresses hepatitis B virus by interrupting interactions between HBV enhancer I and cellular transcription factors. *European Journal of Clinical Investigation*, *27*(11), 908–915. doi:10.1046/j.1365-2362.1997.2020749.x PMID:9395786

Peng, W., Qin, R., Li, X., & Zhou, H. (2013). Botany, phytochemistry, pharmacology, and potential application of Polygonum cuspidatum Sieb. et Zucc.: A review. *Journal of Ethnopharmacology*, *148*(3), 729–745. doi:10.1016/j.jep.2013.05.007 PMID:23707210

Peterson, D. L. (1981). Isolation and characterization of the major protein and glycoprotein of hepatitis B surface antigen. *The Journal of Biological Chemistry*, *256*(13), 6975–6983. PMID:7240257

Porres, J. C., Carreño, V., Ruíz, M., Marrón, J., & Bartolomé, J. (1989). Interferon antibodies in patients with chronic HBV infection treated with recombinant interferon. *Journal of Hepatology*, *8*(3), 351–357. doi:10.1016/0168-8278(89)90034-2 PMID:2732449

Qi, F., Wang, Z., Cai, P., Zhao, L., Gao, J., Kokudo, N., ... Tang, W. (2013). Traditional Chinese medicine and related active compounds: A review of their role on hepatitis B virus infection. *Drug Discoveries & Therapeutics*, *7*(6), 212–224. doi:10.5582/ddt.2013.v7.6.212 PMID:24423652

Qi, F. H., Wang, Z. X., Cai, P. P., Zhao, L., Gao, J. J., Kokudo, N., ... Tang, W. (2013). Traditional Chinese medicine and related active compounds: A review of their role on hepatitis B virus infection. *Drug Discoveries & Therapeutics*, *7*(6), 212–224. doi:10.5582/ddt.2013.v7.6.212 PMID:24423652

Rahmani, Z., Huh, K.-W., Lasher, R., & Siddiqui, A. (2000). Hepatitis B virus X protein colocalizes to mitochondria with a human voltage-dependent anion channel, HVDAC3, and alters its transmembrane potential. *Journal of Virology*, *74*(6), 2840–2846. doi:10.1128/JVI.74.6.2840-2846.2000 PMID:10684300

Rechtman, M. M., Har-Noy, O., Bar-Yishay, I., Fishman, S., Adamovich, Y., Shaul, Y., ... Shlomai, A. (2010). Curcumin inhibits hepatitis B virus via down-regulation of the metabolic coactivator PGC-1α. *FEBS Letters*, *584*(11), 2485–2490. doi:10.1016/j.febslet.2010.04.067 PMID:20434445

Rios, J., & Waterman, P. (1997). A review of the pharmacology and toxicology of Astragalus. *Phytotherapy Research: An International Journal Devoted to Medical and Scientific Research on Plants and Plant Products*, *11*(6), 411–418. doi:10.1002/(SICI)1099-1573(199709)11:6<411::AID-PTR132>3.0.CO;2-6

Sarin, B., Verma, N., Martín, J. P., & Mohanty, A. (2014). An overview of important ethnomedicinal herbs of Phyllanthus species: Present status and future prospects. *The Scientific World Journal*. PMID:24672382

Shanmugam, B., Shanmugam, K. R., Ravi, S., Subbaiah, G. V., Ramakrishana, C., Mallikarjuna, K., & Reddy, K. S. (2017). Exploratory studies of (-)-Epicatechin, a bioactive compound of Phyllanthus niruri, on the antioxidant enzymes and oxidative stress markers in D-galactosamine-induced hepatitis in rats: A study with reference to clinical prospective. *Pharmacognosy Magazine*, *13*(49, Suppl 1), S56. doi:10.4103/0973-1296.203973 PMID:28479727

Shin, M. S., Kang, E. H., & Lee, Y. I. (2005). A flavonoid from medicinal plants blocks hepatitis B virus-e antigen secretion in HBV-infected hepatocytes. *Antiviral Research, 67*(3), 163–168. doi:10.1016/j.antiviral.2005.06.005 PMID:16118024

Singh, D. V., Agarwal, S., Kesharwani, R. K., & Misra, K. (2013). 3D QSAR and pharmacophore study of curcuminoids and curcumin analogs: Interaction with thioredoxin reductase. *Interdisciplinary Sciences, Computational Life Sciences, 5*(4), 286–295. doi:10.100712539-013-0177-6 PMID:24402822

Singh, K. P., Crane, M., Audsley, J., Avihingsanon, A., Sasadeusz, J., & Lewin, S. R. (2017). HIV-hepatitis B virus coinfection: Epidemiology, pathogenesis, and treatment. *AIDS (London, England), 31*(15), 2035–2052. doi:10.1097/QAD.0000000000001574 PMID:28692539

Summers, J., Smith, P. M., & Horwich, A. L. (1990). Hepadnavirus envelope proteins regulate covalently closed circular DNA amplification. *Journal of Virology, 64*(6), 2819–2824. doi:10.1128/JVI.64.6.2819-2824.1990 PMID:2335817

Summers, J., Smith, P. M., Huang, M., & Yu, M. (1991). Morphogenetic and regulatory effects of mutations in the envelope proteins of an avian hepadnavirus. *Journal of Virology, 65*(3), 1310–1317. doi:10.1128/JVI.65.3.1310-1317.1991 PMID:1995945

Sun, Y., Li, L., Li, J., & Li, Z. (2007). Inhibition of hepatitis B virus replication by Rheum palmatum L. ethanol extract in a stable HBV-producing cell line. *Virologica Sinica, 22*(1), 14–20. doi:10.100712250-007-0056-6

Tai, M. C., Tsang, S. Y., Chang, L. Y., & Xue, H. (2005). Therapeutic potential of wogonin: A naturally occurring flavonoid. *CNS Drug Reviews, 11*(2), 141–150. doi:10.1111/j.1527-3458.2005.tb00266.x PMID:16007236

Teng, C.-F., Yu, C.-H., Chang, H.-Y., Hsieh, W.-C., Wu, T.-H., Lin, J.-H., Wu, H.-C., Jeng, L.-B., & Su, I.-J. (2019). Chemopreventive effect of phytosomal curcumin on hepatitis b virus-related hepatocellular carcinoma in a transgenic mouse model. *Scientific Reports, 9*(1), 1–13. doi:10.103841598-019-46891-5 PMID:31316146

Tian, Y., Chen, W., & Ou, J.-J. (2011). Effects of interferon-α/β on HBV replication determined by viral load. *PLoS Pathogens, 7*(7), e1002159. doi:10.1371/journal.ppat.1002159 PMID:21829354

Tseng, Y. P., Wu, Y. C., Leu, Y. L., Yeh, S. F., & Chou, C. K. (2010). Scutellariae radix suppresses hepatitis B virus production in human hepatoma cells. *Frontiers in Bioscience (Elite Edition), 2*, 1538–1547. PMID:20515825

Upadhyaya, J., Kesharwani, R. K., & Misra, K. (2009). Metabolism, pharmacokinetics and bioavailability of ascorbic acid; synergistic effect with tocopherols and curcumin. *J Comput Intell Bioinform, 2*(1), 77–84.

Venkateswaran, P., Millman, I., & Blumberg, B. S. (1987). Effects of an extract from Phyllanthus niruri on hepatitis B and woodchuck hepatitis viruses: In vitro and in vivo studies. *Proceedings of the National Academy of Sciences of the United States of America, 84*(1), 274–278. doi:10.1073/pnas.84.1.274 PMID:3467354

Wang, B. E. (2000). Treatment of chronic liver diseases with traditional Chinese medicine. *Journal of Gastroenterology and Hepatology*, *15*(5 (Suppl.)), E67–E70. doi:10.1046/j.1440-1746.2000.02100.x PMID:10921385

Wang, B.-Q. (2010). Salvia miltiorrhiza: Chemical and pharmacological review of a medicinal plant. *Journal of Medicinal Plants Research*, *4*(25), 2813–2820.

Wang, Y.-P., Zhao, W., Xue, R., Zhou, Z.-X., Liu, F., Han, Y.-X., ... Chen, H.-S. (2011). Oxymatrine inhibits hepatitis B infection with an advantage of overcoming drug-resistance. *Antiviral Research*, *89*(3), 227–231. doi:10.1016/j.antiviral.2011.01.005 PMID:21277330

Waris, G., Huh, K.-W., & Siddiqui, A. (2001). Mitochondrially associated hepatitis B virus X protein constitutively activates transcription factors STAT-3 and NF-κB via oxidative stress. *Molecular and Cellular Biology*, *21*(22), 7721–7730. doi:10.1128/MCB.21.22.7721-7730.2001 PMID:11604508

Wei, Z.-Q., Zhang, Y.-H., Ke, C.-Z., Chen, H.-X., Ren, P., He, Y.-L., Hu, P., Ma, D.-Q., Luo, J., & Meng, Z.-J. (2017). Curcumin inhibits hepatitis B virus infection by down-regulating cccDNA-bound histone acetylation. *World Journal of Gastroenterology*, *23*(34), 6252. doi:10.3748/wjg.v23.i34.6252 PMID:28974891

Wu, Y., Lu, Y., Li, S.-y., Song, Y., Hao, Y., & Wang, Q. (2015). Extract from Phyllanthus urinaria L. inhibits hepatitis B virus replication and expression in hepatitis B virus transfection model in vitro. *Chinese Journal of Integrative Medicine*, *21*(12), 938–943. doi:10.100711655-015-2076-7 PMID:25869593

Wu, Y.-H. (2016). Naturally derived anti-hepatitis B virus agents and their mechanism of action. *World Journal of Gastroenterology*, *22*(1), 188. doi:10.3748/wjg.v22.i1.188 PMID:26755870

Xiong, L. (1993). Therapeutic effect of combined therapy of Salvia miltiorrhizae and Polyporus umbellatus polysaccharide in the treatment of chronic hepatitis B. *Zhongguo Zhong xi yi jie he za zhi Zhongguo Zhongxiyi jiehe zazhi= Chinese journal of integrated traditional and Western medicine, 13*(9), 533.

Yang, H., Zhou, Z., He, L., Ma, H., Qu, W., Yin, J., Jia, M., Zhao, X., Shan, J., & Gao, Y. (2018). Hepatoprotective and inhibiting HBV effects of polysaccharides from roots of Sophora flavescens. *International Journal of Biological Macromolecules*, *108*, 744–752. doi:10.1016/j.ijbiomac.2017.10.171 PMID:29111266

Yarnell, E., & Abascal, K. (2010). Herbal medicine for viral hepatitis. *Alternative and Complementary Therapies*, *16*(3), 151–157. doi:10.1089/act.2010.16308

Ye, G., Zhu, H. Y., Li, Z. X., Ma, C. H., Fan, M. S., Sun, Z. L., & Huang, C. G. (2007). LC-MS characterization of efficacy substances in serum of experimental animals treated with Sophora flavescens extracts. *Biomedical Chromatography*, *21*(6), 655–660. doi:10.1002/bmc.805 PMID:17370298

Zacharakis, G., Koskinas, J., Kotsiou, S., Papoutselis, M., Tzara, F., Vafeiadis, N., Archimandritis, A. J., & Papoutselis, K. (2005). Natural history of chronic HBV infection: A cohort study with up to 12 years follow-up in North Greece (part of the Interreg I-II/EC-project). *Journal of Medical Virology*, *77*(2), 173–179. doi:10.1002/jmv.20434 PMID:16121378

Zhang, H., Li, C., Kwok, S.-T., Zhang, Q.-W., & Chan, S.-W. (2013). A review of the pharmacological effects of the dried root of Polygonum cuspidatum (Hu Zhang) and its constituents. *Evidence-Based Complementary and Alternative Medicine*. PMID:24194779

Zhang, H., Yu, C.-H., Jiang, Y.-P., Peng, C., He, K., Tang, J.-Y., & Xin, H.-L. (2012). Protective effects of polydatin from Polygonum cuspidatum against carbon tetrachloride-induced liver injury in mice. *PLoS One*, *7*(9), e46574. doi:10.1371/journal.pone.0046574 PMID:23029551

Zhang, L., Wang, G., Hou, W., Li, P., Dulin, A., & Bonkovsky, H. L. (2010). Contemporary clinical research of traditional Chinese medicines for chronic hepatitis B in China: An analytical review. *Hepatology (Baltimore, Md.)*, *51*(2), 690–698. doi:10.1002/hep.23384 PMID:20101751

Zhang, Y.-B., Luo, D., Yang, L., Cheng, W., He, L.-J., Kuang, G.-K., Li, M.-M., Li, Y.-L., & Wang, G.-C. (2018). Matrine-type alkaloids from the roots of Sophora flavescens and their antiviral activities against the hepatitis B virus. *Journal of Natural Products*, *81*(10), 2259–2265. doi:10.1021/acs.jnatprod.8b00576 PMID:30298740

Zhang, Y.-B., Zhan, L.-Q., Li, G.-Q., Wang, F., Wang, Y., Li, Y.-L., Ye, W.-C., & Wang, G.-C. (2016). Dimeric matrine-type alkaloids from the roots of Sophora flavescens and their anti-hepatitis B virus activities. *The Journal of Organic Chemistry*, *81*(15), 6273–6280. doi:10.1021/acs.joc.6b00804 PMID:27352066

Zhang, Y. Y., & Hu, K. Q. (2015). Rethinking the pathogenesis of hepatitis B virus (HBV) infection. *Journal of Medical Virology*, *87*(12), 1989–1999. doi:10.1002/jmv.24270 PMID:25989114

Zhao, Q., Chen, X.-Y., & Martin, C. (2016). Scutellaria baicalensis, the golden herb from the garden of Chinese medicinal plants. *Science Bulletin*, *61*(18), 1391–1398. doi:10.100711434-016-1136-5 PMID:27730005

Zhao, T., Tang, H., Xie, L., Zheng, Y., Ma, Z., Sun, Q., & Li, X. (2019). Scutellaria baicalensis Georgi. (Lamiaceae): A review of its traditional uses, botany, phytochemistry, pharmacology and toxicology. *The Journal of Pharmacy and Pharmacology*, *71*(9), 1353–1369. doi:10.1111/jphp.13129 PMID:31236960

Zhao, Y., Geng, C.-A., Chen, H., Ma, Y.-B., Huang, X.-Y., Cao, T.-W., He, K., Wang, H., Zhang, X.-M., & Chen, J.-J. (2015). Isolation, synthesis and anti-hepatitis B virus evaluation of p-hydroxyacetophenone derivatives from Artemisia capillaris. *Bioorganic & Medicinal Chemistry Letters*, *25*(7), 1509–1514. doi:10.1016/j.bmcl.2015.02.024 PMID:25737008

Zhao, Y., Geng, C.-A., Ma, Y.-B., Huang, X.-Y., Chen, H., Cao, T.-W., He, K., Wang, H., Zhang, X.-M., & Chen, J.-J. (2014). UFLC/MS-IT-TOF guided isolation of anti-HBV active chlorogenic acid analogues from Artemisia capillaris as a traditional Chinese herb for the treatment of hepatitis. *Journal of Ethnopharmacology*, *156*, 147–154. doi:10.1016/j.jep.2014.08.043 PMID:25219603

Zhao, Y., Geng, C.-A., Sun, C.-L., Ma, Y.-B., Huang, X.-Y., Cao, T.-W., He, K., Wang, H., Zhang, X.-M., & Chen, J.-J. (2014). Polyacetylenes and anti-hepatitis B virus active constituents from Artemisia capillaris. *Fitoterapia*, *95*, 187–193. doi:10.1016/j.fitote.2014.03.017 PMID:24685503

Zhiguo, P., Yanpei, W., & Peizheng, G. (1999). Observation on Effects of Combined Treatment of Chinese Toad Bufotoxin and Salvia Miltiorrhiza in Patients Suffering from Chronic Hepatitis B. *Modern Diagnosis & Treatment, 3*.

Zhong, L., Hu, J., Shu, W., Gao, B., & Xiong, S. (2015). Epigallocatechin-3-gallate opposes HBV-induced incomplete autophagy by enhancing lysosomal acidification, which is unfavorable for HBV replication. *Cell Death & Disease*, *6*(5), e1770–e1770. doi:10.1038/cddis.2015.136 PMID:25996297

Zhou, Z., Zhang, Y., Ding, X.-R., Chen, S.-H., Yang, J., Wang, X.-J., Jia, G.-L., Chen, H.-S., Bo, X.-C., & Wang, S.-Q. (2007). Protocatechuic aldehyde inhibits hepatitis B virus replication both in vitro and in vivo. *Antiviral Research*, *74*(1), 59–64. doi:10.1016/j.antiviral.2006.12.005 PMID:17298850

Chapter 9
Enhancing the Therapeutic Efficacy of Flavonoids as Anticancer Drugs Through Novel Drug Delivery Systems

Anamika Basu
https://orcid.org/0000-0003-4775-5323
Gurudas College, Kolkata, India

ABSTRACT

Flavonoids are a group of heterocyclic compounds that are well-known for their anti-cancer activity. Fruits and vegetables are the main dietary sources of flavonoids. Several mechanisms have been proposed for the effect of flavonoids to combat cancer. But before considering the flavonoids as chemotherapeutic drugs for cancer, a number of problems still need to be addressed before their therapeutic uses. Solubility may play a major role in the therapeutic efficacy of flavonoids. Bioavailability of flavonoids are also affected by several other factors. Nanotechnology is the most efficient tool to solve the problems of solubility, stability, and oral bioavailability. Nanotechnology-based drug delivery has several benefits compared to the traditional drug delivery systems. Different types of nano delivery systems are used for producing nanomedicines such as lipid-based nanomedicines, polymer-based nanomedicines, and inorganic nanoparticles. Different types of flavonoids encapsulated nanoparticles have been developed to improve their effectiveness against different types of cancer.

1. INTRODUCTION

Flavonoids are a group of heterocyclic compounds that consist of two benzene rings (A and B) combined with an oxygen-containing heterocyclic benzopyran ring (C). About 9000 compounds are present in this group with difference ring substitutions and number of unsaturation (Veeramuthu, et al., 2017). The basic chemical structure of flavonoid compounds is shown in Figure 1. Flavonoids are well-known as antioxidant and many other important bioactivities related to human health, curing and preventing many

DOI: 10.4018/978-1-7998-4453-2.ch009

Figure 1. Basic chemical structure of flavonoid compounds

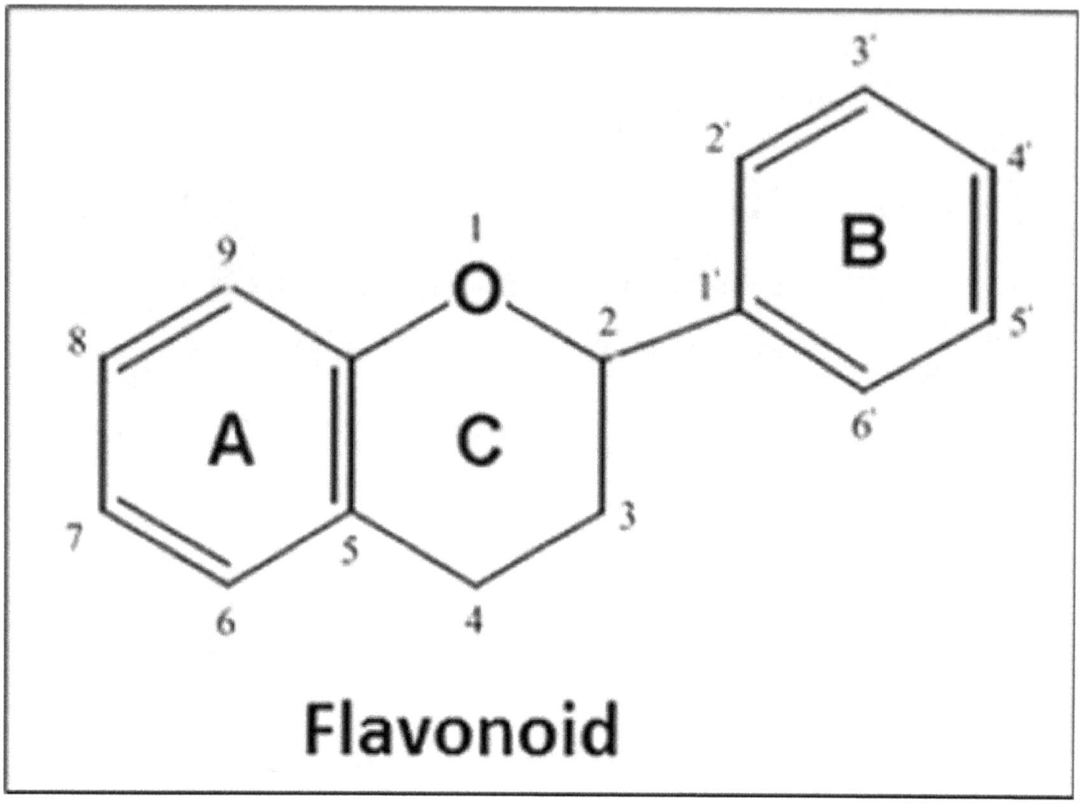

diseases. Flavonoids micronutrients are closely connected with human dietary ingredients and health. Fruits and vegetables are the main dietary sources of flavonoids along with tea, honey. Flavonoids are among the most abundant and most studied phytochemicals in oregano species, citrus fruits, saskatoon berries.

Flavonoids which are plant secondary metabolites, can be classified into four major groups, such as flavanols, flavones, anthocyanidins, and isoflavonoids. Furthermore, they are divided into some subclasses (Kopustinskiene et al., 2020). They are available in dietary foods such as lemon, black tea, chocolate, milk and grape wines etc. and can cure various ailments viz. cancer, diabetes, viral infection, cardiovascular diseases etc. (Keservani, Sharma & Kesharwani, 2018; Amawi et al., 2017; Wang et al., 2018). Fruits and vegetables having flavonoids have been described as cancer nutraceuticals.

1.1 Classification of Flavonoids

The chemical nature of flavonoids can be classified according to their hydroxylation pattern in skeletal structure, conjugation between the aromatic rings, glycosidic moieties (present and absent), methoxy groups and other substituents on their basic chemical structure (Figure 1) (Brodowska, 2017; Santos et al., 2017).

1.1.1 According to Chemical Structure

According to chemical structures the whole group of flavonoids can be classified into fourteen groups e.g. flavanols, flavones, isoflavones, flavanones, flavonols and flavanonols etc. (Neveu et al., 2010) are shown in Table 1.

According to source, flavonoids can be divided into two groups i.e. natural or dietary and synthetic flavonoids. Dietary (natural) flavonoids are present in food resources as shown in Figure 2.

Phenol-Explorer is the first comprehensive database on polyphenol content in foods (Rothwell et al, 2012, 2013). The database contains more than 35,000 content values for 500 different polyphenols in over 400 foods. These data are derived from the systematic collection of more than 60,000 original content values found in more than 1,300 scientific publications. Each of these publications has been critically evaluated before inclusion in the database. The whole data on the polyphenol composition of foods is available for download. Using this database, the mean contents of different classes of flavonoids are enlisted in Table 2.

A novel synthetic sulfur containing tricyclic flavonoid (Babii et al., 2018) with chlorine as halogen substituent at the benzopyran core (ClCl-flav) is synthesized for antibacterial activity against clinically significant microorganisms such as *Staphylococcus aureus*, *Escherichia coli* and *Klebsiella pneumoniae.*

1.2 Biological Role of Flavonoids

Flavonoids are considered as disease preventing dietary supplements. They are now considered as an essential component in a variety of pharmaceutical, nutraceutical, medicinal, as well as cosmetic and other applications. Many flavonoid compounds exhibit an antioxidative activity, free radical scavenging capacity, antidiabetic, cardioprotective, anti-inflammatory, anti-allergic while some other flavonoid compounds display antiviral activities (Kesharwani, Misra & Singh 2019; Karak, 2019). More recently flavonoids are proven to be the most effective as an anti-cancer therapeutics, through apoptosis process by two ways such as induction of cell cycle arrest and inhibition of key enzymes, which are involved in tumor promotion. Several mechanisms have been proposed for the effect of flavonoids to combat the initiation and promotion stages of the different types of cancer. Major molecular mechanisms of action of flavonoids are downregulation of mutant p53 protein, cell cycle arrest, inhibition of heat shock proteins, tyrosine kinase inhibition, estrogen receptor binding capacity and inhibition of expression of Ras proteins.

Different types of flavonoids such as flavones, hydroxy flavonoids, isoflav-2-enes, flavonoid glycosides, O-methylated flavonoids are prevalent in these medicinal plants.

Anticancer effects of flavonoids according to their mode of action are summarized in Figure 3.

1.3 Flavonoids in Activation of Apoptosis

Flavonoids can activate apoptosis or programmed cell death in tumor cells by two mechanisms (Kopustinskiene et al., 2020; Li & Xu, 2007); Genoux et al., 2011)(examples are shown in Table 4). First one by activating anti-apoptotic proteins (Bax, Bak and p53) and in second mechanism by suppressing pro-apoptotic proteins (Bcl-2 and Bcl-xL).

Table 1. Classification of flavonoids

Subgroup	Chemical structure	Examples
Flavanols	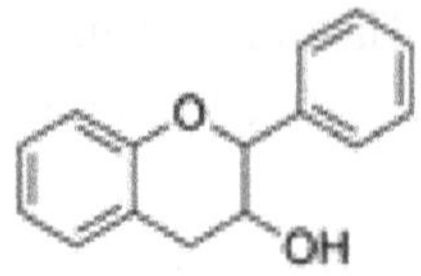 Flavanol	Epicatechin, Catechin, Epigallocatechin
Flavones	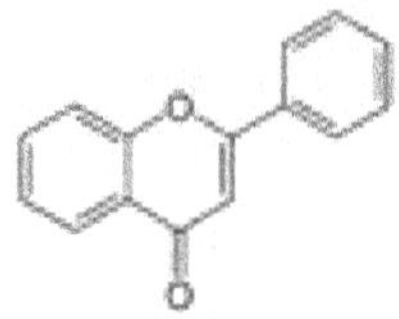 Flavone	Apigenin, Baicalein, Luteolin, Chrysin
Isoflavones	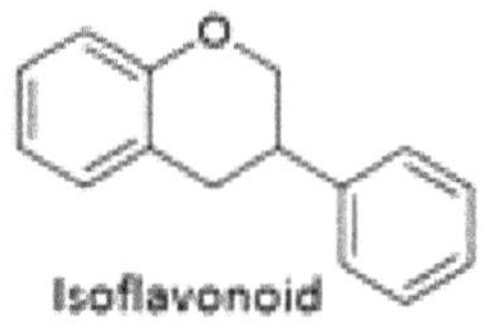 Isoflavonoid	Genistein, Genistin, Glycitein Daidzein
Flavanones	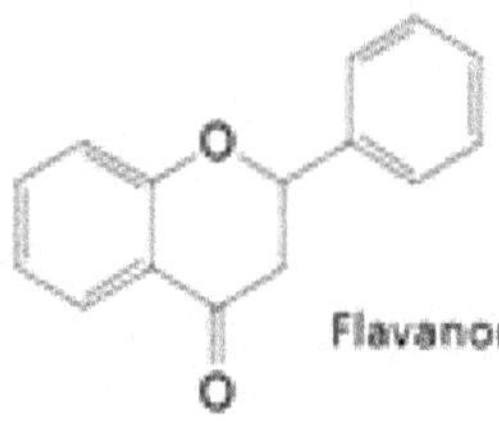 Flavanone	Hesperidin, Naringenin, Hesperetin, Narirutin
Flavonols	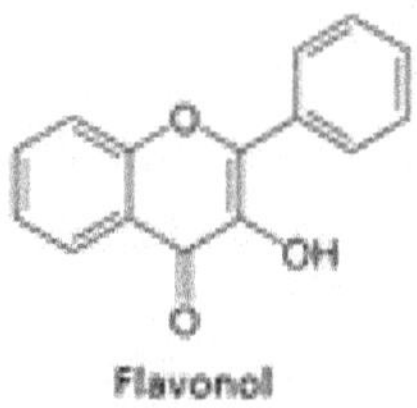 Flavonol	Kaempferol, Myricetin, Quercetin,
Flavanonols	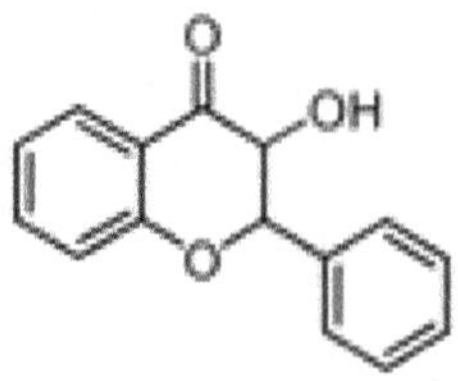 Flavanonol	Taxifolin

continued on following page

Table 1. Continued

Subgroup	Chemical structure	Examples
Anthocyanins	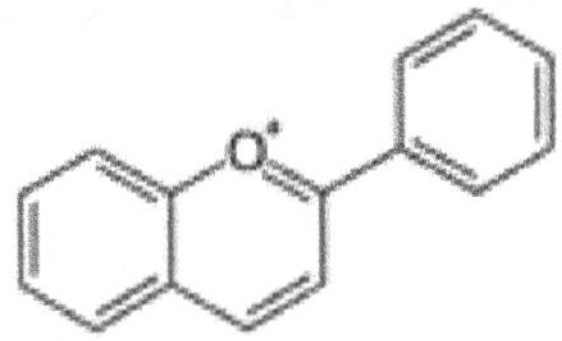 Anthocyanidin	Delphinidin, Malvidin, Pelargonidin, Peonidin, Petunidin
Neoflavonoids	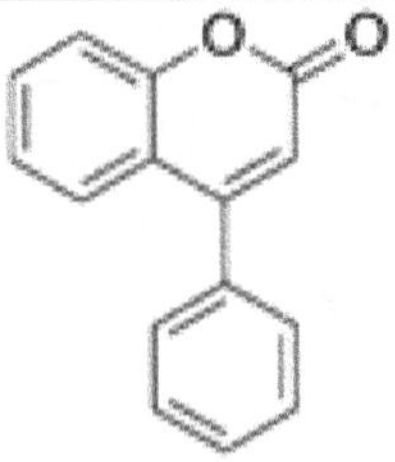 Neoflavonoids	Melannein
Chalcones	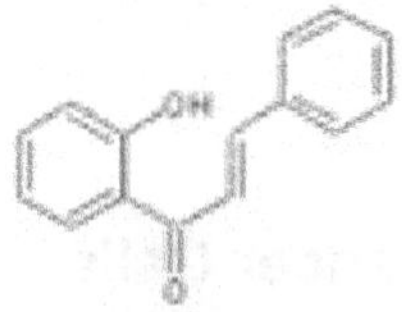 Chalcones	Butein, Xanthohumol
Catechins	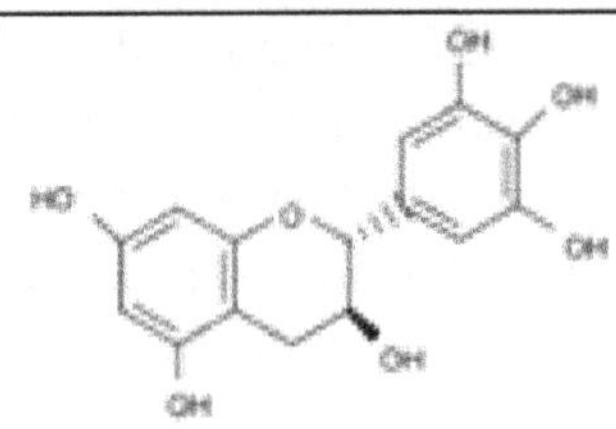 (+) Catechin (C)	Epicatechin, Epigallocatechin gallate
Proanthocyanidins	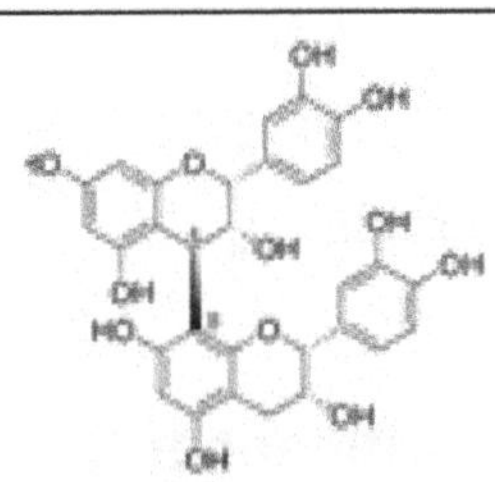 Proanthocyanidin B_2 dimer	Proanthocyanidin A_2 dimer, Proanthocyanidin B_5 dimer, Proanthocyanidin B_2 dimer
Stilbenes	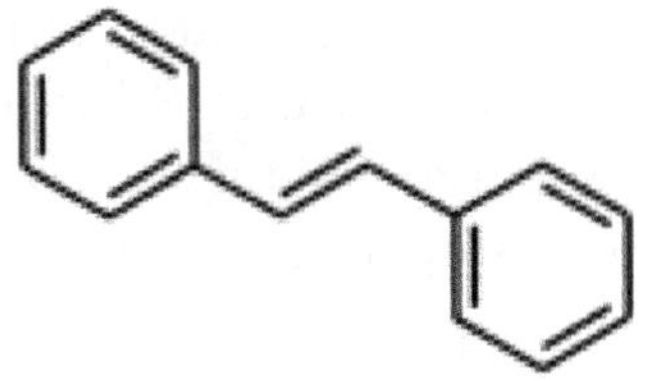 Stilbenes	Resveratrol, Piceatannol, Pinosylvin

continued on following page

Table X. Continued

Subgroup	Chemical structure	Examples
Derivatives of flavonoids		
Flavone glycosides	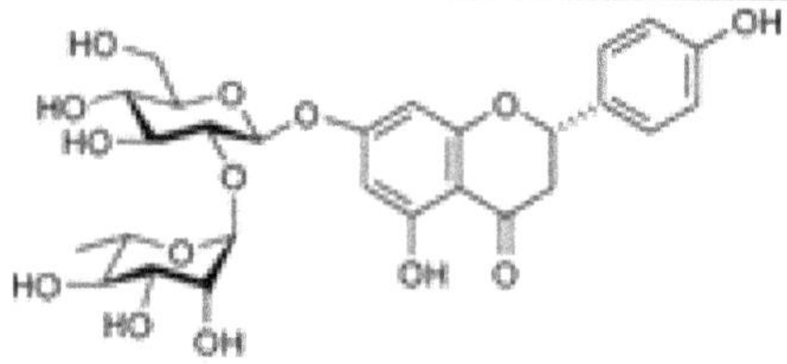 Naringin	Baicalin, Naringin
Flavonol glycosides	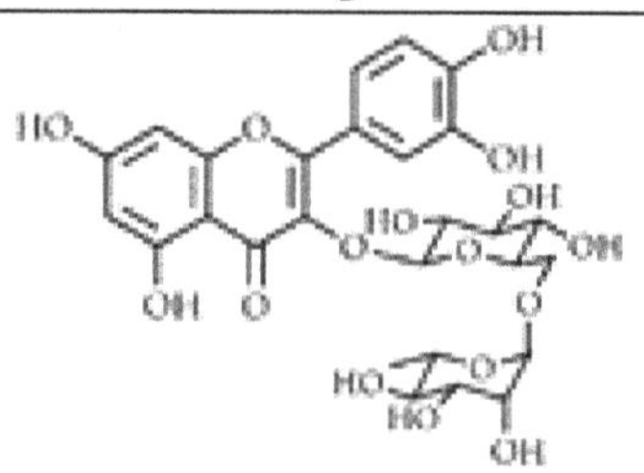 Rutin	Rutin

1.4 Cytotoxic Effects of Flavonoids in Cancer Cells

Cytotoxic effects of flavonoids can be differed with variation in their chemical structures such as the presence of saturation of the C_2-C_3 bond and substitution with hydroxyl groups in the A and B rings (Figure 1) (Sak, 2014). Flavonoids having cytotoxic effect on human blood cancer cells and lung cancer, melanoma and uterine cancer cells, are shown in Table 5 (Abotaleb et al., 2019).

There are several advantages of using flavonoids as anticancer drugs. These are as follows:

i) Chemical diversity
ii) Structural complexity
iii) Various biological activity
iv) Abundant availability in foods and medicinal plants
v) Lack of cytotoxicity to normal cells

1.5 Limitations of Using Flavonoids as Anticancer Drugs

Flavonoid phytochemicals can be considered as chemotherapeutic drugs for cancer. But, a number of problems still need to be addressed before their therapeutic uses. Solubility may play major role in the therapeutic efficacy of flavonoids. Low solubility of flavonoid aglycones in water coupled with its short residence time in the intestine as well as its lower absorption does not allow humans to suffer acute toxic effects from the consumption of flavonoids, with the exception of a rare occurrence of allergy. The low solubility of the flavonoids in water often presents a problem for its medicinal applications.

Biological activity of the phytochemicals presents in food as well as in herbal formulations from medicinal plants, can be affected during their absorption in human body. For example, flavonoids, which are

Figure 2. Different food resources of flavonoids

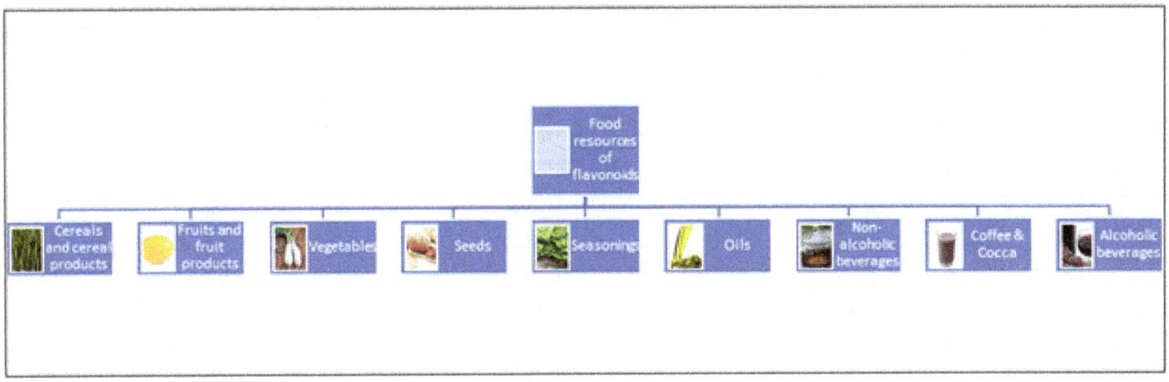

Table 2. The mean contents of different classes of flavonoids present in different foods

Name of food	Subgroup of flavonoids	Examples	mean content
Lemon	Flavanones	Eriodictyol	17.60 mg/100 g FW
		Hesperetin	17.10 mg/100 g FW
		Naringenin	0.55 mg/100 g FW
	Flavones	Luteolin	1.27 mg/100 g FW
	Flavonols	Quercetin	0.37 mg/100 g FW
Radish	Flavonols	Kaempferol	0.63 mg/100 g FW
Peanut	Isoflavones	Biochanin A	0.06 mg/100 g FW
		Daidzein	0.48 mg/100 g FW
		Genistein	0.03 mg/100 g FW
Coriander	Flavonols	Quercetin	2.50 mg/100 g FW
Olive oil	Flavones	Apigenin	0.10 mg/100 g FW
Black Tea	Flavanols	Catechin	2.45 mg/100 ml
		Epigallocatechin	7.19 mg/100 ml
	Flavonols	Kaempferol	6.36e-03 mg/100 ml
		Quercetin	3.64e-03 mg/100 ml
Chocolate, milk	Flavanols	Catechin	4.64 mg/100 g FW
		Epicatechin	14.58 mg/100 g FW
Grape wines	Flavanols	Catechin	6.81 mg/100 ml
		Epicatechin	3.78 mg/100 ml
	Flavanones	Naringin	0.75 mg/100 ml
		Naringenin	0.05 mg/100 ml
	Flavonols	Kaempferol	0.23 mg/100 ml
		Myricetin	0.83 mg/100 ml
		Quercetin	0.83 mg/100 ml

Table 3. Some of the Indian medicinal plants, and specific flavonoids (Mohanraj et al., 2018)

INDIAN MEDICINAL PLANT	PHYTOCHEMICAL IDENTIFIER	PHYTOCHEMICAL NAME	REFERENCES
Aloe vera	CID:5280443	apigenin	Flavones
Andrographis paniculata	CID:5280443	apigenin	Flavones
Centella asiatica	CID:5280443	apigenin	Flavones
Gmelina arborea	CID:5280443	apigenin	Flavones
Pogostemon cablin	CID:5280443	apigenin	Flavones
Oroxylum indicum	CID:5281605	baicalein	Flavones
Oroxylum indicum	CID:5281607	chrysin	Flavones
Catharanthus roseus	CID:128861	Cyanidin	Hydroxyflavonoids
Hibiscus rosa-sinensis	CID:128861	Cyanidin	Hydroxyflavonoids
Catharanthus roseus	CID:128853	Delphinidin	Hydroxyflavonoids
Mucuna pruriens	CID:5280961	genistein	Isoflav-2-enes
Valeriana jatamansi	CID:10621	hesperidin	Flavonoid glycosides
Cassia angustifolia	CID:5281654	Isorhamnetin	Flavones
Catharanthus roseus	CID:5281654	Isorhamnetin	Flavones
Azadirachta indica	CID:5280863	kaempferol	Flavones
Cassia angustifolia	CID:5280863	kaempferol	Flavones
Catharanthus roseus	CID:5280863	kaempferol	Flavones
Centella asiatica	CID:5280863	kaempferol	Flavones
Phyllanthus amarus	CID:5280863	kaempferol	Flavones
Smilax china	CID:5280863	kaempferol	Flavones
Centella asiatica	CID:5280445	luteolin	Flavones
Gmelina arborea	CID:5280445	luteolin	Flavones
Centella asiatica	CID:5281672	myricetin	Flavones
Catharanthus roseus	CID:442428	naringin	Flavonoid glycosides
Catharanthus roseus	CID:440832	Pelargonidin	Hydroxyflavonoids
Catharanthus roseus	CID:5280343	quercetin	Flavones
Centella asiatica	CID:5280343	quercetin	Flavones
Gmelina arborea	CID:5280343	quercetin	Flavones
Hibiscus rosa-sinensis	CID:5280343	quercetin	Flavones
Phyllanthus amarus	CID:5280343	quercetin	Flavones
Saraca asoca	CID:5280343	quercetin	Flavones
Withania somnifera	CID:5280343	quercetin	Flavones
Phyllanthus amarus	CID:5280459	quercitrin	Flavonoid glycosides
Andrographis paniculata	CID:5281703	Wogonin	O-methylated flavonoids

Figure 3. Anticancer effects of flavonoids

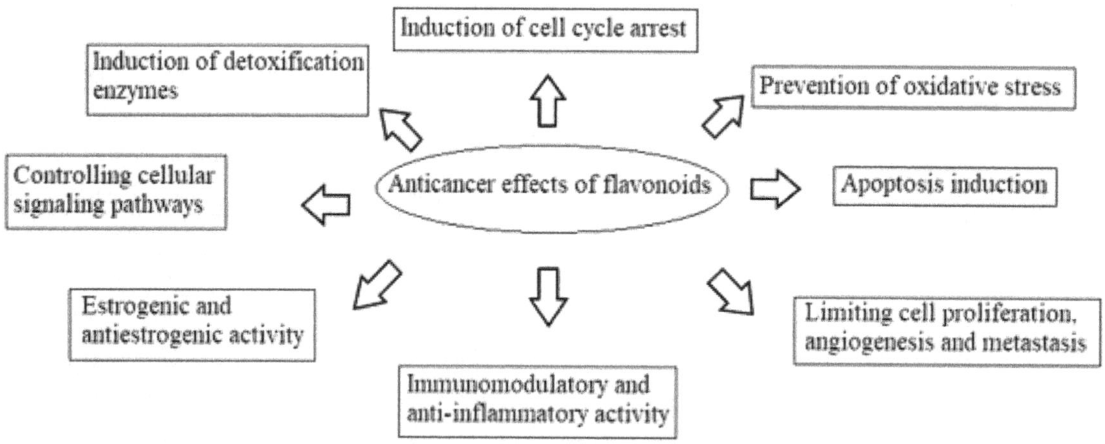

Table 4. List of flavonoids in apoptosis induction

Subgroup of flavonoids	Name of flavonoids
Isoflavones	Genistein, daidzein
Flavanones	Hesperitin, naringenin
Flavanols	Catechins, epigallocatechin gallate
Flavonols	Quercetin, kaempferol
Flavones	Apigenin, chrysin
Anthocyanidin	Pelargonidin, cyanidin, delphinidin

aglycone and hydrophilic in nature, are absorbed through the epithelial cell layer of our gastrointestinal tract by diffusion method (Karaś et al., 2017). But flavonoids which are present in nature in glycosidic form (e.g. hesperidin) are not readily absorbed in the intestine and is hydrolyzed to hespertitin by microflora β-glucosidase in the colon prior to absorption (Sacco et al., 2013).

Because, the bioavailability of flavonoids is affected by their molecular weight and chemical structure and food matrix. According to National Agricultural Library, USDA, the parameter food matrix is defined as the nutrient and non-nutrient components of foods and their molecular relationships, for example chemical bonds present in them.

After absorption in small intestine flavonoids are subjected to metabolism in liver and metabolic products are available in circulatory system. For other flavonoids, which are not absorbed in small intestine are structurally modified in colon, by microorganisms. After that microbial metabolic products

Table 5. List of flavonoids having cytotoxic effect

Flavonoids having cytotoxic effect on human blood cancer cells	Flavonoids having cytotoxic effect on lung cancer, melanoma and uterine cancer cells
Quercetin	Quercetin
Fisetin	Fisetin
Galangin	Galangin
Kaempferol	Kaempferol
Myricetin	Quercitrin
Rutin	Rutin
Naringenin	Naringenin
Apigenin	Hesperidin
Baicalein	Apigenin
Chrysin	Baicalein
Luteolin	Chrysin
Wogonin	Luteolin
Baicalin	Nobiletin
Hesperitin	Baicalin
Quercitrin	Hesperitin

Table 6. Bioavailability table for following flavonoids

Name of flavonoids	Molar weight	logP	Polar surface area
Genistein	270.24	2.58	90.90
Daidzein	254.24	2.78	67
Hesperetin	302.28	2.90	96
Naringenin	272.25	3.19	87
Catechins	290.27	0.49	110
Epigallocatechin gallate	458.37	2.08	197
Quercetin	302.24	1.99	131.36
Kaempferol	286.24	2.28	111.13
Apigenin	270.24	2.58	90.90
Chrysin	254.24	2.87	70.67
Pelargonidin	271.25	3.20	92.92
Cyanidin	287.25	2.91	112.45
Fisetin	286.24	2.52	107
Galangin	270.24	2.83	87
Myricetin	318.24	1.69	151.59
Rutin	610.52	1.76	266
Baicalein	270.24	2.58	90.90
Luteolin	286.24	2.28	111.13
Wogonin	284.27	2.88	79.90
Baicalin	446.361	0.31	183
Quercitrin	448.38	0.49	190.28
Hesperidin	610.57	-1.16	234.29
Nobiletin	402.39	2.48	82

are reached the circulatory system. Maximal plasma concentration (T_{max}) is a key parameter to express bioavailability of phytochemicals for example flavonoids.

Following physiochemical properties of phytochemicals are considered as important during their absorption in small intestine-

1. Molecular mas
2. Lipophilicity, is expressed as the logarithm of the partition coefficient between water and 1-octanol, i.e. log P)
3. Number of hydrogen donor atoms and acceptor atoms
4. Polar surface area (PSA)
5. Number of freely-rotatable bonds
6. Molecular volume
7. Dietary intake forms

Among them, three phytochemical properties, such as molecular mass, lipophilicity and polar surface area, are selected (Table 6) to predict maximal plasma concentration (T_{max}) using model by statistical analysis (Selby-Pham et al., 2017). Not only that flavonoids when consumed in liquid form, dissolved faster into gastro intestinal tract. Similarly, when flavonoids are consumed as a whole in form of fruits and vegetables, their food matrices, are also considered to determine bioavailability. Bioavailability of flavonoids are also affected by several other factors in our GI tract. Different pH environment, enzymatic degradation, mechanistic action, cause degradation of phytochemicals. To solve these problems, suitable delivery systems must be considered to protect phytochemicals during their medicinal uses (Xiao et al., 2017).

1.6 Overcoming Limitations

Different approaches are used to increase bioavailability of flavonoids as anticancer agents. These are enlisted here as follows:

a) Protection of labile flavonoids in different physiochemical environments of GI tract
b) Extension of gastric retention time to increase amount of absorption of phytochemicals
c) Increasing hydrophilicity of compound to improve their solubility
d) Controlled release system to maintain constant level in circulatory system
e) Modification of metabolic activity by inhibiting metabolic enzymes

Figure 4. Comparison between the traditional and nanotechnology-based drug delivery systems

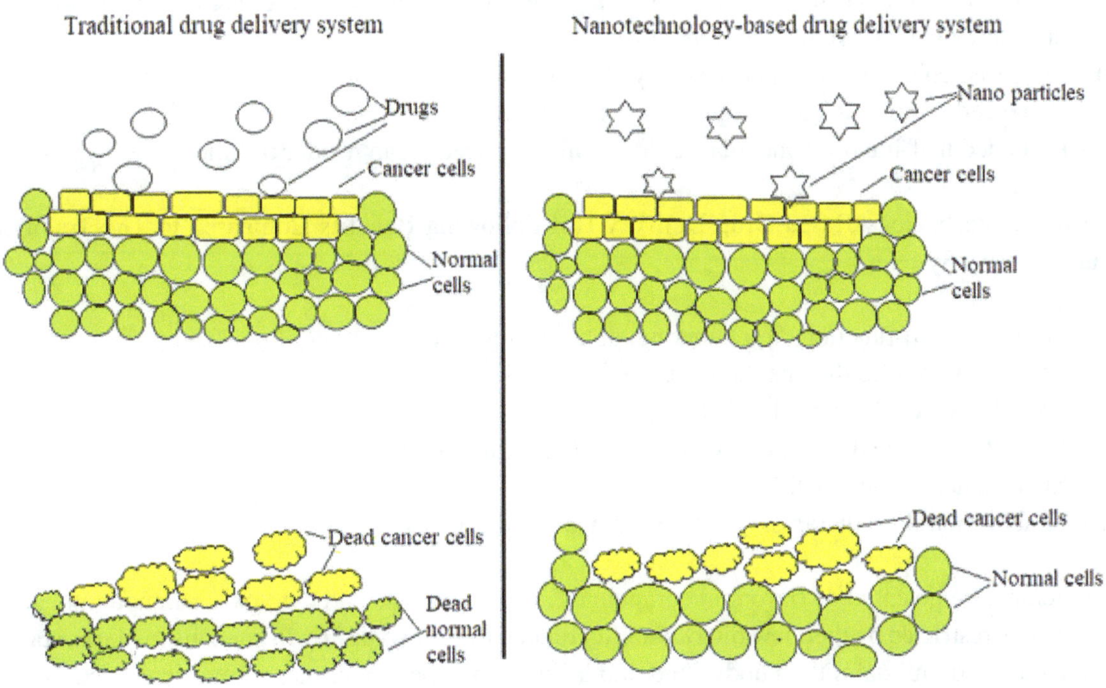

Nanomedicine is a combination of nanotechnology to medicine and pharmaceutical formulations. Thus, the limitations of phytochemicals and the associated health concerns, such as improving solubility, improvement of bioavailability, specific targeting of tumour cells or tissues without affecting the healthy cells, improved cellular uptake of phytochemicals, reducing doses of phytochemicals and achieving steady-state therapeutic concentration of the phytochemicals over an extended period, can be achieved. Nanotechnology is the most efficient tool to solve the problems of solubility, stability and oral bioavailability in delivery of flavonoid compounds. Moreover, a nanotechnology-based delivery of chemotherapeutic medicines for phytochemicals, show numerous advantages to traditional delivery methods (Keservani, 2016). The advantages are facilitated transport across biological barriers in gastrointestinal tract by enhancing bioavailability, targeted delivery of phytochemicals, protection from biological and/or environmental degradation in stomach and controlled release of phytochemicals, in and around tumor. In oncology, targeted drug delivery systems suggest several potential benefits, such as protecting the entrapped therapeutic drug from degradation in acidic environment of GIT, reducing toxicity to normal cells, modifying the pharmacokinetic and tissue distribution profile to increase drug distribution in the tumour, preventing the side effects of clinical formulations for improving solubility and increasing cellular uptake and internalization in cancer cells.

1.7 Advantages of Nanotechnology are as Follows

(i) Nanotechnology may help in increasing the solubility & bioavailability of drugs.
(ii) New dosage forms and better exploration of less-used drug administration routes for efficient therapeutic outcomes.
(iii) Nanoparticles with diameter less than 200 nm, are not screened out of circulation by liver and spleen causing extended circulation time.
(iv) Nanotechnology is better suited for drug targeting of individual tissues either by active and passive drug targeting with minimized side effects.
(v) Improved epithelium cell permeability along gastro intestinal tract.
(vi) Enhanced stability in adverse gastric environment.
(vii) Extended half-life of antineoplastic drug with enhanced mean residence time

1.8 Nanotechnology-Based Drug Delivery Has Following Benefits Compared to The Traditional Drug Delivery Systems

i. Provides multi-functionality: targeting, delivery, reporting
ii. Provides improved therapeutic index
iii. Provides lowered toxic side effects
iv. Delivers multiple drugs directly to tumor site (Figure 4)
v. Enables nucleic acid delivery
vi. Enables non-drug therapies (photothermal, photodynamic)

The therapeutic potential of flavonoid compounds as antiapoptotic and cytotoxic compound in cancer treatment is restricted by their low bioavailability related to poor solubility in aqueous medium, stability in aqueous medium, stability in body fluid and lastly absorbance in our gastrointestinal tract. To solve

Table 7. Different nano delivery systems for flavonoids, used as anticancer agents

Name of flavonoid	Types of nano delivery systems
Genistein	i) Nanoemulsions loaded with genistein developed in the form of a lozenge (Irimie et al., 2017) ii) genistein-loaded polymeric nanomicelles (Kwon et al., 2007) iii) genistein loaded in solid lipid nanoparticles (Kim et al., 2017) iv) genistein into small (~33 nm) PEGylated silica nanoparticles (Pool et al., 2018)
Daidzein	i) Daidzein self-assembled into micelles (Zhang et al., 2011)
Epigallocatechin gallate (EGCG)	i) EGCG-loaded solid lipid nanoparticles (Frias et al., 2016) ii) EGCG-loaded polymeric nanoparticles (Zhang & Zhang, 2018) iii) nanotransfersomes containing EGCG (Avadhani et al., 2017)
Quercetin	i) quercetin-loaded poly (lactic-co-glycolic acid) nanoparticles with size about 180 nm (Chitkara et al., 2012) ii) quercetin-loaded nanorods (Alam et al., 2016) iii) quercetin-loaded silica nanoparticles (Lee et al., 2016) iv) nano graphene oxide-a novel carrier for quercetin (Rahmanian et al., 2014)
Hesperidin	i) hesperidin nanoparticles loaded by poly lactic co-Glycolic acid for improved therapeutic efficiency and cytotoxicity (Ali et al., 2019) ii) hesperidin with silver nanoparticles (Sahu et al., 2014) iii) hesperidin in zinc oxide nanoparticle (Ansar et al., 2018)
Naringenin	i) Hyaluronic acid (HA) decorated naringenin loaded poly caprolactone (PCL) nanoparticles (Parashar et al., 2018) ii) PVP- coated naringenin nanoparticles (Kumar & Abraham, 2016)
Hesperetin	i) effectively encapsulated into poly (d,l-lactic-co-glycolic acid) nanoparticles (Duranoğlu et al., 2018) ii) hesperetin conjugated PEGylated gold nanoparticles (Krishnan et al., 2017) iii) hesperetin-loaded solid lipid nanoparticles (Fathi et al., 2013) iv) hesperetin loaded nanostructure lipid carriers (NLC) were coated with different biopolymers (chitosan, alginate, and low methoxypectin) (Fathi & Varshosaz, 2013)
Catechin	i) nano-encapsulation of catechin in starch nanoparticles (Ahmad et al., 2019) ii) catechin-loaded folate-conjugated chitosan nanoparticles (Liu et al., 2018) iii) catechins-loaded nanoparticles prepared from chitosan and an edible polypeptide (Tang et al., 2013) iv) self-assembled tea catechin/gelatin nanoparticles (Chen et al., 2010) v) molecular assembly of size-controlled nanoparticles (30–230 nm) with catechin and keratin (Yi et al., 2018)
Kaempferol	i) PLGA nanoparticles incorporating kaempferol (Luo et al., 2012) ii) kaempferol loaded lecithin/chitosan nanoparticles (Ilk et al., 2017) iii) nanoparticles of Kaempferol with PLGA (50:50) as the polymer iv) kaempferol nanoparticle formulation (Tzeng et al., 2011) v) kaempferol loaded gelatin nanoparticles (Chuang et al., 2019)
Apigenin	i) apigenin loaded lipid nanocapsules (Ding et al., 2013) ii) apigenin loaded in poly (lactic-co-glycolide) nanoparticles (Das et al., 2013) iii) apigenin-loaded polymeric micelles (Zhai et al., 2013) iv) carbon nanopowder (CNP) drug carrier for apigenin (Ding et al., 2014) v) Apigenin loaded PEGylate PLGA nanoparticles (Feng et al., 2015)
Chrysin	i) chrysin loaded chitosan nanoparticles (Sangeetha et al, 2017) ii) chrysin encapsulated into poly (D, L-lactic-co-glycolic acid) poly (ethylene glycol) (PLGA-PEG) (Mohammadinejad et al, 2015) iii) chrysin-phospholipid complex loaded solid lipid nanoparticles (Zheng et al., 2019) iv) chrysin-loaded nanofibrous mats (Deldar et al., 2018) v) chrysin-loaded PLGA-PEG nanoparticles (Firouzi-Amandi et al., 2018)
Pelargonidin	i) pelargonidin-PLGA nanoparticles (Roy et al, 2017) ii) silica-coated magnetite nanoparticles for pelargonidin (Yari & Rashnoo, 2017)
Cyanidin	i) silica-coated magnetite nanoparticles for cyanidin (Yari & Rashnoo, 2017) ii) caseins nanoparticles for cyanidin (Ouyang, et al, 2020) iii) TiO2 nanoparticles with cyanidin (Kurepa et al, 2014)
Fisetin	i) albumin based nanoparticles for fisetin (Ghosh et al, 2016) ii) poly (lactic acid) nanoparticles loaded with fisetin (Feng et al, 2019) iii) fisetin encapsulated into PLGA NPs (poly-lactide-co-glycolic acid nanoparticles) (Kadari et al, 2017) iv) fisetin loaded α-tocopherol-poly (lactic acid)-based polymeric micelles (Wang et al, 2017)
Galangin	i) selenium nanoparticles with galangin (Li et al, 2018) ii) Galangin and Gold nanoparticles iii) galangin-loaded PEGylated liposomes (Yao et al, 2019)
Myricetin	i) myricetin-mediated gold nanoparticles (Sathishkumar et al, 2017) ii) myricetin solid lipid nanoparticles (Gaber et al, 2019) iii) chitosan encapsulated myricetin nanoparticles iv) ZnO nanoparticles (NPs) and myricetin v) myricetin–nicotinamide nanococrystals (Liu et al, 2016)
Rutin	i) rutin-loaded PLGA nanoparticles (Kadriye, 2019) ii) rutin-encapsulated-chitosan nanoparticles (Ahmed et al, 2016) iii) rutin-loaded chitosan nanoparticles (Patil et al, 2019) iv) rutin-modified silver nanoparticles (Coutinho et al, 2019)
Baicalein	i) baicalein loaded iron oxide nanoparticles (Kavithaa et al, 2017) ii) baicalein loaded chitosan nanoparticles (Babu et al, 2012) iii) baicalein-loaded mesoporous silica nanoparticles iv) baicalein loaded chitosan nanoparticles v) baicalein-loaded nanoliposomes (Li et al, 2016)
Luteolin	i) polymer-encapsulated luteolin nanoparticle (Majumdar et al, 2014) ii) luteolin-loaded solid lipid nanoparticles (Dang et al, 2014) iii) luteolin loaded into biodegradable diblock copolymer micelles of methoxy polyethylene glycol-polycaprolactone, methoxy polyethylene glycol-polylactide-co-glycolide, and methoxy polyethylene glycol-polylactide (Qing et al, 2017)

continued on following page

Table 7. Continued

Name of flavonoid	Types of nano delivery systems
Wogonin	i) wogonin-loaded solid lipid nanoparticles (Baek et al, 2018) ii) magnetic nanoparticles of wogonin (Wang et al, 2012) iii) encapsulation of wogonin with albumin or lipid nanoparticles (Sharma et al, 2017)
Baicalin	i) use of baicalin-conjugated gold nanoparticles (Lee et al, 2016) ii) baicalin-loaded PEGylated lipid nanoparticles (Zhang et al, 2016) iii) solid lipid nanoparticles of baicalin (Li et al, 2018)
Quercitin	i) quercitin impregnated silver nanoparticle ii) quercitin loaded PLGA-MNPs (Verma et al, 2013)
Hesperidin	i) hesperidin nanoparticles loaded by poly lactic co-Glycolic acid (Ali et al, 2019) ii) silver nanoparticles for hesperidin (Sahoo et al, 2016) iii) hesperidin in zinc oxide nanoparticle (Ansar et al, 2018) iv) hesperidin nanoparticles with Poly (D, L-lactic-co-glycolic acid) (Ali et al, 2018) v) hesperidin nanoparticle with a chitosan solution
Nobiletin	i) nobiletin-loaded chitosan nanoparticles (Luque-Alcaraz et al, 2012) ii) magnetic iron oxide nanoparticles for nobiletin (Goh et al, 2019)

these problems novel nanotechnology-based drug delivery systems are developed for proper therapeutic use of natural flavonoids with improved bioavailability and optimum efficiency in medicinal uses.

1.9 Different Types of Nano Delivery Systems are Summarized Here

i) Protein and glyconanotechnology e.g. peptide lego, peptide scaffolds, lipid -like self-assembly, peptide nanotubes, lipid-like peptide, nanostructures, surface nanocoating peptide (peptide ink), glyconanoparticles
ii) Lipid nanotechnology e.g. liposomes, solid lipid nanoparticles, nanostructured lipid carriers (NLCs)
iii) Bio-nanomachines e.g. DNA nanomachines, protein nanomachines, biological nanobot (cell), DNA motor, B-2 DNA nanomechanical device, DNA origami
iv) Carbon nanotubes

There are several phytochemical-loaded nanomedicines have been experimentally verified for treatment of cancers. Lipid based nanomedicines, such as liposomes, solid lipid nanoparticles (SLNs), nanostructured lipid carriers (NLCs) and lipid micelles have shown some optimistic results for use of this type of nanomedicine in anticancer drug delivery. Lipid-based nanomedicines can enhance a specific drug accumulation into the tumour site, improving the pharmacokinetic profile (short biological plasma half-life, non-uniform oral absorption, etc.) and safety (reduced formation of toxic degradation compounds and localized activity) of such molecules e.g. genistein, epigallocatechin gallate, hesperetin etc. (Table 7).

Liposomes are self-assembled vesicular drug delivery systems which are obtained spontaneously by dispersion of phospholipids into an aqueous medium, as similar to biological membrane formation in living cells. These are biocompatible and biodegradable micro vesicles in nature. Liposomes can be used to incorporate highly lipophilic antitumor molecules into their lipid bilayer(s) and at the same time hydrophilic chemotherapeutic agents can be carried through their internal aqueous compartments. Liposomes have excellent potential for delivering various types of molecules e.g. baicalein.

Solid lipid nanoparticles (SLNs) an efficient, nontoxic, and versatile colloidal drug carrier system for chrysin, luteolin and wogonin, are composed of solid lipids (i.e. fatty acids; mono, di and triglycerides; phospholipids; etc.), to exhibit high compatibility and biodegradability.

Polymer-based nanomedicines, such as polymeric nanoparticles, polymeric micelles, polymer drug conjugates and dendrimers can be used for improvement in therapeutic efficacy of anticancer drugs such as quercetin, hesperidin, naringenin, hesperetin, kaempferol, apigenin, chrysin, pelargonidin, fisetin, rutin and baicalin (as shown in Table 7). poly(lactideco-glycolide) (PLGA), polylactide (PLA), polycaprolactone (PCL), polyglycolide, poly (d, l-lactide) and chitosan are the examples of polymeric nanoparticles, used for anticancer drugs.

Inorganic nanoparticles, including gold nanoparticles, carbon nanotubes, magnetic nanoparticles and multifunctional inorganic nanoparticle-based cancer therapy are studied extensively in cancer treatment. Silver nanoparticles conjugated with hesperidin and quercitin phytochemicals are used in treatment of cancer cells, which have cytotoxic effect on cancerous cells and biocompatible with normal cells. Similarly, carbon nanotube conjugated apigenin proven to be more cytotoxic in cancer treatment.

2. CONCLUSION

Different types of flavonoids encapsulated nanoparticles have been developed to improve their effectiveness against different types of cancer. Limitations of flavonoids as therapeutic agents in anti-cancer drug can be overcome by applying different techniques of nanotechnology.

REFERENCES

Abotaleb, M., Samuel, S. M., Varghese, E., Varghese, S., Kubatka, P., Liskova, A., & Büsselberg, D. (2019). Flavonoids in cancer and apoptosis. *Cancers (Basel), 11*(1), 28. doi:10.3390/cancers11010028 PMID:30597838

Ahmad, M., Mudgil, P., Gani, A., Hamed, F., Masoodi, F. A., & Maqsood, S. (2019). Nano-encapsulation of catechin in starch nanoparticles: Characterization, release behavior and bioactivity retention during simulated in-vitro digestion. *Food Chemistry, 270*, 95–104. doi:10.1016/j.foodchem.2018.07.024 PMID:30174096

Ahmad, N., Ahmad, R., Naqvi, A. A., Alam, M. A., Ashafaq, M., Samim, M., Iqbal, Z., & Ahmad, F. J. (2016). Rutin-encapsulated chitosan nanoparticles targeted to the brain in the treatment of Cerebral Ischemia. *International Journal of Biological Macromolecules, 91*, 640–655. doi:10.1016/j.ijbiomac.2016.06.001 PMID:27264648

Alam, M. M., Abdullah, K. M., Singh, B. R., Naqvi, A. H., & Naseem, I. (2016). Ameliorative effect of quercetin nanorods on diabetic mice: Mechanistic and therapeutic strategies. *RSC Advances, 6*(60), 55092–55103. doi:10.1039/C6RA04821H

Ali, S. H., Sulaiman, G. M., & Al-Halbosiy, M. M. (2018). In Vitro study for hesperidin nanoparticles effect on phagocytic activity against Staphylococcus aureus. *Magallat Markaz Buhut al-Tiqniyyat al-Ahya'iyyat, 12*(2), 36–39.

Ali, S. H., Sulaiman, G. M., Al-Halbosiy, M. M., Jabir, M. S., & Hameed, A. H. (2019). Fabrication of hesperidin nanoparticles loaded by poly lactic co-Glycolic acid for improved therapeutic efficiency and cytotoxicity. *Artificial Cells, Nanomedicine, and Biotechnology*, *47*(1), 378–394. doi:10.1080/21691401.2018.1559175 PMID:30691314

Ali, S. H., Sulaiman, G. M., Al-Halbosiy, M. M., Jabir, M. S., & Hameed, A. H. (2019). Fabrication of hesperidin nanoparticles loaded by poly lactic co-Glycolic acid for improved therapeutic efficiency and cytotoxicity. *Artificial Cells, Nanomedicine, and Biotechnology*, *47*(1), 378–394. doi:10.1080/21691401.2018.1559175 PMID:30691314

Amawi, H., Ashby, C. R. Jr, & Tiwari, A. K. (2017). Cancer chemoprevention through dietary flavonoids: What's limiting? *Chinese Journal of Cancer*, *36*(1), 50. doi:10.118640880-017-0217-4 PMID:28629389

Ansar, S., Abudawood, M., Alaraj, A. S., & Hamed, S. S. (2018). Hesperidin alleviates zinc oxide nanoparticle induced hepatotoxicity and oxidative stress. *BMC Pharmacology & Toxicology*, *19*(1), 65. doi:10.118640360-018-0256-8 PMID:30340509

Ansar, S., Abudawood, M., Alaraj, A. S., & Hamed, S. S. (2018). Hesperidin alleviates zinc oxide nanoparticle induced hepatotoxicity and oxidative stress. *BMC Pharmacology & Toxicology*, *19*(1), 65. doi:10.118640360-018-0256-8 PMID:30340509

Avadhani, K. S., Manikkath, J., Tiwari, M., Chandrasekhar, M., Godavarthi, A., Vidya, S. M., Hariharapura, R. C., Kalthur, G., Udupa, N., & Mutalik, S. (2017). Skin delivery of epigallocatechin-3-gallate (EGCG) and hyaluronic acid loaded nano-transfersomes for antioxidant and anti-aging effects in UV radiation induced skin damage. *Drug Delivery*, *24*(1), 61–74. doi:10.1080/10717544.2016.1228718 PMID:28155509

Babii, C., Mihalache, G., Bahrin, L. G., Neagu, A. N., Gostin, I., Mihai, C. T., Sârbu, L.-G., Birsa, L. M., & Stefan, M. (2018). A novel synthetic flavonoid with potent antibacterial properties: In vitro activity and proposed mode of action. *PLoS One*, *13*(4), e0194898. doi:10.1371/journal.pone.0194898 PMID:29617411

Babu, V. N., & Kannan, S. (2012). Enhanced delivery of baicalein using cinnamaldehyde cross-linked chitosan nanoparticle inducing apoptosis. *International Journal of Biological Macromolecules*, *51*(5), 1103–1108. doi:10.1016/j.ijbiomac.2012.08.038 PMID:22981825

Baek, J. S., Na, Y. G., & Cho, C. W. (2018). Sustained cytotoxicity of wogonin on breast cancer cells by encapsulation in solid lipid nanoparticles. *Nanomaterials (Basel, Switzerland)*, *8*(3), 159. doi:10.3390/nano8030159 PMID:29533979

Brodowska, K. M. (2017). Natural flavonoids: Classification, potential role, and application of flavonoid analogues. *European Journal of Biological Research*, *7*(2), 108–123.

Chen, Y. C., Yu, S. H., Tsai, G. J., Tang, D. W., Mi, F. L., & Peng, Y. P. (2010). Novel technology for the preparation of self-assembled catechin/gelatin nanoparticles and their characterization. *Journal of Agricultural and Food Chemistry*, *58*(11), 6728–6734. doi:10.1021/jf1005116 PMID:20476739

Chitkara, D., Nikalaje, S. K., Mittal, A., Chand, M., & Kumar, N. (2012). Development of quercetin nanoformulation and in vivo evaluation using streptozotocin induced diabetic rat model. *Drug Delivery and Translational Research*, *2*(2), 112–123. doi:10.100713346-012-0063-5 PMID:25786720

Chuang, Y. L., Fang, H. W., Ajitsaria, A., Chen, K. H., Su, C. Y., Liu, G. S., & Tseng, C. L. (2019). Development of Kaempferol-loaded gelatin nanoparticles for the treatment of corneal neovascularization in mice. *Pharmaceutics*, *11*(12), 635. doi:10.3390/pharmaceutics11120635 PMID:31795237

Coutinho, M. S., Latocheski, E., Neri, J. M., Neves, A. C., Domingos, J. B., Cavalcanti, L. N., Gasparotto, L. H. S., Moraes, E. P., & Menezes, F. G. (2019). Rutin-modified silver nanoparticles as a chromogenic probe for the selective detection of Fe 3+ in aqueous medium. *RSC Advances*, *9*(51), 30007–30011. doi:10.1039/C9RA06653E

Dang, H., Meng, M. H. W., Zhao, H., Iqbal, J., Dai, R., Deng, Y., & Lv, F. (2014). Luteolin-loaded solid lipid nanoparticles synthesis, characterization, & improvement of bioavailability, pharmacokinetics in vitro and vivo studies. *Journal of Nanoparticle Research*, *16*(4), 2347. doi:10.100711051-014-2347-9

Das, S., Das, J., Samadder, A., Paul, A., & Khuda-Bukhsh, A. R. (2013). Strategic formulation of apigenin-loaded PLGA nanoparticles for intracellular trafficking, DNA targeting and improved therapeutic effects in skin melanoma in vitro. *Toxicology Letters*, *223*(2), 124–138. doi:10.1016/j.toxlet.2013.09.012 PMID:24070738

Deldar, Y., Pilehvar-Soltanahmadi, Y., Dadashpour, M., Montazer Saheb, S., Rahmati-Yamchi, M., & Zarghami, N. (2018). An in vitro examination of the antioxidant, cytoprotective and anti-inflammatory properties of chrysin-loaded nanofibrous mats for potential wound healing applications. *Artificial Cells, Nanomedicine, and Biotechnology*, *46*(4), 706–716. doi:10.1080/21691401.2017.1337022 PMID:28595461

Ding, B., Chen, H., Wang, C., Zhai, Y., & Zhai, G. (2013). Preparation and in vitro evaluation of apigenin loaded lipid nanocapsules. *Journal of Nanoscience and Nanotechnology*, *13*(10), 6546–6552. doi:10.1166/jnn.2013.7763 PMID:24245113

Ding, S. M., Zhang, Z. H., Song, J., Cheng, X. D., Jiang, J., & Jia, X. B. (2014). Enhanced bioavailability of apigenin via preparation of a carbon nanopowder solid dispersion. *International Journal of Nanomedicine*, *9*, 2327. doi:10.2147/IJN.S60938 PMID:24872695

Duranoğlu, D., Uzunoglu, D., Mansuroglu, B., Arasoglu, T., & Derman, S. (2018). Synthesis of hesperetin-loaded PLGA nanoparticles by two different experimental design methods and biological evaluation of optimized nanoparticles. *Nanotechnology*, *29*(39), 395603. doi:10.1088/1361-6528/aad111 PMID:29972381

Fathi, M., & Varshosaz, J. (2013). Novel hesperetin loaded nanocarriers for food fortification: Production and characterization. *Journal of Functional Foods*, *5*(3), 1382–1391. doi:10.1016/j.jff.2013.05.006

Fathi, M., Varshosaz, J., Mohebbi, M., & Shahidi, F. (2013). Hesperetin-loaded solid lipid nanoparticles and nanostructure lipid carriers for food fortification: Preparation, characterization, and modeling. *Food and Bioprocess Technology*, *6*(6), 1464–1475. doi:10.100711947-012-0845-2

Feng, C., Yuan, X., Chu, K., Zhang, H., Ji, W., & Rui, M. (2019). Preparation and optimization of poly (lactic acid) nanoparticles loaded with fisetin to improve anti-cancer therapy. *International Journal of Biological Macromolecules*, *125*, 700–710. doi:10.1016/j.ijbiomac.2018.12.003 PMID:30521927

Feng, W. M., Guo, H. H., Xue, T., Wang, X., Tang, C. W., Ying, B., Gong, H., & Cui, G. (2015). Anti-inflammation and anti-fibrosis with PEGylated, apigenin loaded PLGA nanoparticles in chronic pancreatitis disease. *RSC Advances*, *5*(102), 83628–83635. doi:10.1039/C5RA17686G

Firouzi-Amandi, A., Dadashpour, M., Nouri, M., Zarghami, N., Serati-Nouri, H., Jafari-Gharabaghlou, D., Karzar, B. H., Mellatyar, H., Aghebati-Maleki, L., Babaloo, Z., & Pilehvar-Soltanahmadi, Y. (2018). Chrysin-nanoencapsulated PLGA-PEG for macrophage repolarization: Possible application in tissue regeneration. *Biomedicine and Pharmacotherapy*, *105*, 773–780. doi:10.1016/j.biopha.2018.06.037 PMID:29909345

Frias, I., Neves, A. R., Pinheiro, M., & Reis, S. (2016). Design, development, and characterization of lipid nanocarriers-based epigallocatechin gallate delivery system for preventive and therapeutic supplementation. *Drug Design, Development and Therapy*, *10*, 3519–3528. doi:10.2147/DDDT.S109589 PMID:27826184

Gaber, D. M., Nafee, N., & Abdallah, O. Y. (2017). Myricetin solid lipid nanoparticles: Stability assurance from system preparation to site of action. *European Journal of Pharmaceutical Sciences*, *109*, 569–580. doi:10.1016/j.ejps.2017.08.007 PMID:28818532

Genoux, E., Nicolle, E., & Boumendjel, A. (2011). Flavonoids as anticancer agents: Recent progress and state of the art? *Current Organic Chemistry*, *15*(15), 2608–2615. doi:10.2174/138527211796367363

Ghosh, P., Roy, A. S., Chaudhury, S., Jana, S. K., Chaudhury, K., & Dasgupta, S. (2016). Preparation of albumin-based nanoparticles for delivery of fisetin and evaluation of its cytotoxic activity. *International Journal of Biological Macromolecules*, *86*, 408–417. doi:10.1016/j.ijbiomac.2016.01.082 PMID:26820351

Goh, J. X. H., Tan, L. T. H., Goh, J. K., Chan, K. G., Pusparajah, P., Lee, L. H., & Goh, B. H. (2019). Nobiletin and derivatives: Functional compounds from citrus fruit peel for colon cancer chemoprevention. *Cancers (Basel)*, *11*(6), 867. doi:10.3390/cancers11060867 PMID:31234411

Ilk, S., Saglam, N., & Özgen, M. (2017). Kaempferol loaded lecithin/chitosan nanoparticles: Preparation, characterization, and their potential applications as a sustainable antifungal agent. *Artificial Cells, Nanomedicine, and Biotechnology*, *45*(5), 907–916. doi:10.1080/21691401.2016.1192040 PMID:27265551

Irimie, A. I., Sonea, L., Jurj, A., Mehterov, N., Zimta, A. A., Budisan, L., Braicu, C., & Berindan-Neagoe, I. (2017). Future trends and emerging issues for nanodelivery systems in oral and oropharyngeal cancer. *International Journal of Nanomedicine*, *12*, 4593–4606. doi:10.2147/IJN.S133219 PMID:28721037

Kadari, A., Gudem, S., Kulhari, H., Bhandi, M. M., Borkar, R. M., Kolapalli, V. R. M., & Sistla, R. (2017). Enhanced oral bioavailability and anticancer efficacy of fisetin by encapsulating as inclusion complex with HPβCD in polymeric nanoparticles. *Drug Delivery*, *24*(1), 224–232. doi:10.1080/10717544.2016.1245366 PMID:28156161

Karak, P. (2019). Biological activities of flavonoids: An overview. *International Journal of Pharmaceutical Sciences and Research*, *10*(4), 1567–1574.

Karaś, M., Jakubczyk, A., Szymanowska, U., Złotek, U., & Zielińska, E. (2017). Digestion and bioavailability of bioactive phytochemicals. *International Journal of Food Science & Technology*, *52*(2), 291–305. doi:10.1111/ijfs.13323

Kavithaa, K., Sumathi, S., & Padma, P. R. (2017). Intracellular uptake of PEG-funtionalized baicalein loaded iron oxide nanoparticles regulates apoptotic genes in triple negative breast cancer cells: Mitochondrial pathway targeted therapy for breast cancer. *Journal of Cluster Science*, *28*(4), 2057–2073. doi:10.100710876-017-1204-2

Keservani, R. K., Kesharwani, R. K., Sharma, A. K., & Jarouliya, U. (2015). Dietary supplements, nutraceutical, and functional foods in immune response (immunomodulators). In D. Bagchi, A. Swaroop, & H. G. Preuss (Eds.), *Nutraceutical and Functional Foods in Human Life and Disease Prevention* (pp. 343–360). CRC Press, Taylor and Francis.

Keservani, R. K., Sharma, A. K., & Kesharwani, R. K. (2017). An overview and therapeutic applications of nutraceutical and functional foods. In *Recent Advances in Drug Delivery Technology* (pp. 160–201). IGI Global.

Kim, J. T., Barua, S., Kim, H., Hong, S. C., Yoo, S. Y., Jeon, H., Cho, Y., Gil, S., Oh, K., & Lee, J. (2017). Absorption study of genistein using solid lipid microparticles and nanoparticles: Control of oral bioavailability by particle sizes. *Biomolecules & Therapeutics*, *25*(4), 452–459. doi:10.4062/biomolther.2017.095 PMID:28605834

Kızılbey, K. (2019). Optimization of rutin-loaded PLGA nanoparticles synthesized by single-emulsion solvent evaporation method. *ACS Omega*, *4*(1), 555–562. doi:10.1021/acsomega.8b02767

Kopustinskiene, D. M., Jakstas, V., Savickas, A., & Bernatoniene, J. (2020). Flavonoids as anticancer agents. *Nutrients*, *12*(2), 457. doi:10.3390/nu12020457 PMID:32059369

Krishnan, G., Subramaniyan, J., Subramani, P. C., Muralidharan, B., & Thiruvengadam, D. (2017). Hesperetin conjugated PEGylated gold nanoparticles exploring the potential role in anti-inflammation and anti-proliferation during diethylnitrosamine-induced hepatocarcinogenesis in rats. *Asian Journal of Pharmaceutical Sciences*, *12*(5), 442-455.

Kumar, R. P., & Abraham, A. (2016). PVP-coated naringenin nanoparticles for biomedical applications–In vivo toxicological evaluations. *Chemico-Biological Interactions*, *257*, 110–118. doi:10.1016/j.cbi.2016.07.012 PMID:27417253

Kurepa, J., Nakabayashi, R., Paunesku, T., Suzuki, M., Saito, K., Woloschak, G. E., & Smalle, J. A. (2014). Direct isolation of flavonoids from plants using ultra-small anatase TiO 2 nanoparticles. *The Plant Journal*, *77*(3), 443–453. doi:10.1111/tpj.12361 PMID:24147867

Kwon, S. H., Kim, S. Y., Ha, K. W., Kang, M. J., Huh, J. S., Kim, Y. M., ... Lee, J. (2007). Pharmaceutical evaluation of genistein-loaded pluronic micelles for oral delivery. *Archives of Pharmacal Research*, *30*(9), 1138–1143. doi:10.1007/BF02980249 PMID:17958332

Lee, D., Ko, W. K., Hwang, D. S., Heo, D. N., Lee, S. J., Heo, M., Lee, K.-S., Ahn, J.-Y., Jo, J., & Kwon, I. K. (2016). Use of baicalin-conjugated gold nanoparticles for apoptotic induction of breast cancer cells. *Nanoscale Research Letters*, *11*(1), 381. doi:10.118611671-016-1586-3 PMID:27576521

Lee, G. H., Lee, S. J., Jeong, S. W., Kim, H. C., Park, G. Y., Lee, S. G., & Choi, J. H. (2016). Antioxidative and antiinflammatory activities of quercetin-loaded silica nanoparticles. *Colloids and Surfaces. B, Biointerfaces, 143*, 511–517. doi:10.1016/j.colsurfb.2016.03.060 PMID:27038916

Li, K., Zhang, H., Gao, L., Zhai, Y., Shi, M., Li, J., Xiu, C., Cao, J., Cheng, S., Jiang, L., & Di, H. (2016). Preparation and Characterization of Baicalein-Loaded Nanoliposomes for Antitumor Therapy. *Journal of Nanomaterials, 2016*, 2016. doi:10.1155/2016/2861915

Li, N., Han, Z., Li, L., Zhang, B., Liu, Z., & Li, J. (2018). The anti-cataract molecular mechanism study in selenium cataract rats for baicalin ophthalmic nanoparticles. *Drug Design, Development and Therapy, 12*, 1399–1411. doi:10.2147/DDDT.S160524 PMID:29872263

Li, Y., Fang, H., & Xu, W. (2007). Recent advance in the research of flavonoids as anticancer agents. *Mini-Reviews in Medicinal Chemistry, 7*(7), 663–678. doi:10.2174/138955707781024463 PMID:17627579

Li, Y., Guo, M., Lin, Z., Zhao, M., Xia, Y., Wang, C., Xu, T., & Zhu, B. (2018). Multifunctional selenium nanoparticles with Galangin-induced HepG2 cell apoptosis through p38 and AKT signalling pathway. *Royal Society Open Science, 5*(11), 180509. doi:10.1098/rsos.180509 PMID:30564384

Liu, B., Wang, Y., Yu, Q., Li, D., & Li, F. (2018). Synthesis, characterization of catechin-loaded folate-conjugated chitosan nanoparticles and their anti-proliferative effect. *CYTA: Journal of Food, 16*(1), 868–876. doi:10.1080/19476337.2018.1491625

Liu, M., Hong, C., Li, G., Ma, P., & Xie, Y. (2016). The generation of myricetin-nicotinamide nanococrystals by top down and bottom up technologies. *Nanotechnology, 27*(39), 395601–395601. doi:10.1088/0957-4484/27/39/395601 PMID:27535365

Luo, H., Jiang, B., Li, B., Li, Z., Jiang, B. H., & Chen, Y. C. (2012). Kaempferol nanoparticles achieve strong and selective inhibition of ovarian cancer cell viability. *International Journal of Nanomedicine, 7*, 3951–3959. doi:10.2147/IJN.S33670 PMID:22866004

Luque-Alcaraz, A. G., Lizardi, J., Goycoolea, F. M., Valdez, M. A., Acosta, A. L., Iloki-Assanga, S. B., ... Argüelles-Monal, W. (2012). Characterization and antiproliferative activity of nobiletin-loaded chitosan nanoparticles. *Journal of Nanomaterials.*

Majumdar, D., Jung, K. H., Zhang, H., Nannapaneni, S., Wang, X., Amin, A. R., ... Shin, D. M. (2014). Luteolin nanoparticle in chemoprevention: In vitro and in vivo anticancer activity. *Cancer Prevention Research (Philadelphia, Pa.), 7*(1), 65–73.

Mohammadinejad, S., Akbarzadeh, A., Rahmati-Yamchi, M., Hatam, S., Kachalaki, S., Zohreh, S., & Zarghami, N. (2015). Preparation and evaluation of chrysin encapsulated in PLGA-PEG nanoparticles in the T47-D breast cancer cell line. *Asian Pacific Journal of Cancer Prevention, 16*(9), 3753–3758.

Mohanraj, K., Karthikeyan, B. S., Vivek-Ananth, R. P., Chand, R. B., Aparna, S. R., Mangalapandi, P., & Samal, A. (2018). IMPPAT: A curated database of I ndian M edicinal P lants, P hytochemistry A nd T herapeutics. *Scientific Reports, 8*(1), 1–17.

Neveu, V., Perez-Jiménez, J., Vos, F., Crespy, V., Du Chaffaut, L., Mennen, L., & Scalbert, A. (2010). *Phenol-Explorer: an online comprehensive database on polyphenol contents in foods. Database. Journal of Biological Database Biocuration.*

Ouyang, Y., Chen, L., Qian, L., Lin, X., Fan, X., Teng, H., & Cao, H. (2020). Fabrication of caseins nanoparticles to improve the stability of cyanidin 3-O-glucoside. *Food Chemistry, 317*, 126418.

Parashar, P., Rathor, M., Dwivedi, M., & Saraf, S. A. (2018). Hyaluronic acid decorated naringenin nanoparticles: Appraisal of chemopreventive and curative potential for lung cancer. *Pharmaceutics, 10*(1), 33.

Patil, A. G., & Jobanputra, A. H. (2015). Rutin-chitosan nanoparticles: Fabrication, characterization and application in dental disorders. *Polymer-Plastics Technology and Engineering, 54*(2), 202–208.

Pool, H., Campos-Vega, R., Herrera-Hernández, M. G., García-Solis, P., García-Gasca, T., Sánchez, I. C., ... Vergara-Castañeda, H. (2018). Development of genistein-PEGylated silica hybrid nanomaterials with enhanced antioxidant and antiproliferative properties on HT29 human colon cancer cells. *American Journal of Translational Research, 10*(8), 2306.

Qing, W., Wang, Y., Li, H., Ma, F., Zhu, J., & Liu, X. (2017). Preparation and characterization of copolymer micelles for the solubilization and in vitro release of luteolin and luteoloside. *AAPS PharmSciTech, 18*(6), 2095–2101.

Rahmanian, N., Hamishehkar, H., Dolatabadi, J. E. N., & Arsalani, N. (2014). Nano graphene oxide: A novel carrier for oral delivery of flavonoids. *Colloids and Surfaces. B, Biointerfaces, 123*, 331–338.

Rajesh, K. (2019). Kesharwani, K Misra, DB Singh, Perspectives and challenges of tropical medicinal herbs and modern drug discovery in the current scenario. *Asian Pacific Journal of Tropical Medicine, 12*(1), 1–7.

Rothwell, J. A., Perez-Jimenez, J., Neveu, V., Medina-Remon, A., M'Hiri, N., García-Lobato, P., ... Scalbert, A. (2013). Phenol-Explorer 3.0: A major update of the Phenol-Explorer database to incorporate data on the effects of food processing on polyphenol content. *Database (Oxford).*

Rothwell, J. A., Urpi-Sarda, M., Boto-Ordonez, M., Knox, C., Llorach, R., Eisner, R., ... Andres-Lacueva, C. (2012). Phenol-Explorer 2.0: A major update of the Phenol-Explorer database integrating data on polyphenol metabolism and pharmacokinetics in humans and experimental animals. *Database (Oxford),* ●●●, 2012.

Roy, M., Pal, R., & Chakraborti, A. S. (2017). Pelargonidin-PLGA nanoparticles: Fabrication, characterization, and their effect on streptozotocin induced diabetic rats. *Indian Journal of Experimental Biology, 55*, 819–830.

Sacco, S. M., Horcajada, M. N., & Offord, E. (2013). Phytonutrients for bone health during ageing. *British Journal of Clinical Pharmacology, 75*(3), 697–707.

Sahu, N., Soni, D., Chandrashekhar, B., Satpute, D. B., Saravanadevi, S., Sarangi, B. K., & Pandey, R. A. (2016). Synthesis of silver nanoparticles using flavonoids: Hesperidin, naringin and diosmin, and their antibacterial effects and cytotoxicity. *International Nano Letters, 6*(3), 173–181.

Sahu, N., Soni, D., Chandrashekhar, B., Satpute, D. B., Saravanadevi, S., Sarangi, B. K., & Pandey, R. A. (2016). Synthesis of silver nanoparticles using flavonoids: Hesperidin, naringin and diosmin, and their antibacterial effects and cytotoxicity. *International Nano Letters*, *6*(3), 173–181.

Sak, K. (2014). Cytotoxicity of dietary flavonoids on different human cancer types. *Pharmacognosy Reviews*, *8*(16), 122.

Sangeetha, K. S. S., Umamaheswari, S., Reddy, C. U. M., & Kalkura, S. N. (2017). Chrysin loaded chitosan nanoparticle: Formulation and in-vitro characterization. *International Journal of Pharmaceutical Sciences and Research*, *8*(3), 1102–1109. doi:10.13040/IJPSR.0975-8232.8(3).1102-09

Santos, E. L., Maia, B. H. L. N. S., Ferriani, A. P., & Teixeira, S. D. (2017). *Flavonoids: Classification, biosynthesis and chemical ecology* (Vol. 6). InTech.

Sathishkumar, P., Li, Z., Huang, B., Guo, X., Zhan, Q., Wang, C., & Gu, F. L. (2019). Understanding the surface functionalization of myricetin-mediated gold nanoparticles: Experimental and theoretical approaches. *Applied Surface Science*, *493*, 634–644.

Selby-Pham, S. N., Miller, R. B., Howell, K., Dunshea, F., & Bennett, L. E. (2017). Physicochemical properties of dietary phytochemicals can predict their passive absorption in the human small intestine. *Scientific Reports*, *7*(1), 1–15.

Sharma, N., Singh, A. K., & Sodhi, S. S., Zhang, J. J., Mongre, R. K., Ghosh, M., ... Jeong, D. K. (2017). Anti-tumor activity of wogonin, an extract from Scutellaria baicalensis, through regulating different signaling pathways. *Chinese Journal of Natural Medicines*, *15*(1), 15–40.

Tang, D. W., Yu, S. H., Ho, Y. C., Huang, B. Q., Tsai, G. J., Hsieh, H. Y., ... Mi, F. L. (2013). Characterization of tea catechins-loaded nanoparticles prepared from chitosan and an edible polypeptide. *Food Hydrocolloids*, *30*(1), 33–41.

Tzeng, C. W., Yen, F. L., Wu, T. H., Ko, H. H., Lee, C. W., Tzeng, W. S., & Lin, C. C. (2011). Enhancement of dissolution and antioxidant activity of kaempferol using a nanoparticle engineering process. *Journal of Agricultural and Food Chemistry*, *59*(9), 5073–5080.

Veeramuthu, D., Raja, W. R. T., Al-Dhabi, N. A., & Savarimuthu, I. (2017). Flavonoids: anticancer properties. *Flavonoids: From Biosynthesis to Human Health, 287.*

Verma, N. K., Crosbie-Staunton, K., Satti, A., Gallagher, S., Ryan, K. B., Doody, T., ... Volkov, Y. (2013). Magnetic core-shell nanoparticles for drug delivery by nebulization. *Journal of Nanobiotechnology*, *11*(1), 1.

Wang, L., Zhang, D. Z., & Wang, Y. X. (2017). Bioflavonoid fisetin loaded α-tocopherol-poly (lactic acid)-based polymeric micelles for enhanced anticancer efficacy in breast cancers. *Pharmaceutical Research*, *34*(2), 453–461.

Wang, L., Zhang, H., Chen, B., Xia, G., Wang, S., Cheng, J., ... Ren, Y. (2012). Effect of magnetic nanoparticles on apoptosis and cell cycle induced by wogonin in Raji cells. *International Journal of Nanomedicine*, *7*, 789.

Wang, T. Y., Li, Q., & Bi, K. S. (2018). Bioactive flavonoids in medicinal plants: Structure, activity and biological fate. *Asian Journal of Pharmaceutical Sciences*, *13*(1), 12–23.

Xiao, J., Cao, Y., & Huang, Q. (2017). Edible nanoencapsulation vehicles for oral delivery of phytochemicals: A perspective paper. *Journal of Agricultural and Food Chemistry*, *65*(32), 6727–6735.

Yao, H., Lu, H., Zhang, J., Xue, X., Yin, C., Hu, J., ... Xu, H. (2019). Preparation of Prolonged-Circulating Galangin-Loaded Liposomes and Evaluation of Antitumor Efficacy In Vitro and Pharmacokinetics In Vivo. *Journal of Nanomaterials*.

Yari, A., & Rashnoo, S. (2017). Optimization of a new method for extraction of cyanidin chloride and pelargonidin chloride anthocyanins with magnetic solid phase extraction and determination in fruit samples by HPLC with central composite design. *Journal of Chromatography. B, Analytical Technologies in the Biomedical and Life Sciences*, *1067*, 38–44.

Yi, Z., Sun, Z., Chen, G., Zhang, H., Ma, X., Su, W., ... Li, X. (2018). Size-controlled, colloidally stable and functional nanoparticles based on the molecular assembly of green tea polyphenols and keratins for cancer therapy. *Journal of Materials Chemistry. B, Materials for Biology and Medicine*, *6*(9), 1373–1386.

Zhai, Y., Guo, S., Liu, C., Yang, C., Dou, J., Li, L., & Zhai, G. (2013). Preparation and in vitro evaluation of apigenin-loaded polymeric micelles. *Colloids and Surfaces. A, Physicochemical and Engineering Aspects*, *429*, 24–30.

Zhang, G., & Zhang, J. (2018). Enhanced oral bioavailability of EGCG using pH-sensitive polymeric nanoparticles: Characterization and in vivo investigation on nephrotic syndrome rats. *Drug Design, Development and Therapy*, *12*, 2509.

Zhang, S., Wang, J., & Pan, J. (2016). Baicalin-loaded PEGylated lipid nanoparticles: Characterization, pharmacokinetics, and protective effects on acute myocardial ischemia in rats. *Drug Delivery*, *23*(9), 3696–3703.

Zhang, Z., Huang, Y., Gao, F., Gao, Z., Bu, H., Gu, W., & Li, Y. (2011). A self-assembled nanodelivery system enhances the oral bioavailability of daidzein: In vitro characteristics and in vivo performance. *Nanomedicine (London)*, *6*(8), 1365–1379.

Zheng, G., Zheng, M., Yang, B., Fu, H., & Li, Y. (2019). Improving breast cancer therapy using doxorubicin loaded solid lipid nanoparticles: Synthesis of a novel arginine-glycine-aspartic tripeptide conjugated, pH sensitive lipid and evaluation of the nanomedicine in vitro and in vivo. *Biomedicine and Pharmacotherapy*, *116*.

Chapter 10
Phytosomes as a Novel Approach for Herbal Phytoconstituents

Shweta Gedam
Sandip Institute of Pharmaceutical Science, Nasik, India

Akshada Atul Bakliwal
Sandip Institute of Pharmaceutical Science, Nasik, India

Swati Gokul Talele
Sandip Institute of Pharmaceutical Science, Nasik, India

Vijay Sharadkumar Chudiwal
Sun Pharma, Mumbai, India

ABSTRACT

Phytosomes are a new approach for delivery of drugs. Phytosomes mean herbal drugs loaded in vesicles, which are available in the nano form. The phytosome offers an envelope like coating around the active moieties of drug, and due to this, the main constituent of herbal extract remains safe from degradation by bacteria and digestive secretion. It is a patented technology which is advantageous in delivering the herbal drugs. Phytosomes have better pharmacological and pharmacokinetic parameters. It is used for development of delivery system with improved bioavailability of phytoconstituents present in herbal extracts. Phytosomes are prepared by the use of phospholipids by forming the complex between phospholipids and phytoconstituent. Phytosomes have a vast scope in pharma-industries and good research space for industry, scholars, students. Phospholipids are use as carriers for water soluble and lipid soluble nutrients and natural digestive aids.

DOI: 10.4018/978-1-7998-4453-2.ch010

1. INTRODUCTION

Phytosomes are modern natural products that are formed by binding of individual component of herbal extract to phosphatidylcholine. and gives a improved conventional herbal extracts. It is advantageous in delivering the herbal drug at predetermined rate, Increase in bioavailability of drugs, delivery of drug at the targeted site, minimizes the toxic effects, Control of the distribution of drug is achieved by incorporate the drug in carrier system or in changing the structure of the drug at molecular level. Herbal drug are becoming more popular in the modern world for their applications and safety aspects which has enhanced absorption and bioavailability (Semalty et al., 2010; Gandhi et al., 2012). The bioavailability can be markedly superior with the utilization of different novel combined form of two words i.e. 'Phyto' means plant & 'somes' means cell like. The pharma world constantly works and struggle to make such type of formulations which can show greater absorption and bioavailability in comparison to the previous one, specially for phytoconstituents (Kalita et al., 2013). In this recently developed technology, the water-soluble phytoconstituents are incorporated into lipid compatible moiety to cross the lipid biomembranes and enters into systemic circulations, which shows better absorption because they can easily cross the various membranes (Jadhav et al., 2014). This technology is widely use for some compounds like terpenoids and flavonoids.The phytosome operation gives birth to a little cell whereby the precious plant extracts are preserved from deadening bydigestive enzymes and gut bacteria. Phytosomes are healthier to shift from a hydrophilic domain into the lipid-friendly domain of the enterocyte cell membrane and from there into the cell finally accomplishing the blood the molecular organization of liposomes and phytosomes is shown in figure 1. (Jain et al., 2010)

Figure 1. Molecular organization of liposomes and phytosomes

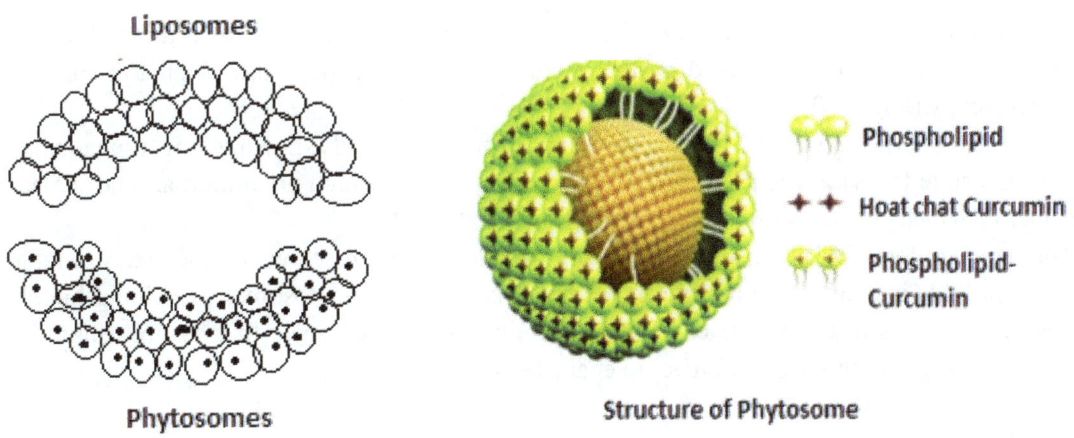

1.1 Background

In 1989, the term phytosome was firstly introduced. Italian scientist focused on the poorly bioavailable polyphenols as it is weakly bind to the phospholipids present in the plant tissue. This polyphenols then converted into phytosomes increased their bioavailability (Bombardelli et al., 1989). In the preparation of phytosomes, polyphenols is reacted with phosphatidylcholine which is main constituent of phospholipid present in the cell membrane. The clinical usefulness of botanical polyphenol was verified by phytosome technology because of its better bioavailability which also enhance the efficacy (Kidd, 2019).

1.2 Phytosome Technology

Phytosomes is link between traditional and novel drug delivery system. It consists of phytoconstituents of herbal extract complexed with phospholipids. This technology is an innovative model to enhance bioavailability and solubility of the drug without withdrawing the nutrient safety (Amit et al., 2013; Venkatesan et al., 2000). Up to now, this technology has been effective with herbal extracts forinstance curcumin, *Ginkgo biloba*, grape seed, ginseng, milk thistle, and other goods used aswidespread nutritional. This technology permitted the compound to be appropriately assimilated into the body and be carried tothe target site. For the herbal formulation to have good bioavailability, they need tohave a proper equilibrium among hydrophilicity and lipophilicity. In addition, they need to be ableto be soluble into fluid present in the intestines besides cross biomembranes. This is the reason why phytosomes have extra bioavailability than simple herbal medicines (Verma et al., 2013; Tripathy et al., 2013).

1.3 Properties of Phytosomes

Phytosomes characterstics are;

1.4 Physicochemical Properties

- Magnitude of phytosomes ranges from 50 nm to few hundreds of micrometer (Tripathy et al., 2013).
- The reaction of phytosomes with water forms micellar shaped structure same as that of liposomes. The liposomal structure occupied by the phytosomes is revealed by use of photon correlation spectroscopy (Jain, 2005).
- From the ^{1}H NMR and ^{13}C NMR, it was concluded that fatty acids showing long aliphatic chains is responsible for both free phospholipid and complex form which are attired around the active principle which generates lipophilic cover (Dayan et al., 2000).
- The complex forms of phytosomes are freely soluble in aprotic solvents, moderately soluble in fats, insoluble in water and unstable in alcohol. But the some phytosomes containing lipophilic phytoconstituents when they react with phospholipid forms a complex that has maximum water solubility, E.g. Curcumin (MaffeiFacino et al., 1994).

1.5 Biological Properties

- Phytosomes improve absorption.
- Enhance the bioavailability.
- Pharmacokinetic and pharmacodynamics studies in experimental animals it was observed that phytosomes showed excellent results and outcomes than the other traditional formulation (Valenzuela et al., 1989; Saraf et al., 2010).

1.6 Benefits Of Phytosomes

- To enhance the bioavailability of herbal drugs.
- Phytosomes of most of the non-lipophilic herbal drug improves the absorption in the intestinal tract (Saha et al., 2013; War et al., 2015).
- Phytosomes are safe and has both pharmaceutical and cosmetic use.
- Phytosomes are hepatoprotective in nature (Patel et al., 2009).
- Phytosomes when used in cosmetics protects the skin from both exgeneous and endogeneous hazards in stressful environmental conditions providing synergistic effects.
- They also used in drug delivery of proteins and peptides.
- Phytosomes shows better entrapment efficiency as drug itself forms vesicles when bond with lipid (Kumar et al., 2010; Moscarella et al., 1993) .
- They had less toxicological effects.
- Phytosomes are also easy to prepare (Awasthi et al., 2011).

1.7. Drawbacks of Phytosomes

Phytoconstituent are rapidly eliminated from phytosomes. The duration of action is short.

2. MECHANISM OF PHYTOSOME FORMATION

The polyphenolic elements of herbal essence made themselves relatively healthy for straightconjugation with phosphatidylcholine. Phytosome ensues from the response of a stoichiometric quantity of the phospholipid-like phosphatidylcholine with the polyphenolic ingredients like simple flavonoids (some e.g. shown in the table. 4) in an aprotic solvent. Phosphatidylcholine is a multifunctional complex, the phosphatide part being lipophilic and thecholine part being hydrophilic in behaviour. The choline head of the phosphatidylcholine conjugate tothese compounds while lipid-soluble phosphatide part containing the body and tail which thencovers the choline bound material. Hence, the Phytomolecules yield a lipid soluble molecular compound with phospholipids named as phyto-phospholipid complex (Murray, 2008). Phytomolecules are anchored through chemical bonds to the polar choline head of phospholipids, as can be confirmed by precise spectroscopic methods. Frequently, detailed chemical examination designates that, the unit phytosome is typically a flavonoid molecule connected with not less thanone phosphatidylcholine molecule. The outcome is a tiny microsphere or cell is formed. In the blue phytosome spectrum, the spectrum from the polyphenol (red) is obscured by the orange spectrum from phosphatidylcholine (Aggarwal et al., 2012).

3. METHODS OF PREPARATION OF PHYTOSOMES

3.1 Rotary Evaporator Vacuum Method

In this, the phytosomal complex is mixed with anhydrous ethanol in 250 ml of round bottom flask. This flask is then attached to rotary evaporator. The solvent is evaporated at 60°C temperature and there is formation of thin film layer around the flask. In phosphate buffer at pH 7.4, film is hydrated and lipid layer will peel off to form a vesicle suspension. The phytosomal suspension is then endangered to probe sonication which is then stored in the refrigerator for 24 hrs before the characterization.

In this method, phospholipid i.e. soya lecithin reacts with polyphenolic extract.This is then added to 5ml of dicloromethane with continuous stirring. When dicloromethane gets evaporated there is formation of thin film. To this, 5ml of n-hexane was added with stirring and kept in fume hood for complete removal of solvent. After complete removal of n-hexane, the film was hydrated and sonicated to get preferred phytosomal complex.

In this, accurately weighed phospholipid and polyphenolic extract together placed in 100 ml of round bottom flask. Reflux it with 30 ml of dichloromethane at 60°C for 3 hours to decrease it up to 5-10ml. Then add 30ml of n-hexane with continuous stirring to form a precipitate. Collect the precipitate and stored it in a vacuum desiccator for overnight. The dried precipitate is then passed through the mesh size of #100 and stored it in ambered coloured well closed container (Xiao et al., 2006).

3.2 Reflux Method

Polyphenolic extract and phospholipid were placed in 100ml of round bottom flask and refluxed with dichloromethane for 1 hour at a temperature not exceeding 40°C. The obtained clear solution is then evaporated. Add 15 ml of n-hexane to it until precipitate was obtained. Place the obtained precipitate in the desiccator (Sikarwar et al., 2008).

4. EVALUATION OF PHYTOSOMES

4.1 Physicochemical Evaluation

This is responsible for stability as well as therapeutic efficacy of phytosomes. It enhance absorption and bioavailability of the product. Some of the essential physicochemical properties are as follows:

4.1.1 Vesicle Stability

For the determination of vesicle stability, the size and shape of vesicles is very important. The mean size and shape is determined using DLS and TEM analysis respectively (Cevc et al., 1995).

4.1.2 Vesicle Size and Zeta Potential

Vesicle size is determined by using Dynamic Light Scattering (DLS) while Photon Correlation Spectroscopy (PCS) can be used for the zeta potential determination (Kumari et al., 2011).

4.1.3 Transition Temperature

The transition temperature of the vesicular lipid systems can be determined using Differential scanning calorimetry.

4.1.4 Visualization

Scanning electron microscopy (SEM) and Transmission electron microscopy (TEM) analysis can be used for visualization.

4.1.5 Surface Tension Activity Measurement

The surface tension of the drug can be measured by the ring method in a Du Nouy ring tensiometer in aqueous solution (Varde et al., 2012).

4.2 Spectroscopic Evaluation

The interaction between the phytoconstituent molecule and the phospholipid molecule is very important which can be determined with the help of following spectroscopic methods (Gabetta et al., 2000):

4.2.1 ^{1}H-NMR

There are several examples whose NMR spectra can helps to determine the interaction between the phosoplipid and phytoconstituent. One of them, the interaction between the distearoyl phosphatidylcholine with (+)-catechin and its stoichiometric complex studied by Bombardelli *et al.* By NMR evaluation a marked change can be seen in ^{1}H-NMR signal of those particular atoms which take part in the complex formation. The protons of flavonoids can be identified by their broad signals. Signals of phospholipids are singlet corresponding to the N-$(CH_3)_3$ of choline and broad.

4.2.2 ^{13}C-NMR

All the flavonoid carbons are clearly invisible in the ^{13}C-NMR spectrum of (+)- catechin and its stoichiometric complex with distearoyl phosphatidylcholine, particularly when recorded in C6D6 atroom temperature. Most of the resonances of the fatty acid chains retain their original sharp line shape and the signals corresponding to the glycerol and choline portion of the lipid (between 60–80 ppm) are broadened and some are shifted.

4.3 Characterization Techniques of Phytosomes

4.3.1 Differential scanning calorimeter (DSC)

In this, the samples Drug polyphenolic extract, phosphatidylcholine, a physical mixture of drug extract and Phosphatidylcholine, and drug-phospholipid complex were placed in an aluminium cell and heated to a temperature of 50-250°C/minutes from 0 to 400°C in the atmosphere of nitrogen (Maryana et al., 2015).

4.3.2 Scanning Electron Microscopy (SEM)

SEM was used to determine the size of the particle and its appearance. Dry sample was placed on electron microscope brass stub coated withgold in an ion sputter. Random scanning of the complex at 100.

4.3.3 Transition Electron Microscopy (TEM)

TEM was used to characterize the size of phytosomal vesicles with 1000magnification (Singh et al., 2016).

4.3.4 Drug Entrapment and Loading Capacity

Drug phytosomal complex was centrifuged at 10000 rpm for90 minutes at 4°C to separate phytosome from the untrapped drug.The concentration of free drug can be measured by doing ultraviolet spectroscopy. The percentage drug entrapment can be calculated as given formula:

$$Entapment\ efficiency(\%) = \frac{Actual\ drug\ loading}{Theoretical\ drug\ loading} X100.$$

4.3.5 Fourier Transform Infrared Spectroscopy (FTIR) Analysis

FTIR analysis will be done for checking the structure as well as chemicalstability of drug, phospholipid. The phytosomal drug will be crushed with potassium bromide to obtain pellets at 600 kg/cm^2 pressure. Scanning will be done between the ranges of 4000-400 $cm\text{-}^{1}$.

4.3.6 Size analysis and Zeta Potential

Malvern Zeta sizer is used to check the particle size and zeta size of phytosomal complex. Argon laser is used for this particle size and zeta sizer characterization.

4.3.7 In Vitro and In Vivo Evaluations

In vivo and *In vitro* evaluation of phytosomes can be done on the different models depending on the phytoconstituents present in that particular phytosome formulation. Various models like beagle dogs, rodents, wistar rats can be used forthe in vivo study and for comparison of pharmacokinetic parameters of pure extract with its phytosomal formulations (Nagpal et al., 2016R).

5. SOME PATENTED TECHNOLOGY OF PHYTOSOME

There is abundant work has been done for commercialization of Phytosome, out of which few patents technology is given below:

6. RECENT RESEARCH WORK ON PHYTOSOMES

Researcher studied phytosomes abundantly because it is innovative process used to enhance solubility and bioavailability of herbal medicines. Some of the research work on phytosomes are listed below:

Table 1. Patented technologies of Phytosomes

S. N.	Patent No.	Patent Title	Description of Innovation
1	EP1813280	Compositions comprising *Gingko biloba* derivatives for the treatment of asthmatic and allergic conditions	Useful for asthma and allergic condition
2	WO/2004/045541	Soluble isoflavone compositions	Exhibit improved Solubility
3	EP1690862	Fatty acid monoesters of sorbityl furfural and composition for cosmetic and dermatological use	Fatty acid monoester of sorbitol furfural selected from two different series of compounds
4	EP0283713	Complex of saponin with phospholipid and pharmaceutical and cosmetic compositions containing them	High lipophilic and improved bioavilability and suitable for use in pharmaceutical cosmetic compositions
5	EP1214084	An antioxidant preparation based on plant extract for the treatment of aging or photo damaged skin	Used in circulation problems, arteriosclerosisand high blood pressure
6	EP1640041	Cosmetic and dermatological compositions for the treatment of aging and photo damaged skin	Cosmetic/dermatological composition fortopical treatment
7	EP2228062A1	Phospholipid curcumin complex and piperine as chemo sensitizing agent	Treatment of drug resistant
8	US/2007/0015698	Treatment of skin and wound repair with thymosin beta-4	Composition of thymosin for treatment of skin
9	EP/1844785	Phospholipid complexes of olive fruits or leaves extracts having improved bioavailability	Having improved bioavailability

- In 2014, Giorgio, et al formulated curcumin phytosomes which is used in surgical decompression of the median nerve. This treatment has better compatibility and it has high fulfilment.
- In 2013, Gianni et al., prepared a phytosomes containing caffeine free green tea catechin. It is useful globally in health profile.
- In 2011, Cuomo et al., formulated the curcuminoid phytosomes which enhanced absorption and increase plasma profile.
- In 2009, Forster et al., mentioned in their review herbal topical drug delivery formulations which is used in cosmetics.
- In 2006, Banyu et al., formulated silymarin phytosomes and examined its pharmacokinetics in rats. This phytosomes are formulated to increase the lipophilic property and also enhance the biological effect of sallying.
- In 2005, Marti et al., established the Quercetin-phospholipid complex by easy and reproducible technique and also presented that the preparation expressed improved therapeutic efficiency than the molecule in rat liver injury made by carbon tetrachloride.
- In 2002, Busby et al., described that the practice of a silymarin phytosome displayed a better photoprotectant action from ethanol-induced behavioural deficits than uncomplexedsilymarin.

7. COMMERCIAL PRODUCTS ON PHYTOSOMES

Commercial products available in the market are listed below:

- Silybin phytosomes: Used as an antioxidant and hepatoprotective.
- Grape seed phytosomes: Used as an anticancer and antioxidant agent.
- Ginseng phytosomes: Used as an immunomodulator.
- Hawthorn phytosomes: Acts as an antihypertensive, cardioprotective.
- Ginko select phytosomes: Acts as an anti-aging agent and protects brain.
- Green select phytosomes: Used as an anticancer and antioxidant agent.
- Esculoside phytosomes: Used as an anti-cellulite and acts as microcirculation improver.

8. CONCLUSION

Now-a-days, the phytoconstituents have great importance and used worldwide due to its less side effects. Their is necessity of suitable drug delivery for the ideal delivery of active constituents. Phytosomes is novel drug delivery which is safe, effective and releases the drug at site of action. Considering that most of the herbal medicaments have poor aqueous solubility and bioavailability, to enhance the solubility and bioavailability of herbal extract, phytosomes is an innovative approach which is utilized successfully. Because of various prospective benefits, these advances build interest of industrialist in phytosomes formulation.

REFERENCES

Aggarwal, K. V., Gupta, A., & Chaturvedi, S. (2012). Improvement in bioavailability of class III drug: Phytolipid delivery system. *International Journal of Pharmacy and Pharmaceutical Sciences*, *4*(1), 38.

Amin, T., & Bhat, S. (2012). A Review on phytosome technology as a novel approach to improve the bioavailability of neutraceuticals. *International Journal of Advancements in Research and Technology*, *1*, 1–15.

Amit, P., Tanwar, Y. S., Rakesh, S., & Poojan, P. (2013). Phytosome: Phyto lipid drug delivery system for improving the bioavailability of the herbal drug. *J Pharm Sci Biosci Res.*, *3*(2), 51–57.

Awasthi, R., Kulkarni, T. G., & Pawar, K. V. (2011). Phytosomes an approach to increase the bioavailability of plant extract. *International Journal of Pharmacy and Pharmaceutical Sciences*, *3*(2), 2.

Bombardelli, E., Curtis, B., & Della, L. R. (1989). Complexes between phospholipids and vegetal derivatives of biological interest. *Fitoterapia*, *90*(Suppl.1), 1–9.

Bombardelli, E., & Mustich, G. (1991). *Bilobalide-phospholipid complex, their uses and formulation containing them*. U. S. Patent No. EPO-275005.

Cevc, G., Schatzlein, A., & Blume, G. (1995). Transdermal drug carriers: Basic properties, optimization and transfer efficiency in case of epicutaneously applied peptides. *Journal of Controlled Release*, *36*(1-2), 3–16. doi:10.1016/0168-3659(95)00056-E

Dayan, N., & Touitou, E. (2000). Carriers for skin delivery of trihexyphenidyl HCl: Ethosomes vs. liposomes. *Biomaterials*, *21*(18), 1879–1885. doi:10.1016/S0142-9612(00)00063-6 PMID:10919691

Gabetta, B., Fuzzati, N., Griffini, A., Lolla, E., Pace, R., Ruffilli, T., & Peterlongo, F. (2000). Characterization of proanthocyanidins from grape seeds. *Fitoterapia, 71*(2), 162–175. doi:10.1016/S0367-326X(99)00161-6 PMID:10727813

Gandhi, A., Dutta, A., Pal, A., & Bakshi, P. (2012). Recent trend of phytosomes for delivering herbal extract with improved bioavailability. *Journal of Pharmacognosy and Phytochemistry, 1*(4), 6.

Jadhav, I. A., Wadhave, A. A., Arsul, V. A., & Sawarkar, H. S. (2014). Phytosome a novel approach in herbal drug. *Int J Pharm Anal, 2*(5), 478.

Jain, N., Gupta, P. B., Thakur, N., Jain, R., & Banweer, J. (2010). Phytosome a novel drug delivery system for herbal medicine. *International Journal of Pharmaceutical Sciences and Drug Research, 2*(4), 224.

Jain, N. K. (2005). *Liposomes as drug carriers, controlled and novel drug delivery* (1st ed.). CBS publisher.

Kalita, B., Das, K. M., & Sharma, K. A. (2013). Novel phytosome formulation making herbal extract more effective. *The Journal of Pharmacy Technology, 6*(11), 1295.

Kidd, P. M. (2009). Bioavailability and activity of phytosome complexes from botanical polyphenols: The silymarin, curcumin, green tea, and grape seed extracts. *Alternative Medicine Review, 14*(3), 226–246. PMID:19803548

Kumar, P., Yadav, S., Agarwal, A., & Kumar, N. (2010). Phytosomes a novel phyto- phospholipid carrier: An overview. *Int J Pharm Res Dev, 2*(6), 1–7.

Kumari, P., Singh, N., & Cheriyan, P., & Neelam. (2011). Phytosome: A novel approach for phytomedicine. *International Journal of Institutional Pharmacy and Life Sciences, 1*, 89–100.

Maffei Facino, R., Carini, M., Aldini, G., Bombardelli, E., & Morazzoni, P. (1994). Free radicals scavenging action and anti-enzyme activities of procyanidins from Vitisvinifera. A mechanism for their capillary protective action. *Arzneimittel-Forschung, 44*, 592–601. PMID:8024628

Maryana, W., Rahma, A., Mudhakir, D., & Rachmawati, H. (2015). Phytosome containing silymarin for oral administration: Formulation and physical evaluation. *Journal of Biomedical Science and Engineering, 25*, 56.

Moscarella, S., Giusti, A., Marra, F., Marena, C., Lampertico, M., Relli, P., Gentilini, P., & Buzzelli, G. (1993). Therapeutic and anti lipoperoxidant effect of silybin phosphatidylcholine complex in chronic liver disease: Preliminary result. *Current Therapeutic Research, Clinical and Experimental, 53*(1), 98–102. doi:10.1016/S0011-393X(05)80160-2

Murray, D. (2008). *Phytosomes-Increase the absorption of herbal extract.* Available at: www.doctormurray.com/articles/silybin.htm

Nagpal, N., Arora, M., & Swami, G., Rageeb, & Kapoor, R. (2016). Designing of a phytosome dosage form with *Tecomellaundulata*as a noveldrug delivery for better utilization. *Pakistan Journal of Pharmaceutical Sciences, 29*(4), 1231–1235. PMID:27393436

Patel, J., Patel, R., Khambolja, K., & Patel, N. (2009). An overview of phytosomes as an advanced herbal drug delivery system. *Asian J Pharm Sci, 4*(6), 363–371.

Saha, S., Sarma, A., Saikia, P., & Chakraarty, T. (2013). Phytosome: A brief overview. *Scholars Academic Journal of Pharmacy*, *2*, 12–20.

Saraf, S., & Kaur, C. D. (2010). Phytoconstituents as photoprotective novel cosmetic formulations. *Pharmacognosy Reviews*, *4*(7), 1–11. doi:10.4103/0973-7847.65319 PMID:22228936

Semalty, A., Semalty, M., Rawat, M. S., & Franceschim, F. (2010). Supramolecular phospholipids-polyphenolics interactions: The phytosome strategy toimprove the bioavailability of phytochemicals. *Fitoterapia*, *81*(5), 306–314. doi:10.1016/j.fitote.2009.11.001 PMID:19919847

Sikarwar, M. S., Sharma, S., Jain, A. K., & Parial, S. D. (2008). Preparation, characterization and evaluation of marsupsin phospholipid complex. *AAPS PharmSciTech*, *9*(1), 129–137. doi:10.120812249-007-9020-x PMID:18446473

Singh, R. P., Gangadharappa, V. H., & Mruthunjaya, K. (2016). Phytosome loaded novel herbal drug delivery system: A review. *Int Res J Pharm*, *7*(6), 15–21. doi:10.7897/2230-8407.07656

Tripathy, S., Patel, D., Baro, L., & Nair, S. (2013). A review on phytosomes, their characterization, advancement and potential for transdermal application. *Journal of Drug Delivery and Therapeutics*, *3*(3), 147–152. doi:10.22270/jddt.v3i3.508

Valenzuela, A., Aspillaga, M., Vial, S., & Guerra, R. (1989). Selectivity of silymarin on the increase of the glutathione content in different tissues of the rat. *Planta Medica*, *55*(05), 420–422. doi:10.1055-2006-962056 PMID:2813578

Varde, N., Mehta, N., Thakor, N., Shah, V., & Upadhyay, U. (2012). Phytosomes a potential phospholipid nanoparticulate carrier for the bioavailability enhancement of herbal extracts. *International Journal of Comprehensive Pharmacy*, *10*, 1-7.

Venkatesan, N., Babu, B. S., & Vyas, S. P. (2000). Protected particulate drug carriers for prolonged systemic circulation. *Indian Journal of Pharmaceutical Sciences*, *62*, 327–333.

Verma, H., Prasad, S. B., & Yashwant, S. H. (2013). Herbal drug delivery system: A modern era prospective. *Int J Current Pharma Rev Res*, *4*, 88–101.

War, P. A., Bhang, A. H., & Ale, D. B. (2015). Phytsome as a novel biomedicine: A microencapsulated drug delivery system. *Journal of Bioanalysis & Biomedicine*, *7*(1), 8.

Xiao, Y., Song, Y., Chen, Z., & Ping, Q. (2006). The preparation of silybin–phospholipid complex and the study on its pharmacokinetics in rats. *International Journal of Pharmaceutics*, *37*, 77–82. PMID:16300915

Chapter 11
Novel Approaches in Nutraceuticals

Bhushan Rajendra Rane
https://orcid.org/0000-0002-1482-1884
Shri D.D. Vispute College of Pharmacy and Research Center, Raigad, India

Mounika Shankaraiah Bharath
Shri D.D. Vispute College of Pharmacy and Research Center, Raigad, India

Rutuja Raju Patil
Shri D.D. Vispute College of Pharmacy and Research Center, Raigad, India

Raj K. Keservani
Faculty of B. Pharmacy, CSM Group of Institutions, Prayagraj, India

Ashish S. Jain
Shri D. D. Vispute College of Pharmacy and Research Center, India

ABSTRACT

Nutraceuticals have both wholesome and therapeutic properties. In recent years, there are many research works accessible in writing which recommend the utilization of nutraceuticals in treatment of different maladies like diabetes, malignancy, Alzheimer's, etc. It is additionally demonstrated that they are protected to utilize and have potential medical advantages. Yet, the fundamental interest in building up a nutraceutical detailing is its low bio-availability, substance flimsiness, and poor bioavailability. Because of these reasons, nutraceuticals are not misused appropriately and not generally acknowledged in pharma divisions for relief and treatment. In any case, with progression in science and innovation, it is conceivable to create systems or methodologies that can be utilized to define the nutraceuticals to its greatest use. In this chapter, the authors examine different advances in methodologies and procedures accessible for building up nutraceuticals.

DOI: 10.4018/978-1-7998-4453-2.ch011

1. INTRODUCTION

Hippocrates (460–377 BC), the notable father of current medicine, expressed "Let food be thy medicine and medicine be the food", to anticipate the relationship between suitable food and health and their restorative guides. Human ways of life have changed drastically in the course of the most recent couple of decades because of industrialization and changing work cultures which have constrained individuals into different quick eating societies with increasingly moment and mouth-watering dinners, however diminished the amount and quality in supplements. Simultaneously, industrialization has all the while caused air and water contamination, and soil and nourishment contaminated in view of broad utilization of different synthetic chemicals, substantial metals, electromagnetic waves, and other possibly unsafe man-made things. These issues have prompted an expanded frequency of diabetes, obesity, malignant growths, vascular ailments, physiological issues, just as other degenerative infections prompting extreme dysfunction (Saktivel et al., 2012).

In couple of late years, another eating routine health model is advancing which places more weight on the positive parts of eating routine. The new way of life accepted by individuals today has adjusted the fundamental nourishment. Ingestion of the low-quality nourishment has expanded complex prompting various infections caused because of ill-advised food life–style. The patients being unfulfilled with the excessive, new, antimicrobial strategy are looking for adjusting or substitute advantageous items and the fulfillment of accomplished criteria makes nutraceuticals especially engaging (Das et al., 2011). Stephen Defelice MD, founder and chairman of the Foundation for innovation in medicine (FIM) Cranford, New Jersy, founded the term nutraceuticals from food and pharmaceutical in 1989. Rendering to Defelice nutraceuticals are nourishment or part of a nourishment that conveys medicinal or health helps including the mitigation as well as checking the activity of a disease (Ansari et al., 2013; Rane et al., 2020).

A Nutraceuticals is an entire term which characterizes any substance separated from food nutrition sources with extra health benefits alongside the essential dietary benefit officially present in them. They act nonspecifically to advance general health of the people and furthermore to switch and counteract harmful conditions. The expression "nutraceutical" joins two words – "supplement" (a feeding food segment) and "pharmaceutical" (a therapeutic medication) (Ganpathy et al., 2016). In the US, the expression "nutraceutical" items are controlled as medications, food nutrients and dietary supplements. The term isn't characterized the equivalent in various nations, however is normally characterized as an item beyond supplements that is generally sold in therapeutic agents not more often than not connected with food. A nutraceutical item might be defined as a substance, which has physiological preferred position or gives assurance against endless difficulty (Nasri et al., 2014).

1.2 Classification and Categorization of Nutraceuticals

The term nutraceuticals, itself is a wide class which contain numerous classifications and subcategories under it. To know the applications, the nutraceuticals are required to be classified. The grouping into different classes relying upon their uses is:

a. *Conventional nutraceuticals*: Under the category of customary Nutraceuticals infers nourishment in which no adjustment to the food is made; it is basically common, entire supplements with new significant about their potential health abilities (Chintale et al., 2013), e.g. lycopene in tomatoes, omega-3 unsaturated fats in salmon (Sapkale et al., 2012).

Figure 1. Classification of Nutraceuticals
(Sharma et al., 2017; Tiwari et al., 2019)

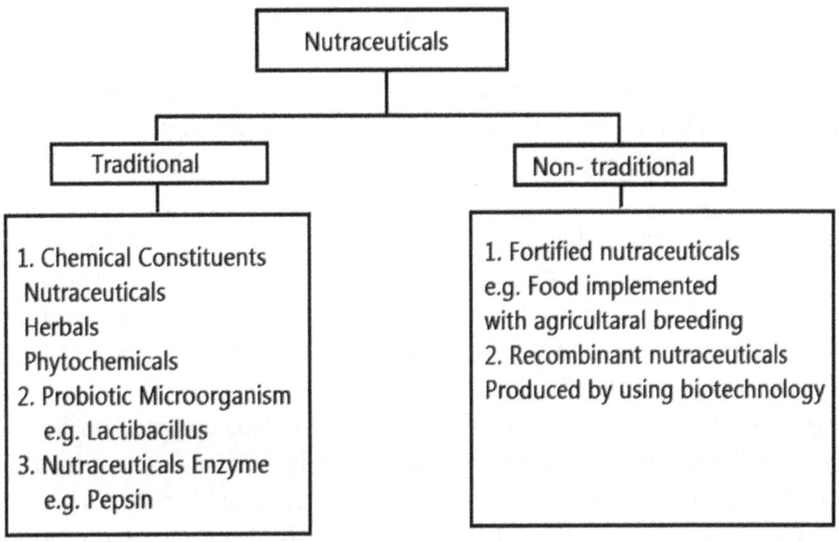

b. *Nontraditional nutraceuticals:* They are the result from crude refinement or extra supplements as well as actives, e.g., squeezed orange sustained with calcium, grains with included nutrients or minerals and flour with extra folic acid are non-customary nutraceutical (Chintale et al., 2013). Examples - β-carotene rich rice, soybeans, and oats.
c. *Strengthened nutraceuticals:* It creates revitalized nourishment from crude state or extra supplements or potentially nutrients, e.g. squeezed orange empowered with calcium, oats with included nutrients or minerals and flour with beneficial folic acid. A few cases are milk sustained with cholecalciferol utilized in nutrient D deficiency (Singh et al., 2012).
d. *Recombinant nutraceuticals:* Energy-giving supplement, for example, butter, alcohol, matured starch, yogurt, cheddar, vinegar, and others are produced with the guide of biotechnology. The production of probiotics and the extraction of bioactive parts by compound/active ingredients just as genetically building blocks are accomplished through biotechnology (Singh et al., 2012). Gold Kiwi fruit is genetically modified for an unusual state of ascorbic acid, Carotenoids, and Lutein and Zeaxanthin (Sharma et al., 2017).

e. *Potential and built up nutraceuticals:* A potential nutraceutical is one that holds a guarantee of a specific health or health advantage; such a potential nutraceutical just turns into a trustworthy one after there is sufficient clinical information to demonstrate such a benefit. The nourishment products utilized as nutraceutical are described as - Prebiotic, Dietary fiber, Omega-3 fatty acid, antioxidant (Pandey et al., 2010).
f. *Phytochemicals:* These are the substance constituents of plants with particular organic activity. These have been accounted for active fractions which applies their activities toward the digestion and biochemical responses in living creatures and in this manner, give health benefits (Sharma et al., 2017) E.g. Carotenoids and Flavonoid etc.
g. *Herbals:* The herbs possessing medicinal values to be utilized in treatment and prevention of ailments are been included in the class. Natural items may comprise of whole plant utilized or any part thereof, e.g. dried leaf, organic product, stem, seeds, roots, or focused extract (Sharma et al., 2017).
h. *Functional substances:* Nutraceuticals somewhat distinguish from practical supplements. At the point when nourishment is being prepared or prepared utilizing "logical insight" with or without data of how or why it is being utilized, the food is called Functional nourishment. Therefore, useful nourishment offers the body with the required sum of nutrients, fats, proteins, sugars, and so on required for its sound existence (Sapkale et al., 2012).
i. *Dietary supplements and dietary filaments:* A dietary enhancement is an item which involves a strengthening dietary fixing added as a solution for insufficiencies or ailments. Nutrients and minerals as dietary supplements exist in various nutrients or single fixing items in the market. Its sources incorporate dark colored rice, banana, grains, oats, dry beans, and vegetables.
j. *Probiotics and prebiotics:* Probiotics, as per an accord definition, are 'living small scale life forms (microorganism), which upon ingestion in specific numbers, apply medical advantages past innate fundamental nourishment on the other hand probiotics are inexactly known as live microorganisms having a place with regular biota with low or no pathogenicity, yet with elements of significance to the health and prosperity of the host. New genera and strains of probiotics are rising; some with high medical advantages as in *Lactobacillus plantarum* disconnects (PCS20, PCS22, PCS25 and PCS26) from *Slovenian cheddar* with high antimicrobial and immunomodulatory abilities (Sapkale et al., 2012).

1.3 Advantages

1. More advantageous life
2. Better temperament and fearlessness
3. Better working limit
4. Better social condition
5. May increment the health estimation of our eating routine
6. Provides more advantageous life and help us live more.
7. May assist us with avoiding specific ailments.
8. May have a mental profit by accomplishing something for oneself.
9. May be seen to be progressively "normal" than conventional medication and more unwilling to deliver terrible symptoms

10. May give food for populaces extraordinary needs (for example supplement thick supplements for the elderly (Rane et al., 2020; Tank et al., 2010)
11. The society wins lower health consumption, lower social use and progressively gainful supplements can promote better-quality strong resource, continuance and in general physical appearance. For this rationale, they are typically taken by competitors to advance their presentation. Nourishment supplements can likewise stop an assortment of ailments and health conditions. For instance, pregnant ladies are directed to take folic acid to stay away from birth issues. Different supplements are utilized in blend with medications as a technique for corresponding or elective treatment for health conditions.

1.4 Disadvantage

1. Bioavailability improvement is one of the principle tasks in finding genuine nutraceutical items. The bioavailability of supplements is mind boggling in food eaten in its ordinary state. Nutraceuticals with low bioavailability rates results in supplements being likely from the body without giving any dietary or therapeutic benefit.
2. Effect of placebo: Similar to pharmaceuticals, some portion of the adequacy of nutraceuticals might be agreed to the misleading impact. Customers consuming nutraceuticals may loosely credit their utilization of nutraceuticals for healing disease/ disorder when the body is frequently ready to recover without anyone else.
3. Item quality issues: Nutraceuticals from the worldwide market may ideal to utilize natural or unusual elements, yet the absence of guideline may bargain the safety and efficacy of items.
4. Health and Interactions with different medications: The peril is that a large number of these items don't give purchasers strong data about their safety and efficacy, conceivable symptoms, connections with professionally prescribed drugs or the effect they may have on existing restorative conditions (Tank et al., 2010).
5. Since dietary supplements are not as carefully controlled as medications, their efficacy may not be as trustworthy. Additionally, when taken in amounts that surpass the proposed dietary admission, a few supplements might be dangerous and cause adverse symptoms. Nutrient's harmfulness, for instance, can begin as liver damage, hazy vision, pain, bone irregularities and inflammation, drowsiness and nausea. Supplements can likewise collaborate with drugs, which can cause undesirable symptoms and decline the adequacy of the medicine.

1.5 Novel Approaches in Nutraceuticals

The expanding inclinations of purchasers to eat well food items and the nutraceuticals appearing at be positive in averting just as relieving numerous sicknesses instigated researchers and analysts to search for proficient conveyance frameworks. The utilization of novel drug delivery approaches to formulate in order to deal with the efficacy issues of the substance is drawing increasingly more consideration of the researchers (Sharma et al., 2017).

Nano emulsion is the nano-sized formulation in which two immiscible liquids are mixed to form a single phase with the help of an emulsifier. These are thermodynamically stable isotropic system with the help of an emulsifying agent. The droplet size of emulsion ranges between 20 to 200 nm. For instance, resveratrol which is a characteristic compound found in red grape skin, peanuts, and blueberries

Figure 2. Novel Approaches in Nutraceuticals

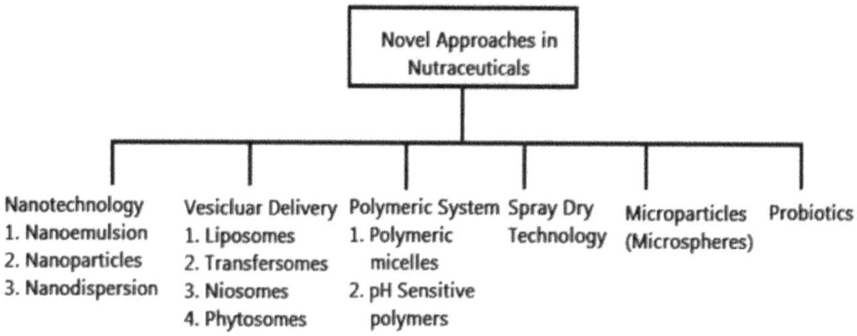

have been found to possess powerful antioxidant properties. But resveratrol has poor bioavailability. To overcome this disadvantage, it has been encapsulated into the nano emulsion. This method has resulted in better retention and enhanced properties of the system. Similarly, researchers have demonstrated that curcumin is effective as nano emulsion for the treatment of inflammation in mice by inhibition of inflammatory mediator (Sharma at al., 2017).

1.5.1. Excipient Nano Emulsions

Nano emulsions have been described as excellent transporters for lipophilic bioactive compound with enhanced properties in contrast to conventional emulsions. Excipients diets certainly do not have functionality themselves but have the capacity to improve the functional value of supplements present in normal foods by changing their bio accessibility, absorption, and chemical transformation (Salvia et al., 2016).

1.5.2 Nanocarriers

The encapsulation of nutraceutical into nanocarriers based platforms decreases pharmacokinetic limitations after oral administration of nutraceuticals (Siddiqui et al., 2009). Different kinds of nanocarriers, e.g. polymeric nanoparticles, solid lipid nanoparticles, polymeric conjugates, liposome's, micelles, carbon nanotubes and others have been investigated in recent years so as to modulate the pharmacokinetics. eg - magnetic nanoparticles of curcumin (MNP-CUR) were created so as to improve its bioavailability and efficacy (Yellapu et al., 2013). The formulation exhibited 2.5 fold increase in improvement in serum bioavailability as compare to local curcumin.

1.5.3 Liposomes

A liposome is a spherical vesicle with a membrane composed of a phospholipid bilayer used to deliver drug or genetic material into a cell. Liposomes can be made composed of naturally derived phospholipids with mixed lipid chain like egg phosphatidyl ethanolamine or of pure components like DOPE (dioleoyl phosphatidyl ethanolamine). Due to their size and hydrophobic and hydrophilic characteristics (besides biocompatibility), liposomes are promising systems for delivery of medication (Akbarzadeh et al., 2013; Godin et al., 2004). Intranasal quercetin liposomes are one of the examples which have been accounted to enhance the penetration of quercetin through blood brain barriers and increase the therapeutic anticancer efficacy of the product (Manach et al., 2004). Similarly, buccal liposomal formulation of silymarin has likewise been demonstrated to offer hepatoprotective impact with improved bioavailability of the product resulting in better therapeutic response (Bombardelli et al., 1989; Bhattacharya, 2009). The anti-gout topical liposomal planning of colchicine has additionally been demonstrated exceptionally effective in the treatment of gout (Maiti et al., 2005).

1.5.4 Phytosomes

Phytosomes are the complex of phospholipids and the biologically active ingredients (Maiti et al., 2007). Phytosomes are the novel formulation technology which overcomes the problems of associated with phytopharmaceuticals degradation (You et al., 2006). Oral formulation of Ginseng phytosomes, prepared using phospholipid complexation has been found to overcome the problem related to the low solubility of Ginseng and results in the increased absorption in the body which enhances the therapeutic effect of Ginseng as an immunomodulator (Machida et al., 2000). Oral phytosomal formulation of Hawthorn (flavonoid) having cardio protective and antihypertensive properties have additionally been accounted to offer improved efficacy. Quercetin, possessing the properties of an anticancer as well as an antioxidant compound was also subjected to the oral preparation of Quercetin phytosomes providing better therapeutic efficacy of the drug (Chao et al., 2010). Furthermore, curcumin phytosomal oral preparation, utilizing curcumin-phospholipid complexation technique has additionally been researched on, and it has offered elevated bioavailability and increased antioxidant activity (Gavini et al., 2005).

1.5.5 Microspheres

Microspheres are the spherical vesicular particles falling within the diameter range of 1-1000 μm. Because of their little size, microspheres can be ingested or infused, can be changed in accordance with any ideal release profile and can exhibit site-specific as well as organ targeted drug delivery (Cevc et al., 2002). Intravenous formulation of camptothecin (natural product) loaded microspheres, formulated using oil-in-water evaporation method has been reported to provide prolonged anticancer effect (Cevc et al., 2002; Zheng et al., 2006; Patel et al., 2009; Garti & McClements, 2012).

1.5.6 Transfersomes

Transfersomes are called as ultra-deformable vesicles comprising of an aqueous phase as a core surrounded by the lipid bilayer complex which makes the formulation self-optimizing and self-regulating. Therefore, the transfersomes are capable of crossing several transport barriers conveniently and acts as the carrier in the non-invasive techniques of delivery (Forst & Sullivan, 2009). The scientists have demonstrated topical arrangement of capsaicin transfersomes to enhanced skin penetration with improved analgesic effect (Zhang et al., 2016). Colchicine transfersomal formulation has additionally been studied to provide better penetration and thus advanced treatment of Gout (Zeeb et al., 2015). Similarly, *in vitro* preparation of vincristine transfersomes exhibits increased entrapment efficiency and improved skin permeation and results into the better therapeutic effect of the anticancer drug. Transdermal formulation of curcumin transfersomes has been also reported to deliver enhanced entrapment efficiency with intensified permeation through the skin which improvises the anti-inflammatory effect of curcumin on the body (Shibamoto et al., 2008).

1.5.7 Hydrogel

Hydrogel beads have great potential for binding, protecting and releasing nutraceuticals within the food industry. Hydrophilic nutraceuticals can often be simply mixed with a biopolymer solution, and then hydrogel beads can be formed however, some kind of attractive interaction is required between the nutraceuticals and the biopolymer molecules to ensure that the bioactive agents are retained. Hydrophobic nutraceuticals are usually trapped in lipid droplets first by forming an emulsion or nano emulsion, and then they are mixed with the biopolymer solution used to form the hydrogel beads. Hydrogel beads therefore have considerable potential for overcoming some of the challenges currently limiting the utilization of nutraceuticals in functional foods. E.g.: - chemical stability of curcumin-enriched lipid droplets can be improved by trapping them within polysaccharide-based hydrogel beads (Pegg & Shahidi, 2007). Curcumin-loaded lipid droplets could also be trapped within calcium alginate beads, and that their release rate depended on the hydrogel pore size, which was controlled by altering the alginate and calcium concentrations (Srinivas et al., 2009).

2. TECHNOLOGIES AVAILABLE IN NUTRACEUTICALS

2.1 Nanotechnology

Nanotechnology is a technology that provides powerful energy to transform food systems. Nanomaterials possess extraordinary features, as well as the development of technologies offer potential opportunities for the world of science, technology, and commercial opportunities. Nanoscale control over food molecules can lead to alterations in many macroscale factors, such as texture, taste, other sensory features, processing, and stability between shelf life. The use of nanotechnology in food and agriculture systems is growing rapidly.

One of the most important uses of nanotechnology in food and nutrition is the design and construction of functional food ingredients with improved water solubility, thermal stability, oral availability, sensory and physiological properties. (Solans et al., 2001, Sharma et al., 2018). Due to its low solubility, many phytoconstituents are poorly absorbed by the human body. One of the most important and interesting applications is to increase the availability of phytochemicals by altering pharmacokinetics (PK) and biodistribution (BD) (Keservani et al., 2017; Wang et al., 2008). The integrated amalgamation and production of active food ingredients are important applications in food and nutrition that can be achieved through nanotechnological methods (Wandrey et al., 2009).

The administration of active phytochemicals in the human body requires the use of a suitable vehicle to deliver the effective amount of the active component to the desired location in the body. Overcoming instability, moderate water dissolution, and improving the bioavailability of nutraceuticals. Another way to incorporate a combination of interest into a food matrix is to use nano emulsion. Nano emulsions are the smallest substrate emulsions that appear transparent or dark blue (Vos et al., 2010). Curcumin nano emulsions with MCT (medium chain triglycerides) had significantly better bioactivity than curcumin solution (Kim et al., 1996).

2.2 Encapsulation Technology

The process of entrapping one substance (active agent) within another substance (coating material) is known as encapsulation. In the food industry, the encapsulation process can be used for a variety of reasons. Encapsulation is a useful tool to improve the delivery of bioactive molecules (e.g. antioxidants, minerals, vitamins, phytosterols, lutein, fatty acids, lycopene) and living cells (e.g. probiotic) in food. In most instances, encapsulation is referring to a technology in which the bioactive components are completely covered, and protected by a barrier (Milanovc et al., 2010; Parris et al., 2005).

Several important reasons for the incorporation of functional materials include improved stability in the final products and during processing. For instance, probiotics are extremely sensitive to changes in pH, mechanical stress, mobility conditions, and digestive enzymes in the stomach. Probiotic bacteria are defined as living microorganisms and organic foods with significant health benefits in the host, if present in sufficient amounts (Parris et al., 2005). Encapsulation increases not only its availability, but more importantly performance. The choice of an encapsulation system remains important because it should be effective and easily incorporated into the diet without compromising the structure and taste of the food. (Parris et al., 2005). Another advantage of encapsulation is the low viscosity and degradation of flexible materials, such as odors, which often contain a mixture of flexible and fragrant organic molecules (Zuidam & Heinrich, 2009). The incorporation of essential oil into various nanospheres has been used as a controlled release medium with specific delivery sites to enhance the anti-microbial activity of the oil (Voilley & Etievant, 2006). In addition to the functions mentioned above, many other ingredients and dietary supplements have been incorporated into encapsulation, such as vitamins, micronutrients, fish oil, peptides, etc. (Hall, 2003).

2.3 Nutrigenomics

Genome science and technology have been put together to discover a new food concept with a new anti-microbial function, now called Nutraceuticals, in furtherance of a genetic program called Nutrigenomics (nourishment genome science). Nutrigenomics contains three categories of genomics that regulate genes, proteins, and metabolites (transcriptomics, proteomics, and metabolomics) as used in the field of nutrition and health. Nutrigenomics forms the scientific basis for developing nutritional needs that are tailored to the needs of groups of consumers, in order to be healthy, vulnerable, or ill. RO Brennan in 1975 defined the term 'nutrigenetics' in his book Nutrigenetics. Nutrigenomics is a newly developed method that combines many genomic techniques with molecular biology techniques. Nutrigenomics is a technology involved in various fields of education as shown below, in scientific analysis of the relationship between diet and dietary supplements and health care and disease prevention (Hayashi, 1989). Studies of yeast have shown that by increasing the activity of one type, SIR2 can extend their life span. Genetically modified, SIRT1 was found in humans. Polyphenol-like Quercetin derived from apples and tea, and Resveratrol (found in grapes and red wine) have been found to increase SRT1 activity in laboratory tests. Interestingly, Resveratrol has been found to increase SRT1 13-fold activity (Re, 1998). Dietary cholesterol has a significant effect on the gene expression of β-hydroxy-β-methyl-glutaryl (HMG) - CoA reductase.

2.4 Spray Drying Technology

Spray suspension has also been used for a few minor configurations because the product may be sealed with a specific carrier used in the feed slurry by a practice known as alternative selection. Typical carriers of these synthesis processes include carbohydrates, gums, and esters cellulose and ether. Consolidation of carrier companies is also used to provide strong and stable agents for certain feed elements (Mehta et al., 2018). The condition shows a well-formed powder with moisture content suitable for storage and use. The bioactive substance has also been found to be present within fiber carriers, thus indicating the release of fiber encapsulation as possible instead of maltodextrin-carrying substances. The presence of organisms does not seem to change the particle size or shape. Crystallization behavior was monitored and may be present in all prescribed amorphous spray powders (Naksuriya et al., 2014)

2.5 Phytoconstituents Based Dry Powder Inhalers

The phytoconstituent drug delivery system is a unique drug delivery strategy and has become very popular in the field of drug delivery research due to its simple production process. It possesses therapeutic potential for various pulmonary and non-pulmonary diseases. There are various programs for the delivery of new Phytoconstituents, inhaled drugs available. - Resveratrol, Curcumin, Quercetin, Baicalein (Feng et al., 2017).

Curcumin has a wide range of pharmaceutical activity ranging from anti-inflammatory to anti-carcinogenic (Sherbiny & Smyth, 2012; Misra et. al., 2018; Kesharwani et. al., 2019). Few researchers have studied the effect of curcumin in the treatment chronic lung diseases (Taki et al., 2016). In addition, it also shows strong anti-cancer activity in various lung cancer lines such as human lung adenocarcinoma cell line (A549), lung adenocarcinoma (Calu-3), lung metastasis cell line (B16BL6) (Yang et al., 2007) and the cell line of the macrophage mouse (RAW 264.7) (Kurniawansyh et al., 2015). The biopharmaceutical and pharmacokinetic properties of curcumin have been thoroughly investigated, high protein binding, rapid metabolism, and rapid removal from the body (Sherbiny & Smyth, 2012). Curmin loaded microparticles are produced using hydroxy-propyl-beta-cyclodextrin (HP-β-CD) and polyvinyl pyrrolidone (PVP) using an atomized injection solvent extraction (ARISE) system. The ARISE system has shown a better yield of 80%, a satisfactory particle size with a smooth surface and open practice. Microparticles have shown a 70-fold increase in the solubility and dissolution of curcumin in saline solution (Yang et al., 2015).

2.6 Two-Dimensional NMR for Exploring Plant Metabolome

NMR spectroscopy is a powerful analytical technique to compare metabolite formation in the field of plant metabolomics. Various 2D NMR technologies are available for effort detection.eg - J solved test (JRES NMR), distribution of NMR spectroscopy (DOSY). While both JRES and DOSY are two-dimensional

Figure 3. Relation Between Nutragenomic and Life Sciences

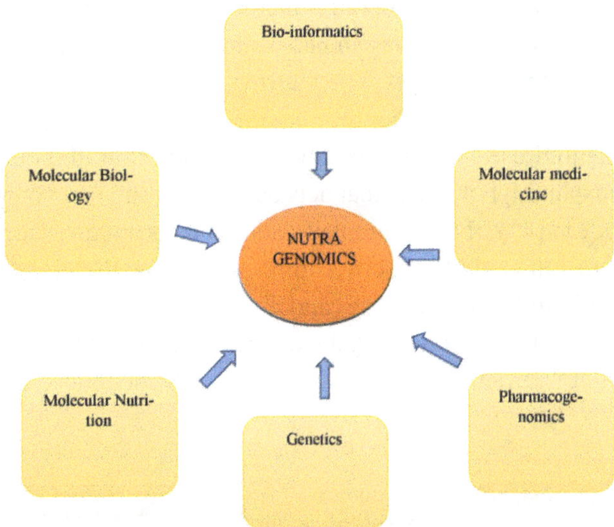

modes, the most useful features of both experiments are the ability to extract a simplified proton display with minimal distortion rather than a collection of information displayed in the second dimension such as combining continuous coef translation and translation, respectively (Ali et al., 2006).

2D JRES NMR is also used to assist in the differentiation of different ginseng commercial arrangements and to assist in the supply of various phenolic chemicals found in different Greek grape varieties (Price et al., 1997; Novoa et al., 2011).

The severity of the ordered spectroscopy or DOSY depends on the difference in the temporal separation between molecules of different cell sizes (Politi et al., 2009). DOSY tests appear to be particularly relevant in plant extraction analysis as the proton spectrum of each compound (or actually compounds of the same molecular weight) can be labeled separately to achieve what can be described as "NMR chromatography" (Ivan, 2016). This simple concept was used for direct NMR analysis of commercial herbal extracts of *Echinacea purpurea, Hypericum perforatum, Ginkgo biloba* and *Valeriana cinalis* (Jaganathan and Supriyanto, 2012).

2.7 Lycosome Technology

Lycosome technology represents a new development in modern technology aimed at improving the availability of nutraceuticals and synthetic drugs and the delivery of certain organs. Lycosome technology demonstrates a nano-microencapsulation method that uses different natural lycopene methods as a living compound. Lycopene is a compound of non-polar tetraterpene containing eight units of isoprene with 13 double bindings that are important in its antioxidant activity. Lycopene gains unity and the ability to interact with phospholipids in cis isomerization caused by heat, light exposure, and pH changes. It promotes the production of highly stable and strong lycopene-phospholipid biofilms that need to be covered and microencapsulation of various amphiphilic chemicals and ultimately the formation of lysosomes - nano-micro dimensional particles that have a natural resistance in the gut. Lycosome particles are made up of the outer layer and the inner layer. The internal domain contains a bioactive compound that needs to be delivered and distributed to the human body. It is protected by an outer layer containing lycopene, a hydrophobic carotenoid used as a basic structure. In addition, the outer layer contains an amphiphilic phospholipid (phosphatidyl choline) that acts as a chaperone for lycopene, an emulsifying and hydrophilizing agent. A wide variety of micro emulsification modus operandi including spray drying, ultrasound, supercritical CO2 fusion, and other body components allow the discovery of various lycosome formations of nutraceuticals and synthetic drugs and dietary products that are useful in preventing and controlling cardiovascular disease and type 2 diabetes mellitus. In addition, lycosome technology can be used for the production of fortified foods such as active black chocolate, margarine and butter.

3. APPLICATIONS

3.1 Nutraceuticals in Disease Management

Nutraceutical are associated with treatment and mitigation of different infections, for example, cancer, Diabetes, Parkinson's, hyperacidity, asthma, hypertension etc. (Ahmed et al., 2011). The utilizations of nutraceuticals alongside their source and use are described in Table 1.

3.2 Nutraceuticals in Geriatric

Ginkgo biloba for neuroprotection - Ginkgo is generally known for its health benefits for the older population in Chinese medicine (Zou et al., 2012). Extract of *Ginkgo biloba* is well known to prevent Alzheimer's disease. The herbal extract EGb761 prepared from *G. biloba* are rich in phytochemicals, for example, flavonoids and terpenoids. These phytonutrients improve the functions of platelets and nerve cells and the blood flow to the nervous system and cerebrum, because of their antioxidant properties (Cohen, 2008).

Cranberry are obtained from evergreen dwarf shrubs of subgenus *oxycoccus* and genus *vaccinium* family Ericaceae and oregano are obtained from dried leaves and flowering tops of *Origanum vulgare* belonging to mint family lamiaceae possess multiple medicinal properties, such as antimicrobial, antiviral, antimutagenic, antiangiogenic, and antioxidative functions. This herb was known to increase life span activity of human beings. Cranberries are high in antioxidants properties which decreases oxidative damage and phytochemicals, likely proanthocyanins and vitamin C, which neutralize free radicals (Neto, 2007; He & Rui, 2006).

Olive oil as a phenolics supplement: Scientific studies proved that olive oil has beneficial effects on health and life span activity in humans (Zaveri, 2006; Sagar et al., 2006). This is due to the presence of

Figure 4. Various Application of Nutraceuticals

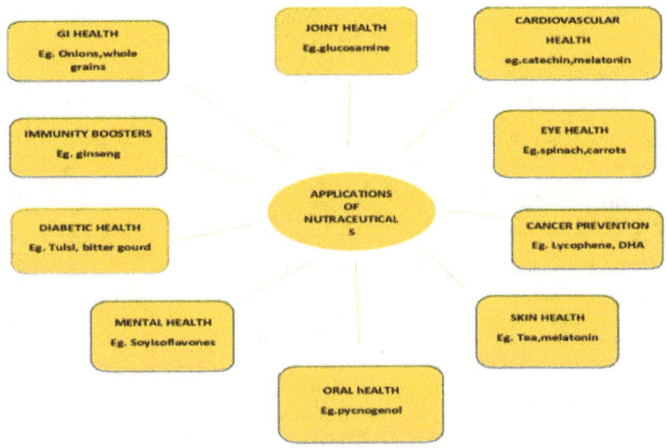
APPLICATIONS OF NUTRACEUTICAL S
GI HEALTH Eg. Onions,whole grains
JOINT HEALTH Eg.glucosamine
CARDIOVASCULAR HEALTH eg.catechin,melatonin
IMMUNITY BOOSTERS Eg. ginseng
EYE HEALTH Eg.spinach,carrots
DIABETIC HEALTH Eg. Tulsi, bitter gourd
CANCER PREVENTION Eg. Lycophene, DHA
MENTAL HEALTH Eg. Soyisoflavones
SKIN HEALTH Eg. Tea,melatonin
ORAL hEALTH Eg.pycnogenol

abundant amount of phenolic compounds. Pre- clinical studies revealed that tyrosol, are the main phenols present in olive oil, significantly increase of life span activity, and also provide resistance to thermal and oxidative stress (Zarse et al., 2012). The essentially increment of life expectancy action and furthermore gives protection from warm and oxidative stress (Bryan, 2008). Phenolic compound of olive oil have also been used to study its affects for treatment of different types of cancer. They also had known for to prevent carcinogenesis process initiation.

Green tea as health supplement: Green tea contains polyphenolic catechins which have a number of health benefits i.e. prevention of Parkinson's disease, and heart diseases (Bryan, 2008). Green tea can prevent angiogenesis and tumor formation (Kim et al., 2009). The health benefits of green tea are due its phytoconstituents such as polyphenolic catechins, like epicatechin, epicatechin-3-gallate, epigallocatechin, Epigallocatechin gallate (EGCG), catechin, and gallocatechin (Kim et al., 2009). Among these, EGCG is the abundant catechin in green tea, and knowm to induce antioxidant enzymes, including glutathione peroxidase, catalase, and glutathione S-transferase, in mice (Aggarwal & Harikumar, 2009). l-theanine present in green tea has health benefits, such as antitumor, Alzheimer's disease prevention, and blood pressure reduction. (Prakash & Gupta, 2014; Lee et al., 2010) green tea increases longitivity action and stress resistance through its antioxidant properties.

Curcumin and thioflavin T are the pharmacologically active substance in turmeric (Curcuma longa), and also use as health supplement and has been widely used as an herbal medicine. Curcumin possesses many biological activities, such as antioxidative, anti-inflammatory, anticancer, and anti neurodegenerative properties (Kesharwani et. al., 2018; Liao et al., 2011; Rajasekaran et al., 2008). With its multiple unrelated activities, curcumin has been considered as a potential aging intervention compound (Miyashita et al., 2011; Fasano et al., 2010).

Table 1. Nutraceutical and their Therapeutic Benefits

Phytochemicals	Source	Chemicals classification	Therapeutic benefits
Eugenol	*Eugenia caryophyllus*	Terpenoid (Monoterpenoid)	analgesic, dental protective, flavouring agent (Wahab & Aziz, 2012)
Quinine	*Cinchona succirubra*	Alkaloids (Quinoline)	Antimalarial,bitter stomachic (Ahmad et al., 2011)
Ephedrine	*Ephedra Gerardiana*	Alkaloids (Amines)	Bronchial asthma,joint ache(Ahmad et al., 2011)
Reserpine	*Rauwolfiaserpentina*	Alkaloids (Indole)	Hypertension(Ahmad et al., 2011)
Taxol	*Taxusbrevifolia*	Terpenoid (Diterpenoids)	Anticancer drug. (Ahmad et al., 2011)
Beta carotene	Carrots, Green leafy vegetables	Carotenoids	Antioxidants, pro-vitamins (Ahmad et al., 2011)
Luteolin	*Reseda lutea*	Flavonoids	Antioxidant, Anticarcinogenic (Ahmad et al., 2011)
Digitalis	*Digitalis purpurea*	Glycosides (Cardiac)	Congestive Heart Failure (Zou et al., 2010)
Senna	*Cassia augustifolia*	Glycosides (Anthraquinones)	Laxatives (Zou et al., 2010)

The mainstream of the nutraceuticals owns manifold therapeutic aids and have been demanded to have physiological aids (Henrotin et al., 2011) or provide defense against various illnesses as the following Products:

- Cardiovascular agents: - Spirulina (*Spirulina maxima*)
- Anti-obese agents: - Curcumin (*Curcumin longa*)
- Anti-diabetic agents: - Androghrolide (*Andrographis paniculata*)
- Anti-cancer agent: -Vincristine (*Vinca rosea*)
- Immune boosters: - Resveratol (*Fallopia japonica*)

3.4 Nutraceutical in Diabetes

Omega-3-fatty acids are recommended to decrease glucose tolerance and stimulate insulin sensitivity in diabetic patients. Insulin is mandatory for the synthesis of long chain n-3 fatty acids, which comprises of ethyl esters that may be possibly advantageous in diabetic patients. Lipoic acid is a universally used antioxidant, may be more effective as a long-term dietary supplement aimed at the prophylactic protection of diabetic patients. Dietary fibers from psyllium help in decrease in weight, glucose control in diabetic patients and to reduce lipid levels in hyperlipidemia (Gera Jemimah et al., 2019).

3.5 Use of Customary Nutraceutical in Chronic Disease Control

Table 2. Nutraceuticals and its Effect

Nutraceuticals	Effects
Allenssl allenic carotenoid fucoxanthin (brown seaweeds)	Improves insulin resistance and decreases blood glucose levels through the regulation of cytokine secretion from WAT(white adipose tissue) (Macredmond et al., 2010)
Polyunsaturated fatty acid	Prevent several disorders affecting lungs and always (Ganesan et al., 2010).
Unsaponiflable residues of avocado and soybean oils)	Stimulates synthesis of aggrecan and extracellular .matrix components as type 2collagen and by reducing the production of catabolic (MMP-3) and pro –inflammatory (IL-8and IL-6) mediators in OA (osteoarthritis) (Marotta et al., 2011)
Conjugated linoleic acid	Significantly improves AHR (airway hyper responsiveness) associated with a reduction in leptin/ adiponectin ratio in mild asthma (Kastorini et al., 2011)
Siphonaxanthin, a marine carotenoid (green algae)	Induce apoptosis in HL-60 cells by decreases BCI -2, and increases activation of caspase (Bulathsinghala et al., 2010)
FPP (fermented papaya preparation)	Unregulated TNF and thioredoxin (trx) in liver and cirrhosis (Gupta et al., 2011)
MUFAS (monounsaturated fats)	Lowers CVD (cardiovascular disease) risk and MS (metabolic syndrome). (Berry et al.,2011)
1,25(oh)D, or Calcitriol	Regulates the level of p21 and p27 and increases expression of BRCA -1 and -2 tumor suppressor genes contributing in the DNA repair mechanism
Resveratrol	Chemosensitizes tumor by modulating drug transporters cell survival proteins, cell proliferative protein, and members of the NF–kB and STAT3 signaling pathways (Ferrucci et al.,2016)
Fortified wheat flour	Reduces prevalence of NTDs (neutral tube defect) at birth and increases blood folate concentrations (Winters, 2006)

3.6 Nutraceutical use In Certain Ailments

Glucosamine and Chondroitin Glucosamine is a precursor to a particle called a glycosamino glycan, this particle is used in the creation and repair of gristle. Glucosamine sulphate in numerous European nations used as primary line of action for stiffness. Glucosamine sulphate stimulates the manufacture of hyaluronic cutting in joint unsolidified. Hyaluronic acid relieves pain and improves mobility by repairing damaged cartilage. In vitro trial of Glucosamine has exposed a dose dependent increase in proteoglycan after managing it. It is marketed usually as hydrochloride or sulfate salt. Both compounds have anti-inflammatory effects. Mixture of Glucosamine and Chondroitin are obtainable.

Methylsulfonyl Methane (MSM) is sold as nutritional and dietary supplement often used in combination with glucosamine and Chondroitin for helping to treat or prevent some disease or disorders. MSM is the oxidized form of dimethylsulfoxied; a natural organic form of sulfur. Both of these are used for discomfort and inflammation. MSM has benefit over DSMO as it is unscented and does not cause skin irritation. MSM provide source of Sulphur for the formation of the cartilage matrix or the antioxidant system (Palliyaguru et al., 2015).

3.7 Cancer Treatment

There is a tremendous need in clinics to impair cancer progression through non-invasive therapeutic approaches as all the currently available cancer therapeutic options are expensive but none of them are safe. The use of natural compounds to achieve this is of importance to improve the quality of life of young patients during their treatments. Some natural mix ups that have shown outstanding results in vitro and in vivo are: Chebulagic acid Apigenin, Nor cantharidin, Saffron/Crocin, Parthenolide, Longikaurin E Lupeol, Spongistatin 1, Deoxy-variolin B (Assi et al., 2016).

Withania somnifera commonly known as Ashwagandha, is one of the most powerful plants. The effectiveness of radiation therapy has been shown to enhance and the side effects of chemotherapeutic agents have been reduced when its extract was used in combination and moreover, the constituents do not interfere with their tumor-reducing actions (Fraser et al., 2015). Recently, it has been found that the plant contains withanolides which have anti-tumorigenic properties and this property has been demonstrated in experimental models (Vue et al., 2015). Chemotherapy induced peripheral neuropathy (CIPN) is a sincere dose-limiting lateral result. Vitamin E may help prevent CIPN. l-glutamine, and omega-3 are also promising in the prevention of the effects of CIPN (Aswathy et al., 2015). Caffeic acid phenethyl ester (CAPE) is a normal bioactive molecule which has been stated to have anti-cancer property. Synergistic effects of various combinations of dietary natural products including curcumin, quercetin, soybean isoflavones and silibinin have been described that have potential for the treatment of prostate cancer. Various factors have been suggested which help in the decrease of cancer cell replication and increase in the chance of remission. For the prevention and successful treatment of cancers, it is necessary that dietary supplements with high doses of vitamin C are consumed in at-risk populations along with some changes in lifestyle (Pandey et al., 2005).

4. LATEST RESEARCH WORK ON NUTRACEUTICALS

Recent research emphasized on use of Microwave pretreatment as a promising strategy for increase of nutraceutical content. He investigated the microwave pretreatment of milk thistle on oil extraction yield and its physicochemical properties, nutraceuticals content, and fatty acids profile and found that chlorophyll content, saponification value, and total phenolic content increased. Moreover, he also found that the number of nutraceuticals including tocopherols and phytosterols increased remarkably in treated seeds oil. Lastly it was concluded that microwave pretreatment can be successfully used (B Fathi et al., 2019).

Literature reveals the information on enhancing immunity in viral infection with special emphasis in COVID-19 virus. It was suggested that the balanced nutrition is essential for maintaining immunity and management of viral infections. It's summarized that some vitamins (A, D, E & C), nutraceuticals (green tea, turmeric, blueberry etc.) and probiotics could help in prevention of viral infection (Ranil et al., 2020).

In worldwide concern regarding the recent outbreak of a deadly novel strain of coronavirus, Mark et al discovered that Nutraceuticals have potential for boosting the Type 1 Interferon Response to RNA Viruses including Influenza and Coronavirus. The anti-inflammatory impact of antioxidant nutraceuticals might also be expected to quell the excessive inflammatory reaction within lung parenchyma evoked by viral infections whose lethality is mediated by an acute respiratory distress syndrome. These nutraceuticals could decrease such as response both by suppressing viral spread, and by dampening pro-inflammatory signaling endothelial cells that promotes influx of inflammatory cells (Mark et al., 2020).

Table 3. Marketed products available for Nutraceuticals

S. No.	Brand name	Generic name	Manufacturer	Uses
1.	Nicholas Nutraceuticals Calcitrex-F	Calcium citrate, Vitamin D3 and Folic acid	Nicholas pharmaceuticals	Supplement for strong bones and teeth
2.	Healthvit Clove 470 mg	Clove Bud Powder (*SyzigiumAromaticum*) – 470 mg	DF pharmacy LTD.	Helps Regulate Blood Sugar Levels, Promotes Bone Health, Improves Liver Health, Improves Digestion
3.	Echinacea Immunity 400mg Capsule	*ChinaceaPurpurea* Extract (Aerial) (Standardized for 4% Echinacoside) as a major ingredient.	Allen Nutraceuticals	First-choice treatment for colds, flu, infections and for generally boosting the immune system.
4.	Swisse Beauty Grape Seed Tablets	Grapeseed; Vitamin C; Vitamin E	Health & Happiness (H&H) Inc.	Improve circulation & cardiovascular health Support collagen production Immune system support
5.	Organic Spirulina Tablets	Organic Spirulina powder	Sea nutrition	Strengthen daily immunity and metabolism. improve haemoglobin levels, fight allergies, reduce stress levels, boost stamina, reduces fatigue and aid in body detox.

5. CONCLUSION

Nutraceuticals provide all the important substances that should be present in a healthy diet for humans. Nutraceuticals provide energy and nutrient supplements to body, which are required for maintaining good health. Nutraceutical industry is growing at a much faster rate in comparison to food and pharmaceutical industry. Nutraceutical and functional food play an important role in the promotion and care of human health to prevent diseases. The use of nutraceuticals is a key to obtain therapeutic outcomes with reduced side effects. And with advancement and availability of technology it is possible to formulate nutraceuticals with maximum stability and high efficacy.

6. FUTURE PROSPECTIVE

Tremendous requests of nutraceuticals endeavor the pharmaceutical enterprises to create herbals nourishing supplements. Expanding mindfulness levels about wellness and health, impelled by media inclusion are provoking most of individuals to lead more advantageous ways of life, practice more, and practice good eating habits. Developing field in nutraceuticals are Nano-nutraceuticals, Nutrigenomics, Nutrigenetics, Molecular nourishment and health and adequacy of nutraceuticals (Parasuram et al., 2011). The total nutraceutical commercial center demonstrates that end administrators are searching for insignificantly treated nourishment with extra wholesome aids and organoleptic esteem. This recent development pushes the next development in the nutraceutical market which places internationally. The rising nutraceuticals mechanical appears to be bound to lodge the set in the new period. Its huge advancement has suggestions for the food, pharmaceutical, medicinal services, and crude preparations many researchers believe that catalysts mean another energizing wilderness in nutraceuticals. Catalysts have been underemployed they are effective to be a hot part in the upcoming. Fermentation expertise utilizing microorganisms to make new nourishment crops likewise implies potential. Worldwide propensities to sound products cannot be upset. Organizations dazzling the lead by underwriting deliberately in order, item development and showcasing and client instruction will not go unrewarded. (Shukla et al., 2014).

REFERENCES

Aggarwal, B., & Harikumar, K. (2009). Potential therapeutic effects of curcumin, the anti-inflammatory agent, against neurodegenerative, cardiovascular, pulmonary, metabolic, autoimmune and neoplastic diseases. *The International Journal of Biochemistry & Cell Biology*, *41*(1), 40–59. doi:10.1016/j.biocel.2008.06.010 PMID:18662800

Ahmad, F., Ahmad, F. A., Azad, A., Alam, S., & Ashraf, A. (2013). Nutraceuticals is the need of hour. *World J PharmSci*, *2*(25), 16–25.

Akbarzadeh, A., Sadabady, A., Davaran, S., Sang, W. J., Zarghami, N. Z., Hanifehpour, M., Kouhiand, M. K., & Nejati, K. (2013). Liposome:classification, preparation, and applications. *Nanoscale Research Letters*, *8*(1), 102. doi:10.1186/1556-276X-8-102 PMID:23432972

Ali, K., Maltese, F., Zyprian, E., Rex, M., Choi, Y. H., & Verpoorte, R. (2009). NMR metabolic fingerprinting based identification of grapevine metabolites associated with downy mildew resistance. *Journal of Agricultural and Food Chemistry*, *57*(20), 9599–9606. doi:10.1021/jf902069f PMID:19785416

Ansari, S., Chauhan, B., Kalam, N., & Kumar, G. (2013). Current ideas and forecasts of herbal nutraceutical: A review. *Journal of Advanced Pharmacy and Research*, *4*(1), 4–8.

Anwekar, H., Patel, S., & Singhai, A. K. (2011). Liposome- as drug carriers. *IJPLS*, *2*(7), 951–945.

Assi, M., Derbré, F., Lefeuvre, L., & Rebillard, A. (2016). Antioxidant supplementation accelerates cachexia development by promoting tumor growth in C26 tumor-bearing mice. *Free Radical Biology & Medicine*, *91*, 204–214. doi:10.1016/j.freeradbiomed.2015.12.019 PMID:26708754

Aswathy, R. G., Sivakumar, B., Maekawa, T., & Kumar, D. (2015). Prospects of nano-nutraceuticals for better and healthier future. *Journal of Nutrition & Food Sciences*, *5*(4).

Babili, F., Bouajila, J., Souchard, J., Bertrand, C., Bellvert, F., Fouraste, I., Moulis, C., & Valentin, A. (2011). Oregano: Chemical analysis and evaluation of its antimalarial, antioxidant, and cytotoxic activities. *Journal of Food Science*, *76*(3), 12–18. doi:10.1111/j.1750-3841.2011.02109.x PMID:21535822

Berry, R. J., Bailey, L., Mulinare, J., Bower, C., & Dary, O. (2011). Folic Acid Working Group, Fortification of flour with folic acid. *Food and Nutrition Bulletin*, *31*(1_suppl1), S22–S35. doi:10.1177/15648265100311S103 PMID:20629350

Bhattacharya, S. (2009). Phytosomes: Emerging strategy in delivery of herbal drugs and nutraceuticals. *Pharmacy Times*, *4*(1), 9–12.

Bombardelli, E., Curri, S. B., Loggia, D. R., Del, N. P., Tubaro, A., & Gariboldi, P. (1989). Complexes between phospholipids and vegetal derivatives of biological interest. *Fitoterapia*, *60*, 1–9.

Bryan, J. (2008). Psychological effects of dietary components of tea: Caffeine and Ltheanine. *Nutrition Reviews*, *66*(2), 82–90. doi:10.1111/j.1753-4887.2007.00011.x PMID:18254874

Bulathsinghala, P., Syrigos, K. N., & Saif, M. W. (2010). Role of vitamin D in the prevention of pancreatic cancer. *Journal of Nutrition and Metabolism*, *2010*, 1–9. doi:10.1155/2010/721365 PMID:21274445

Cevc, G., Schätzlein, A., & Richardsen, H. (2002). Ultradeformable lipid vesicles can penetrate the skin and other semi-permeable barriers unfragmented. Evidence from double label CLSM experiments and direct size measurements. *Biochimica et Biophysica Acta*, *1564*(1), 21–30. doi:10.1016/S0005-2736(02)00401-7 PMID:12100992

Chao, P., Deshmukh, M., Kutscher, H. L., Gao, D., Rajan, S. S., Hu, P., Laskin, D. L., Stein, S., & Sinko, P. J. (2010). Pulmonary targeting microparticulate camptothecin delivery system: Anticancer evaluation in a rat orthotopic lung cancer model. *Anti-Cancer Drugs*, *21*(1), 65–76. doi:10.1097/CAD.0b013e328332a322 PMID:19966540

Chintale, A. G., Kadam, V. S., Sakhare, R. S., Birajdar, G. O., & Nalwad, D. N. (2013). Role of Nutraceuticals – a comphrensive review. *IJRPC*, *3*(2), 2231–2781.

Chiou, D., & Langrish, T. (2007). Development and characterization of novel nutraceuticals with spray dry technology. *Journal of Food Engineering*, *82*(1), 84–91. doi:10.1016/j.jfoodeng.2007.01.021

Cohen, E., & Dillin, A. (2008). The insulin paradox: Aging, proteotoxicity and neurodegeneration. *Nature Reviews. Neuroscience*, *9*(10), 759–767. doi:10.1038/nrn2474 PMID:18769445

Das, L., Bhaumik, E., Raychaudhuri, U., & Chakraborty, R. (2011). Role of nutraceuticals in human health. *Journal of Food Science and Technology*, *49*(2), 173–183. doi:10.100713197-011-0269-4 PMID:23572839

El-Sherbiny, & Smyth, H. (2012). Controlled release pulmonary administration of curcumin using swellable biocompatible microparticles. *Journal of Molecular Pharmaceutics & Organic Process Research*, *9*, 269–280. PMID:22136259

Engy, A. M., & Mohamed, A. F. (2015). Two-dimensional NMR spectroscopic approaches for exploring plant metabolome: A review. *Journal of Advanced Research*, *6*(1), 3–15. doi:10.1016/j.jare.2014.10.003 PMID:25685540

Fasano, E., Serini, S., Piccioni, E., Innocenti, I., & Calviello, G. (2010). Chemoprevention of lung pathologies by dietary n-3 polyunsaturated fatty acids. *Current Medicinal Chemistry*, *17*(29), 3358–3376. doi:10.2174/092986710793176401 PMID:20712568

Fathi-Achachloueia, B. (2019). Microwave pretreatment as a promising strategy for increment of nutraceutical content and extraction yield of oil from milk thistle seed. *Industrial Crops and Products*, *128*, 527–533. doi:10.1016/j.indcrop.2018.11.034

Feng, T., Wei, Y., Lee, R., & Zhao, L. (2017). Liposomal curcumin and its application in cancer. *International Journal of Nanomedicine*, *12*, 6027–6044. doi:10.2147/IJN.S132434 PMID:28860764

Ferrucci, V., Boffa, I., De Masi, G., & Zollo, M. (2016). Natural compounds for pediatric cancer treatment. *Naunyn-Schmiedeberg's Archives of Pharmacology, 389*(2), 131–149. doi:10.100700210-015-1191-5 PMID:26650503

Forst & Sullivan. (n.d.). Global Nutraceutical Industry Investing in Healthy Life. *FICCI*, 5-26.

Fraser, S. P., Hemsley, F., & Djamgoz, M. B. (2015). Caffeic acid phenethyl ester: Inhibition of metastatic cell behaviours via voltage-gated sodium channel in human breast cancer in vitro. *The International Journal of Biochemistry & Cell Biology, 71*, 111–118. doi:10.1016/j.biocel.2015.12.012 PMID:26724521

Ganapathy, M., & Bhunia, S. (2016). Nutraceuticals: The New Generation Therapeutics. *Adv. Tech Bio Med, 4*(2), 2-5.

Ganesan, P., Noda, K., Manabe, Y., Ohkubo, T., Tanaka, Y., Maoka, T., Sugawara, T., & Hirata, T. (2010). Siphonaxanthin, a marine carotenoid from green algae, effectively induces apoptosis in human leukemia (HL-60) cells. *Biochimica et Biophysica Acta, 1810*(5), 497–503. doi:10.1016/j.bbagen.2011.02.008 PMID:21371530

Garti, N., & McClements, D. J. (2012). Encapsulation technologies and delivery systems for food ingredients and nutraceuticals. florida: Woodhead publishing series in food sciences. *Technology and Nutrition, 1*, 23–30.

Gavini, E., Alamanni, M. C., Cossu, M., & Giunchedi, P. (2005). Tabletted microspheres containing *Cynarascolymus* (var. Spinososardo) extract for the preparation of controlled release nutraceutical matrices. *Journal of Microencapsulation, 22*(5), 487–499. doi:10.1080/02652040500099919 PMID:16361192

Godin, B., & Touitou, E. (2004). Mechanism of bacitracin permeation enhancement through the skin and cellular membranes from an ethosomal carrier. *Journal of Controlled Release, 94*(2-3), 365–379. doi:10.1016/j.jconrel.2003.10.014 PMID:14744487

Gopi, S., Amalraj, A., & Józef, T. (2016). Introduction of nanotechnology in herbal drugs and nutraceutical: A review. *Journal of Nanomedicine & Biotherapeutic Discovery, 6*(2), 1–8. doi:10.4172/2155-983X.1000143

Gupta, S. C., Kannappan, R., Reuter, S., Kim, J. H., & Aggarwal, B. B. (2011). Chemosensitization of tumors by resveratrol. *Annals of the New York Academy of Sciences, 215*(1), 150–160. doi:10.1111/j.1749-6632.2010.05852.x PMID:21261654

Hall, S. S. (2003). Longevity research. In vivo vitalis? Compounds activate life-extending genes. *Science, 301*(5637), 1165.

Hamid, N., Azar, B., Hedayatollah, S., & Mahmoud, R. K. (2014). New Concepts in Nutraceuticals as Alternative for Pharmaceuticals. *International Journal of Preventive Medicine, 5*(12), 1487–1499. PMID:25709784

Hayashi, H. (1989). Drying technologies of foods – their history and future. *Drying Technology, 7*(2), 315–369. doi:10.1080/07373938908916590

He, X., & Rui, H. L. (2006). Cranberry phytochemicals: Isolation, structure elucidation, and their antiproliferative and antioxidant activities. *Journal of Agricultural and Food Chemistry, 54*(19), 7069–7074. doi:10.1021/jf061058l PMID:16968064

Henrotin, Y., Lambert, C., Couchourel, D., Ripoll, C., & Chiotelli, E. (2011). Nutraceuticals: Do they represent a new era in the management of osteoarthritis? – A narrative review from the lessons taken with five products. *OsCar, 19*(1), 1–21. doi:10.1016/j.joca.2010.10.017 PMID:21035558

Ivan, M. P. (2016). Lycosome technology: Advances and perspectives. *American Journal of Food Science and Nutrition, 3*(1), 18–23.

Jaganathan, S., & Supriyanto, E. (2012). Ant proliferative and molecular mechanism of eugenol-induced apoptosis in cancer cells. *Molecules (Basel, Switzerland), 17*(6), 290–304. doi:10.3390/molecules17066290 PMID:22634840

Jayawardena, R., Sooriyaarachchi, P., Chourdakis, M., Jeewandara, C., & Ranasinghef, P. (2020). Enhancing immunity in viral infections, with special emphasis on COVID-19: A review. *Diabetes & Metabolic Syndrome: Clinical Research & Reviews*, 1-54.

Kastorini, C. M., Milionis, H. J., Esposito, K., Giugliano, D., Goudevenos, J. A., & Panagiotakos, D. B. (2011). The effect of mediterranean diet on metabolic syndrome and its components: A meta-analysis of 50 studies and 534,906 individuals. *Journal of the American College of Cardiology, 57*(11), 1299–1313. doi:10.1016/j.jacc.2010.09.073 PMID:21392646

Keservani, R., Sharma, A., & Kesharwani, R. (Eds.). (2017). Drug Delivery Approaches and Nanosystems, Volume 1 (Novel Drug Carriers). CRC Press.

Kesharwani, R., Misra, K., & Singh, D. (2019). Perspectives and challenges of tropical medicinal herbs and modern drug discovery in the current scenario. *Asian Pacific Journal of Tropical Medicine, 12*(1), 1–7. doi:10.4103/1995-7645.250337

Kim, K. I., Yoon, Y. H., & Baek, Y. J. (1996). Effects of rehydration media and immobilization in Ca-alginate on the survival of Lactobacillus casei and Bifido bacterium bifidum. *Korean J Dairy Sci, 18*, 193–198.

Kim, T. I., Lee, Y. K., Park, S. G., Choi, I. S., Ban, J. O., Park, H. K., Nam, S.-Y., Yun, Y. W., Han, S. B., Oh, K. W., & Hong, J. T. (2009). l-Theanine, an amino acid in green tea, attenuates b-amyloid-induced cognitive dysfunction and neurotoxicity: Reduction in oxidative damage and inactivation of ERK/p38 kinase and NF-kB pathways. *Free Radical Biology & Medicine, 47*(11), 1601–1610. doi:10.1016/j.freeradbiomed.2009.09.008 PMID:19766184

Kurniawansyah, F., Mammucari, R., & Foster, N. (2015). Inhalable curcumin formulations by supercritical technology. *Powder Technology, 284*, 289–298. doi:10.1016/j.powtec.2015.04.083

Lee, K. S., Lee, B. S., Semnani, S., Avanesian, A., Um, C.-Y., Jeon, H.-J., Seong, K.-M., Yu, K., Min, K.-J., & Jafari, M. (2010). Curcumin extends life span, improves health span, and modulates the expression of age-associated aging genes in Drosophila melanogaster. *Rejuvenation Research, 13*(5), 561–570. doi:10.1089/rej.2010.1031 PMID:20645870

Liao, V. H., Yu, C. W., Chu, Y. J., Li, W. H., Hsieh, Y. C., & Wang, T. T. (2011). Curcumin-mediated lifespan extension in Caenorhabditiselegans. *Mechanisms of Ageing and Development*, *132*(10), 480–487. doi:10.1016/j.mad.2011.07.008 PMID:21855561

Machida, Y., Onishi, H., Kurita, A., Hata, H., Morikawa, A., & Machida, Y. (2000). Pharmacokinetics of prolonged-release CPT-11-loaded microspheres in rats. *Journal of Controlled Release*, *66*(2-3), 159–175. doi:10.1016/S0168-3659(99)00267-9 PMID:10742577

MacRedmond, R., Singhera, G., Attridge, S., Bahzad, M., Fava, C., Lai, Y., Hallstrand, T. S., & Dorscheid, D. (2010). Conjugated linoleic acid improves airway hyper-reactivity in overweight mild asthmatics. *Clinical and Experimental Allergy*, *40*(7), 1071–1078. doi:10.1111/j.1365-2222.2010.03531.x PMID:20642580

Maiti, K., Mukherjee, K., Gantait, A., Ahamed, H., Saha, B., & Mukherjee, P. (2005). Enhanced therapeutic benefit of quercetin-phospholipid complex in carbon tetrachloride induced acute liver injury in rats: A comparative study. *Int J Pharm Technol*, *4*, 84–90.

Maiti, K., Mukherjee, K., Gantait, A., Saha, B., & Mukherjee, P. (2007). Curcumin-phospholipid complex: Preparation, therapeutic evaluation and pharmacokinetic study in rats. *International Journal of Pharmaceutics*, *330*(1-2), 155–163. doi:10.1016/j.ijpharm.2006.09.025 PMID:17112692

Manach, C., Scalbert, A., Morand, C., Rémésy, C., & Jiménez, L. (2004). Polyphenols: Food sources and bioavailability. *The American Journal of Clinical Nutrition*, *79*(5), 727–747. doi:10.1093/ajcn/79.5.727 PMID:15113710

Marotta, F., Chui, D. H., Jain, S., Polimeni, A., Koike, K., Zhou, L., Lorenzetti, A., Shimizu, H., & Yang, H. (2011). Effect of a fermented nutraceutical on thioredoxin level and TNF-alpha signaling in cirrhotic patients. *Journal of Biological Regulators and Homeostatic Agents*, *25*, 37–45. PMID:21382272

McCarty, M., & DiNicolantonio, J. (2020). Nutraceuticals have potential for boosting the type 1 interferon response to RNA viruses including influenza and coronavirus. *Progress in Cardiovascular Diseases*, *63*(3), 1–8. doi:10.1016/j.pcad.2020.02.007 PMID:32061635

Milanovic, J., Manojlovic, V., Levic, S., Rajic, N., Nedovic, V., & Bugarski, B. (2010). Microencapsulation of flavors in carnauba wax. *Sensors (Basel)*, *10*(1), 901–912. doi:10.3390100100901 PMID:22315575

Mishra, H., Kesharwani, R., Singh, D., Tripathi, S., Dubey, S., & Misra, K. (2018). Computational study of curcumin, retinoic acid and its conjugates against GSK-3 beta. *Network Modeling and Analysis in Health Informatics and Bioinformatics*, *8*, 3. doi:10.100713721-018-0177-x

Miyashita, K., Nishikawa, S., Beppu, F., Tsukui, T., Abe, M., & Hosokawa, M. (2011). The allenic carotenoid fucoxanthin, a novel marine nutraceutical from brown seaweeds. *Journal of the Science of Food and Agriculture*, *91*(7), 1166–1174. doi:10.1002/jsfa.4353 PMID:21433011

Naksuriya, O., Okonogi, S., Schielers, R., & Hennink, W. (2014). Curcumin nanoformulations: A review of pharmaceutical properties and preclinical studies and clinical data related to cancer treatment. *Biomaterials*, *35*(10), 3365–3383. doi:10.1016/j.biomaterials.2013.12.090 PMID:24439402

Neto, C. (2007). Cranberry and blueberry: Evidence for protective effects against cancer and vascular diseases. *Molecular Nutrition & Food Research, 51*(6), 652–664. doi:10.1002/mnfr.200600279 PMID:17533651

Novoa-Carballal, R., Fernandez-Megia, E., Jimenez, C., & Riguera, R. (2011). NMR methods for unravelling the spectra of complex mixtures. *Natural Product Reports, 28*(1), 78–98. doi:10.1039/C005320C PMID:20936238

Palliyaguru, D. L., Singh, S. V., & Kensler, T. W. (2016). Withania somnifera: From prevention to treatment of cancer. *Molecular Nutrition & Food Research, 60*(6), 1342–1353. doi:10.1002/mnfr.201500756 PMID:26718910

Pandey, M., Verma, R., & Sara, S. (2010). Nutraceuticals: new era of medicine and health. *AJPCR, 3*(1).

Pandey, N., Prasad, M., Rai, S., & Rai, S. (2011). Medicinal plants derived nutraceuticals: A re-emerging health aid. *Int J Pharm Bio Sci, 2*(4), 20–41.

Parasuram, R., Rawat, B., & Thangvel, S. (2011). Nutraceuticals: An area of tremendous scope. *International Journal of Research in Ayurveda and Pharmacy, 2*(4), 10–15.

Parris, N., Cooke, P., & Hicks, K. (2005). Encapsulation of essential oils in zeinnano spherical particles. *Journal of Agricultural and Food Chemistry, 53*(12), 4788–4792. doi:10.1021/jf040492p PMID:15941317

Patel, R., Singh, S., Singh, S., Sheth, N., & Gendle, R. (2009). Development and characterization of curcumin loaded transfer some for transdermal delivery. *J Pharm Sci Res, 1*, 71–80.

Pegg, R., & Shahidi, F. (2007). Encapsulation, stabilization, and controlled release of food ingredients and bioactives. In M. S. Rahman (Ed.), *Handbook of food preservation* (2nd ed., pp. 1–1088). CRC Press.

Piyush, M., Bothiraja, C., Kakasaheb, M., Shivajirao, K., & Atmaram, P. (2018). Phytoconstituent based dry powder inhalers as biomedicine for the management of pulmonary disease. *Biomedicine and Pharmacotherapy, 108*, 828–837. doi:10.1016/j.biopha.2018.09.094 PMID:30372894

Politi, M., Zloh, M., Pintado, M., Castro, P., Heinrich, M., & Prieto, J. M. (2009). Direct metabolic fingerprinting of commercial herbal tinctures by nuclear magnetic resonance spectroscopy and mass spectrometry. *Phytochem Anal: PCA, 20*(4), 328–334. doi:10.1002/pca.1131 PMID:19405164

Prakash, D., & Gupta, C. (2014). Phytochemicals of nutraceutical importance from Curcuma longa L. and their role in human health. In Phytochemicals of Nutraceutical Importance. Wallingford: CABI.

Price, W. S., Nara, M., & Arata, Y. (1997). A pulsed field gradient NMR study of the aggregation and hydration of parvalbumin. *Biophysical Chemistry, 65*(2–3), 179–187. doi:10.1016/S0301-4622(97)00003-3 PMID:17029854

Rajasekaran, A., Sivagnanam, G., & Xavier, R. (2008). Nutraceuticals as therapeutic agents: A review. *Res J Pharm Tech, 3*, 28–40.

Rane, B., & Kesarwani, R. (2020). *Introduction to nutraceuticals and dietary supplements.* CRC Press. doi:10.1201/9780367821517-4

Re, M. I. (1998). Microencapsulation by spray drying. *Drying Technology*, *16*(6), 1195–1236. doi:10.1080/07373939808917460

Sagar, S., Yance, D., & Wong, R. (2006). Natural health products that inhibit angiogenesis: A potential source for investigational new agents to treat cancer-part 1. *Current Oncology (Toronto, Ont.)*, *13*, 14–26. PMID:17576437

Sakthivel, L., Timmakondu, N., Chellappan, D., & Subramaniam, S. (2012). Nutraceuticals and their medicinial importance. *IJHAS*, *1*(2), 47–53.

Salvia-Trujillo, L., Olga, M., & McClements, D. (2016). Excipient Nanoemulsions for Improving Oral Bioavailability of Bioactives. *Nanomaterials MDPI*, *6*(17), 1–16. doi:10.3390/nano6010017 PMID:28344274

Sanli, O., Karaca, I., & Isiklan, N. (2009). Preparation, characterization, and salicylic acid release behaviour of chitosan/ poly (vinyl alcohol) blend microspheres. *Journal of Applied Polymer Science*, *111*(6), 2731–2740. doi:10.1002/app.29319

Sapkale, A., Thorat, M., VirPrasad, R., & Singh, M. (2012). Nutraceuticals –Global status and applications: A review. *IJPCS*, *1*(3).

Sarin, R., Sharma, M., Singh, R., & Kumar, S. (2012). Nutraceuticals: A review. *Int Res J Pharm*, *3*, 95–99.

Sharma, A., Keservani, R., & Kesharwani, R. (Eds.). (2018). *Nanobiomaterials: applications in drug delivery*. CRC Press. doi:10.1201/9781315204918

Sharma, R., Kaur, A., Thakur, S., Bhardwaj, K., & Bose, S. (2017). Role of nutraceuticals in health care. *IJGP*, *11*(3), S385.

Sharma, R., & Singh, R. B. (2013). Bioactive foods and nutraceutical supplementation criteria in cardiovascular protection. *The Open Nutraceuticals Journal*, *3*, 141–153.

Shibamoto, T., Kanazawa, K., Shahidi, F., & Ho, C. (2008). Functional food and health: an overview. In T. Shibamoto, K. Kanazawa, F. Shahidi, & C.-T. Ho (Eds.), ACS symposium series: Vol. 993. *Functional food and health* (pp. 1–6). Oxford Univ. Press. doi:10.1021/bk-2008-0993.ch001

Shukla, G., Kumari, S., Maguddayao, A., Prashar, S., & Kumar, C. (2014). Nutraceuticals: The future therapeutics. *Int J Pharm Technol*, *4*(1), 46–50.

Siddiqui, I. A., Adhami, V., Bharali, D., Hafeez, B., Asim, M., Khwaja, S., Ahmad, N., Cui, H., Mousa, S. A., & Mukhtar, H. (2009). Introducing nanochemoprevention as a novel approach for cancer control: Proof of principle with green tea polyphenol epigallocatechin-3-gallate. *Cancer Research*, *2*(7), 1712–1716. doi:10.1158/0008-5472.CAN-08-3978 PMID:19223530

Singh, J., & Sinha, S. (2012). Classification and regulatory acts and applications of nutraceuticals for health. *IJPBS*, *2*(1), 177–187.

Solans, C., Izquierdo, P., Nolla, J., Azemar, N., & Garcia-Celma, M. J. (2005). Nano-emulsions. *Curr Opin Colloid In*, *10*(3–4), 102–110. doi:10.1016/j.cocis.2005.06.004

Srinivas, P., Philbert, M., Vu, T., Huang, Q., Kokini, J., Saltos, E., Chen, H., & Ross, S. (2009). Nanotechnology research: Applications in nutrition sciences. *The Journal of Nutrition, 140*(1), 119–124. doi:10.3945/jn.109.115048 PMID:19939997

Taki, M., Tagami, T., Fukushige, K., & Ozeki, T. (2016). Fabrication of nanocomposite particles using a two-solution mixing-type spray nozzle for use in an inhaled curcumin formulation. *International Journal of Pharmaceutics, 511*(1), 104–110. doi:10.1016/j.ijpharm.2016.06.134 PMID:27374204

Tank, D., Gandhi, S., & Shah, M. (2010). Nutraceuticals-portmanteau of science and nature. *IJPSR, 5*(3), 33–38.

Tiwari, R., Kumar, A., & Singh, K. (2019). Nutraceuticals Inspiring the Current Therapy for Lifestyle Diseases. *Advances in Pharmacological Sciences*, 1–5. PMID:30755770

Voilley, A., & Etievant, P. (2006). *Flavor in food*. Woodhead Publishing Limited. doi:10.1533/9781845691400

Vos, P., Faas, M., Spasojevic, M., & Sikkema, J. (2010). Review: Encapsulation for preservation of functionality and targeted delivery of bioactive food components. *International Dairy Journal, 20*(4), 292–302. doi:10.1016/j.idairyj.2009.11.008

Vue, B., Zhang, S., & Chen, Q. (2015). Synergistic effects of dietary natural products as anti-prostate cancer agents. *Natural Product Communications, 10*(12), 2179–2188. doi:10.1177/1934578X1501001241 PMID:26882694

Wahab, B., & Abd, S. (2012). Ginkgo biloba protects against intermittent hypoxia-induced memory deficits and hippocampal DNA damage in rats. *Phytomedicine, 19*(5), 444–450. doi:10.1016/j.phymed.2011.11.011 PMID:22265820

Wandrey, C., Bartkowiak, A., & Harding, S. (2009). Materials for Encapsulation. In N. J. Zuidam & V. A. Nedovic (Eds.), Encapsulation Technologies for Food Active Ingredients and Food Processing, Springer: Dordrecht (pp. 31–100). Academic Press.

Wang, X., Jiang, Y., Wang, Y., Huang, M., Ho, C., & Huang, Q. (2008). Enhancing anti inflammation activity of curcumin through o/w nanoemulsions. *Food Chemistry, 108*(2), 419–424. doi:10.1016/j.foodchem.2007.10.086 PMID:26059118

Winters, M. (2006). Ancient medicine, modern use: Withania somnifera and its potential role in integrative oncology. *Alternative Medicine Review, 11*, 269–277. PMID:17176166

Yallapu, M., Ebeling, M., Khan, S., Sundram, V., Chauhan, N., Gupta, B., Puumala, S., Jaggi, M., & Chauhan, S. (2013). Novel curcumin-loaded magnetic nanoparticles for or pancreatic cancer treatment. *NIH Public Access, 12*(8), 1471–1480. doi:10.1158/1535-7163.MCT-12-1227 PMID:23704793

Yang, K., Lin, L., Tseng, T., Wang, S., & Tsai, T. (2007). Oral bioavailability of curcumin in rat and the herbal analysis from Curcuma longa by LC-MS/MS. *Journal of Chromatography. B, Analytical Technologies in the Biomedical and Life Sciences, 853*(1-2), 183–189. doi:10.1016/j.jchromb.2007.03.010 PMID:17400527

Yang, S., Kim, H., Lefeber, A., Erkelens, C., Angelova, N., Choi, Y., & Verpoorte, R. (2006). Application of two-dimensional nuclear magnetic resonance spectroscopy to quality control of ginseng commercial products. *Planta Medica*, *72*(4), 364–369. doi:10.1055-2005-916240 PMID:16557479

You, J., Cui, F., Han, X., Wang, Y., Yang, L., Yu, Y., & Li, Q. (2006). Study of the preparation of sustained-release microspheres containing zedoary turmeric oil by the emulsion-solvent-diffusion method and evaluation of the self-emulsification and bioavailability of the oil. *Colloids and Surfaces. B, Biointerfaces*, *48*(1), 35–41. doi:10.1016/j.colsurfb.2005.12.011 PMID:16480856

Zarse, K., Jabin, S., & Ristow, M. L. (2012). Theanine extends lifespan of adult Caenorhabditis elegans. *European Journal of Nutrition*, *51*(6), 765–768. doi:10.100700394-012-0341-5 PMID:22422488

Zaveri, N. T. (2006). Green tea and its polyphenolic catechins: Medicinal uses in cancer and non-cancer applications. *Life Sciences*, *78*(18), 2073–2080. doi:10.1016/j.lfs.2005.12.006 PMID:16445946

Zeeb, B., Saberi, A., Weiss, J., & McClements, D. (2015). Formation and characterization of filled hydrogel beads based on calcium alginate: Factors influencing nanoemulsion retention and release. *Food Hydrocolloids*, *50*, 27–36. doi:10.1016/j.foodhyd.2015.02.041

Zhang, Z., Zhang, R., Zou, L., Chen, L., Ahmed, Y., Bisri, W., Balamash, K., & McClements, D. (2016). Encapsulation of curcumin in polysaccharide-based hydrogel beads: Impact of bead type on lipid digestion and curcum in bioaccesibility. *Food Hydrocolloids*, *58*, 160–170. doi:10.1016/j.foodhyd.2016.02.036

Zheng, Y., Hou, S., Chen, T., & Lu, Y. (2006). Preparation and characterization of transfersomes of three drugs *in vitro*. *Zhongguo Zhongyao Zazhi*, *31*, 728–731. PMID:17048677

Zou, S., Carey, J., Liedo, P., Ingram, D., Yu, B., & Ghaedian, R. (2010). Prolongevity effects of an oregano and cranberry extract are diet dependent in the Mexican fruit fly (Anastrephaludens). *Journal of Gerontology*, *65*, 41–50. PMID:19906819

Zou, S., Carey, J., Liedo, P., Ingram, D., Yu, B., & Ghaedian, R. (2012). Prolongevity effects of a botanical with oregano and cranberry extracts in Mexican fruit flies: Examining interactions of diet restriction and age. *Age Jordor*, *34*(2), 269–279. doi:10.100711357-011-9230-8 PMID:21455602

Zuidam, N., & Heinrich, J. (2009). Encapsulation of aroma. In N. Zuidam & V. Nedovic (Eds.), Encapsulation technologies for food active ingredients and food processing; Springer: Dordrecht (pp. 127–160). Academic Press.

Chapter 12
Medicinal Plants and Their Bioactive Compounds for the Management and Treatment of Gout

Bui Thanh Tung
University of Medicine and Pharmacy, Vietnam National University, Hanoi, Vietnam

ABSTRACT

Gout is a complex form of arthritis which is characterized by sudden, severe attacks of pain, swelling, redness, and tenderness in the joints. Gout is a type of inflammatory arthritis that is triggered by the crystallization of uric acid within the joints and is often associated with hyperuricemia. Natural products offer many options to reduce the progress and symptoms of diseases, including gout. Natural compound structure including lignans, flavonoids, tannins, polyphenols, triterpenes, sterols, and alkaloids have anti-inflammatory, antioxidant, and XO activities. In this chapter, the authors present medicinal plants and isolated compounds which are used to prevent and reduce the pathogenesis of gout.

1. INTRODUCTION

Gout, a common form of chronic arthritis, is characterized by a persistent increase in serum urate concentration exceeding normal levels (hyperuricemia), followed by the formation of urate crystals and the deposition of these molecules in the affected joints or other tissues. It is a complex disease typically described with four periods, including an asymptomatic phase of hyperuricemia, critical gouty arthritis, intercritical period and chronic gout with tophi. Acute gout occurs suddenly, which produces severe symptoms like erythema, pain leading to swelling of the diseased joints and activity limitation in individuals (Choi, Mount, & Reginato, 2005). After an acute gouty episode is treated, patients can reenter another period of this disease without symptoms of inflammatory joints called intercritical phase. Gout may be similar to rheumatoid arthritis, which has the presence of tophaceous deposition on extensor tendon surfaces as rheumatoid nodules related to small and symmetric joints (Riches, Wright,

DOI: 10.4018/978-1-7998-4453-2.ch012

& Ralston, 2009). Characteristic gouty hyperuricemic, an asymptomatic period with the absence of arthritis or nephrolithiasis, occurs after urate concentration in serum is persistently higher than 7mg/mL (416 μmol/L). Xanthine oxidase (XO), an enzyme abundantly presents in the liver and intestine, is able to catalyze the oxidation of hypoxanthine, xanthine and then to acid uric, with the involvement in a catabolic sequence of purine metabolism in humans (Ojha et al., 2017).

Gout management recommends a limitation of the acute inflammatory symptoms, recurrent prevention and reduction of the chronic complications in joints, kidneys or other affected sites as well as achievement of a target serum urate level for all patients (Rees, Hui, & Doherty, 2014). The acute gouty treatment has four therapeutic options including colchicine, corticosteroids, non-steroidal anti-inflammatory drugs (NSAIDs) and analgesics. NSAIDs are not only effectively treated acute attacks but also generally used for patients who have no complications such as piroxicam, indomethacin, ketoprofen, ibuprofen and sulindac. Corticosteroids, indicated orally, intravenously, intramuscularly or intraarticular, are also effective therapy of acute flares with minimal side effects as triamcinolone hexacetonide, triamcinolone acetonide or methylprednisolone. Colchicine, known as a pharmacologically active component obtained from roots of *Colchicum autumnale*, is administered widely for the treatment of gout. However, the use of colchicine also induces several gastrointestinal side effects such as diarrhea, nausea and vomiting (Sarawate et al., 2006).

Medicinal plants have been showed may decrease the development of the various disease, including gout. Many studies were carried out to investigate the effect of medicinal plant extracts on gout and to isolate and identify their bioactive compounds. These compounds, including alkaloids, flavonoids, saponins polyphenols, sterols and triterpenes, have shown various beneficial pharmacology activities such as anti-inflammatory, and antioxidant, anti-XO enzyme (Bansal, Gupta, Singh, & Chaudhary, 2010). Some compounds such as colchicine, resveratrol curcumin, epigallocatechin-3-gallate, quercetin, luteolin have been administered in individuals with Gout's disease and provided positive results. Below we will summarize relevant medicinal plants and bioactive compounds are used for the treatment of gout.

2. MEDICINAL PLANTS ARE USED FOR THE TREATMENT OF GOUT WITH XO INHIBITORY ACTIVITY IN THE WORLD

Many researchers have tried to find out medicinal plants that may be a potential candidate for the treatment of gout base on inhibitory XO enzyme. Fazleen I. Abu Bakar has reviewed 85 Malaysian anti-gout plants which possess significant inhibition of XO activity with higher proportions, especially, *Cinnamomum cassia, Momordica charantia, Kaempferia galanga, Morinda elliptica, Artemisia vulgaris* and *Chrysanthemum indicum*, by the presence of their varied active phytoconstituents such as coumarins, flavonoids, apigenin, luteolin and tannin (Abu Bakar et al., 2018). Azmi has also studied natural products in Malaysia as remedies inspired by the local folks for gout treatment and found that *Carica papaya* aqueous leave extract effectively prevents the activity of XO enzyme (Azmi, Jamal, & Amid, 2012). Kong et al., have evaluated 122 different Chinese plants based on clinical applications of traditional administrations for the improvement of gout as well as some diseases related to increased urate concentration as potent XO inhibitors. They have found that the most promising plants are *Chrysanthemum indicum (Asteraceae), Polygonum cuspidatum (Polygonaceae), Cinnamomum cassia (Lauraceae) and Lycopus europaeus (Lamiatae)* which show the strongest inhibition of the XO enzyme (Kong, Cai, Huang, Cheng, & Tan, 2000). Mai Thanh Thi Nguyen evaluated 288 herbal extracts, obtained from 96 species used as traditional therapies for gout in Vietnam, among them, *Chrysanthemum sinense, Artemisia vulgaris, Blumea balsamifera, Caesalpinia sappan* and *Tetracera scandens* reduced significantly XO activity with IC_{50} below 20 µg/ml. They furthermore reviewed the concentration-dependent inhibitory effect on this enzyme of some bioactive components from *Chrysanthemum sinense* flower extract, namely, caffeic acid, 1,5-di-O-caffeoylquinic acid, eriodictyol and luteolin (Nguyen et al., 2004). Patrick et al. assayed 26 varied species, which belong to 18 different families, known as anti-gout agents for Indigenous people in America, among these plants, *Larix laricina* was the strongest XO inhibitor (Owen & Johns, 1999). Jaroslav Havlik conducted an *in vitro* study to investigate the XO inhibitions of 27 medicinal plants which were able to decrease the complicated symptoms of gout, rheumatism and arthritis as a traditional treatment in the Central-East Europe region and the Czech Republic. It was revealed that *Populus nigra* and *Betula pendula* had the highest inhibitory effect on XO, correlated with clinical data of phytotherapy in Central European region (Havlik et al., 2010). Karmella L. Apaya also studied several Philippine selected plants based on their anti-inflammation in herbal remedies, which might be associated with preventing XO activity; including *Antegonon leptopus, Adenanthena payonina, Blumea balsamifera, Calophyllum inophyllum, Cassia fistula, Cassia alata, Gliricidia sepium, Mimosa pudica, Michelia alba, Pogostemon cablin, Portulaca olercea, Solanum tornum, Vitex negundo* and *Tinosphora rumphii.* Among of studied species, *B. balsamifera* and *M. pudica* have highest XO inhibitory activity (Apaya & Chichioco-Hern, 2011). Yasser Bustanji investigated the eighteen Jordanian plants for pharmacological aspects against enzyme XO and then, found *Achillea fragrantissima* (Forssk.) Sch. Bip., *Origanum vulgare* L., *Origanum syriacum* L., *Pimpinella anisum* L. and *Hyoscyamus reticulatus* L., which might be potential for isolating new natural active components as XO effective inhibitors (Bustanji et al., 2011). Similarly, Agustin Yumita assayed XO inhibitory activity of 13 traditional plants that have been traditionally used in Indonesia for gout treatment. They found that *Woodfordia floribunda* has the greatest XO inhibitory activity (Yumita, Suganda, & Sukandar, 2013). Moreover, from the screening data on inhibitory XO enzyme activity, some medicinal plant has been deeper study the effect on the treatment of gout. Here we present in detail several valuable medicinal plants for gout treatment.

2.1 Acacia Confuse

Acacia confusa Merr. (Leguminosae) has been widely administered in South-East Asia and Taiwan folklore, containing many phytochemicals as phenolic compounds and their derivatives, flavonoids, flavonol glycoside have responsibility for its significant pharmacological properties, such as abilities to inhibit XO, semicarbazide-sensitive amine oxidase and angiotensin I converting enzyme, antioxidant and radical scavenging activity as well as prevention of hyperuricemia and inflammatory progress (Lin, Chang, & Chang, 2018). Yu-Tang Tung extensively carried out an *in vivo* experiment in hyperuricemic mice induced by potassium oxonate (PO) and reported the antihyperuricemic property of *Acacia confusa* heartwood extracts via significant reduction of serum uric acid concentrations after administration of these extracts as well as the presence of main constituents such as (−)-2,3-cis-3,4-cis-4′-methoxy-3,3′,4,7,8-pentahydroxyflavan, (−)-2,3-cis-3,4-cis-3,3′,4,4′,7,8-hexahydroxyflavan, okanin, transilitin and melanoxetin. All of them were able to strongly inhibit enzyme XO, especially, melanoxetin exhibited a more considerable inhibition in comparison with allopurinol (Tung & Chang, 2010; Tung et al., 2010).

2.2 Cinnamomum Cassia

Cinnamomum cassia bark or cinnamomi cortex, a common spice, is known as a traditional remedy for treating diarrhea, gastritis, immune-related diseases, cancer and diabetes as well as important ingredients in many prescriptions to enhance hyperuricemia and gout disorder in Chinese medicine. Woo-Young Shin showed that *Cinnamomum cassia* administration resulted in the improvement in the life of mice with septic shock induced by lipopolysaccharide or gout caused by monosodium urate as well as the inhibition of interleukin-1β (IL-1β) secretion via the reduction of inflammasome activities including AIM2, NLRC4 and NLRP3, concurrently, the attenuation of ASC oligomerization and its speck formation in cytosol (Shin et al., 2017). *Chrysanthemum indicum* is well-known in Korean and China as traditional therapy for hypertension, several inflammatory and infectious disorders. In addition, its flowers are also administered like herbal teas to treat headaches and eye diseases and present various pharmacological capabilities against oxidation and cancer. The combined extracts of *Cinnamomum cassia* and *Chrysanthemum indicum* have synergism antihyperuricemic effects compared to *Cinnamomum cassia* or *Chrysanthemum indicum* alone, which are evaluated by the significant reduction of uric acid concentrations in rats with normal conditions and hyperuricemia caused by PO as well as the increase in renal uric acid excretion in diseased rats. The main components of this mixture including o-methoxycinnamaldehyde, cinnamaldehyde, chlorogenic acid, trans-cinnamic acid, isochlorogenic acid and coumarin, show XO inhibitory activities in *in vitro* study (Y.-S. Lee et al., 2017).

2.3 Cinnamomum Osmophloeum

Cinnamomum osmophloeum belonging to genus Cinnamomum of family Lauraceae as indigenous cinnamon or pseudocinnamomum, has been widely used to cook or treat varied diseases like gout, arthritis, nerve pains, cold and relieve fever. Wang et al. reviewed that the *Cinnamomum osmophloeum* leaf oil exhibited remarkably XO inhibition and cinnamaldehyde, the major constituent in the *Cinnamomum osmophloeum* leaves, showed potent XO inhibition with an IC_{50} value of 8.4 μg/ml. Furthermore, hyperuricemic mice treated with cinnamaldehyde decreased the levels of uric acid in comparison with the hyperuricemic control mice (S. Wang et al., 2008).

2.4 Chatuphalatika Extract

Chatuphalatika is known as an herbal combination of the same parts of *Terminalia belerica* Linn. *T. Chebula, Phyllanthus emblica Linn* and *T. arjuna* (Roxb.) Wight & Arn. Vilasinee Hirunpanich Sato showed the capability against inflammation of this extract via the measure of inflammatory intermediary formation caused by LPS in RAW 264.7 macrophages, which was demonstrated by the significant downregulation of iNOS and TNF-α gene expression. An *in vivo* study reviewed that Chatuphalatika extracts presented as a noncompetitive XO inhibitor and its oral administration at a dose of 1000 mg/kg resulted in the efficacious suppression of uric acid generation by XO inhibition in the liver as well as the decrease in plasma uric acid concentrations in hyperuricemic mouse induced by oxonate (Sato et al., 2018).

2.5 Dimocarpus Longan

Dimocarpus longan Lour., an evergreen fruit tree that belongs to the Sapindaceae family, is native to temperate and tropical Asia and widely grows in Southeast Asia and Southern China. *Dimocarpus longan* contains many phenolic components, which provide this plant have many therapeutic activities as antifungal, antimicrobial, anti-inflammatory, antioxidant, antiobesity, hypolipidemic, antifatigue, anticancer, antitumor, neuroprotective, immunomodulatory, anti-tyrosinase, memory-ameliorating and urate-decreasing effect. Shi-Yuan Sheu et al., isolated ten components from longan flower, such as corilagin, geraniin, chebulinic acid, gallic acid, chebulagic acid, protocatechuic acid, acetonylgeraniin A, (-)-epicatechin, proanthocyanidin A2 and procyanidin B2; and showed these compounds had strong *in vitro* XO inhibition. Furthermore, the *Dimocarpus longan* extract at a dose of 50–100 mg/kg markedly decreased plasma uric acid concentrations in hyperuricemic mice (Sheu et al., 2016).

2.6 Dioscorea Collettii

Dioscorea collettii has been frequently used in China as a therapeutic folklore for improving inflammatory symptoms related to hyperuricemia and gouty arthritis. It was also reported that total saponin isolated from *Dioscorea* (TSD) possessed several considerable effects as analgesic, anti-hyperuricemia and anti-inflammation. Keeping in view the pharmacological potential of *Dioscorea* saponin, Guang-Liang Chen et al, experimented on hyperuricemic rats and then showed that total saponin from this plant significantly reduces the concentrations of uric acid in plasma as well as the activities of serum and hepatic XO enzyme, concurrently, increase the urine uric acid levels and the excretion of 24-hour total uric acid (G.-L. Chen, Wei, & Xu, 2006). For a similar purpose, Lu Wang conducted an *in vitro* study on inflammatory THP-1 macrophages caused by MSU crystals. The results revealed that TSD was able to reduce the concentrations of inflammatory cytokines created by THP-1 cells such as IL-1β, IL-18 and TNF-α and the significant number of NALP3 proteins as well as apoptosis-related speck-like, which played prominent roles in the NALP3 inflammasome aggregation. In addition, TSD treatment exhibited the reduction of proteins related to NALP3 inflammasome in rotenone caused THP-1 cells and suppressed caspase-1 activity as well as the stimulation of rotenone-caused NALP3 inflammasome in THP-1 macrophages (L. Wang, Zhu, Duan, Li, & Chen, 2020).

2.7 Hibiscus Sabdariffa

Hibiscus sabdariffa Linn. (roselle) belongs to the Malvaceae family and has enormous promise in pharmacological effects due to the presence of various phytochemicals like polysaccharides, organic acids, polyphenols and anthocyanins (Riaz & Chopra, 2018). The *Hibiscus sabdariffa* have been used in Indonesian traditional therapy for hyperuricemia status. Sri Wahyuningsih et al. reported that the water fraction of *Hibiscus sabdariffa* at doses 37.5 and 75 mg/kg bw and ethyl acetate at doses 6.25 and 12.5 mg/kg bw was effective as an anti-hyperuricemic agent. The ethanol extract of *Hibiscus sabdariffa* and its fraction had a uricosuric effect similar to probenecid (S Wahyuningsih, Sukandar, & Sukrasno, 2016). Moreover, the ethanol extract, water and ethyl acetate fractions also had strong inhibitory XO enzyme activity (Sri Wahyuningsih & Sukandar, 2016). Chih-Yi Kuo showed that the treatment with *Hibiscus sabdariffa* extracts inhibited oxonic acid –caused hyperuricemia, with a greater uric acid, decreased effect than allopurinol administration. They also indicated that *Hibiscus sabdariffa* extract effectively suppressed oxonic acid-induced hyperuricemia by decreasing uric acid and stimulating uricase activity but not by interacting with XO (Kuo et al., 2012). Vitoon Prasongwatana has studied the uricosuric effect of *Hibiscus sabdariffa* in a human model with nine subjects with no history of renal stones and nine with a history of renal stones. Their results showed that the mean levels of uric acid clearance and excretion and fractional excretion of uric acid were all enhanced significantly after the intake of *Hibiscus sabdariffa* tea (Prasongwatana, Woottisin, Sriboonlue, & Kukongviriyapan, 2008).

2.8 Jatropha Isabellei

Jatropha isabellei Müll Arg. (Euphorbiaceae) has been used as a South American therapeutic folklore for symptomatic enhancement of gout and other arthritic diseases. Cássia R.Silva showed that *Jatropha isabellei* crude extract and a rich alkaloid fraction was able to ameliorate inflammatory and hypouricemic status, which resulted from the prevention of neutrophil infiltration, mechanical allodynia, edema and thermal hyperalgesia in rats injected intra-articularly MSU (Silva et al., 2013). Moreover, another *in vivo* study of Janaina Kieling Fröhlich on acute arthritis mouse model reviewed the antiedematogenic and antinociceptive potential after both oral and intravenous administrations of *Jatropha isabellei,* which might be presented by terpenes detected in this plant, especially diterpene jatrophone (Fröhlich et al., 2017).

2.9 Legumes

Chrysoula Spanou has assayed the flavonoids in Legumes for the XO inhibitory potential and published pharmacological features as XO inhibitors of the fractions obtained from both *Lotus edulis* and *Vicia faba* extracts with IC_{50} values ranging from 40–135 μg/mL and 55–260 μg/mL, respectively. XO enzyme was inhibited by all phenolic compounds, which gave Ki values in the range of 13–767 μM. Ten compounds acted as non-competitive inhibitors, meanwhile, one of them exhibited competitive inhibition. Their results indicated that flavonoids extracted from legume plants might be a novel source for possible XO inhibitors (Spanou et al., 2012).

2.10 Lychnophora Species

Lychnophora species, the Brazil folk medicinal herb, have been used for symptomatic treatments of inflammation, rheumatism and bruise and contain many active plants namely *Lychnophoriopsis candelabrum, Lychnophora ericoides, Lychnophora trichocarpha* and *Lychnophora staavioides,* all of them showed excellent XO inhibitory activity (Ferraz Filha, Vitolo, Fietto, & Lombardi, 2006). Ana Catharina Fernandes reviewed that sesquiterpene lactones detected in these species such as goyazensolide, eremantholide C and lychnopholide possessed hyperuricemic property in mice with effective mechanims based on XO inhibition in liver and uricosuric effect (Bernardes, Coelho, & Araújo, 2019). Maíra Ribeirode Souza that the ethanolic extract and ethyl acetate fraction of *Lychnophora trichocarpha, as well as its major bioactive constituents including apigenin, luteolin, eremantholide C, lupeol* and *lychnopholide,* had promised in hypouricemic and inflammatory activities due to the significant decrease in urate levels and the strong hepatic XO inhibition. Especially, an *in vivo* study was conducted to evaluate XO inhibitory potential of apigenin (de Souza et al., 2012).

2.11 Mangifera Indica

Mangifera indica L. *(M. indica)*, a major tropical fruit originated from Asia, has been widely used for anti-inflammatory, anticancer, antidiabetic, antihyperlipidemic, antioxidant, antifungal, antibacterial, anthelmintic, hepatoprotective, gastroprotective, antiplasmodial and immunomodulatory purposes. It was reported that *Mangifera indica* and its ethanol extract might be a promising agent for clinical application as a symptomatic therapy for gouty arthritis due to inhibitory effects on expression of IL-1β and TNF-α in the synovial tissues. Oral administration of *Mangifera indica* extract at the doses of 100 and 200 mg/kg for 9 days could reduce swelling in the diseased ankle as well as the levels of synovial protein, IL-1β mRNA and TNF-α caused by MSU (Y. Jiang, You, Fu, & Yin, 2012). Mangiferin, a glucosyl xanthone extracted from *Mangifera indica* leaves, could inhibit XO activity associated with hypouricemic potential, leading to reduce plasma urate concentrations in a dose and time-dependent manner, concurrently, enhance renal urate levels and fractional excretion of uric acid in hyperuricemic mice treated with mangiferin. Interestingly, the suppression of protein and mRNA expression related to downregulating renal urate transporters such as glucose transporter 9 (GLUT9), renal urate-anion transporter 1 (URAT1), organic anion transporter 10 (OAT10) after mangiferin administration might be responsible for urate excretory promotion by inhibiting urate absorption (H. Yang et al., 2015).

2.12 Morinda Citrifolia

Morinda citrifolia L. is a medicinal plant which is known as a natural nutritional food supplement worldwide for centuries. The fruit of *Morinda citrifolia* plant has a history of use in the pharmacopeias of pacific islands and south East Asia. Several phytoconstituents have been isolated from *Morinda citrifolia* containing polysaccharides amino acids, lignans, anthraquinones, flavonoids, coumarins, iridoids, and fatty acids. *Morinda citrifolia* has promised in alternative medicine for different kind of disorders such as arthritis, diabetes, blood vessel problems, high blood pressure, heart disease, muscle aches and pains, menstrual irregularities, mental depression, headache, cancers, sprains, gastric ulcer, senility, arteriosclerosis, poor digestion, and drug addiction (Pawlus & Kinghorn, 2007). *Morinda citrifolia* extract reduced XO concentration-dependently. Concentrations of 1 and 5 mg/mL *Morinda citrifolia* extract inhibited XO in vitro by 184% and 159%, respectively. Inhibition XO enzymes of *Morinda citrifolia* is the mechanism to explain the ameliorates of gout and gout-like diseases (Palu, Deng, West, & Jensen, 2009).

2.13 Momordica Charantia

Momordica charantia has many pharmacological properties including laxative, antidiabetic, anthelmintic, abortifacient, antimalarial and contraceptive and is applied to treat gout, dysmenorrhea, leprosy, eczema, galactagogue, jaundice, emmenagogue, kidney (stone). *Momordica charantia* extract has the presence of various biologically active chemicals that include fixed oils, glycosides, alkaloids, saponins, triterpenes, steroids and proteins. Intisar Reehem Alsultanee showed that *Momordica charantia* extract possessed prominent therapeutic properties and can be exploited as drug candidate to treat diseases associated with free radical formation, oxidative stress and XO activity such as gout (Alsultanee, Ewadh, & Mohammed, 2014).

2.14 Phyllanthus Niruri

Based on the use of *Phyllanthus niruri* Linn. (Euphorbiaceae) (*P. niruri*) in South America as a medicinal herb for treating excess uric acid, Vikneswaran Murugaiyah investigated the anti-hyperuricemic effect of methanol leaf extracts from this plant on hyperuricemic rats induced by uric acid and PO. Also, they isolated several bioactive constituents, such as hypophyllanthin phyltetralin, phyllanthin and lignans, which had responsibility for the significant enhancement of uric acid levels in plasma towards physiological conditions with a dose-dependent manner, when compared to that of probenecid, allopurinol and benzbromarone used widely in clinical therapy for gout and hyperuricemia (Murugaiyah & Chan, 2006). Furthermore, the treatment by *Phyllanthus niruri* showed *in vitro* XO inhibition as well as a moderate *in vivo* inhibitory activity against this enzyme. Additionally, the intraperitoneal administration with *Phyllanthus niruri* methanol extracts and their active compounds resulted in the higher excretion and clearance of urinary uric acid in comparison with increased uric acid control rats (Murugaiyah & Chan, 2009).

2.15 Pistacia Integerrima

Pistacia integerrima Stew ex. Brandis has widely used in commonly dispensed traditional dosage forms. Naseem Saud Ahmad has investigated the XO inhibitory activity assay in vitro and fructose-induced hyperuricemic animal model to assess the serum uric acid lowering effect by this plant. They found that n-BuOH and EtOAc fraction of this plant showed strong XO inhibitory activity. In addition, ethyl acetate extract had a dose-dependent uric acid-lowering effect in hyperuricemic mice (Ahmad, Farman, Najmi, Mian, & Hasan, 2008).

2.16 Salvia Miltiorrhiza

Salvia miltiorrhiza is a well-known as Chinese herb frequently used in traditional therapy for the treatment of stroke and other cardiovascular disorders, as well as the blood circulative promotion, anti- platelet aggregation, anti-cancer, antioxidant and antiviral. Also, *Salvia miltiorrhiza* has therapeutic effects on gouty-related symptoms, which is demonstrated by the competitive XO inhibition of magnesium lithospermate B isolated from this plant. Interestingly, this pharmacological phytoconstituent also presented the hypouricemic capability in mouse model with PO- caused hyperuricemia through the remarkable reduction of urate concentrations in plasma compared to the hyperuricemia control at different doses of 10, 20 and 30 mg/kg (X. Liu, Chen, Shang, Jiao, & Huang, 2009). For the same purpose of treating gouty-associated disorders, Xinlin Wu investigated the therapeutic potential of another main compound from *Salvia miltiorrhiza,* tanshinone IIA, in rat model with uric acid- caused nephropathy. They demonstrated similar therapeutic properties of tanshinone IIA as allopurinol as well as the effects on renal production and anti-inflammation in a dose-dependent manner. Moreover, both *in vitro* and *in vivo* studies showed that the overproduction of IL-1β and MCP-1 caused by urate and the translocation of NF-κB from cytosome to nucleus was inhibited by this natural compound. Therefore, tanshinone IIA could be a promising candidate for the improvement of kidney dysfunction induced by uric acid in rats via inflammatory attenuation (X. Wu et al., 2012). Another study of Hongjin Tang et al. reported that several active phytochemicals from *Salvia miltiorrhiza* interacted with XO in the active binding site called the molybdenum-pterin center domain. Especially, Salvianolic acid C, a potent XO inhibitor, enhanced significantly the hyperuricemic status in mice models caused by PO (Tang, Yang, Li, Li, & Chen, 2016).

2.17 Selaginella Labordei

Selaginella labordei Hieron, a plant from Selaginella genus, Selaginellaceae, is an herbal medicine treating hepatitis B and gout in China. The extract of *Selaginella labordei* showed inhibitory activities against XO enzyme. Wen-Jie Tan et al., have isolated four flavone compounds from the effective fractions inhibiting XO of *Selaginella labordei* and the structures were elucidated as 4'-methylether robustaflavone, robustaflavone, eriodictyol and amentoflavone. All of these compounds could strongly inhibit XO enzyme (Tan, Xu, Li, & Chen, 2009).

2.18 Selaginella Moellendorffii

Selaginella moellendorffii Hieron, which belongs to the family Selaginellaceae, is a traditional Chinese folk herb with extremely abundant resources. It has been used as an ethnic drug for the treatment of bleeding and chronic inflammation, such as arthritis, gonorrhea, hepatitis, and mastitis. Ping Zhao evaluated the effects of *Selaginella moellendorffii* on gouty arthritis and showing an insight of the possible mechanisms. *Selaginella moellendorffii* aqueous extract has proved to be active in reducing hyperuricemia in a dose-dependent manner, and the levels of blood urea nitrogen and creatinine in high dose group were decreased significantly as compared with hyperuricemic control group. The high dose of *Selaginella moellendorffii* extract could significantly prevent the paw swelling, reduce gouty joint inflammatory features, reduce the release of IL-1β and TNF-α, lower malondialdehyde and myeloperoxidase levels, and increase superoxide dismutase level in a gouty arthritis rat model (Zhao, Chen, Zhang, Deng, & Li, 2017).

2.19 Smilax Riparia

Inspired by the effective gouty and hyperuricemic treatment of the stem and roots of *Smilax riparia* in Chinese medicine, Xiao-Hui Wu conducted an *in vivo* experiment on mouse with hyperuricemia to evaluate a promising uricosuric ability of pallidifloside D via the reduction of GLUT9 and renal mURAT1, leading to the increased excretion of uric acid associated with improvement of renal damage caused by a high level of serum uric acid (X.-H. Wu, Ruan, Zhang, Wang, & Zhang, 2014).

2.20 Smilax China

Smilax china L., a traditional Chinese medicine, which is frequently used for the improvement of diuretic and rheumatic arthritic conditions, as well as for detoxication, and to treat gout, lumbago, tumors, and inflammatory diseases. *Smilax china* contains glycoside, saponin, tannin, fat, smilacin, sugar, coloring matter, gum, starch and cinchonin and it exhibits anti-inflammatory, anti-psoriatic, diuretic, digestive and anti-diabetic, properties (Bhati, Singh, Saharan, Ram, & Bhandari, 2011). Lvyi Chen showed that the orally administration of *Smilax china* presented stronger anti-hyperuricemic potential in hyperuricemic mice. Moreover, *Smilax china* extract markedly reversed the serum uric acid level, fractional excretion of urate and blood urea nitrogen to their normal states, and prevented the renal dysfunction against tubulointerstitial pathologies in hyperuricemic rats. Rutin, caffeic acid, oxyresveratrol and resveratrol extracted from *Smilax china* showed different inhibitory activities on XO in vitro, and exhibited competitive or mixed inhibitory actions (Lvyi Chen et al., 2011). Their data were in agreement with Lee, Sang-Il (S.-I. Lee et al., 2014). Xiao-Hui Wu et al., also observed that the total saponins of *Smilax riparia*, which belongs the same family Smilacaceae of *Smilax china*, could down-regulate renal mURAT1, resulting in the enhancement of urate excretion in the kidney of potassium oxonate-induced hyperuricemic mice (X.-H. Wu, Yu, Zhang, Anderson, & Zhang, 2014). Moreover, anti-hyperuricemia effects of allopurinol are improved by Smilax riparia coadministration. Xiao-Hui Wu showed that compared with allopurinol alone, the combination of allopurinol and SRS significantly decreased the level of uric acid, creatinine, XO, mURAT1, mGLUT9 and mOAT1 in a hyperuricemic mouse model (X.-H. Wu et al., 2015).

2.21 Stauntonia Brachyanthera

Stauntonia brachyanthera, which belongs the family of Lardizabalaceae, has been used in traditional for arthralgia syndrome and rheumatism arthritis in the south-east of China. Xuan-li Liu has isolated several nor-oleanane triterpenoids. These nor-oleanane triterpenoids exhibited inhibitory activities on XO and their potential possibilities as the candidate compounds for the treatment of gout (X.-l. Liu, Li, & Meng, 2016).

2.22 Vitex Negundo

Vitex negundo, an ethnobotanical plant, has valuable therapeutic properties due to the antimicrobial, anti-oxidant, anticancer, anti-inflammatory and antidiabetic exhibition of various active components obtained from volatile oils of different plant parts such as lignans, terpenes, flavonoids, steroids and iridoids. In addition, *Vitex negundo* plays an important role in modulating cellular mechanisms like menstrual cycle, cell cycle, apoptosis, polycystic ovary disease and motility of sperms (Tandon, 2005). Umamaheswari studied the hypouricaemic capability of different fractions from *Vitex negundo* hydromethanolic leaf extract and then, which were investigated by a considerable decrease in plasma urate concentrations and activities against XO enzyme in mice with hyperuricemic symptoms (Umamaheswari, Asokkumar, Sudalaivelmurugiah, Sivashnmugam, & Subhadradevi, 2009).

3 NATURAL PRODUCT COMPOUND FOR THE TREATMENT OF GOUT

3.1 Colchicine

Colchicine, an efficacious phytoconstituent isolated from plants of the genus *Colchicum (autumn crocus),* has been widely used for gouty treatment because of its important effects on the management of acute gouty arthritis with low-dose administration demonstrated in clinical experiments.

3.2 Curcumin

Turmeric of *Curcuma longa,* a rhizomatous perennial plant belongs to the ginger family, Zingiberaceae. The active phytochemicals are curcuminoids, such as curcumin, demethoxycurcumin and bis-demethoxyc-urcumin (Aggarwal, Sundaram, Malani, & Ichikawa, 2007; Upadhyaya, Kesharwani & Misra, 2009;

Kesharwani & Misra, 2011). Curcuminoids has anti-inflammatory, antioxidant, antitumor, antibacterial activities, etc (Singh et al., 2013; Carvalho, Gomes, Pereira-Wilson, & Lima, 2016; Jiang et al., 2017). Turmeric nanoparticles have been showed in vivo anti-gout activity in mice model by reduced the joint diameter and significantly reduced biochemical parameters, including cholesterol, triglycerides, low-density lipoprotein, urea, uric acid, and creatinine, alanine aminotransferase, and aspartate aminotransferase (Mustafa Kiyani et al., 2019; Kesharwani et al., 2020). Baofeng Chen reported that curcumin had the enormous ability to degrade IκBα and stimulate NF-κB signaling pathway, concurrently, expression of NF-κB downstream genes related to inflammation such as COX-2, IL-6, IL-1β, PGE2 and TNF-α in the MSU-promoted THP-1-derived macrophages. Treatment with curcumin also presented the inhibitory effect on MSU-induced mitochondrial dysfunction in RAW264.7 and THP-1 cells via activities as NLRP3 inflammasome inhibitor resulting from suppressing mitochondrial membrane potential decrease as well as mitochondria ROS (Singh et al., 2013; Kesharwani et al., 2015; Chen et al., 2019). James W. Daily has reviewed the randomized clinical trials to provide scientific evidence that supports the use of turmeric and its curcumin-enriched (about 1000 mg/day of curcumin) for treating arthritis (Daily, Yang, & Park, 2016). Gui-Zhen Ao has synthesized a series of curcumin derivatives as potent dual inhibitors of XO and URAT1 which can be served as anti-hyperuricemic agents. These compounds proved efficient effects on anti-hyperuricemic activity and uricosuric activity *in vivo* (Ao et al., 2017).

3.3 Epigallocatechin-3-Gallate

Epigallocatechin-3-gallate (EGCG), a major constituent of green tea catechin, has been used for antioxidants. Chuang Zhu showed that EGCG exhibited a decrease in the serum uric acid and serum creatinine level in manner dose-dependence, reduction of hepatic adenosine deaminase and XO activities in mice treated high EGCG dose compared to control mice group, accompanied with downregulation of renal mRNA expression related to concentrations of GLUT9 and URAT1 on mice with increased uric acid levels (C. Zhu et al., 2018). The nucleotide-binding oligomerization domain (NOD)-like receptor (NLR) family pyrin domain containing 3 (NLRP3) inflammasome is responsible for the gout inflammatory symptoms induced by monosodium urate crystal. Hye Eun Lee showed that EGCG inhibited caspase-1 and IL-1β formation in mouse macrophages, which indicated its inhibitory effect on NLRP3 inflammasome is responsible for inflammation in gout disorder caused by MSU crystals. Another *in vivo* study on acute gouty rat model showed that mice with oral EGCG administration exhibited fewer inflammatory signals in MSU-caused gouty foot tissues, concurrently, inhibited de novo mitochondrial DNA synthesis and ROS formation in mouse macrophages associated with NLRP3 inflammasome suppression (H. E. Lee et al., 2019). Chen also showed that EGCG attenuates UA-induced injury in NRK-49F cells by up-regulation of miR-9 and might by inactivation of NF-κB and JAK-STAT signal pathways (LL Chen & Xu, 2018). Fang Li demonstrated that EGCG significantly reduced the high level of serum uric acid and inhibited XOD activity in the serum and liver tissues; EGCG significantly increased OAT1 expression in the kidney tissues and decreased GLUT9 expression in rats induced hyperuricemia by oxonic acid potassium salt combined with ethylamine pyrimidine (Fang Li, Liu, Xie, Liu, & Zou, 2020). Ohishi Tomokazu also reviewed favorable suppressive effects on inflammatory diseases based on the capability of EGCG/ green tea against nuclear factor-κB activation via antioxidant mechanisms related to ROS scavengers (Ohishi, Goto, Monira, Isemura, & Nakamura, 2016).

3.4 Luteolin

Luteolin is a natural flavonoid found in a variety of plants with a variety of pharmacological activities such as anti-inflammatory, anti-oxidation, immune regulation, angiogenesis and neuroprotection (El-Raey, Ibrahim, & Eldahshan, 2013). Jiakai Yan et al., have shown that luteolin exhibits a significant inhibitory activity on XO in a competitive manner (Yan, Zhang, Hu, & Ma, 2013). Moreover, Rui-Ming Shen reported the anti-inflammatory effect of luteolin on rats with acute gout arthritis. Luteolin improved the ankle swelling index of rats with acute gout arthritis, and significantly down-regulated the levels of IL-1β, IL-17, TNF-α, IL-6 in acute gout arthritis rats induced by monosodium urate (Shen, Zhong, & Li, 2019). Yan Lin also demonstrated that the two flavones, luteolin and luteolin-4′-O-glucoside, possess a potent effect in hyperuricemia mice by decreasing the level of mURAT1 and inhibiting XO activity, which contributes to enhancing uric acid excretion and improving hyperuricemia-induced renal dysfunction. In addition, luteolin and luteolin-4′-O-glucoside also alleviated paw swelling and inflammation induced by monosodium urate crystals (Y. Lin et al., 2018).

3.5 Quercetin

Quercetin is one of the most abundant flavonoids in the daily diet and can be a potent nutritional supplement for inhibiting gout and peroxidative damage (Keservani et al., 2010; Kesharwani et al., 2019). Quercetin could inhibit reversibly the formation of uric acid and superoxide radicals (O_2-) catalyzed by XO in a mixed-type manner (Zhang, Wang, Zhang, & Gong, 2018). Kenji et al., have studied the anti-inflammatory and analgesic abilities of quercetin in monosodium urate crystal-induced gout arthritis in mice. They found that quercetin inhibited monosodium urate -induced mechanical hyperalgesia, superoxide anion formation, leukocyte recruitment, inflammasome components mRNA expression, TNFα and IL-1β production, inflammasome stimulation, a decrease of antioxidants levels and NFκB activation (Ruiz-Miyazawa et al., 2017). Moreover, the combination between quercetin and rutin also reduce serum urate levels in hyperuricemic mice induced by oxonate, may be explained by the inhibition of XDH/XO activities in mouse liver (J. X. Zhu, Wang, Kong, Yang, & Zhang, 2004). Jingqun Huang also found that quercetin treatment attenuated edema in a dose-dependent manner and decreased histological signs of acute inflammation on MSU crystal-induced inflammation in rats. In addition, quercetin treatment suppressed leucocyte recruitment, decreased chemokine levels, decreased levels of the lipid peroxidation end-product malondialdehyde, and increased antioxidant enzyme activity in treated gouty arthritis rats (Huang et al., 2012). In a clinical trial, Synytsia showed that quercetin has a positive result in patients with hyperuricemia. Patients with gout and hypertension received quercetin: 2 grams 3 times per day during 6 weeks, and after that with 2 grams per night, for a further 12 weeks. Quercetin significantly reduces the level of the uric acid level and can reduce systolic BP to 6.3% and diastolic - to 11.5% without adding or increasing the dose of antihypertensive drugs (Synytsia, 2016). Yuanlu Shi et al., have shown the effects of 4 weeks of oral supplementation of quercetin on plasma uric acid, blood pressure and fasting glucose in healthy males. The intervention included one tablet containing 500 mg quercetin daily for 4 weeks could reduce elevated plasma uric acid concentrations without affecting fasting glucose, urinary excretion of uric acid or blood pressure (Y. Shi & Williamson, 2016).

3.6 Resveratrol

Resveratrol, a polyphenolic component belongs to stilbenes group, is found in the skin of grapes, red wine and other nuts or fruits (Bhat, Kosmeder, & Pezzuto, 2001) and possesses prominent therapeutic features including cardiovascular protection, serum glucose decrease, antioxidant, anti-inflammation, anti-cancer as well as neuroprotection (Fei Li, Gong, Dong, & Shi, 2012). Additionally, this natural active compound displays effective activities as ROS scavengers, increase in the level of gluthatione and amelioration of antioxidant endogenous (Kumar, Naidu, Seghal, & Padi, 2006). Resveratrol has a potent antioxidant by scavenging ROS, increasing gluthatione level and improving the antioxidant endogenous. Haiyan Chen et al., have shown that resveratrol could reduce the gouty arthritis. They demonstrated that resveratrol inhibited articular inflammation in gouty arthritis- mice induced by MSU and down-regulation of serum uric acid in hyperuricemia-Kunming mice induced by yeast polysaccharide and potassium oxonate (H. Chen et al., 2016). Yun-Wei Shi et al., also showed that stilbenes, including resveratrol, trans-4-hydroxystilbene, pterostilbene, polydatin, and mulberroside A have antihyperuricemic activities in Potassium oxonate-induced hyperuricemic mice. They have indicated that the number and position, methoxylation and glycosylation of hydroxyl groups in these trans-stilbenes were required for their effects (Y. W. Shi et al., 2012). Moreover, Qi-Bin Yang showed the anti-inflammatory potiential via downregulation of SIRT1 mRNA and protein levels in peripheral blood mononuclear from gouty individuals when compared to healthy controls. Also, resveratrol treatment with a dose-dependent manner produced the downregulation of SIRT1 protein concentrations in blood mononuclear cells from individuals with intercritical gout caused by MSU crytals, accompanied by the amelioration of inflammatory cytokine release and stimulation of MSU-induced autophagy. In addition, the mRNA levels of NLR family pyrin domain containing 3 and NF-κB p65 were regulated by resveratrol (Q.-B. Yang, He, Zhong, Xie, & Zhou, 2019). Hongmei Li also showed that resveratrol could act as TAK1 inhibitor related to MAPK and NF-Kb pathways, which contributed to the therapeutic potential for gout disease (H. Li et al., 2019). Wang P et al. reviewed that concurrent use of resveratrol and sodium alginate were able to be more effective acute gouty treatment than colchicine in mice, which was explained by the remarkable decrease in symovial levels of CXCL10, IL-1β and CCR5 in comparison with colchicine administration. Additionally, the obvious reduction of NLRP3 expression in synovial tissues resulted from treatment with resveratrol in the presense or absence of sodium alginate (P. Wang et al., 2015).

4. CONCLUSION

Medicinal plants have been shown may be applied to reduce signals and towards the treatment of gouts. The main chemical compounds such as resveratrol, quercetin, curcumin epigallocatechin-3-gallate, luteolin have shown a strong effect against gout. Therefore, it is necessary to study deeper details about medicinal plants and find new bioactive compounds against gout disease.

Abbreviation

MSU: monosodium urate; XO: xanthine oxidase; NLRP3: (NOD)-like receptor (NLR) family pyrin domain containing 3; URAT1: renal urate-anion transporter 1; OAT1: organic anion transporter 1; GLUT9: glucose transporter 9; TNF-α: tumor necrosis factor α; IL-1β: Interleukin 1 beta; ROS: Reactive oxygen species; EGCG: Epigallocatechin-3-gallate; CCR5: chemokine receptor type 5; CXCL10: C–X–C motif chemokine 10 (CXCL10) (interferon γ-induced protein 10); TAK1: Transforming growth factor beta-activated kinase 1; NF-κB: Nuclear factor kappa-light-chain-enhancer of activated B; MAPK: Mitogen-activated protein kinase.

REFERENCES

Abu Bakar, F. I., Abu Bakar, M. F., Rahmat, A., Abdullah, N., Sabran, S. F., & Endrini, S. (2018). Anti-gout potential of Malaysian medicinal plants. *Frontiers in Pharmacology*, *9*, 261. doi:10.3389/fphar.2018.00261 PMID:29628890

Aggarwal, B. B., Sundaram, C., Malani, N., & Ichikawa, H. (2007). *Curcumin: the Indian solid gold. In The molecular targets and therapeutic uses of curcumin in health and disease*. Springer. doi:10.1007/978-0-387-46401-5

Ahmad, N. S., Farman, M., Najmi, M. H., Mian, K. B., & Hasan, A. (2008). Pharmacological basis for use of Pistacia integerrima leaves in hyperuricemia and gout. *Journal of Ethnopharmacology*, *117*(3), 478–482. doi:10.1016/j.jep.2008.02.031 PMID:18420362

Alsultanee, I. R., Ewadh, M. J., & Mohammed, M. F. (2014). Novel natural anti gout medication extract from Momdica Charantia. *J Nat Sci Res*, *4*(17), 16–23.

Ao, G.-Z., Zhou, M.-Z., Li, Y.-Y., Li, S.-N., Wang, H.-N., Wan, Q.-W., Li, H.-Q., & Hu, Q.-H. (2017). Discovery of novel curcumin derivatives targeting xanthine oxidase and urate transporter 1 as anti-hyperuricemic agents. *Bioorganic & Medicinal Chemistry*, *25*(1), 166–174. doi:10.1016/j.bmc.2016.10.022 PMID:28340987

Apaya, K. L., & Chichioco-Hern, C. L. (2011). Xanthine oxidase inhibition of selected Philippine medicinal plants. *Journal of Medicinal Plants Research*, *5*(2), 289–292.

Azmi, S., Jamal, P., & Amid, A. (2012). Xanthine oxidase inhibitory activity from potential Malaysian medicinal plant as remedies for gout. *International Food Research Journal*, *19*(1), 159.

Bansal, P., Gupta, V., Singh, R., & Chaudhary, A. K. (2010). Pharmacological potential of medicinal plant used in treatment of gout. *Drug Invention Today, 2*(10).

Bernardes, A. C. F. P. F., Coelho, G. B., Araújo, M. C. P. M., & Saúde-Guimarães, D. A. (2019). In vivo anti-hyperuricemic activity of sesquiterpene lactones from Lychnophora species. *Revista Brasileira de Farmacognosia*, *29*(2), 241–245. doi:10.1016/j.bjp.2018.12.008

Bhat, K. P., Kosmeder, J. W. II, & Pezzuto, J. M. (2001). Biological effects of resveratrol. *Antioxidants & Redox Signaling*, *3*(6), 1041–1064. doi:10.1089/152308601317203567 PMID:11813979

Bhati, R., Singh, A., Saharan, V. A., Ram, V., & Bhandari, A. (2011). Pharmacognostical standardization, extraction and anti-diabetic activity of Smilax china L. rhizome. *Asian Journal of Traditional Medicines*, *6*(5), 218–223.

Bustanji, Y., Hudaib, M., Tawaha, K., Mohammad, M., Almasri, I., Hamed, S., & Oran, S. (2011). In vitro xanthine oxidase inhibition by selected Jordanian medicinal plants. *Jordan Journal of Pharmaceutical Sciences*, *4*, 1.

Carvalho, A. C., Gomes, A. C., Pereira-Wilson, C., & Lima, C. F. (2016). Mechanisms of Action of Curcumin on Aging: Nutritional and Pharmacological Applications A2 - Malavolta, Marco. In E. Mocchegiani (Ed.), *Molecular Basis of Nutrition and Aging* (pp. 491–511). Academic Press. doi:10.1016/B978-0-12-801816-3.00035-2

Chen, B., Li, H., Ou, G., Ren, L., Yang, X., & Zeng, M. (2019). Curcumin attenuates MSU crystal-induced inflammation by inhibiting the degradation of IκBα and blocking mitochondrial damage. *Arthritis Research & Therapy*, *21*(1), 193. doi:10.118613075-019-1974-z PMID:31455356

Chen, G.-L., Wei, W., & Xu, S.-Y. (2006). Effect and mechanism of total saponin of Dioscorea on animal experimental hyperuricemia. *The American Journal of Chinese Medicine*, *34*(01), 77–85. doi:10.1142/S0192415X06003655 PMID:16437741

Chen, H., Zheng, S., Wang, Y., Zhu, H., Liu, Q., Xue, Y., Qiu, J., Zou, H., & Zhu, X. (2016). The effect of resveratrol on the recurrent attacks of gouty arthritis. *Clinical Rheumatology*, *35*(5), 1189–1195. doi:10.100710067-014-2836-3 PMID:25451618

Chen, L., & Xu, Y. (2018). Epigallocatechin gallate attenuates uric acid-induced injury in rat renal interstitial fibroblasts NRK-49F by up-regulation of miR-9. *European Review for Medical and Pharmacological Sciences*, *22*(21), 7458–7469. PMID:30468495

Chen, L., Yin, H., Lan, Z., Ma, S., Zhang, C., Yang, Z., Li, P., & Lin, B. (2011). Anti-hyperuricemic and nephroprotective effects of Smilax china L. *Journal of Ethnopharmacology*, *135*(2), 399–405. doi:10.1016/j.jep.2011.03.033 PMID:21420478

Choi, H. K., Mount, D. B., & Reginato, A. M. (2005). Pathogenesis of gout. *Annals of Internal Medicine*, *143*(7), 499–516. doi:10.7326/0003-4819-143-7-200510040-00009 PMID:16204163

Daily, J. W., Yang, M., & Park, S. (2016). Efficacy of turmeric extracts and curcumin for alleviating the symptoms of joint arthritis: A systematic review and meta-analysis of randomized clinical trials. *Journal of Medicinal Food*, *19*(8), 717–729. doi:10.1089/jmf.2016.3705 PMID:27533649

de Souza, M. R., de Paula, C. A., de Resende, M. L. P., Grabe-Guimarães, A., de Souza Filho, J. D., & Saúde-Guimarães, D. A. (2012). Pharmacological basis for use of Lychnophora trichocarpha in gouty arthritis: Anti-hyperuricemic and anti-inflammatory effects of its extract, fraction and constituents. *Journal of Ethnopharmacology*, *142*(3), 845–850. doi:10.1016/j.jep.2012.06.012 PMID:22732730

El-Raey, M. A., Ibrahim, G. E., & Eldahshan, O. A. (2013). Lycopene and Lutein; A review for their Chemistry and Medicinal Uses. *Journal of Pharmacognosy and Phytochemistry*, *2*(1).

Ferraz Filha, Z., Vitolo, I., Fietto, L., Lombardi, J., & Saúde-Guimarães, D. A. (2006). Xanthine oxidase inhibitory activity of Lychnophora species from Brazil ("Arnica"). *Journal of Ethnopharmacology*, *107*(1), 79–82. doi:10.1016/j.jep.2006.02.011 PMID:16621372

Fröhlich, J. K., Stein, T., da Silva, L. A., Biavatti, M. W., Tonussi, C. R., & Lemos-Senna, E. (2017). Antinociceptive and anti-inflammatory activities of the Jatropha isabellei dichloromethane fraction and isolation and quantitative determination of jatrophone by UFLC-DAD. *Pharmaceutical Biology, 55*(1), 1215–1222. doi:10.1080/13880209.2017.1295999 PMID:28249559

Havlik, J., de la Huebra, R. G., Hejtmankova, K., Fernandez, J., Simonova, J., Melich, M., & Rada, V. (2010). Xanthine oxidase inhibitory properties of Czech medicinal plants. *Journal of Ethnopharmacology, 132*(2), 461–465. doi:10.1016/j.jep.2010.08.044 PMID:20800669

Huang, J., Zhu, M., Tao, Y., Wang, S., Chen, J., Sun, W., & Li, S. (2012). Therapeutic properties of quercetin on monosodium urate crystal-induced inflammation in rat. *The Journal of Pharmacy and Pharmacology, 64*(8), 1119–1127. doi:10.1111/j.2042-7158.2012.01504.x PMID:22775215

Jiang, S., Han, J., Li, T., Xin, Z., Ma, Z., Di, W., Hu, W., Gong, B., Di, S., Wang, D., & Yang, Y. (2017). Curcumin as a potential protective compound against cardiac diseases. *Pharmacological Research, 119*, 373–383. doi:10.1016/j.phrs.2017.03.001 PMID:28274852

Jiang, Y., You, X.-Y., Fu, K.-L., & Yin, W.-L. (2012). Effects of extract from Mangifera indica leaf on monosodium urate crystal-induced gouty arthritis in rats. *Evidence-Based Complementary and Alternative Medicine*. PMID:23304232

Keservani, Sharma, & Kesharwani, Vyas, & Chadoker. (2010). Nutritional Supplements: An Overview. *International Journal of Current Pharmaceutical Review and Research, 1*(1), 59–75.

Kesharwani, Misra, & Singh. (2019). Perspectives and challenges of tropical medicinal herbs and modern drug discovery in the current scenario. *Asian Pacific Journal of Tropical Medicine, 12*(1), 1–7.

Kesharwani, S., & Singh, R. Adeppa, & Misra. (2015). A novel approach for overcoming drug resistance in breast cancer chemotherapy by targeting new synthetic curcumin analogues against Aldehyde Dehydrogenase 1 (ALDH1A1) and Glycogen Synthase Kinase-3 β (GSK-3β). *Applied Biochemistry and Biotechnology*. Advance online publication. doi:10.100712010- 015-1696-x

Kesharwani & Misra. (2011). Prediction of binding site for Curcuminoids at human Topoisomerase II α protein; an in silico approach. *Current Science, 101*(8), 1060–1064.

Kesharwani & Misra. (2021). *Biotechnology in the Modern Medicinal System: Advances in Gene Therapy, Immunotherapy, and Targeted Drug Delivery*. Apple Academic Press.

Kong, L., Cai, Y., Huang, W., Cheng, C. H., & Tan, R. (2000). Inhibition of xanthine oxidase by some Chinese medicinal plants used to treat gout. *Journal of Ethnopharmacology, 73*(1-2), 199–207. doi:10.1016/S0378-8741(00)00305-6 PMID:11025157

Kumar, A., Naidu, P., Seghal, N., & Padi, S. (2006). Neuroprotective effects of resveratrol against intracerebroventricular colchicine-induced cognitive impairment and oxidative stress in rats. *Pharmacology, 79*(1), 17–26. doi:10.1159/000097511 PMID:17135773

Kuo, C.-Y., Kao, E.-S., Chan, K.-C., Lee, H.-J., Huang, T.-F., & Wang, C.-J. (2012). Hibiscus sabdariffa L. extracts reduce serum uric acid levels in oxonate-induced rats. *Journal of Functional Foods, 4*(1), 375–381. doi:10.1016/j.jff.2012.01.007

Lee, H. E., Yang, G., Park, Y. B., Kang, H. C., Cho, Y.-Y., Lee, H. S., & Lee, J. Y. (2019). Epigallocatechin-3-gallate prevents acute gout by suppressing NLRP3 inflammasome activation and mitochondrial DNA synthesis. *Molecules (Basel, Switzerland)*, *24*(11), 2138. doi:10.3390/molecules24112138 PMID:31174271

Lee, S.-I., Lee, Y.-K., Kim, S.-D., Cheng, J., Yang, S. H., & Suh, J.-W. (2014). Xanthine and aldehyde oxidase inhibitory activities, and antihyperuricemic effects of fermented Smilax china L. Leaf extracts and fractions. *Journal of Applied Biological Chemistry*, *57*(1), 53–59. doi:10.3839/jabc.2014.009

Lee, Y.-S., Son, E., Kim, S.-H., Lee, Y. M., Kim, O. S., & Kim, D.-S. (2017). Synergistic uric acid-lowering effects of the combination of Chrysanthemum indicum linne flower and Cinnamomum cassia (L.) J. Persl Bark Extracts. *Evidence-Based Complementary and Alternative Medicine*, *2017*, 2017. doi:10.1155/2017/9764843 PMID:28769989

Li, F., Gong, Q., Dong, H., & Shi, J. (2012). Resveratrol, a neuroprotective supplement for Alzheimer's disease. *Current Pharmaceutical Design*, *18*(1), 27–33. doi:10.2174/138161212798919075 PMID:22211686

Li, F., Liu, Y., Xie, Y., Liu, Z., & Zou, G. (2020). Epigallocatechin gallate reduces uric acid levels by regulating xanthine oxidase activity and uric acid excretion in vitro and in vivo. *Annals of Palliative Medicine*, *9*(2), 331–338. doi:10.21037/apm.2019.11.28 PMID:32008337

Li, H., Ou, G., He, Y., Ren, L., Yang, X., & Zeng, M. (2019). Resveratrol attenuates the MSU crystal-induced inflammatory response through the inhibition of TAK1 activity. *International Immunopharmacology*, *67*, 62–68. doi:10.1016/j.intimp.2018.12.004 PMID:30537632

Lin, H.-Y., Chang, T.-C., & Chang, S.-T. (2018). A review of antioxidant and pharmacological properties of phenolic compounds in Acacia confusa. *Journal of Traditional and Complementary Medicine*, *8*(4), 443–450. doi:10.1016/j.jtcme.2018.05.002 PMID:30302324

Lin, Y., Liu, P.-G., Liang, W.-Q., Hu, Y.-J., Xu, P., Zhou, J., Pu, J.-B., & Zhang, H.-J. (2018). Luteolin-4′-O-glucoside and its aglycone, two major flavones of Gnaphalium affine D. Don, resist hyperuricemia and acute gouty arthritis activity in animal models. *Phytomedicine*, *41*, 54–61. doi:10.1016/j.phymed.2018.02.002 PMID:29519319

Liu, X., Chen, R., Shang, Y., Jiao, B., & Huang, C. (2009). Superoxide radicals scavenging and xanthine oxidase inhibitory activity of magnesium lithospermate B from Salvia miltiorrhiza. *Journal of Enzyme Inhibition and Medicinal Chemistry*, *24*(3), 663–668. doi:10.1080/14756360802323829 PMID:18686136

Liu, X., Li, S., & Meng, D. (2016). Anti-gout nor-oleanane triterpenoids from the leaves of Stauntonia brachyanthera. *Bioorganic & Medicinal Chemistry Letters*, *26*(12), 2874–2879. doi:10.1016/j.bmcl.2016.04.048 PMID:27133595

Murugaiyah, V., & Chan, K.-L. (2006). Antihyperuricemic lignans from the leaves of Phyllanthus niruri. *Planta Medica*, *72*(14), 1262–1267. doi:10.1055-2006-947224 PMID:16953466

Murugaiyah, V., & Chan, K.-L. (2009). Mechanisms of antihyperuricemic effect of Phyllanthus niruri and its lignan constituents. *Journal of Ethnopharmacology*, *124*(2), 233–239. doi:10.1016/j.jep.2009.04.026 PMID:19397979

Mustafa Kiyani, M., Sohail, M. F., Shahnaz, G., Rehman, H., Akhtar, M. F., Nawaz, I., ... Imran Bokhari, S. A. (2019). Evaluation of turmeric nanoparticles as anti-gout agent: Modernization of a traditional drug. *Medicina*, *55*(1), 10. doi:10.3390/medicina55010010 PMID:30642012

Nguyen, M. T. T., Awale, S., Tezuka, Y., Le Tran, Q., Watanabe, H., & Kadota, S. (2004). Xanthine oxidase inhibitory activity of Vietnamese medicinal plants. *Biological & Pharmaceutical Bulletin*, *27*(9), 1414–1421. doi:10.1248/bpb.27.1414 PMID:15340229

Ohishi, T., Goto, S., Monira, P., Isemura, M., & Nakamura, Y. (2016). Anti-inflammatory action of green tea. *Anti-Inflammatory & Anti-Allergy Agents in Medicinal Chemistry (Formerly Current Medicinal Chemistry-Anti-Inflammatory and Anti-Allergy Agents)*, *15*(2), 74-90.

Ojha, R., Singh, J., Ojha, A., Singh, H., Sharma, S., & Nepali, K. (2017). An updated patent review: Xanthine oxidase inhibitors for the treatment of hyperuricemia and gout (2011-2015). *Expert Opinion on Therapeutic Patents*, *27*(3), 311–345. doi:10.1080/13543776.2017.1261111 PMID:27841045

Owen, P. L., & Johns, T. (1999). Xanthine oxidase inhibitory activity of northeastern North American plant remedies used for gout. *Journal of Ethnopharmacology*, *64*(2), 149–160. doi:10.1016/S0378-8741(98)00119-6 PMID:10197750

Palu, A., Deng, S., West, B., & Jensen, J. (2009). Xanthine oxidase inhibiting effects of noni (Morinda citrifolia) fruit juice. *Phytotherapy Research*, *23*(12), 1790–1791. doi:10.1002/ptr.2842 PMID:19434757

Pawlus, A. D., & Kinghorn, A. D. (2007). Review of the ethnobotany, chemistry, biological activity and safety of the botanical dietary supplement Morinda citrifolia (noni). *The Journal of Pharmacy and Pharmacology*, *59*(12), 1587–1609. doi:10.1211/jpp.59.12.0001 PMID:18053321

Prasongwatana, V., Woottisin, S., Sriboonlue, P., & Kukongviriyapan, V. (2008). Uricosuric effect of Roselle (Hibiscus sabdariffa) in normal and renal-stone former subjects. *Journal of Ethnopharmacology*, *117*(3), 491–495. doi:10.1016/j.jep.2008.02.036 PMID:18423919

Rees, F., Hui, M., & Doherty, M. (2014). Optimizing current treatment of gout. *Nature Reviews. Rheumatology*, *10*(5), 271–283. doi:10.1038/nrrheum.2014.32 PMID:24614592

Riaz, G., & Chopra, R. (2018). A review on phytochemistry and therapeutic uses of Hibiscus sabdariffa L. *Biomedicine and Pharmacotherapy*, *102*, 575–586. doi:10.1016/j.biopha.2018.03.023 PMID:29597091

Riches, P. L., Wright, A. F., & Ralston, S. H. (2009). Recent insights into the pathogenesis of hyperuricaemia and gout. *Human Molecular Genetics*, *18*(R2), R177–R184. doi:10.1093/hmg/ddp369 PMID:19808794

Ruiz-Miyazawa, K. W., Staurengo-Ferrari, L., Mizokami, S. S., Domiciano, T. P., Vicentini, F. T., Camilios-Neto, D., ... Teixeira, M. M. (2017). Quercetin inhibits gout arthritis in mice: Induction of an opioid-dependent regulation of inflammasome. *Inflammopharmacology*, *25*(5), 555–570. doi:10.100710787-017-0356-x PMID:28508104

Sarawate, C. A., Brewer, K. K., Yang, W., Patel, P. A., Schumacher, H. R., Saag, K. G., & Bakst, A. W. (2006). Gout medication treatment patterns and adherence to standards of care from a managed care perspective. *Mayo Clinic Proceedings*. 10.4065/81.7.925

Sato, V. H., Sungthong, B., Rinthong, P.-O., Nuamnaichati, N., Mangmool, S., Chewchida, S., & Sato, H. (2018). Pharmacological effects of Chatuphalatika in hyperuricemia of gout. *Pharmaceutical Biology, 56*(1), 76–85. doi:10.1080/13880209.2017.1421235 PMID:29298537

Shen, R.-M., Zhong, L.-B., & Li, G.-Q. (2019). Anti-inflammatory effect of luteolin in acute gouty arthritis rat model. *Hainan Yixueyuan Xuebao, 25*(17), 20–24.

Sheu, S.-Y., Fu, Y.-T., Huang, W.-D., Chen, Y.-A., Lei, Y.-C., Yao, C.-H., ... Kuo, T.-F. (2016). Evaluation of xanthine oxidase inhibitory potential and in vivo hypouricemic activity of Dimocarpus longan Lour. extracts. *Pharmacognosy Magazine, 12*(46, Suppl 2), S206. doi:10.4103/0973-1296.182176 PMID:27279708

Shi, Y., & Williamson, G. (2016). Quercetin lowers plasma uric acid in pre-hyperuricaemic males: A randomised, double-blinded, placebo-controlled, cross-over trial. *British Journal of Nutrition, 115*(5), 800–806. doi:10.1017/S0007114515005310 PMID:26785820

Shi, Y. W., Wang, C. P., Liu, L., Liu, Y. L., Wang, X., Hong, Y., Li, Z., & Kong, L. D. (2012). Antihyperuricemic and nephroprotective effects of resveratrol and its analogues in hyperuricemic mice. *Molecular Nutrition & Food Research, 56*(9), 1433–1444. doi:10.1002/mnfr.201100828 PMID:22865646

Shin, W.-Y., Shim, D.-W., Kim, M.-K., Sun, X., Koppula, S., Yu, S. H., Kim, H.-B., Kim, T.-J., Kang, T.-B., & Lee, K.-H. (2017). Protective effects of Cinnamomum cassia (Lamaceae) against gout and septic responses via attenuation of inflammasome activation in experimental models. *Journal of Ethnopharmacology, 205*, 173–177. doi:10.1016/j.jep.2017.03.043 PMID:28347828

Silva, C. R., Fröhlich, J. K., Oliveira, S. M., Cabreira, T. N., Rossato, M. F., Trevisan, G., ... Athayde, M. L. (2013). The antinociceptive and anti-inflammatory effects of the crude extract of Jatropha isabellei in a rat gout model. *Journal of Ethnopharmacology, 145*(1), 205–213. doi:10.1016/j.jep.2012.10.054 PMID:23127654

Singh, Agarwal, Kesharwani, & Misra. (2013). Atom based QSAR and pharmacophore study of curcuminoids and curcumin analogs: Interaction with thioredoxin reductase. *Interdisciplinary Sciences, Computational Life Sciences, 5*, 286–295.

Singh, Gupta, Kesharwani, & Misra. (n.d.). Comparative docking and ADMET study of some curcumin derivatives and herbal congeners targeting β-amyloid. *Network Modeling and Analysis in Health Informatics and Bioinformatics*. Advance online publication. doi:10.100713721-012-0021-7

Spanou, C., Veskoukis, A. S., Kerasioti, T., Kontou, M., Angelis, A., Aligiannis, N., Skaltsounis, A.-L., & Kouretas, D. (2012). Flavonoid glycosides isolated from unique legume plant extracts as novel inhibitors of xanthine oxidase. *PLoS One, 7*(3), e32214. doi:10.1371/journal.pone.0032214 PMID:22396752

Synytsia, I. (2016). Evaluation of using quercetin in patients with gout and hypertension. *Ukrainian Scientific Medical Youth Journal*, (4 (98)), 54–58.

Tan, W.-J., Xu, J.-C., Li, L., & Chen, K.-L. (2009). Bioactive compounds of inhibiting xanthine oxidase from Selaginella labordei. *Natural Product Research, 23*(4), 393–398. doi:10.1080/14786410802228736 PMID:19296380

Tandon, V. R. (2005). Medicinal uses and biological activities of Vitex negundo. *Natural Product Radiance, 4*(3), 162–165.

Tang, H., Yang, L., Li, W., Li, J., & Chen, J. (2016). Exploring the interaction between Salvia miltiorrhiza and xanthine oxidase: Insights from computational analysis and experimental studies combined with enzyme channel blocking. *RSC Advances, 6*(114), 113527–113537. doi:10.1039/C6RA24396G

Tung, Y.-T., & Chang, S.-T. (2010). Inhibition of xanthine oxidase by Acacia confusa extracts and their phytochemicals. *Journal of Agricultural and Food Chemistry, 58*(2), 781–786. doi:10.1021/jf901498q PMID:20047272

Tung, Y.-T., Hsu, C.-A., Chen, C.-S., Yang, S. C., Huang, C.-C., & Chang, S.-T. (2010). Phytochemicals from Acacia confusa heartwood extracts reduce serum uric acid levels in oxonate-induced mice: Their potential use as xanthine oxidase inhibitors. *Journal of Agricultural and Food Chemistry, 58*(18), 9936–9941. doi:10.1021/jf102689k PMID:20806936

Umamaheswari, M., Asokkumar, K., Sudalaivelmurugiah, M., Sivashnmugam, A., & Subhadradevi, V. (2009). Hypouricaemic and antioxidant activities of the fractions of Vitex negundo L. leaf extract. *Phytopharmacology and Therapeutic Values V*, 59-70.

Upadhyaya, Kesharwani, & Misra. (2009). Metabolism, Pharmacokinetics and Bioavailability of Ascorbic Acid; Synergistic Effect in presence of Tocopherols and Curcumin. *Journal of Computational Intelligence in Bioinformatics, 2*(1), 77–84.

Wahyuningsih, S., & Sukandar, E. (2016). In vitro xanthine oxidase inhibitor activity of ethanol extract and fraction roselle calyx (Hibiscus sabdariffa L.). *Int. J. Pharma. Clin. Res., 94*, 5–35.

Wahyuningsih, S., Sukandar, E. Y., & Sukrasno, L. D. (2016). Antihyperuricemia activity of the ethanol extract of Roselle calyx and its fraction (Hibiscus sabdariffa Linn) on male wistar rats. *International Journal of Pharmacy and Pharmaceutical Sciences, 8*, 278–280.

Wang, L., Zhu, L., Duan, C., Li, L., & Chen, G. (2020). Total saponin of Dioscorea collettii attenuates MSU crystal-induced inflammation via inhibiting the activation of the NALP3 inflammasome and caspase-1 in THP-1 macrophages. *Molecular Medicine Reports, 21*(6), 2466–2474. doi:10.3892/mmr.2020.11035 PMID:32236574

Wang, P., Ren, D., Chen, Y., Jiang, M., Wang, R., & Wang, Y.-G. (2015). Effect of sodium alginate addition to resveratrol on acute gouty arthritis. *Cellular Physiology and Biochemistry, 36*(1), 201–207. doi:10.1159/000374064 PMID:25967960

Wang, S., Yang, C., Liao, J., Zhen, W., Chu, F., & Chang, S. (2008). Essential oil from leaves of Cinnamomum osmophloeum acts as a xanthine oxidase inhibitor and reduces the serum uric acid levels in oxonate-induced mice. *Phytomedicine, 15*(11), 940–945. doi:10.1016/j.phymed.2008.06.002 PMID:18693097

Wu, X., Liu, L., Xie, H., Liao, J., Zhou, X., Wan, J., Yu, K., Li, J., & Zhang, Y. (2012). Tanshinone IIA prevents uric acid nephropathy in rats through NF-κB inhibition. *Planta Medica, 78*(09), 866–873. doi:10.1055-0031-1298487 PMID:22588836

Wu, X.-H., Ruan, J.-L., Zhang, J., Wang, S.-Q., & Zhang, Y.-W. (2014). Pallidifloside D, a saponin glycoside constituent from Smilax riparia, resist to hyperuricemia based on URAT1 and GLUT9 in hyperuricemic mice. *Journal of Ethnopharmacology*, *157*, 201–205. doi:10.1016/j.jep.2014.09.034 PMID:25267580

Wu, X.-H., Wang, C.-Z., Wang, S.-Q., Mi, C., He, Y., Zhang, J., Zhang, Y.-W., Anderson, S., & Yuan, C.-S. (2015). Anti-hyperuricemia effects of allopurinol are improved by Smilax riparia, a traditional Chinese herbal medicine. *Journal of Ethnopharmacology*, *162*, 362–368. doi:10.1016/j.jep.2015.01.012 PMID:25617746

Wu, X.-H., Yu, C.-H., Zhang, C.-F., Anderson, S., & Zhang, Y.-W. (2014). Smilax riparia reduces hyperuricemia in mice as a potential treatment of gout. *The American Journal of Chinese Medicine*, *42*(01), 257–259. doi:10.1142/S0192415X14200018 PMID:24467548

Yan, J., Zhang, G., Hu, Y., & Ma, Y. (2013). Effect of luteolin on xanthine oxidase: Inhibition kinetics and interaction mechanism merging with docking simulation. *Food Chemistry*, *141*(4), 3766–3773. doi:10.1016/j.foodchem.2013.06.092 PMID:23993547

Yang, H., Gao, L., Niu, Y., Zhou, Y., Lin, H., Jiang, J., Kong, X., Liu, X., & Li, L. (2015). Mangiferin inhibits renal urate reabsorption by modulating urate transporters in experimental hyperuricemia. *Biological & Pharmaceutical Bulletin*, *38*(10), b15–b00402. doi:10.1248/bpb.b15-00402 PMID:26228630

Yang, Q.-B., He, Y.-L., Zhong, X.-W., Xie, W.-G., & Zhou, J.-G. (2019). Resveratrol ameliorates gouty inflammation via upregulation of sirtuin 1 to promote autophagy in gout patients. *Inflammopharmacology*, *27*(1), 47–56. doi:10.100710787-018-00555-4 PMID:30600470

Yumita, A., Suganda, A. G., & Sukandar, E. Y. (2013). Xanthine oxidase inhibitory activity of some Indonesian medicinal plants and active fraction of selected plants. *International Journal of Pharmacy and Pharmaceutical Sciences*, *5*, 293–296.

Zhang, C., Wang, R., Zhang, G., & Gong, D. (2018). Mechanistic insights into the inhibition of quercetin on xanthine oxidase. *International Journal of Biological Macromolecules*, *112*, 405–412. doi:10.1016/j.ijbiomac.2018.01.190 PMID:29410028

Zhao, P., Chen, K., Zhang, G., Deng, G., & Li, J. (2017). Pharmacological basis for use of Selaginella moellendorffii in gouty arthritis: Antihyperuricemic, anti-inflammatory, and xanthine oxidase inhibition. *Evidence-Based Complementary and Alternative Medicine*, *2017*, 2017. doi:10.1155/2017/2103254 PMID:28250791

Zhu, C., Xu, Y., Liu, Z.-H., Wan, X.-C., Li, D.-X., & Tai, L.-L. (2018). The anti-hyperuricemic effect of epigallocatechin-3-gallate (EGCG) on hyperuricemic mice. *Biomedicine and Pharmacotherapy*, *97*, 168–173. doi:10.1016/j.biopha.2017.10.013 PMID:29091862

Zhu, J. X., Wang, Y., Kong, L. D., Yang, C., & Zhang, X. (2004). Effects of Biota orientalis extract and its flavonoid constituents, quercetin and rutin on serum uric acid levels in oxonate-induced mice and xanthine dehydrogenase and xanthine oxidase activities in mouse liver. *Journal of Ethnopharmacology*, *93*(1), 133–140. doi:10.1016/j.jep.2004.03.037 PMID:15182918

Compilation of References

Abboud, Y., Saffaj, T., Chagraoui, A., El Bouari, A., Brouzi, K., Tanane, O., & Ihssane, B. (2014). Biosynthesis, characterization and antimicrobial activity of copper oxide nanoparticles (CONPs) produced using brown alga extract (*Bifurcaria bifurcata*). *Applied Nanoscience*, *4*(5), 571–576. doi:10.100713204-013-0233-x

Abdulbaqi, I. M., Darwis, Y., Khan, N. A. K., Assi, R. A., & Khan, A. A. (2016). Ethosomal nanocarriers: The impact of constituents and formulation techniques on ethosomal properties, in vivo studies, and clinical trials. *International Journal of Nanomedicine*, ***•••***, 11.

Abotaleb, M., Samuel, S. M., Varghese, E., Varghese, S., Kubatka, P., Liskova, A., & Büsselberg, D. (2019). Flavonoids in cancer and apoptosis. *Cancers (Basel)*, *11*(1), 28. doi:10.3390/cancers11010028 PMID:30597838

Abou El Wafa, A. A., Mursi, N. M., & El-Shaboury, K. M. (2003). *A pharmaceutical study on certain ocular drug delivery systems* (Doctoral dissertation). Cairo University, Cairo, Egypt.

Abu Bakar, F. I., Abu Bakar, M. F., Rahmat, A., Abdullah, N., Sabran, S. F., & Endrini, S. (2018). Anti-gout potential of Malaysian medicinal plants. *Frontiers in Pharmacology*, *9*, 261. doi:10.3389/fphar.2018.00261 PMID:29628890

Acharya, N., Parihar, G., & Acharya, S. (2011). Phytosomes: Novel approach for delivering herbal extract with improved bioavailability. *Pharma Science Monitor*, *2*(1), 144–160.

Afrin, S., Jahan, I., Hasan, A. N., & Deepa, K. N. (2018). Novel Approaches of Herbal Drug Delivery. *Journal of Pharmaceutical Research International*, *21*(5), 1–11. doi:10.9734/JPRI/2018/39143

Aggarwal, B. B., Sundaram, C., Malani, N., & Ichikawa, H. (2007). *Curcumin: the Indian solid gold. In The molecular targets and therapeutic uses of curcumin in health and disease*. Springer. doi:10.1007/978-0-387-46401-5

Aggarwal, B., & Harikumar, K. (2009). Potential therapeutic effects of curcumin, the anti-inflammatory agent, against neurodegenerative, cardiovascular, pulmonary, metabolic, autoimmune and neoplastic diseases. *The International Journal of Biochemistry & Cell Biology*, *41*(1), 40–59. doi:10.1016/j.biocel.2008.06.010 PMID:18662800

Aggarwal, K. V., Gupta, A., & Chaturvedi, S. (2012). Improvement in bioavailability of class III drug: Phytolipid delivery system. *International Journal of Pharmacy and Pharmaceutical Sciences*, *4*(1), 38.

Ahmad, F., Ahmad, F. A., Azad, A., Alam, S., & Ashraf, A. (2013). Nutraceuticals is the need of hour. *World J Pharm-Sci*, *2*(25), 16–25.

Ahmad, M., Mudgil, P., Gani, A., Hamed, F., Masoodi, F. A., & Maqsood, S. (2019). Nano-encapsulation of catechin in starch nanoparticles: Characterization, release behavior and bioactivity retention during simulated in-vitro digestion. *Food Chemistry*, *270*, 95–104. doi:10.1016/j.foodchem.2018.07.024 PMID:30174096

Ahmad, N. S., Farman, M., Najmi, M. H., Mian, K. B., & Hasan, A. (2008). Pharmacological basis for use of Pistacia integerrima leaves in hyperuricemia and gout. *Journal of Ethnopharmacology, 117*(3), 478–482. doi:10.1016/j.jep.2008.02.031 PMID:18420362

Ahmad, N., Ahmad, R., Naqvi, A. A., Alam, M. A., Ashafaq, M., Samim, M., Iqbal, Z., & Ahmad, F. J. (2016). Rutin-encapsulated chitosan nanoparticles targeted to the brain in the treatment of Cerebral Ischemia. *International Journal of Biological Macromolecules, 91*, 640–655. doi:10.1016/j.ijbiomac.2016.06.001 PMID:27264648

Ahmmad, B., Leonard, K., Islam, M. S., Kurawaki, J., Muruganandham, M., Ohkubo, T., & Kuroda, Y. (2013). Green synthesis of mesoporous hematite (a-Fe2O3) nanoparticles and their photocatalytic activity. *Advanced Powder Technology, 24*(1), 160–167. doi:10.1016/j.apt.2012.04.005

Ajazuddin Saraf, S. (2010). Applications of novel drug delivery system for herbal formulations. *Fitoterapia, 81*(7), 680–689. doi:10.1016/j.fitote.2010.05.001 PMID:20471457

Akbarzadeh, A., Sadabady, A., Davaran, S., Sang, W. J., Zarghami, N. Z., Hanifehpour, M., Kouhiand, M. K., & Nejati, K. (2013). Liposome:classification, preparation, and applications. *Nanoscale Research Letters, 8*(1), 102. doi:10.1186/1556-276X-8-102 PMID:23432972

Akiladevi, D., & Sachinandan, D. (2010). Ethosomes: A noninvasive approach for transdermal drug delivery. *International Journal of Current Pharmaceutical Research, 2*, 1–4.

Akram, M., Shahab-Uddin, A. A., Usmanghani, K., Hannan, A., Mohiuddin, E., & Asif, M. (2010). Curcuma longa and curcumin: A review article. *Rom J Biol Plant Biol, 55*(2), 65–70.

Alam, M. M., Abdullah, K. M., Singh, B. R., Naqvi, A. H., & Naseem, I. (2016). Ameliorative effect of quercetin nanorods on diabetic mice: Mechanistic and therapeutic strategies. *RSC Advances, 6*(60), 55092–55103. doi:10.1039/C6RA04821H

Alberti, A., & Caporaso, N. (2011). HBV therapy: Guidelines and open issues. *Digestive and Liver Disease, 43*, S57–S63. doi:10.1016/S1590-8658(10)60693-7 PMID:21195373

Alexander, A., Patel, R. J., Saraf, S., & Saraf, S. (2016). Recent expansion of pharmaceutical nanotechnologies and targeting strategies in the field of phytopharmaceuticals for the delivery of herbal extracts and bioactives. *Journal of Controlled Release, 241*, 110–124. doi:10.1016/j.jconrel.2016.09.017 PMID:27663228

Alexis, F., Basto, P., Levy-Nissenbaum, E., Radovic-Moreno, A. F., Zhang, L., Pridgen, E., & Farokhzad, O. C. (2008). HER-2-targeted nanoparticle-affibody bioconjugates for cancer therapy. *ChemMedChem, 3*(12), 1839–1843. doi:10.1002/cmdc.200800122 PMID:19012296

Alexis, F., Pridgen, E., Molnar, L. K., & Farokhzad, O. C. (2008). Factors affecting the clearance and bio distribution of polymeric nanoparticles. *Molecular Pharmaceutics, 5*(4), 505–515. doi:10.1021/mp800051m PMID:18672949

Ali, A., & Ahmed, S. (2018). A review on chitosan and its nanocomposites in drug delivery. *International Journal of Biological Macromolecules, 109*, 273–286. doi:10.1016/j.ijbiomac.2017.12.078 PMID:29248555

Ali, D. M., Sasikala, M., Gunasekaran, M., & Thajuddin, N. (2011). Biosynthesis and characterization of silver nanoparticles using marine cyanobacterium, *Oscillatoria willei. Digest Journal of Nanomaterials and Biostructures, 6*, 385–390.

Ali, J., Akhtar, N., Sultana, Y., Baboota, S., & Ahuja, A. (2008). Antipsoriatic microemulsion gel formulations for topical drug delivery of babchi oil (Psoralea corylifolia). *Methods and Findings in Experimental and Clinical Pharmacology, 30*(4), 277–285. doi:10.1358/mf.2008.30.4.1185802 PMID:18773122

Ali, K., Maltese, F., Zyprian, E., Rex, M., Choi, Y. H., & Verpoorte, R. (2009). NMR metabolic fingerprinting based identification of grapevine metabolites associated with downy mildew resistance. *Journal of Agricultural and Food Chemistry, 57*(20), 9599–9606. doi:10.1021/jf902069f PMID:19785416

Ali, S. H., Sulaiman, G. M., & Al-Halbosiy, M. M. (2018). In Vitro study for hesperidin nanoparticles effect on phagocytic activity against Staphylococcus aureus. *Magallat Markaz Buhut al-Tiqniyyat al-Ahya'iyyat, 12*(2), 36–39.

Ali, S. H., Sulaiman, G. M., Al-Halbosiy, M. M., Jabir, M. S., & Hameed, A. H. (2019). Fabrication of hesperidin nanoparticles loaded by poly lactic co-Glycolic acid for improved therapeutic efficiency and cytotoxicity. *Artificial Cells, Nanomedicine, and Biotechnology, 47*(1), 378–394. doi:10.1080/21691401.2018.1559175 PMID:30691314

Allen, T., & Cullis, P. (2013). Liposomal drug delivery systems: From concept to clinical applications. *Advanced Drug Delivery Reviews, 65*(1), 36–48. doi:10.1016/j.addr.2012.09.037 PMID:23036225

Allmendinger, A., Spavieri, J., Kaiser, M., Casey, R., Hingley-Wilson, S., Lalvani, A., Guiry, M., Blunden, G., & Tasdemir, D. (2010). Antiprotozoal, anti-mycobacterial and cytotoxic potential of twenty-three British and Irish red algae. *Phytotherapy Research, 24*(7), 1099–1103. doi:10.1002/ptr.3094 PMID:20077438

Alsultanee, I. R., Ewadh, M. J., & Mohammed, M. F. (2014). Novel natural anti gout medication extract from Momdica Charantia. *J Nat Sci Res, 4*(17), 16–23.

Amawi, H., Ashby, C. R. Jr, & Tiwari, A. K. (2017). Cancer chemoprevention through dietary flavonoids: What's limiting? *Chinese Journal of Cancer, 36*(1), 50. doi:10.118640880-017-0217-4 PMID:28629389

Amin, T., & Bhat, S. (2012). A Review on phytosome technology as a novel approach to improve the bioavailability of neutraceuticals. *International Journal of Advancements in Research and Technology, 1*, 1–15.

Amit, J., Sunil, C., Vimal, K., & Anupam, P. (2008). The pharma review. New Delhi: Kongposh Publications Pvt, Ltd.

Amit, P., Tanwar, Y. S., Rakesh, S., & Poojan, P. (2013). Phytosome: Phyto lipid drug delivery system for improving the bioavailability of the herbal drug. *J Pharm Sci Biosci Res., 3*(2), 51–57.

Ammon, H. P. T., & Anazodo, M. L. (1991). Curcumin: A potent inhibitor of leukotriene B4 formation in rat peritoneal polymorphonuclear neutrophils (PMNL). *Planta Medica, 58*, 226.

Ammon, H. P. T., Safayhi, H., Mack, T., & Sabieraj, J. (1993). Mechanism of. *Medica (Stuttgart), 57*, 1–7.

Amruthraj, N. J., Raj, J. P. P., & Lebel, A. (2015). Capsaicin-capped silver nanoparticles: Its kinetics, characterization and biocompatibility assay. *Applied Nanoscience, 5*(4), 403–409. doi:10.100713204-014-0330-5

Anand, P., Kunnumakkara, A. B., Newman, R. A., & Aggarwal, B. B. (2007). Bioavailability of Curcumin: Problems and Promises. *Molecular Pharmaceutics, 4*(6), 807–818. doi:10.1021/mp700113r PMID:17999464

Ande, M.P., Syamala, K., Rao, P.S., Mohan, K.M. & Lingam, S.S. (2017). Marine Nutraceuticals. *Aquaculture Times, 3*(2), 6-9.

Aneiros, A., & Garateix, A. (2004). Bioactive peptides from marine sources: Pharmacological properties and isolation procedures. *Journal of Chromatography. B, Analytical Technologies in the Biomedical and Life Sciences, 803*(1), 41–53. doi:10.1016/j.jchromb.2003.11.005 PMID:15025997

Anju, D., & Arun, N. (2012). Novel Herbal Drug Delivery System (NHDDS): The need of Hour, 2012, International Conference on Environment. *Chemistry and Biology IPCBEE, 49*, 34. doi:10.7763/IPCBEE

Ankamwar, B., Daml, C., Ahmad, A., & Sastry, M. (2005). Biosynthesis of Gold and Silver Nanoparticles Using *Emblica Officinalis* Fruit Extract, Their Phase Transfer and Trans metallationinan Organic Solution. *Journal of Nanoscience and Nanotechnology*, *5*(10), 1665–1671. doi:10.1166/jnn.2005.184 PMID:16245525

Ansari, S. H., Islam, F., & Sameem, M. (2012). Influence of nanotechnology on herbal drugs: A Review. *Journal of Advanced Pharmaceutical Technology & Research*, *3*(3), 142–146. doi:10.4103/2231-4040.101006 PMID:23057000

Ansari, S., Chauhan, B., Kalam, N., & Kumar, G. (2013). Current ideas and forecasts of herbal nutraceutical: A review. *Journal of Advanced Pharmacy and Research*, *4*(1), 4–8.

Ansar, S., Abudawood, M., Alaraj, A. S., & Hamed, S. S. (2018). Hesperidin alleviates zinc oxide nanoparticle induced hepatotoxicity and oxidative stress. *BMC Pharmacology & Toxicology*, *19*(1), 65. doi:10.118640360-018-0256-8 PMID:30340509

Anwekar, H., Patel, S., & Singhai, A. K. (2011). Liposome- as drug carriers. *IJPLS*, *2*(7), 951–945.

Ao, G.-Z., Zhou, M.-Z., Li, Y.-Y., Li, S.-N., Wang, H.-N., Wan, Q.-W., Li, H.-Q., & Hu, Q.-H. (2017). Discovery of novel curcumin derivatives targeting xanthine oxidase and urate transporter 1 as anti-hyperuricemic agents. *Bioorganic & Medicinal Chemistry*, *25*(1), 166–174. doi:10.1016/j.bmc.2016.10.022 PMID:28340987

Apaya, K. L., & Chichioco-Hern, C. L. (2011). Xanthine oxidase inhibition of selected Philippine medicinal plants. *Journal of Medicinal Plants Research*, *5*(2), 289–292.

Arena, A., Gugliandolo, C., Stassi, G., Pavone, B., Iannello, D., Bisignano, G., & Maugeri, T. L. (2009). An exopoly-saccharide produced by *Geobacillus thermodenitrificans* strain B3-72: Antiviral activity on immunocompetent cells. *Immunology Letters*, *123*(2), 132–137. doi:10.1016/j.imlet.2009.03.001 PMID:19428560

Armendariz, V., Gardea-Torresdey, J. L., Jose-Yacaman, M., Gonzalez, J., Herrera, I., & Parsons, J. G. (2002). Gold nanoparticles formation by oat and wheat biomasses. *Proceedings –Waste Research Technology Conference at the Kansas City*.

Armendariz, V., Herrera, I., Peralta-videa, J. R., Jose-yacaman, M., Troiani, H., Santiago, P., & Gardea-Torresdey, J. L. (2004). Size controlled gold nanoparticle formation by *Avena sativa* biomass: Use of plants in nanobiotechnology. *Journal of Nano Research*, *6*(4), 377–382. doi:10.100711051-004-0741-4

Arockiya, F., Parthiban, C., Ganesh-Kumar, V., & Anantharaman, P. (2012). Biosynthesis of antibacterial gold nanoparticles using brown alga, *Stoechospermum marginatum* (kützing). *Spectrochimica Acta. Part A: Molecular and Biomolecular Spectroscopy*, *99*, 166–173. doi:10.1016/j.saa.2012.08.081 PMID:23063860

Aroonsri, P., Jintanaporn, W., Saengrawee, S., Wathita, P., & Supaporn, M. (2008). Applications of novel drug delivery system for herbal formulations. *Nanomedicine; Nanotechnology, Biology, and Medicine*, *4*, 70–78.

Arthri Blend, S. R. (2009). A formulation containing herbal extracts and nutrients to support healthy joints and connective tissues in the body. *Nutraceuticals World*. Retrieved from http://findarticles.com/particles/mi_hb223/is_6_7/ai_n29102045/

Arthri, B. S. (n.d.). A formulation containing herbal extracts and nutrients to support healthy joints and connective tissues in the body. *Nutraceuticals World*. Available from: http://findparticles.com/particles/mi_hb223/is_6_7/ai_n29102045/

Arulanandraj, N., Dhivya, S., & Gopal, V. (2018). A review on Herbal Nanoparticles. *PharmaTutor.*, *6*(5), 32–37. doi:10.29161/PT.v6.i5.2018.32

Ashokkumar, S., Ravi, S., Kathiravan, V., & Velmurugan, S. (2014). Rapid biological synthesis of silver nanoparticles using *Leucas martinicensis* leaf extract for catalytic and antibacterial activity. *Environmental Science and Pollution Research International*, *21*(19), 11439–11446. doi:10.100711356-014-3012-7 PMID:24906826

Ashwani, G., & Kumar, S. (2011). Potential of novel drug delivery systems for herbal drugs. *Indian Journal of Pharmaceutical Education and Research*, *45*(3), 225–235.

Assi, M., Derbré, F., Lefeuvre, L., & Rebillard, A. (2016). Antioxidant supplementation accelerates cachexia development by promoting tumor growth in C26 tumor-bearing mice. *Free Radical Biology & Medicine*, *91*, 204–214. doi:10.1016/j.freeradbiomed.2015.12.019 PMID:26708754

Aswathy, R. G., Sivakumar, B., Maekawa, T., & Kumar, D. (2015). Prospects of nano-nutraceuticals for better and healthier future. *Journal of Nutrition & Food Sciences*, *5*(4).

Atmakuri, L. R., & Dathi, S. (2010). Current trends in herbal medicines. *Journal of Pharmacy Research*, *3*(1), 109–113.

Atram, S. (2014). Recent development of herbal formulation- a novel drug delivery system. *International Ayurvedic Medical Journal*, *2*, 953–958.

Atram, S. (2014). Recent development of herbal formulation. A novel drug delivery system. InternationalAyurveda. *Medical Journal*, *2*(6), 952–958.

Avadhani, K. S., Manikkath, J., Tiwari, M., Chandrasekhar, M., Godavarthi, A., Vidya, S. M., Hariharapura, R. C., Kalthur, G., Udupa, N., & Mutalik, S. (2017). Skin delivery of epigallocatechin-3-gallate (EGCG) and hyaluronic acid loaded nano-transfersomes for antioxidant and anti-aging effects in UV radiation induced skin damage. *Drug Delivery*, *24*(1), 61–74. doi:10.1080/10717544.2016.1228718 PMID:28155509

Awasthi, R., Kulkarni, G. T., & Pawar, V. K. (2011). Phytosomes: An approach to increase the bioavailability of plant extracts. *International Journal of Pharmacy and Pharmaceutical Sciences*, *3*(2), 1–3.

Awasthi, R., Kulkarni, T. G., & Pawar, K. V. (2011). Phytosomes an approach to increase the bioavailability of plant extract. *International Journal of Pharmacy and Pharmaceutical Sciences*, *3*(2), 2.

Azmin, M. N., Florence, A. T., Handjani-Vila, R. M., Stuart, J. F. B., Vanlerberghe, G., & Whittaker, J. S. (1985). The effect of non-ionic surfactant vesicle (niosome) entrapment on the absorption and distribution of methotrexate in mice. *The Journal of Pharmacy and Pharmacology*, *37*(4), 237–242. doi:10.1111/j.2042-7158.1985.tb05051.x PMID:2860220

Azmi, S., Jamal, P., & Amid, A. (2012). Xanthine oxidase inhibitory activity from potential Malaysian medicinal plant as remedies for gout. *International Food Research Journal*, *19*(1), 159.

Babii, C., Mihalache, G., Bahrin, L. G., Neagu, A. N., Gostin, I., Mihai, C. T., Sârbu, L.-G., Birsa, L. M., & Stefan, M. (2018). A novel synthetic flavonoid with potent antibacterial properties: In vitro activity and proposed mode of action. *PLoS One*, *13*(4), e0194898. doi:10.1371/journal.pone.0194898 PMID:29617411

Babili, F., Bouajila, J., Souchard, J., Bertrand, C., Bellvert, F., Fouraste, I., Moulis, C., & Valentin, A. (2011). Oregano: Chemical analysis and evaluation of its antimalarial, antioxidant, and cytotoxic activities. *Journal of Food Science*, *76*(3), 12–18. doi:10.1111/j.1750-3841.2011.02109.x PMID:21535822

Babu, V. N., & Kannan, S. (2012). Enhanced delivery of baicalein using cinnamaldehyde cross-linked chitosan nanoparticle inducing apoptosis. *International Journal of Biological Macromolecules*, *51*(5), 1103–1108. doi:10.1016/j.ijbiomac.2012.08.038 PMID:22981825

Baek, J. S., Na, Y. G., & Cho, C. W. (2018). Sustained cytotoxicity of wogonin on breast cancer cells by encapsulation in solid lipid nanoparticles. *Nanomaterials (Basel, Switzerland)*, *8*(3), 159. doi:10.3390/nano8030159 PMID:29533979

Baiguera, C., Boschetti, A., Raffetti, E., Zanini, B., Puoti, M., & Donato, F. (2018). Phyllanthus niruri versus Placebo for Chronic Hepatitis B Virus Infection: A Randomized Controlled Trial. *Complementary Medicine Research*, *25*(6), 376–382. doi:10.1159/000484927 PMID:30372693

Bajpai, V. K., Shukla, S., Kang, S. M., Hwang, S. K., Song, X., Huh, Y. S., & Han, Y. K. (2018). Developments of Cyanobacteria for Nano-Marine Drugs: Relevance of Nano-formulation s in Cancer Therapies. *Marine Drugs*, *16*(6), E179. doi:10.3390/md16060179 PMID:29882898

Baker, P. W., Kennedy, J., Dobson, A. D. W., & Marchesi, J. R. (2009). Phylogenetic Diversity and Antimicrobial Activities of Fungi Associated with *Haliclona simulans* Isolated from Irish Coastal Waters. *Marine Biotechnology (New York, N.Y.)*, *11*(4), 540–547. doi:10.100710126-008-9169-7 PMID:19083060

Bakliwal A. A., & Talele S. G. (2018). Formulation and evaluation of nateglinide nanosponges. *Indian Drugs, 55*(2), 27-35.

Banerjee, J., & Narendhirakannan, R. (2011). Biosynthesis of silver nanoparticles from *Syzygium cumini* (L.) seed extract and evaluation of their in vitro antioxidant activities. *Digest Journal of Nanomaterials and Biostructures*, *6*, 961–968.

Bangham, A., & Horne, R. (1964). Negative staining of phospholipids and their structured modification by surface active agents as observed in the electron microscope. *Journal of Molecular Biology*, *8*(5), 660–668. doi:10.1016/S0022-2836(64)80115-7 PMID:14187392

Banker, G. S., Lieberman, H. A., & Rieger, M. M. (Eds.). (1996). Pharmaceutical dosage forms: disperse systems. Academic Press.

Banker, G. S., & Rhodes, C. T. (1990). *Modern pharmaceutics* (3rd ed.). Marcel Dekkar, Inc.

Bansal, P., Gupta, V., Singh, R., & Chaudhary, A. K. (2010). Pharmacological potential of medicinal plant used in treatment of gout. *Drug Invention Today, 2*(10).

Bansal, V., Rautray, D., Ahamd, A., & Sastry, M. (2004). Biosynthesis of zirconia nanoparticles using the fungus *Fusarium oxysporum*. *Journal of Materials Chemistry*, *14*(22), 3303–3305. doi:10.1039/b407904c

Bansal, V., Rautray, D., Bharde, A., Ahire, K., Sanyal, A., Ahmad, A., & Sastry, M. (2005). Fungus-mediated biosynthesis of silica and titania particles. *Journal of Materials Chemistry*, *15*(26), 2583–2589. doi:10.1039/b503008k

Bar, H., Bhui, D. K., Sahoo, G. P., Sarkar, P., Pyne, S., & Misra, A. (2009). Green synthesis of silver nanoparticles using seed extract of *Jatropha curcas*. *Colloids and Surfaces. A, Physicochemical and Engineering Aspects*, *348*(1-3), 212–216. doi:10.1016/j.colsurfa.2009.07.021

Barragan-Montero, V., Winum, J. Y., Molès, J. P., Juan, E., Clavel, C., & Montero, J. L. (2005). Synthesis and properties of isocannabinoid and cholesterol derivatized rhamnosurfactants: Application to liposomal targeting of keratinocytes and skin. *European Journal of Medicinal Chemistry*, *40*(10), 1022–1029. doi:10.1016/j.ejmech.2005.04.009 PMID:15950324

Barzaghi, N., Crema, F., Gatti, G., Pifferi, G., & Perucca, E. (1990). Pharmacokinetic studies on IdB 1016, a silybin-phosphatidylcholine complex, in healthy human subjects. *European Journal of Drug Metabolism and Pharmacokinetics*, *15*(4), 333–338. doi:10.1007/BF03190223 PMID:2088770

Basavaraja, S., Balaji, S. D., Lagashetty, A., Rajasab, A. H., & Venkataraman, A. (2007). Extracellular biosynthesis of silver nanoparticles using the fungus *Fusarium semitectum*. *Materials Research Bulletin*, *43*(5), 1164–1170. doi:10.1016/j.materresbull.2007.06.020

Basavegowda, N., Sobczak-Kupiec, A., Malina, D., Yathirajan, H. S., Keerthi, V. R., Chandrashekar, N., Dinkar, S., & Liny, P. (2013). Plant mediated synthesis of gold nanoparticles using fruit extracts of *ananas comosus* (L.) (pineapple) and evaluation of biological activities. *Advanced Materials Letters*, *4*(5), 332–337. doi:10.5185/amlett.2012.9423

Baskaralingam, V., Sargunar, C. G., Lin, Y. C., & Chen, J. C. (2012). Green synthesis of silver nanoparticles through *Calotropis gigantea* leaf extracts and evaluation of antibacterial activity against *Vibrio alginolyticus*. *Nanotech Dev.*, *2*(1), e3. doi:10.4081/nd.2012.e3

Belofsky, G. N., Jensen, P. R., Renner, M. K., & Fenical, W. (1998). New cytotoxic sesquiterpenoid nitrobenzoyl esters from a marine isolate of the fungus *Aspergillus versicolor. Tetrahedron, 54*(9), 1715–1724. doi:10.1016/S0040-4020(97)10396-9

Benson, H. A. E. (2005). Transdermal drug delivery: Penetration enhancement techniques. *Current Drug Delivery, 2*(1), 23–33. doi:10.2174/1567201052772915 PMID:16305405

Benson, H. E., & Watkinson, A. C. (2011). *Topical and transdermal drug delivery: Principles and practice*. Wiley Online Library. doi:10.1002/9781118140505

Bernardes, A. C. F. P. F., Coelho, G. B., Araújo, M. C. P. M., & Saúde-Guimarães, D. A. (2019). In vivo anti-hyperuricemic activity of sesquiterpene lactones from Lychnophora species. *Revista Brasileira de Farmacognosia, 29*(2), 241–245. doi:10.1016/j.bjp.2018.12.008

Berry, R. J., Bailey, L., Mulinare, J., Bower, C., & Dary, O. (2011). Folic Acid Working Group, Fortification of flour with folic acid. *Food and Nutrition Bulletin, 31*(1_suppl1), S22–S35. doi:10.1177/15648265100311S103 PMID:20629350

Bhadury, P., Mohammad, B. T., & Wright, P. C. (2006). The current status of natural products from marine fungi and their potential as anti-infective agents. *Journal of Industrial Microbiology & Biotechnology, 33*(5), 325–337. doi:10.100710295-005-0070-3 PMID:16429315

Bhagavathy, S., Sumathi, P., & Bell, I. J. B. (2011). Green algae chlorococcumhumicola-a new source of bioactive compounds with antimicrobial activity. *Asian Pacific Journal of Tropical Biomedicine, 1*(1), S1–S7. doi:10.1016/S2221-1691(11)60111-1

Bhainsa, K. C., & D'Souza, S. F. (2006). Extracellular biosynthesis of silver nanoparticles using the fungus *Aspergillus fumigates. Colloids and Surfaces. B, Biointerfaces, 47*(2), 160–164. doi:10.1016/j.colsurfb.2005.11.026 PMID:16420977

Bhardwaj, A., & Kumar, L. (2011). Colloidal drug delivery system: A future prospective for treatment of tuberculosis. *American Journal of PharmTech Research, 1*(3), 102–123.

Bhati, R., Singh, A., Saharan, V. A., Ram, V., & Bhandari, A. (2011). Pharmacognostical standardization, extraction and anti-diabetic activity of Smilax china L. rhizome. *Asian Journal of Traditional Medicines, 6*(5), 218–223.

Bhat, K. P., Kosmeder, J. W. II, & Pezzuto, J. M. (2001). Biological effects of resveratrol. *Antioxidants & Redox Signaling, 3*(6), 1041–1064. doi:10.1089/152308601317203567 PMID:11813979

Bhatnagar, I., & Kim, S.-K. (2010). Immense Essence of Excellence: Marine Microbial Bioactive Compounds. *Marine Drugs, 8*(10), 2673–2701. doi:10.3390/md8102673 PMID:21116414

Bhattacharya, S. (2009). Phytosomes: Emerging strategy in delivery of herbal drugs and nutraceuticals. *Pharmacy Times, 4*(1), 9–12.

Bhattacharya, S. (2009). Phytosomes: Emerging Strategy in Delivery of Herbal Drugs and Nutraceuticals. *Pharmacy Times, 41*, 9–12.

Bhokare, S., Dhongaonkar, C., Lahane, S., Salunke, P., Savale, V., & Thobare, M. (2016). Herbal novel drug delivery- A review. *Wjpps, 5*(6), 593–611.

Bhujbal, S., Kulkarni, P. A., Thatte, V. A., Yeola, R. R., Hadawale, S. S., Bidkar, J. S., & Providencia, C. A. (2011). A novel herbal formulation in the management of diabetes. *International Journal of Pharmaceutical Investigation, 1*(4), 222–226. doi:10.4103/2230-973X.93009 PMID:23071947

Biondi, S., Fornalé, S., Oksman-Caldentey, K. M., Eeva, M., Agostani, S., & Bagni, N. (2000). Jasmonates induce over-accumulation of methylputrescine and conjugated polyamines in Hyoscyamus muticus L. root cultures. *Plant Cell Reports, 19*(7), 691–697. doi:10.1007002999900178 PMID:30754807

Bisht, S., Feldmann, G., Soni, S., Ravi, R., Karikar, C., & Maitra, A. (n.d.). Polymeric nanoparticle-encapsulate curcumin ("nanocurcumin"): A novel strategy for human cancer therapy. *J Nanobiotechnol, 5*, 1-18.

Bisht, S., Feldmann, G., Soni, S., Ravi, R., Karikar, C., Maitra, A., & Maitra, A. (2007). Polymeric nanoparticles-encapsulated curcumin (nanocurcumin): A novel strategy for human cancer therapy. *Journal of Nanobiotechnology, 5*(3), 2–18. doi:10.1186/1477-3155-5-3 PMID:17439648

Blatt, Y., & Kimmelman, E. (1999). *Microencapsulated and controlled-release herbal formulations*. United States Patent 6340478.

Blunt, J. W., Copp, B. R., Munro, M. H. G., Northcote, P. T., & Prinsep, M. R. (2004). Marine Natural products. *Natural Product Reports, 21*(1), 1–49. doi:10.1039/b305250h PMID:15039834

Bombardelli, E., & Mustich, G. (1991). *Bilobalide-phospholipid complex, their uses and formulation containing them.* U. S. Patent No. EPO-275005.

Bombardelli, E., & Curri, S. B., Della Loggia, R., Del Negro, P., Gariboldi, P., & Tubaro, A. (1989). Complexes between phospholipids and vegetal derivates of biological interest. *Fitoterapia, 60*, 1–9.

Bombardelli, E., Curtis, B., & Della, L. R. (1989). Complexes between phospholipids and vegetal derivatives of biological interest. *Fitoterapia, 90*(Suppl.1), 1–9.

Bonifacio, B. V., da Silva, P. B., dos Santos Ramos, M. A., Negri, K. M. S., Bauab, T. M., & Chorilli, M. (2014). Nanotechnology-based drug delivery systems and herbal medicines: A review. *International Journal of Nanomedicine, 9*, 1. PMID:24363556

Bora, K. S., & Sharma, A. (2011). The genus Artemisia: A comprehensive review. *Pharmaceutical Biology, 49*(1), 101–109. doi:10.3109/13880209.2010.497815 PMID:20681755

Borodina, T. N., Rumsh, L. D., Kunizhev, S. M., Sukhorukov, G. B., Vorozhtsov, G. N., & Feldman, B. M. (2008). Entrapment of herbal extracts into biodegradable microcapsules. *Biochemistry (Moscow) Supplement Series B. Biomedical Chemistry, 2*, 176–182.

Brahmankar, D., & Jaiswal, S. (1998). Biopharmaceutics and Pharmacokinetics -A Treatise. Vallabh Prakashan, 61, 359, 362.

Brannon-Peppas, L. (1995). Recent advances on the use of biodegradable microparticles and nanoparticles in controlled drug delivery. *International Journal of Pharmaceutics, 116*(1), 1–9. doi:10.1016/0378-5173(94)00324-X

Breuning, M., Bauer, S., & Goepferich, A. (2008). Polymers and Nanoparticles: Intelligent tools for intracellular targeting. *European Journal of Pharmaceutics and Biopharmaceutics, 68*(1), 112–128. doi:10.1016/j.ejpb.2007.06.010 PMID:17804211

Brodowska, K. M. (2017). Natural flavonoids: Classification, potential role, and application of flavonoid analogues. *European Journal of Biological Research, 7*(2), 108–123.

Brown, K., & Scott, B. M. (2014). *Herbal supplements and methods of use thereof.* US Patent (US 20140141108 A1).

Bruneton, J. (1995). *Pharmacognosy, phytochemistry, medicinal plants.* Lavoisier publishing.

Bryan, J. (2008). Psychological effects of dietary components of tea: Caffeine and Ltheanine. *Nutrition Reviews*, *66*(2), 82–90. doi:10.1111/j.1753-4887.2007.00011.x PMID:18254874

Buckton, G. (1995). Harwood. Interfacial phenomena in Drug Delivery and Targeting. Academic Publishers.

Bulathsinghala, P., Syrigos, K. N., & Saif, M. W. (2010). Role of vitamin D in the prevention of pancreatic cancer. *Journal of Nutrition and Metabolism*, *2010*, 1–9. doi:10.1155/2010/721365 PMID:21274445

Burke, C., Thomas, T., Egan, S., & Kjelleberg, S. (2007). The use of functional genomics for the identification of a gene cluster encoding for the biosynthesis of an antifungal tambjamine in the marine bacterium *Pseudoalteromonas tunicata*. *Environmental Microbiology*, *9*(3), 814–818. doi:10.1111/j.1462-2920.2006.01177.x PMID:17298379

Bustanji, Y., Hudaib, M., Tawaha, K., Mohammad, M., Almasri, I., Hamed, S., & Oran, S. (2011). In vitro xanthine oxidase inhibition by selected Jordanian medicinal plants. *Jordan Journal of Pharmaceutical Sciences*, *4*, 1.

Byun, H. G., Zhang, H., Mochizuki, M., Adachi, K., Shizuri, Y., Lee, W. J., & Kim, S. K. (2003). Novel antifungal diketopiperazine from marine fungus. *The Journal of Antibiotics*, *56*(2), 102–106. doi:10.7164/antibiotics.56.102 PMID:12715868

Cammidge, A. (2003). Dendrimers and other dendritic polymers. John Wiley and Sons Ltd.

Carini, M., Aldini, G., Rossoni, G., Morazzoni, P., & Facino, R. M. (2001). Complexation of Ginkgo biloba extract with phosphatidylcholine improves cardioprotective activity and increases the plasma antioxidant capacity in the rat. *Planta Medica*, *67*(04), 326–330. doi:10.1055-2001-14313 PMID:11458448

Carlson, J. C., Li, S., Burr, D. A., & Sherman, D. H. (2009). Isolation and Characterization of Tirandamycins from a Marine-Derived *Streptomyces* sp. *Journal of Natural Products*, *72*(11), 2076–2079. doi:10.1021/np9005597 PMID:19883065

Carvalho, A. C., Gomes, A. C., Pereira-Wilson, C., & Lima, C. F. (2016). Mechanisms of Action of Curcumin on Aging: Nutritional and Pharmacological Applications A2 - Malavolta, Marco. In E. Mocchegiani (Ed.), *Molecular Basis of Nutrition and Aging* (pp. 491–511). Academic Press. doi:10.1016/B978-0-12-801816-3.00035-2

Castot, A., Djezzar, S., Deleau, N., Guillot, B., & Efthymiou, M. L. (1997). Pharmacovigilance off the beaten track: Herbal surveillance or pharmacovigilance of medicinal plants. *Therapie*, *52*, 97–103. PMID:9231502

Cevc, G., Schatzlein, A., & Blume, G. (1995). Transdermal drug carriers: Basic properties, optimization and transfer efficiency in case of epicutaneously applied peptides. *Journal of Controlled Release*, *36*(1-2), 3–16. doi:10.1016/0168-3659(95)00056-E

Cevc, G., Schätzlein, A., & Richardsen, H. (2002). Ultradeformable lipid vesicles can penetrate the skin and other semi-permeable barriers unfragmented. Evidence from double label CLSM experiments and direct size measurements. *Biochimica et Biophysica Acta*, *1564*(1), 21–30. doi:10.1016/S0005-2736(02)00401-7 PMID:12100992

Chakraborty, K., & Shivakumar, A. (2018). Nano-technology in herbal medicines. *RE:view*. Advance online publication. doi:10.13140/RG.2.2.32261.24808

Chalova, V., Lingbeck, J., Kwon, Y., & Ricke, S. (2008). Extracellular antimutagenic activities of selected probiotic *Bifidobacterium* and *Lactobacillus spp*. as a function of growth phase. *Journal of Environmental Science and Health. Part B, Pesticides, Food Contaminants, and Agricultural Wastes*, *43*(2), 193–198. doi:10.1080/03601230701795262 PMID:18246512

Chanchal, D., & Swarnlata, S. (2008). Novel approaches in herbal cosmetics. *Journal of Cosmetic Dermatology*, *7*(2), 89–95. doi:10.1111/j.1473-2165.2008.00369.x PMID:18482010

Chandel, A. K. S., Kumar, C. U., & Jewrajka, S. K. (2016). Effect of polyethylene glycol on properties and drug encapsulation–release performance of biodegradable/cytocompatible agarose–polyethylene glycol–polycaprolactone amphiphilic co-network gels. *ACS Applied Materials & Interfaces*, *8*(5), 3182–3192. doi:10.1021/acsami.5b10675 PMID:26760672

Chandran, P., Chaudhary, M., Pasricha, R., Ahmad, A., & Sastry, M. (2006). Synthesis of Gold Nanotriangles and Silver Nanoparticles using *Aloe vera* Plant Extract. *Biotechnology Progress*, *22*(2), 577–583. doi:10.1021/bp0501423 PMID:16599579

Chang, C. H., Huang, W. Y., Lai, C. H., Hsu, Y. M., Yao, Y. H., & Chen, T. Y. (2011). Development of novel Nanoparticles shelled with heparin for Berberine delivery to treat *Helicobacter pylori*. *Acta Biomaterialia*, *7*, 593–603.

Chang, C., Huang, W., Lai, C., Hsu, Y., Yao, Y., Chen, T., Wu, J.-Y., Peng, S.-F., & Lin, Y.-H. (2011). Development of novel nanoparticles shelled with heparin for berberine delivery to treat Helicobacter pylori. *Acta Biomaterialia*, *7*(2), 593–603. doi:10.1016/j.actbio.2010.08.028 PMID:20813208

Chang, J.-S., Liu, H.-W., Wang, K.-C., Chen, M.-C., Chiang, L.-C., Hua, Y.-C., & Lin, C.-C. (2005). Ethanol extract of Polygonum cuspidatum inhibits hepatitis B virus in a stable HBV-producing cell line. *Antiviral Research*, *66*(1), 29–34. doi:10.1016/j.antiviral.2004.12.006 PMID:15781129

Chan, J., El Maghraby, G. M., Craig, J. P., & Alany, R. G. (2007). Phase transition water-in-oil microemulsions as ocular drug delivery systems: In vitro and in vivo evaluation. *International Journal of Pharmaceutics*, *328*(1), 65–71. doi:10.1016/j.ijpharm.2006.10.004 PMID:17092668

Chao, P., Deshmukh, M., Kutscher, H. L., Gao, D., Rajan, S. S., Hu, P., Laskin, D. L., Stein, S., & Sinko, P. J. (2010). Pulmonary targeting microparticulate camptothecin delivery system: Anti-cancer evaluation in a rat orthotopic lung cancer model. *Anti-Cancer Drugs*, *21*(1), 65–76. doi:10.1097/CAD.0b013e328332a322 PMID:19966540

Charman, S. A., Charman, W. N., Rogge, M. C., Wilson, T. D., Dutko, F. J., & Pouton, C. W. (1992). Self-emulsifying drug delivery systems: Formulation and biopharmaceutic evaluation of an investigational lipophilic compound. *Pharmaceutical Research*, *9*(1), 87–93. doi:10.1023/A:1018987928936 PMID:1589415

Charman, W. N., Chan, H. K., Finnin, B. C., & Charman, S. A. (1999). Drug delivery: A key factor in realising the full therapeutic potential of drugs. *Drug Development Research*, *46*(3–4), 316–327. doi:10.1002/(SICI)1098-2299(199903/04)46:3/4<316::AID-DDR18>3.0.CO;2-E

Chaturvedi, M. & Kumar, M. (2011). Recent development in novel drug delivery systems of herbal drugs. *International Journal of Green Pharmacy*, 87-94.

Chaturvedi, M., Sinhal, A., Kumar, M., & Saifi, A. (2011). Recent developments in novel drug delivery systems of herbal drugs. *International Journal of Green Pharmacy*, *5*(2), 87–94. doi:10.4103/0973-8258.85155

Chaudhary, G., & Dewakar, K. (2014). Role of Herbs in Preventing Cancer, *Int. Res. J. Pharm*, *5*(4), 264–266.

Chauhan, N. S., Rajan, G., & Gopalakrishna, B. (2009). Phytosomes: A potential phyto-phospholipid carriers for herbal drug delivery. *Journal of Pharmacy Research*, *2*(7), 1267–1270.

Chauhan, R., Kumar, A., & Abraham, J. (2013). A Biological Approach to the Synthesis of Silver Nanoparticles with *Streptomyces* sp JAR1 and its Antimicrobial Activity. *Scientia Pharmaceutica*, *81*(2), 607–621. doi:10.3797cipharm.1302-02 PMID:23833724

Chen, H., & Weng, L. (2000). Comparison on efficacy in treating liver fibrosis of chronic hepatitis B between Astragalus Polygonum anti-fibrosis decoction and jinshuibao capsule. *Zhongguo Zhong xi yi jie he za zhi Zhongguo Zhongxiyi jiehe zazhi= Chinese journal of integrated traditional and Western medicine, 20*(4), 255.

Chen, B., Li, H., Ou, G., Ren, L., Yang, X., & Zeng, M. (2019). Curcumin attenuates MSU crystal-induced inflammation by inhibiting the degradation of IκBα and blocking mitochondrial damage. *Arthritis Research & Therapy*, *21*(1), 193. doi:10.118613075-019-1974-z PMID:31455356

Chen, C., Guo, S., & Liu, B. (2000). A randomized controlled trial of kurorinone versus interferon-alpha2a treatment in patients with chronic hepatitis B. *Journal of Viral Hepatitis*, *7*(3), 225–229. doi:10.1046/j.1365-2893.2000.00216.x PMID:10849265

Chen, G.-L., Wei, W., & Xu, S.-Y. (2006). Effect and mechanism of total saponin of Dioscorea on animal experimental hyperuricemia. *The American Journal of Chinese Medicine*, *34*(01), 77–85. doi:10.1142/S0192415X06003655 PMID:16437741

Chen, H., Chang, X., Weng, T., Zhao, X., Gao, Z., Yang, Y., Xu, H., & Yang, X. (2004). A study of microemulsion systems for transdermal delivery of triptolide. *Journal of Controlled Release*, *98*(3), 427–436. doi:10.1016/j.jconrel.2004.06.001 PMID:15312998

Chen, H., Zheng, S., Wang, Y., Zhu, H., Liu, Q., Xue, Y., Qiu, J., Zou, H., & Zhu, X. (2016). The effect of resveratrol on the recurrent attacks of gouty arthritis. *Clinical Rheumatology*, *35*(5), 1189–1195. doi:10.100710067-014-2836-3 PMID:25451618

Chen, J., Chen, Z., & Wang, W. (2010). Ammonium sulphate gradient loading of brucine into liposome: Effect of phospholipid composition on entrapment efficiency and physicochemical properties in vitro. *Drug Development and Industrial Pharmacy*, *36*(3), 245–253. doi:10.3109/03639040903099736 PMID:19678739

Chen, J., & Siddiqui, A. (2007). Hepatitis B virus X protein stimulates the mitochondrial translocation of Raf-1 via oxidative stress. *Journal of Virology*, *81*(12), 6757–6760. doi:10.1128/JVI.00172-07 PMID:17428866

Chen, L. J., Liu, Y., Li, L., & Gao, F. (2012). Enhanced bioavailability of total paeony glycoside by self-microemulsifying drug delivery system. *Yao Xue Xue Bao*, *47*(12), 1678–1686. PMID:23460976

Chen, L., & Xu, Y. (2018). Epigallocatechin gallate attenuates uric acid-induced injury in rat renal interstitial fibroblasts NRK-49F by up-regulation of miR-9. *European Review for Medical and Pharmacological Sciences*, *22*(21), 7458–7469. PMID:30468495

Chen, L., Yin, H., Lan, Z., Ma, S., Zhang, C., Yang, Z., Li, P., & Lin, B. (2011). Anti-hyperuricemic and nephroprotective effects of Smilax china L. *Journal of Ethnopharmacology*, *135*(2), 399–405. doi:10.1016/j.jep.2011.03.033 PMID:21420478

Chen, L., Zhao, X., Cai, J., Guan, Y., Wang, S., Liu, H., & Li, J. (2013). Triptolide-loaded microemulsion-based hydrogels: Physical properties and percutaneous permeability. *Acta Pharmaceutica Sinica. B*, *3*(3), 185–192. doi:10.1016/j.apsb.2013.05.001

Chen, X., Yi, C., Yang, X., & Wang, X. (2004). Liquid chromatography of active principles in Sophora flavescens root. *Journal of Chromatography. B, Analytical Technologies in the Biomedical and Life Sciences*, *812*(1-2), 149–163. doi:10.1016/S1570-0232(04)00679-8 PMID:15556494

Chen, Y. C., Yu, S. H., Tsai, G. J., Tang, D. W., Mi, F. L., & Peng, Y. P. (2010). Novel technology for the preparation of self-assembled catechin/gelatin nanoparticles and their characterization. *Journal of Agricultural and Food Chemistry*, *58*(11), 6728–6734. doi:10.1021/jf1005116 PMID:20476739

Chen, Y., Lin, X., Park, H., & Greever, R. (2009). Study of artemisinin nanocapsules as anticancer drug delivery systems. *Nanomedicine; Nanotechnology, Biology, and Medicine*, *5*(3), 316–322. doi:10.1016/j.nano.2008.12.005 PMID:19523432

Chen, Y., Yao, F., Ming, K., Shi, J., Zeng, L., Wang, D., Wu, Y., Hu, Y., & Liu, J. (2019). Assessment of the Effect of Baicalin on Duck Virus Hepatitis. *Current Molecular Medicine*, *19*(5), 376–386. doi:10.2174/1566524019666190405095301 PMID:30950349

Chen, Y., & Zhu, J. (2013). Anti-HBV effect of individual traditional C hinese herbal medicine in vitro and in vivo: An analytic review. *Journal of Viral Hepatitis*, *20*(7), 445–452. doi:10.1111/jvh.12112 PMID:23730837

Che, Y., Gloer, J. B., & Wicklow, D. T. (2002). Phomadecalins, A-D Phomapentenone: A New Bioactive Metabolites from *Phoma* sp. NRRL 25697, a Fungal Colonist of *Hypoxylon Stromata. Journal of Natural Products*, *65*(3), 399–402. doi:10.1021/np010519o PMID:11908990

Chien, Y. (1991). *Novel drug delivery systems*. CRC Press. doi:10.1201/9780367805456

Chien, Y. W. (1992). *Novel drug delivery systems, drugs and the Pharmaceutical sciences, 50.* Marcel Dekkar.

Chih-Hung, L., Chun-Han, C., Zih-Chan, L., & Jia-You, F. (2017). Recent advances in oral delivery of drugs and bioactive natural products using solid lipid nanoparticles as the carriers. *Yao Wu Shi Pin Fen Xi*, *25*, 219–234. PMID:28911663

Chintale, A. G., Kadam, V. S., Sakhare, R. S., Birajdar, G. O., & Nalwad, D. N. (2013). Role of Nutraceuticals – a comphrensive review. *IJRPC*, *3*(2), 2231–2781.

Chiou, D., & Langrish, T. (2007). Development and characterization of novel nutraceuticals with spray dry technology. *Journal of Food Engineering*, *82*(1), 84–91. doi:10.1016/j.jfoodeng.2007.01.021

Chisari, F. V., Filippi, P., Buras, J., McLachlan, A., Popper, H., Pinkert, C. A., Palmiter, R. D., & Brinster, R. L. (1987). Structural and pathological effects of synthesis of hepatitis B virus large envelope polypeptide in transgenic mice. *Proceedings of the National Academy of Sciences of the United States of America*, *84*(19), 6909–6913. doi:10.1073/pnas.84.19.6909 PMID:3477814

Chitkara, D., Nikalaje, S. K., Mittal, A., Chand, M., & Kumar, N. (2012). Development of quercetin nanoformulation and in vivo evaluation using streptozotocin induced diabetic rat model. *Drug Delivery and Translational Research*, *2*(2), 112–123. doi:10.100713346-012-0063-5 PMID:25786720

Choi, H. K., Mount, D. B., & Reginato, A. M. (2005). Pathogenesis of gout. *Annals of Internal Medicine*, *143*(7), 499–516. doi:10.7326/0003-4819-143-7-200510040-00009 PMID:16204163

Cho, J. Y., Williams, P. G., Kwon, H. C., Jensen, P. R., & Fenical, W. (2007). Lucentamycins A–D, cytotoxic peptides from the marine-derived actinomycete *Nocardiopsis lucentensis. Journal of Natural Products*, *70*(8), 1321–1328. doi:10.1021/np070101b PMID:17630797

Chowdhury, S., Basu, A., & Kundu, S. (2014). Green synthesis of protein capped silver nanoparticles from phytopathogenic fungus *Macrophomina phaseolina* (Tassi) Goid with antimicrobial properties against multidrug-resistant bacteria. *Nanoscale Research Letters*, *9*(1), 365. doi:10.1186/1556-276X-9-365 PMID:25114655

Chuang, Y. L., Fang, H. W., Ajitsaria, A., Chen, K. H., Su, C. Y., Liu, G. S., & Tseng, C. L. (2019). Development of Kaempferol-Loaded Gelatin Nanoparticles for the Treatment of Corneal Neovascularization in Mice. *Pharmaceutics*, *11*(12), E635. doi:10.3390/pharmaceutics11120635 PMID:31795237

Chu, C., Deng, J., Man, Y., & Qu, Y. (2017). Green tea extracts epigallocatechin-3-gallate for different treatments. *BioMed Research International*, *2017*, 2017. doi:10.1155/2017/5615647 PMID:28884125

Chu, C.-J., Hussain, M., & Lok, A. S. (2002). Quantitative serum HBV DNA levels during different stages of chronic hepatitis B infection. *Hepatology (Baltimore, Md.)*, *36*(6), 1408–1415. doi:10.1002/hep.1840360617 PMID:12447866

Chung, H., & Burk, H. (2001). *Herbal-based oral composition and process for producing the same*. European Patent EP0862446.

Cohen, E., & Dillin, A. (2008). The insulin paradox: Aging, proteotoxicity and neurodegeneration. *Nature Reviews. Neuroscience*, *9*(10), 759–767. doi:10.1038/nrn2474 PMID:18769445

Constantinides, P. P. (1995). Lipid microemulsions for improving drug dissolution and oral absorption: Physical and biopharmaceutical aspects. *Pharmaceutical Research*, *12*(11), 1561–1572. doi:10.1023/A:1016268311867 PMID:8592652

Cornell, B. A., Braach-Maksvytis, V. L., King, L. G., Osman, P. D., Raguse, B., Wieczorek, L., & Pace, R. J. (1997). A biosensor that uses ion-channel switches. *Nature*, *387*(6633), 580–583. doi:10.1038/42432 PMID:9177344

Coutinho, M. S., Latocheski, E., Neri, J. M., Neves, A. C., Domingos, J. B., Cavalcanti, L. N., Gasparotto, L. H. S., Moraes, E. P., & Menezes, F. G. (2019). Rutin-modified silver nanoparticles as a chromogenic probe for the selective detection of Fe 3+ in aqueous medium. *RSC Advances*, *9*(51), 30007–30011. doi:10.1039/C9RA06653E

Cui, F., Wang, Y., Wang, J., Feng, L., & Ning, K. (2007). Preparation of an enteric soluble solid-state emulsion using oily drugs. *International Journal of Pharmaceutics*, *338*(1-2), 152–156. doi:10.1016/j.ijpharm.2007.01.044 PMID:17349753

Cui, S., Zhao, C., Chen, D., & He, Z. (2005). Self-microemulsifying drug delivery systems (SMEDDS) for improving in vitro dissolution and oral absorption of Pueraria lobata isoflavone. *Drug Development and Industrial Pharmacy*, *31*(4-5), 349–356. doi:10.1081/DDC-54309 PMID:16093200

Cui, X., Wang, Y., Kokudo, N., Fang, D., & Tang, W. (2010). Traditional Chinese medicine and related active compounds against hepatitis B virus infection. *Bioscience Trends*, *4*(2). PMID:20448340

Cui, Y., Li, L., Gu, J., Zhang, T., & Zhang, L. (2011). Investigation of microemulsion system for transdermal delivery of ligustrazine phosphate. *African Journal of Pharmacy and Pharmacology*, *5*(14), 1674–1681. doi:10.5897/AJPP11.138

Currier, S. J., Johnston, P. D., & Gorelick, K. J. (2000). Complementary and alternative medicine-herbal medicines. *Science & Medicine*, *7*, 40–43.

Daily, J. W., Yang, M., & Park, S. (2016). Efficacy of turmeric extracts and curcumin for alleviating the symptoms of joint arthritis: A systematic review and meta-analysis of randomized clinical trials. *Journal of Medicinal Food*, *19*(8), 717–729. doi:10.1089/jmf.2016.3705 PMID:27533649

Daisy, P., & Saipriya, K. (2012). Biochemical analysis of Cassia fistula aqueous extracts and phytochemically synthesized gold nanoparticles as hypoglycemic treatment for diabetes mellitus. *International Journal of Nanomedicine*, *7*, 1189–1202. doi:10.2147/IJN.S26650 PMID:22419867

Dang, H., Meng, M. H. W., Zhao, H., Iqbal, J., Dai, R., Deng, Y., & Lv, F. (2014). Luteolin-loaded solid lipid nanoparticles synthesis, characterization, & improvement of bioavailability, pharmacokinetics in vitro and vivo studies. *Journal of Nanoparticle Research*, *16*(4), 2347. doi:10.100711051-014-2347-9

Dang, S.-S., Jia, X.-L., Song, P., Cheng, Y.-A., Zhang, X., Sun, M.-Z., & Liu, E.-Q. (2009). Inhibitory effect of emodin and Astragalus polysaccharide on the replication of HBV. *World journal of gastroenterology. WJG*, *15*(45), 5669. doi:10.3748/wjg.15.5669 PMID:19960563

Das, V., Thomas, R., Varghese, R., Soniya, E. V., Mathew, J. & Radhakrishnan, E. K. (2014). Extracellular synthesis of silver nanoparticles by the Bacillus strain CS 11 isolated from industrialized area. *Biotech*, *4*, 121-126.

Das, L., Bhaumik, E., Raychaudhuri, U., & Chakraborty, R. (2011). Role of nutraceuticals in human health. *Journal of Food Science and Technology*, *49*(2), 173–183. doi:10.100713197-011-0269-4 PMID:23572839

Das, P., Mukherjee, S., & Sen, R. (2008). Improved bioavailability and biodegradation of a model polyaromatic hydrocarbon by a biosurfactant producing bacterium of marine origin. *Chemosphere*, *72*(9), 1229–1234. doi:10.1016/j.chemosphere.2008.05.015 PMID:18565569

Das, P., Mukherjee, S., & Sen, R. (2009). Biosurfactant of marine origin exhibiting heavy metal remediation properties. *Bioresource Technology*, *100*(20), 4887–4890. doi:10.1016/j.biortech.2009.05.028 PMID:19505818

Das, S., Das, J., Samadder, A., Paul, A., & Khuda-Bukhsh, A. R. (2013). Strategic formulation of apigenin-loaded PLGA nanoparticles for intracellular trafficking, DNA targeting and improved therapeutic effects in skin melanoma in vitro. *Toxicology Letters*, *223*(2), 124–138. doi:10.1016/j.toxlet.2013.09.012 PMID:24070738

Dass, S., & Dey, S. K. (2013). A novel approach towards transdermal drug delivery system: A precise review. *Indo American Journal of Pharmaceutical Research*, *3*(6), 4680–4696.

Davidson, S. K., Allen, S. W., Lim, G. E., Anderson, C. M., & Haygood, M. G. (2001). Evidence for the Biosynthesis of Bryostatins by the Bacterial Symbiont "*Candidatus Endobugula sertula*" of the Bryozoan *Bugula neritina. Applied and Environmental Microbiology*, *67*(10), 4531–4537. doi:10.1128/AEM.67.10.4531-4537.2001 PMID:11571152

Davies, G. (2000). *Timetables of Medicine*. Black Dog & Leventhal.

Dayan, N., & Touitou, E. (2000). Carriers for skin delivery of trihexyphenidyl HCl: Ethosomes vs. liposomes. *Biomaterials*, *21*(18), 1879–1885. doi:10.1016/S0142-9612(00)00063-6 PMID:10919691

de Souza, M. R., de Paula, C. A., de Resende, M. L. P., Grabe-Guimarães, A., de Souza Filho, J. D., & Saúde-Guimarães, D. A. (2012). Pharmacological basis for use of Lychnophora trichocarpha in gouty arthritis: Anti-hyperuricemic and anti-inflammatory effects of its extract, fraction and constituents. *Journal of Ethnopharmacology*, *142*(3), 845–850. doi:10.1016/j.jep.2012.06.012 PMID:22732730

Deldar, Y., Pilehvar-Soltanahmadi, Y., Dadashpour, M., Montazer Saheb, S., Rahmati-Yamchi, M., & Zarghami, N. (2018). An in vitro examination of the antioxidant, cytoprotective and anti-inflammatory properties of chrysin-loaded nanofibrous mats for potential wound healing applications. *Artificial Cells, Nanomedicine, and Biotechnology*, *46*(4), 706–716. doi:10.1080/21691401.2017.1337022 PMID:28595461

DeMario, M., & Ratain, M. (1998). Oral chemotherapy: Rationale and future directions. *Journal of Clinical Oncology*, *16*(7), 2557–2567. doi:10.1200/JCO.1998.16.7.2557 PMID:9667278

Desbois, A. P., Mearns-Spragg, A., & Smith, V. J. (2009). A fatty acid from the diatom *Phaeodactylum tricornutum* is antibacterial against diverse bacteria including multi-resistant *Staphylococcus aureus* (MRSA). *Marine Biotechnology (New York, N.Y.)*, *11*(1), 45–52. doi:10.100710126-008-9118-5 PMID:18575935

Devi, V., Jain, N., & Valli, K. (2010). Importance of novel drug delivery systems in herbal medicines. *Pharmacognosy Reviews*, *4*(7), 27–31. doi:10.4103/0973-7847.65322 PMID:22228938

Dewapriya, P., & Kim, S. (2014). Marine microorganisms: An emerging avenue in modern nutraceuticals and functional foods. *Food Research International*, *56*, 115–125. doi:10.1016/j.foodres.2013.12.022

Dewick, P. M. (2002). *Medicinal natural products: a biosynthetic approach.* John Wiley & Sons.

Dhandapani, N. V., & Sumanraj, K. S. (2014). Phytosomes-A review. *International Journal of Pharma Sciences*, *4*(4), 622–625.

Dhiman, R. K., & Chawla, Y. K. (2005). Herbal medicines for liver diseases. *Digestive Diseases and Sciences*, *50*(10), 1807–1812. doi:10.100710620-005-2942-9 PMID:16187178

Dhiman, S., & Thakur, G. S. (2011). Transdermal patches: A recent approch to new drug delivery system. *International Journal of Pharmacy and Pharmaceutical Sciences*, *3*, 26–34.

Dibua, E., & Nnamani, P. (2011). Antimicrobial properties of clove, tobacco and bitter on tooth decay. *Asian Pacific Journal of Tropical Medicine*, *4*(10), 412–420.

Ding, B., Chen, H., Wang, C., Zhai, Y., & Zhai, G. (2013). Preparation and in vitro evaluation of apigenin loaded lipid nanocapsules. *Journal of Nanoscience and Nanotechnology*, *13*(10), 6546–6552. doi:10.1166/jnn.2013.7763 PMID:24245113

Ding, F., Diao, J. X., Sun, Y., & Sun, Y. (2012). Bioevaluation of human serum albumin–hesperidin bioconjugate: Insight into protein vector function and conformation. *Journal of Agricultural and Food Chemistry*, *60*(29), 7218–7228. doi:10.1021/jf300424w PMID:22702966

Ding, P.-L., Liao, Z.-X., Huang, H., Zhou, P., & Chen, D.-F. (2006). (+)-12α-Hydroxysophocarpine, a new quinolizidine alkaloid and related anti-HBV alkaloids from Sophora flavescens. *Bioorganic & Medicinal Chemistry Letters*, *16*(5), 1231–1235. doi:10.1016/j.bmcl.2005.11.073 PMID:16364643

Ding, S. M., Zhang, Z. H., Song, J., Cheng, X. D., Jiang, J., & Jia, X. B. (2014). Enhanced bioavailability of apigenin via preparation of a carbon nanopowder solid dispersion. *International Journal of Nanomedicine*, *9*, 2327. doi:10.2147/IJN.S60938 PMID:24872695

Dixit, N., Baboota, S., Kohli, K., Ahmad, S., & Ali, J. (2007). Silymarin: A review of pharmacological aspects and bioavailability enhancement approaches. *Indian Journal of Pharmacology*, *39*(4), 172. doi:10.4103/0253-7613.36534

Dong, X., Mattingly, C. A., Tseng, M., Cho, M., Adams, V. R., & Mumper, R. J. (2009, May). Development of new lipid based paclitaxel nanoparticles using sequential simplex optimization. *European Journal of Pharmaceutics and Biopharmaceutics*, *72*(1), 9–17. doi:10.1016/j.ejpb.2008.11.012 PMID:19111929

Drexler, K. E. (1992). *Nanosystems: Molecular machinery, manufacturing, and computation*. John Wiley & Sons.

Dua, J. S., & Rana, A. C. (2012). Liposome: Methods Of Preparation And Applications. *IJPSR*, *3*(2), 14–20.

Dubey, S. P., Lahtinen, M., & Sillanpaa, M. (2010). Green synthesis and characterizations of silver and gold nanoparticles using leaf extract of Rosa rugosa. *Colloids and Surfaces. A, Physicochemical and Engineering Aspects*, *364*(1-3), 34–41. doi:10.1016/j.colsurfa.2010.04.023

Du, G., Xiao, M., Yu, S., Wang, M., Xie, Y., & Sang, S. (2018). Phyllanthus urinaria: A potential phytopharmacological source of natural medicine. *International Journal of Clinical and Experimental Medicine*, *11*(7), 6509–6520.

Du, L., Feng, T., Zhao, B., Li, D., Cai, S., Zhu, T., Wang, F., Xiao, X., & Gu, Q. (2010). Alkaloids from a deep ocean sediment-derived fungus *Penicillium* sp. and their antitumor activities. *The Journal of Antibiotics*, *63*(4), 165–170. doi:10.1038/ja.2010.11 PMID:20186171

Du, L., Zhu, T., Fang, Y., Liu, H., Gu, Q., & Zhu, W. (2007). Aspergiolide A, a novel anthraquinone derivative with naphtho(1,2,3-de)chromene-2,7-dione skeleton isolated from a marine-derived fungus *Aspergillus glaucus*. *Tetrahedron*, *63*, 1085–1088. doi:10.1016/j.tet.2006.11.074

Duranoğlu, D., Uzunoglu, D., Mansuroglu, B., Arasoglu, T., & Derman, S. (2018). Synthesis of hesperetin-loaded PLGA nanoparticles by two different experimental design methods and biological evaluation of optimized nanoparticles. *Nanotechnology*, *29*(39), 395603. doi:10.1088/1361-6528/aad111 PMID:29972381

Du, X., Zhao, B., Li, J., Cao, X., Diao, M., Feng, H., Chen, X., Chen, Z., & Zeng, X. (2012). Astragalus polysaccharides enhance immune responses of HBV DNA vaccination via promoting the dendritic cell maturation and suppressing Treg frequency in mice. *International Immunopharmacology*, *14*(4), 463–470. doi:10.1016/j.intimp.2012.09.006 PMID:23006659

Edris, A. E. (2007). Pharmaceutical and therapeutic potentials of essential oils and their individual volatile constituents: A review. *Phytotherapy Research, 21*(4), 308–323. doi:10.1002/ptr.2072 PMID:17199238

Egan, S., James, S., Holmström, C., & Kjelleberg, S. (2002). Correlation between pigmentation and antifouling compounds produced by *Pseudoalteromonas tunicata. Environmental Microbiology, 4*(8), 433–442. doi:10.1046/j.1462-2920.2002.00322.x PMID:12153584

Elena, M. (2003). Mailiohydrin, a cytotoxic chamigrene dibromohydrin from a phillippine *Laurencia* species. *Journal of Natural Products, 64*, 790–791.

El-Gendy, M. M., Hawas, U. W., & Jaspars, M. (2008). Novel bioactive metabolites from a marine derived bacterium *Nocardia* sp. ALAA 2000. *The Journal of Antibiotics, 61*(6), 379–386. doi:10.1038/ja.2008.53 PMID:18667786

El-Raey, M. A., Ibrahim, G. E., & Eldahshan, O. A. (2013). Lycopene and Lutein; A review for their Chemistry and Medicinal Uses. *Journal of Pharmacognosy and Phytochemistry, 2*(1).

El-Ridy, M. S., Badawi, A. A., Safar, M. M., & Mohsen, A. M. (2012). Niosomes as a novel pharmaceutical formulation encapsulating the hepatoprotective drug silymarin. *International Journal of Pharmacy and Pharmaceutical Sciences, 4*(1), 549–559.

El-Sherbiny, & Smyth, H. (2012). Controlled release pulmonary administration of curcumin using swellable biocompatible microparticles. *Journal of Molecular Pharmaceutics & Organic Process Research, 9*, 269–280. PMID:22136259

Engy, A. M., & Mohamed, A. F. (2015). Two-dimensional NMR spectroscopic approaches for exploring plant metabolome: A review. *Journal of Advanced Research, 6*(1), 3–15. doi:10.1016/j.jare.2014.10.003 PMID:25685540

Evans, W. C. (2009). *Trease and Evans Pharmacognosy* (International Edition). E-Book. Elsevier Health Sciences.

Fabiana, T., Thais, R., Jose, O., Nilce, O., Dimitrius, L., & Mamie, M. (2008). Quercetin in w/o microemulsion: In vitro and in vivo skin penetration and efficacy against UVB-induced skin damages evaluated in vivo. *J PharmBiopharm, 69*, 948–957. PMID:18304790

Fahao, C., Wuqing, O., & Yanping, W. (2007). Study of preparation of matrin nanoemulsion and its anti-oxidation on mice. *Journal of Northwest Sci-Tech University of Agriculture and Forestry.*

Fan, Y., & Zhang, Q. (2013). Development of liposomal formulations: From concept to clinical investigations. *Asian Journal of Pharmaceutical Sciences, 8*(2), 81-87.

Fang, J. Y., Hwang, T. L., Huang, Y. L., & Fang, C. L. (2006). Enhancement of the transdermal delivery of catechins by liposomes incorporating anionic surfactants and ethanol. *International Journal of Pharmaceutics, 310*(1-2), 131–138. doi:10.1016/j.ijpharm.2005.12.004 PMID:16413711

Fasano, E., Serini, S., Piccioni, E., Innocenti, I., & Calviello, G. (2010). Chemoprevention of lung pathologies by dietary n-3 polyunsaturated fatty acids. *Current Medicinal Chemistry, 17*(29), 3358–3376. doi:10.2174/092986710793176401 PMID:20712568

Fathi-Achachloueia, B. (2019). Microwave pretreatment as a promising strategy for increment of nutraceutical content and extraction yield of oil from milk thistle seed. *Industrial Crops and Products, 128*, 527–533. doi:10.1016/j.indcrop.2018.11.034

Fathi, M., & Varshosaz, J. (2013). Novel hesperetin loaded nanocarriers for food fortification: Production and characterization. *Journal of Functional Foods, 5*(3), 1382–1391. doi:10.1016/j.jff.2013.05.006

Fathi, M., Varshosaz, J., Mohebbi, M., & Shahidi, F. (2013). Hesperetin-loaded solid lipid nanoparticles and nanostructure lipid carriers for food fortification: Preparation, characterization, and modeling. *Food and Bioprocess Technology*, *6*(6), 1464–1475. doi:10.100711947-012-0845-2

Fatima Grace, X., & Rahul Raj, S. (2014). Herbal ethosomes—A Novel Approach in Herbal Drug Technology. *American Journal of Ethnomedicine*, *1*(4), 226–230.

Fatima Grace, X., Rahul Raj, S., Reshma, I., Sandeep, T., Shanmuganathan, S., & Chamundeeswari, D. (2014). Herbal ethosomes-A novel approach in herbal drug technology. *American Journal of Ethnomedicine*, *1*(4), 226–230.

Feng, C., Yuan, X., Chu, K., Zhang, H., Ji, W., & Rui, M. (2019). Preparation and optimization of poly (lactic acid) nanoparticles loaded with fisetin to improve anti-cancer therapy. *International Journal of Biological Macromolecules*, *125*, 700–710. doi:10.1016/j.ijbiomac.2018.12.003 PMID:30521927

Feng-Lin, Y., Tzu-Hui, W., Liang-Tzung, L., Thau-Ming, C., & Chun-Chingaa, L. (2009). Preparation of naringenin nanopartciles. *Pharmaceutical Research*, *26*(4), 893–902. PMID:19034626

Feng-Lin, Y., Tzu-Hui, W., Liang-Tzung, L., Thau-Ming, C., & Chun-Ching, L. (2009). Preparation of naringenin nanoparticles. *Pharmaceutical Research*, *26*(4), 893–902. PMID:19034626

Feng, T., Wei, Y., Lee, R., & Zhao, L. (2017). Liposomal curcumin and its application in cancer. *International Journal of Nanomedicine*, *12*, 6027–6044. doi:10.2147/IJN.S132434 PMID:28860764

Feng, W. M., Guo, H. H., Xue, T., Wang, X., Tang, C. W., Ying, B., Gong, H., & Cui, G. (2015). Anti-inflammation and anti-fibrosis with PEGylated, apigenin loaded PLGA nanoparticles in chronic pancreatitis disease. *RSC Advances*, *5*(102), 83628–83635. doi:10.1039/C5RA17686G

Ferraz Filha, Z., Vitolo, I., Fietto, L., Lombardi, J., & Saúde-Guimarães, D. A. (2006). Xanthine oxidase inhibitory activity of Lychnophora species from Brazil ("Arnica"). *Journal of Ethnopharmacology*, *107*(1), 79–82. doi:10.1016/j.jep.2006.02.011 PMID:16621372

Ferrucci, V., Boffa, I., De Masi, G., & Zollo, M. (2016). Natural compounds for pediatric cancer treatment. *Naunyn-Schmiedeberg's Archives of Pharmacology*, *389*(2), 131–149. doi:10.100700210-015-1191-5 PMID:26650503

Firdhouse, M. J., & Lalitha, P. (2013). Biomimetic synthesis of silver nanoparticles using aqueous extract of *amaranthus polygonoides. International Journal of Pharma and Bio Sciences*, *4*, 588–595.

Firouzi-Amandi, A., Dadashpour, M., Nouri, M., Zarghami, N., Serati-Nouri, H., Jafari-Gharabaghlou, D., Karzar, B. H., Mellatyar, H., Aghebati-Maleki, L., Babaloo, Z., & Pilehvar-Soltanahmadi, Y. (2018). Chrysin-nanoencapsulated PLGA-PEG for macrophage repolarization: Possible application in tissue regeneration. *Biomedicine and Pharmacotherapy*, *105*, 773–780. doi:10.1016/j.biopha.2018.06.037 PMID:29909345

Flaten, G. E., Chang, T. T., Phillips, W. T., Brandl, M., Bao, A., & Goins, B. (2013). Liposomal formulations of poorly soluble camptothecin: Drug retention and biodistribution. *Journal of Liposome Research*, *23*(1), 70–81. doi:10.3109/08982104.2012.742537 PMID:23210622

Fleet, M. F., & Southam, G. (2006). Morphology of Gold Nanoparticles Synthesized by Filamentous Cyanobacteria from Gold(I)-Thiosulfate and Gold(III)-Chloride Complexes. *Langmuir*, *22*(6), 2780–2787. doi:10.1021/la052652c PMID:16519482

Fleet, M. F., & Southam, G. (2007). Synthesis of palladium nanoparticles by reaction of filamentous cyanobacterial biomass with a palladium (II) chloride complex. *Langmuir*, *23*(17), 8982–8987. doi:10.1021/la7012446 PMID:17658865

Focsan, M., Ardelean, I. I., Craciun, C., & Astilean, S. (2011). Interplay between gold nanoparticle biosynthesis and metabolic activity of cyanobacterium *Synechocystis* sp. PCC 680. *Nanotechnology*, *22*(48), 485101–485109. doi:10.1088/0957-4484/22/48/485101 PMID:22072064

Forst & Sullivan. (n.d.). Global Nutraceutical Industry Investing in Healthy Life. *FICCI*, 5-26.

Forsythe, P., & Bienenstock, J. (2010). Immunomodulation by commensal and probiotic bacteria. *Immunological Investigations*, *39*(4-5), 429–448. doi:10.3109/08820131003667978 PMID:20450286

Franks, A., Haywood, P., Holmström, C., Egan, S., Kjelleberg, S., & Kumar, N. (2005). Isolation and structure elucidation of a novel yellow pigment from the marine bacterium *Pseudoalteromonas tunicata*. *Molecules (Basel, Switzerland)*, *10*(10), 1286–1291. doi:10.3390/10101286 PMID:18007521

Fraser, S. P., Hemsley, F., & Djamgoz, M. B. (2015). Caffeic acid phenethyl ester: Inhibition of metastatic cell behaviours via voltage-gated sodium channel in human breast cancer in vitro. *The International Journal of Biochemistry & Cell Biology*, *71*, 111–118. doi:10.1016/j.biocel.2015.12.012 PMID:26724521

Freiberg, S., & Zhu, X. X. (2004). Polymer microspheres for controlled drug release. *International Journal of Pharmaceutics*, *282*(1–2), 1–18. doi:10.1016/j.ijpharm.2004.04.013 PMID:15336378

Frias, I., Neves, A. R., Pinheiro, M., & Reis, S. (2016). Design, development, and characterization of lipid nanocarriers-based epigallocatechin gallate delivery system for preventive and therapeutic supplementation. *Drug Design, Development and Therapy*, *10*, 3519–3528. doi:10.2147/DDDT.S109589 PMID:27826184

Fröhlich, J. K., Stein, T., da Silva, L. A., Biavatti, M. W., Tonussi, C. R., & Lemos-Senna, E. (2017). Antinociceptive and anti-inflammatory activities of the Jatropha isabellei dichloromethane fraction and isolation and quantitative determination of jatrophone by UFLC-DAD. *Pharmaceutical Biology*, *55*(1), 1215–1222. doi:10.1080/13880209.2017.1295999 PMID:28249559

Fu, R. Q., He, F. C., Meng, D. S., & Chen, L. (2006). Taxol PLA nanoparticles. *ACTA Academiae medicinae militaris tertiae, 28*, 1573-1574.

Gaber, D. M., Nafee, N., & Abdallah, O. Y. (2017). Myricetin solid lipid nanoparticles: Stability assurance from system preparation to site of action. *European Journal of Pharmaceutical Sciences*, *109*, 569–580. doi:10.1016/j.ejps.2017.08.007 PMID:28818532

Gabetta, B., Fuzzati, N., Griffini, A., Lolla, E., Pace, R., Ruffilli, T., & Peterlongo, F. (2000). Characterization of proanthocyanidins from grape seeds. *Fitoterapia*, *71*(2), 162–175. doi:10.1016/S0367-326X(99)00161-6 PMID:10727813

Gai, Y., Zhao, L. L., Hu, C. Q., & Zhang, H. P. (2007). Fusarielin E, a new antifungal antibiotic from *Fusarium* sp. *Chinese Chemical Letters*, *18*(8), 954–956. doi:10.1016/j.cclet.2007.05.048

Gajbhiye, M., Kesharwani, J., Ingle, A., Gade, A., & Rai, M. (2009). Fungus-mediated synthesis of silver nanoparticles and their activity against pathogenic fungi in combination with fluconazole. *Nanotechnology. Biology and Medicine (Aligarh)*, *5*, 382–386. PMID:19616127

Ganapathy, M., & Bhunia, S. (2016). Nutraceuticals: The New Generation Therapeutics. *Adv. Tech Bio Med*, *4*(2), 2-5.

Gande, S., Kopparam, M., & Vobalaboina, V. (2007). Preparation characterization and in vitro and in vivo evalution of lovastatin solid lipid nanoparticle. *AAPS PharmSciTech*, *8*, 1–8.

Gandhi A., Dutta A., Pal A., & Bakshi P. (2012). Recent Trends of Phytosomes for Delivering Herbal Extract with Improved Bioavailability. *Journal of Pharmacognosy and Phytochemistry*, *1*(4), 6-14.

Gandhi, A., Dutta, A., Pal, A., & Bakshi, P. (2012). Recent trend of phytosomes for delivering herbal extract with improved bioavailability. *Journal of Pharmacognosy and Phytochemistry*, *1*(4), 6.

Gandhimathi, R., Arunkumar, M., Selvin, J., Thangavelu, T., Sivaramakrishnan, S., Kiran, G. S., Shanmughapriya, S., & Natarajaseenivasan, K. (2008). Antimicrobial potential of sponge associated marine actinomycetes. *Journal de Mycologie Médicale*, *18*(1), 16–22. doi:10.1016/j.mycmed.2007.11.001

Ganesan, P., Noda, K., Manabe, Y., Ohkubo, T., Tanaka, Y., Maoka, T., Sugawara, T., & Hirata, T. (2010). Siphonaxanthin, a marine carotenoid from green algae, effectively induces apoptosis in human leukemia (HL-60) cells. *Biochimica et Biophysica Acta*, *1810*(5), 497–503. doi:10.1016/j.bbagen.2011.02.008 PMID:21371530

Ganesan, V., Devi, J. A., Astalakshmi, A., Nima, P., & Thangaraja, A. (2013). Eco- Friendly Synthesis of Silver Nanoparticles using a Sea Weed, *Kappaphycus Alvarezii* (Doty) Doty ex P.C.Silva. *International Journal of Engineering and Advanced Technology*, *2*(5).

Gangwar, S., Singh, S., & Garg, G. (2010). Ethosomes: A novel tool for drug delivery through skin. *Journal of Pharmacy Research*, *3*, 688–691.

Gao, D., Han, I., & Wang, J. (2009). Self micro emulsifying drug delivery system loaded with gentiopicrin phospholipid complex for oral delivery; preparation in vivo characterization and in vivo evaluation abstract 2009. *AAPS Annual meeting and exposition*.

Gardea-Torresdey, J. L., Parsons, J. G., Gomez, E., Peralta-Videa, J., Troiani, H. E., & Santiago, P. (2002). Formation and growth of Au nanoparticles inside live alfalfa plants. American Chemical Society, 2, 397–401. doi:10.1021/nl015673+

Garg, R., & Gupta, G. D. (2010). Gastroretentive floating microspheres of silymarin: Preparation and in vitro evaluation. *Tropical Journal of Pharmaceutical Research*, *9*(1). Advance online publication. doi:10.4314/tjpr.v9i1.52037

Garodia, P., Ichikawa, H., Malani, N., Sethi, G., & Aggarwal, B. B. (2007). From ancient medicine to modern medicine: Ayurvedic concepts of health and their role in inflammation and cancer. *Journal of the Society for Integrative Oncology*, *5*(1), 25–37. doi:10.2310/7200.2006.029 PMID:17309811

Garti, N., & McClements, D. J. (2012). Encapsulation technologies and delivery systems for food ingredients and nutraceuticals. florida: Woodhead publishing series in food sciences. *Technology and Nutrition*, *1*, 23–30.

Gavilanes, F., Gonzalez-Ros, J. M., & Peterson, D. L. (1982). Structure of hepatitis B surface antigen. Characterization of the lipid components and their association with the viral proteins. *The Journal of Biological Chemistry*, *257*(13), 7770–7777. PMID:7085648

Gavini, E., Alamanni, M. C., Cossu, M., & Giunchedi, P. (2005). Tabletted microspheres containing *Cynarascolymus* (var. Spinososardo) extract for the preparation of controlled release nutraceutical matrices. *Journal of Microencapsulation*, *22*(5), 487–499. doi:10.1080/02652040500099919 PMID:16361192

Geckeler, K. E. J., & Stirn, J. (1993). Stirn Polyreaktionen Mechanismen,Systematik, Relevanz. *Naturwissenschaften*, *80*(11), 487–500. doi:10.1007/BF01140804 PMID:8264805

Geethalakshmi, R., & Sarada, D. V. L. (2012). Gold and silver nanoparticles from *Trianthema decandra*: Synthesis, characterization, and antimicrobial properties. *International Journal of Nanomedicine*, *7*, 5375–5384. doi:10.2147/IJN.S36516 PMID:23091381

Geng, C.-A., Yang, T.-H., Huang, X.-Y., Yang, J., Ma, Y.-B., Li, T.-Z., Zhang, X.-M., & Chen, J.-J. (2018). Anti-hepatitis B virus effects of the traditional Chinese herb Artemisia capillaris and its active enynes. *Journal of Ethnopharmacology*, *224*, 283–289. doi:10.1016/j.jep.2018.06.005 PMID:29890315

Genoux, E., Nicolle, E., & Boumendjel, A. (2011). Flavonoids as anticancer agents: Recent progress and state of the art? *Current Organic Chemistry, 15*(15), 2608–2615. doi:10.2174/138527211796367363

Gescher, A. J., Sharma, R. A., & Steward, W. P. (2001). Cancer chemoprevention by dietary constituents: A tale of failure and promise. *The Lancet. Oncology, 2*(6), 371–379. doi:10.1016/S1470-2045(00)00392-2 PMID:11905754

Ge, X., Wei, M., He, S., & Yuan, W. E. (2019). Advances of Non-Ionic Surfactant Vesicles (Niosomes) and Their Application in Drug Delivery. *Pharmaceutics, 11*(2), 55. doi:10.3390/pharmaceutics11020055 PMID:30700021

Ghadi, Z. S., Dinarvand, R., Asemi, N., Amiri, F. T., & Ebrahimnejad, P. (2019). Preparation, characterization and in vivo evaluation of novel hyaluronan containing niosomes tailored by Box-Behnken design to co-encapsulate curcumin and quercetin. *European Journal of Pharmaceutical Sciences, 130*, 234–246. doi:10.1016/j.ejps.2019.01.035 PMID:30711688

Ghinaiya, M. (2013). Formulation and evaluation of transdermal patch of an antihypertensive drug. *International Journal of Pharma Sciences, 4*, 3664–3682.

Ghosh, S., Patil, S., Ahire, M., Kitture, R., Jabgunde, A., Kale, S., Pardesi, K. Bellare, J., Dhavale, D.D. & Chopade, B.A. (2011). Synthesis of gold nano-anisotrops using *Dioscorea bulbifera* tuber extract. *Journal of Nanomaterial.*

Ghosh, P., Roy, A. S., Chaudhury, S., Jana, S. K., Chaudhury, K., & Dasgupta, S. (2016). Preparation of albumin-based nanoparticles for delivery of fisetin and evaluation of its cytotoxic activity. *International Journal of Biological Macromolecules, 86*, 408–417. doi:10.1016/j.ijbiomac.2016.01.082 PMID:26820351

Ghosh, S., Patil, S., Ahire, M., Kitture, R., Kale, S., Pardesi, K., Cameotra, S. S., Bellare, J., Dhavale, D. D., & Chopade, B. A. (2012). Synthesis of silver nanoparticles using Dioscorea bulbifera tuber extract and evaluation of its synergistic potential in combination with antimicrobial agents. *International Journal of Nanomedicine, 7*, 483–496. PMID:22334779

Girhepunje, K., Pal, R., Gevariya, H., Behera, A., & Thirumoorthy, N. (2010). Ethosomes: A novel vesicular carrier for enhanced dermal delivery of Ciclopiroxolamine. *Der Pharmacia Lettre, 2*(1), 360–367.

Godin, B., & Touitou, E. (2004). Mechanism of bacitracin permeation enhancement through the skin and cellular membranes from an ethosomal carrier. *Journal of Controlled Release, 94*(2-3), 365–379. doi:10.1016/j.jconrel.2003.10.014 PMID:14744487

Goh, J. X. H., Tan, L. T. H., Goh, J. K., Chan, K. G., Pusparajah, P., Lee, L. H., & Goh, B. H. (2019). Nobiletin and derivatives: Functional compounds from citrus fruit peel for colon cancer chemoprevention. *Cancers (Basel), 11*(6), 867. doi:10.3390/cancers11060867 PMID:31234411

Gomez-Ordonez, E., Jimenez-Escrig, A., & Ruperez, P. (2010). Dietary fibre and physico-chemical properties of several edible seaweeds from the Northwestern Spanish coast. *Food Research International, 9*(9), 2289–2294. doi:10.1016/j.foodres.2010.08.005

Gopi, S., Amalraj, A., & Józef, T. (2016). Introduction of nanotechnology in herbal drugs and nutraceutical: A review. *Journal of Nanomedicine & Biotherapeutic Discovery, 6*(2), 1–8. doi:10.4172/2155-983X.1000143

Goswami, A. M., Sarkar, T. S., & Ghosh, S. (2013). An Ecofriendly synthesis of silver nano-bioconjugates by *Penicillium citrinum* (MTCC9999) and its antimicrobial effect. *AMB Express, 3*(1), 16. doi:10.1186/2191-0855-3-16 PMID:23433075

Goyal, A., & Kumar, S. (2011). Potential of novel drug delivery system for herbal drugs. *Indian Journal of Pharmaceutical Education and Research, 45*, 225–235.

Goyal, A., Kumar, S., Nagpal, M., Singh, I., & Arora, S. (2011). Potential of novel drug delivery systems for herbal drugs. *Ind J Pharm Edu Res, 45*(3), 225–235.

Goyal, A., Kumar, S., Nagpal, M., Singh, I., & Arora, S. (2011). Potential of novel drug delivery systems for herbal drugs. *Indian J Pharm Educ Res*, *45*, 225–235.

Goyal, C., Ahuja, M., & Sharma, S. K. (2011). Preparation and evaluation of anti-inflammatory activity of gugulipid-loaded proniosomal gel. *Acta Pol Pharm Drug Res*, *68*, 147–150.

Graham, S., & Neil, B. (1990). Controlled drug delivery systems. *La Chimica e l'Industria*, *6*, 25–38.

Grayson, S. M., & Frechet, J. M. (2001). Convergent dendrons and dendrimers: From synthesis to applications. *Chemical Reviews*, *101*(12), 3819–3868. doi:10.1021/cr990116h PMID:11740922

Griffin, J. P., & O'Grady, J. (Eds.). (2006). *The textbook of pharmaceutical medicine*. Blackwell.

Grill, A. E., Johnston, N. W., Sadhukha, T., & Panyam, J. (2009). A review of select recent patents on novel nanocarriers. *Recent Patents on Drug Delivery & Formulation*, *3*(2), 137–142. doi:10.2174/187221109788452276 PMID:19519573

Grobbelaar, J. U., & Bornman, C. H. (2004). Algal biotechnology: Real opportunities for Africa. *South African Journal of Botany*, *70*(1), 140–144. doi:10.1016/S0254-6299(15)30274-X

Guang, C., Yu, L., & Wen, G. (2010). Preparation and anti-inflammatory activity of Triptolide ethosomes in an erythema model. *Journal of Liposome Research*, *20*(4), 297–303. doi:10.3109/08982100903544144 PMID:20102297

Gui, S. Y., Wu, L., Peng, D. Y., Liu, Q. Y., Yin, B. P., & Shen, J. Z. (2008). Preparation and evaluation of a microemulsion for oral delivery of berberine. *Die Pharmazie-An International Journal of Pharmaceutical Sciences*, *63*(7), 516–519. PMID:18717486

Gullett, N. P., Amin, A. R., Bayraktar, S., Pezzuto, J. M., Shin, D. M., Khuri, F. R., ... Kucuk, O. (2010, June). Cancer prevention with natural compounds. *Seminars in Oncology*, *37*(3), 258–281. doi:10.1053/j.seminoncol.2010.06.014 PMID:20709209

Gunalana, S., Sivaraja, R., & Rajendran, V. (2012). Green synthesized ZnO nanoparticles against bacterial and fungal pathogens. *Progress in Natural Science*, *22*(6), 693–700. doi:10.1016/j.pnsc.2012.11.015

Gunasekaran, T., Haile, T., Nigusse, T., & Dhanaraju, M. D. (2014). Nanotechnology: An effective tool for enhancing bioavailability and bioactivity of phytomedicine. *Asian Pacific Journal of Tropical Biomedicine*, *4*, S1–S7. doi:10.12980/APJTB.4.2014C980 PMID:25183064

Guo, Q., Zhao, L., You, Q., Yang, Y., Gu, H., Song, G., Lu, N., & Xin, J. (2007). Anti-hepatitis B virus activity of wogonin in vitro and in vivo. *Antiviral Research*, *74*(1), 16–24. doi:10.1016/j.antiviral.2007.01.002 PMID:17280723

Gupta, L., Sharma, A. K., Gothwal, A., Khan, M. S., Khinchi, M. P., Qayum, A., Singh, S. K., & Gupta, U. (2017). Dendrimer encapsulated and conjugated delivery of berberine: A novel approach mitigating toxicity and improving in vivo pharmacokinetics. *International Journal of Pharmaceutics*, *528*(1-2), 88–99. doi:10.1016/j.ijpharm.2017.04.073 PMID:28533175

Gupta, N., Loona, S., & Khan, M. (2012). Ethosomes as elastic vesicles in transdermal drug delivery: An overview. *International Journal of Current Pharmaceutical Research*, *3*(3), 682–687.

Gupta, S. C., Kannappan, R., Reuter, S., Kim, J. H., & Aggarwal, B. B. (2011). Chemosensitization of tumors by resveratrol. *Annals of the New York Academy of Sciences*, *215*(1), 150–160. doi:10.1111/j.1749-6632.2010.05852.x PMID:21261654

Gupta, S., Singh, R., Lokwani, P., Yadav, S., & Gupta, S. (2011). Vesicular system as targeted drug delivery system: An overview. *Int J Pharm Technol*, *3*, 987–1021.

Gu, X. B., Yang, X. J., Hua, Z., Lu, Z. H., Zhang, B., Zhu, Y. F., ... Pei, H. (2012). Effect of oxymatrine on specific cytotoxic T lymphocyte surface programmed death receptor-1 expression in patients with chronic hepatitis B. *Chinese Medical Journal, 125*(8), 1434–1438. PMID:22613649

Guy, R. H. (1996). Current status and future prospects of transdermal drug delivery. *Pharmaceutical Research, 13*(12), 1765–1769. doi:10.1023/A:1016060403438 PMID:8987069

Guy, R. H., Hadgraft, J., & Bucks, D. A. W. (1987). Transdermal drug delivery and cutaneous metabolism. *Xonobiotica, 7*(3), 325–343. doi:10.3109/00498258709043943 PMID:3107225

Hadziyannis, S., Bramou, T., Makris, A., Moussoulis, G., Zignego, L., & Papaioannou, C. (1990). Interferon alfa-2b treatment of HBeAg negative/serum HBV DNA positive chronic active hepatitis type B. *Journal of Hepatology, 11*, S133–S136. doi:10.1016/0168-8278(90)90180-Y PMID:2079571

Haleemkhan, A.A., Naseem, & Vardhini, B. V. (2015). Synthesis of nanoparticles from Plant Extract. *International Journal of Modern Chemistry and Applied Sciences, 2*(3), 195-203.

Hall, S. S. (2003). Longevity research. In vivo vitalis? Compounds activate life-extending genes. *Science, 301*(5637), 1165.

Hamid, N., Azar, B., Hedayatollah, S., & Mahmoud, R. K. (2014). New Concepts in Nutraceuticals as Alternative for Pharmaceuticals. *International Journal of Preventive Medicine, 5*(12), 1487–1499. PMID:25709784

Hao, Y., Zhao, F., Li, N., Yang, Y., & Li, K. A. (2002). Studies on a high encapsulation of colchicine by a niosome system. *International Journal of Pharmaceutics, 244*(1-2), 73–80. doi:10.1016/S0378-5173(02)00301-0 PMID:12204566

Haratifar, E., Shahverdi, H. R., Shakibaie, M., Moghaddam, K. M., Amini, M., Montazeri, H., & Shahv, A. R. (2009). Semi-Biosynthesis of Magnetite-Gold Composite Nanoparticles Using an Ethanol Extract of *Eucalyptus camaldulensis* and Study of the Surface Chemistry. *Journal of Nanomaterials, 5*, 962021.

Harne, S., Sharma, A., Dhaygude, M., Joglekar, S., Kodam, K., & Hudlikar, M. (2012). Novel route for rapid biosynthesis of copper nanoparticles using aqueous extract of Calotropis procera L. latex and their cytotoxicity on tumor cells. *Colloids and Surfaces. B, Biointerfaces, 95*, 284–288. doi:10.1016/j.colsurfb.2012.03.005 PMID:22483347

Harris, A. M. (2019). Hepatitis B. *Travelers'. Health.*

Havlik, J., de la Huebra, R. G., Hejtmankova, K., Fernandez, J., Simonova, J., Melich, M., & Rada, V. (2010). Xanthine oxidase inhibitory properties of Czech medicinal plants. *Journal of Ethnopharmacology, 132*(2), 461–465. doi:10.1016/j.jep.2010.08.044 PMID:20800669

Hawas, U. W., Shaaban, M., Shaaban, K. A., Speitling, M., Maier, A., Kelter, G., Fiebig, H. H., Meiners, M., Helmke, E., & Laatsch, H. (2009). Mansouramycins A-D, cytotoxic isoquinolinequinones from a marine streptomycete. *Journal of Natural Products, 72*(12), 2120–2124. doi:10.1021/np900160g PMID:19921834

Hayashi, H. (1989). Drying technologies of foods – their history and future. *Drying Technology, 7*(2), 315–369. doi:10.1080/07373938908916590

Heard, C. M., Johnson, S., Moss, G., & Thomas, C. P. (2006). In vitro transdermal delivery of caffeine, theobromine, theophylline and catechin from extract of Guarana, Paullinia cupana. *International Journal of Pharmaceutics, 317*(1), 26–31. doi:10.1016/j.ijpharm.2006.02.042 PMID:16600539

He, H. B., & Tang, X. (2005). Preparation of zedoary oil nano-emulsion and the influence factors on its preparation process. *Journal of Shenyang Pharmaceutical University, 3*, 164–186. http://www.indena.com/pdf/phytosome_int.pdf

Henrotin, Y., Lambert, C., Couchourel, D., Ripoll, C., & Chiotelli, E. (2011). Nutraceuticals: Do they represent a new era in the management of osteoarthritis? – A narrative review from the lessons taken with five products. *OsCar, 19*(1), 1–21. doi:10.1016/j.joca.2010.10.017 PMID:21035558

Hesari, A., Ghasemi, F., Salarinia, R., Biglari, H., Tabar Molla Hassan, A., Abdoli, V., & Mirzaei, H. (2018). Effects of curcumin on NF-κB, AP-1, and Wnt/β-catenin signaling pathway in hepatitis B virus infection. *Journal of Cellular Biochemistry, 119*(10), 7898–7904. doi:10.1002/jcb.26829 PMID:29923222

He, X., Fang, J., Huang, L., Wang, J., & Huang, X. (2015). Sophora flavescens Ait.: Traditional usage, phytochemistry and pharmacology of an important traditional Chinese medicine. *Journal of Ethnopharmacology, 172*, 10–29. doi:10.1016/j.jep.2015.06.010 PMID:26087234

He, X., & Rui, H. L. (2006). Cranberry phytochemicals: Isolation, structure elucidation, and their antiproliferative and antioxidant activities. *Journal of Agricultural and Food Chemistry, 54*(19), 7069–7074. doi:10.1021/jf0610581 PMID:16968064

He, Y., Du, Z., Lv, H., Jia, Q., Tang, Z., Zheng, X., Zhang, K., & Zhao, F. (2013). Green synthesis of silver nanoparticles by *Chrysanthemum morifolium* Ramat extract and their application in clinical ultrasound gel. *International Journal of Nanomedicine, 8*, 1809–1815. doi:10.2147/IJN.S43289 PMID:23687447

He, Z. F., Liu, D. Y., Zeng, S., & Ye, J. T. (2008). Study on preparation of ampelopsin liposomes. Zhongguo Zhong yao za zhi Zhongguo zhongyao zazhi. *Zhongguo Zhongyao Zazhi, 33*(1), 27–30. PMID:18338614

Hirai, S., Kim, Y. I., Goto, T., Kang, M. S., Yoshimura, M., Obata, A., & Kawada, T. (2007). Inhibitory effect of naringenin chalcone on inflammatory changes in the interaction between adipocytes and macrophages. *Life Sciences, 81*(16), 1272–1279. doi:10.1016/j.lfs.2007.09.001 PMID:17915259

Hoet, P. H., Brüske-Hohlfeld, I., Salata, O. V., & Brnske, H. I. (2004). Nano particles known and unknown health risk. *J. Nanobiotecnol, 2*(1), 12. doi:10.1186/1477-3155-2-12 PMID:15588280

Hoffman, A. S. (2008). The origin and evolution of controlled drug delivery systems. *Journal of Controlled Release, 132*(3), 153–163. doi:10.1016/j.jconrel.2008.08.012 PMID:18817820

Holland, A. (1999). *Voices of Qi: an introductory guide to traditional Chinese medicine*. North Atlantic Books.

Holmberg, K., Shah, D. O., & Schwuger, M. J. (2002). *Handbook of applied surface and colloid chemistry* (Vol. 1). John Wiley & Sons.

Honarya, S., Barabadi, H., Gharaeifathaba, D. E., & Naghibi, F. (2012). Green synthesis of copper oxide nanoparticles using *Penicillium aurantiogriseum, Penicillium citrinum* and *Penicillium waksmanii. Digest Journal of Nanomaterials and Biostructures, 7*, 999–1005.

Hong, W., Chen, D. W., Zhao, X. L., Qiao, M. X., & Hu, H. Y. (2008). Preparation and study in vitro of long-circulating nanoliposomes of curcumin. Zhongguo Zhong yao za zhi, Zhongguo zhongyao zazhi. *Zhongguo Zhongyao Zazhi, 33*(8), 889–892. PMID:18619344

Hong, W., Chen, D., Zhao, X., Qiao, M., & Hu, H. (2008). Preparation and study in vitro of long-circulating nanoliposomes of curcumin. *Zhongguo Zhongyao Zazhi, 33*, 889–892. PMID:18619344

Hou, J., & Zhou, S. (2003). Formulation and preparation of glycyrrhizic acid solid lipid nanoparticles. *Journal of Third Military Medical University*, (11).

Huang, H.-C., Tao, M.-H., Hung, T.-M., Chen, J.-C., Lin, Z.-J., & Huang, C. (2014). (−)-Epigallocatechin-3-gallate inhibits entry of hepatitis B virus into hepatocytes. *Antiviral Research*, *111*, 100–111. doi:10.1016/j.antiviral.2014.09.009 PMID:25260897

Huang, J. L., Li, Q. B., Sun, D. H., Lu, Y. H., Su, Y. B., Yang, X., Wang, H., Wang, Y., Shao, W., He, N., Hong, J., & Chen, C. (2007). Biosynthesis of silver and gold nanoparticles by novel sundried Cinnamomum camphora leaf. *Nanotechnology*, *18*(10), 105104. doi:10.1088/0957-4484/18/10/105104

Huang, J., Zhu, M., Tao, Y., Wang, S., Chen, J., Sun, W., & Li, S. (2012). Therapeutic properties of quercetin on monosodium urate crystal-induced inflammation in rat. *The Journal of Pharmacy and Pharmacology*, *64*(8), 1119–1127. doi:10.1111/j.2042-7158.2012.01504.x PMID:22775215

Huang, R.-L., Chen, C.-C., Huang, H.-L., Chang, C.-G., Chen, C.-F., Chang, C., & Hsieh, M.-T. (2000). Anti-hepatitis B virus effects of wogonin isolated from Scutellaria baicalensis. *Planta Medica*, *66*(08), 694–698. doi:10.1055-2000-9775 PMID:11199123

Huang, S.-X., Mou, J.-F., Luo, Q., Mo, Q.-H., Zhou, X.-L., Huang, X., Xu, Q., Tan, X.-D., Chen, X., & Liang, C.-Q. (2019). Anti-Hepatitis B Virus Activity of Esculetin from Microsorium fortunei In Vitro and In Vivo. *Molecules (Basel, Switzerland)*, *24*(19), 3475. doi:10.3390/molecules24193475 PMID:31557836

Huang, X., & Brazel, C. S. (2001). On the importance and mechanisms of burst release in matrix-controlled drug delivery systems. *Journal of Controlled Release*, *73*(2–3), 121–136. doi:10.1016/S0168-3659(01)00248-6 PMID:11516493

Huang, Y., Sun, M., Yang, X., Ma, A., Ma, Y., & Zhao, A. (2019). Baicalin relieves inflammation stimulated by lipopolysaccharide via upregulating TUG1 in liver cells. *Journal of Physiology and Biochemistry*, *75*(4), 463–473. doi:10.100713105-019-00698-0 PMID:31396818

Ilk, S., Saglam, N., & Özgen, M. (2017). Kaempferol loaded lecithin/chitosan nanoparticles: Preparation, characterization, and their potential applications as a sustainable antifungal agent. *Artificial Cells, Nanomedicine, and Biotechnology*, *45*(5), 907–916. doi:10.1080/21691401.2016.1192040 PMID:27265551

Inagaki, F., Nunoura, T., Nakagawa, S., Teske, A., Lever, M., Lauer, A., Suzuki, M., Takai, K., Delwiche, M., Colwell, F. S., Nealson, K. H., Horikoshi, K., D'Hondt, S., & Jorgensen, B. B. (2006). Biogeographical distribution and diversity of microbes in methane hydrate-bearing deep marine sediments on the Pacific Ocean Margin. *Proceedings of the National Academy of Sciences of the United States of America*, *103*(8), 2815–2820. doi:10.1073/pnas.0511033103 PMID:16477011

Ina, M. (2011). Dendrimer: A novel drug delivery system. *Journal of Drug Delivery and Therapeutics*, *1*(2), 70–74.

Inamdar, N. S., Edalat, V. B., Kotwal, V. B., & Pawar, S. S. (2008). Herbal drugs in milieu of modern drugs. *Int J Green Pharm*, *2*(1), 2–8. doi:10.4103/0973-8258.39154

Inoue, K., Kumazawa, E., Kuga, H., Susaki, H., Masubuchi, N., & Kajimura, T. (2004). *CM-dextran-polyalcohol-camptothecin conjugate. In Polymer Drugs in the Clinical Stage*. Springer.

Iosio, T. A. M. A. R. A., Voinovich, D. A. R. I. O., Perissutti, B., Serdoz, F., Hasa, D., Grabnar, I., Acqua, S. D., Zara, G. P., Muntoni, E., & Pinto, J. F. (2011). Oral bioavailability of silymarin phytocomplex formulated as self-emulsifying pellets. *Phytomedicine*, *18*(6), 505–512. doi:10.1016/j.phymed.2010.10.012 PMID:21111585

Iravani, S. (2011). Green synthesis of metal nanoparticles using plants. *Green Chemistry*, *13*(10), 2638–2650. doi:10.1039/c1gc15386b

Irimie, A. I., Sonea, L., Jurj, A., Mehterov, N., Zimta, A. A., Budisan, L., Braicu, C., & Berindan-Neagoe, I. (2017). Future trends and emerging issues for nanodelivery systems in oral and oropharyngeal cancer. *International Journal of Nanomedicine, 12*, 4593–4606. doi:10.2147/IJN.S133219 PMID:28721037

Ishida, K., Cipriano, T. F., Rocha, G. M., Weissmuller, G., Gomes, F., Miranda, K., & Rozental, S. (2013). Silver nanoparticle production by the fungus *Fusarium oxysporum*: Nanoparticle characterisation and analysis of antifungal activity against pathogenic yeasts. *Memorias do Instituto Oswaldo Cruz, 109*(2), 1–9. doi:10.1590/0074-0276130269 PMID:24714966

Isnansetyo, A., & Kamei, Y. (2003). MC21-A, a bactericidal antibiotic produced by a new marine bacterium, *Pseudoalteromonas phenolica* sp. nov. O-BC30T against methicillin-resistant *Staphylococcus aureus. Antimicrobial Agents and Chemotherapy, 47*(2), 480–488. doi:10.1128/AAC.47.2.480-488.2003 PMID:12543647

Isnansetyo, A., & Kamei, Y. (2009). Bioactive substances produced by marine isolates of *Pseudomonas. Journal of Industrial Microbiology & Biotechnology, 36*(10), 1239–1248. doi:10.100710295-009-0611-2 PMID:19582493

Ivan, M. P. (2016). Lycosome technology: Advances and perspectives. *American Journal of Food Science and Nutrition, 3*(1), 18–23.

Iwaki, T., Kakihara, Y., Toda, T., Abdullah, M., & Okuyama, K. (2003). Preparation of high coercivity magnetic fe Pt nanoparticles by liquid process. *Journal of Applied Physics, 94*(10), 6807–6811. doi:10.1063/1.1619577

Iwata, F., Sato, S., Mukai, T., Yamada, S., Takeo, J., Abe, A., Okita, T., & Kawahara, H. (2009). Lorneic Acids, Trialkyl-Substituted Aromatic Acids from a Marine-Derived Actinomycete. *Journal of Natural Products, 72*(11), 2046–2048. doi:10.1021/np900353y PMID:19856955

Jadhav, I. A., Wadhave, A. A., Arsul, V. A., & Sawarkar, H. S. (2014). Phytosome a novel approach in herbal drug. *Int J Pharm Anal, 2*(5), 478.

Jaganathan, S., & Supriyanto, E. (2012). Ant proliferative and molecular mechanism of eugenol-induced apoptosis in cancer cells. *Molecules (Basel, Switzerland), 17*(6), 290–304. doi:10.3390/molecules17066290 PMID:22634840

Jain, S., Jain, V., & Mahajan, S. C. (2014). Lipid based vesicular drug delivery systems. *Advances in Pharmaceutics.*

Jain, H., Patel, J., Joshi, K., Patel, P., & Upadhyay, U. (2011). Ethosomes: A novel drug carrier. *Pharm Globale Int J Compr Pharm, 7*, 1–4.

Jain, N. K. (2005). *Liposomes as drug carriers, controlled and novel drug delivery* (1st ed.). CBS publisher.

Jain, N., Gupta, P. B., Thakur, N., Jain, R., & Banweer, J. (2010). Phytosome a novel drug delivery system for herbal medicine. *International Journal of Pharmaceutical Sciences and Drug Research, 2*(4), 224.

Jain, S., Jain, A. K., Pohekar, M., & Thanki, K. (2013). Novel self-emulsifying formulation of quercetin for improved in vivo antioxidant potential: Implications for drug-induced cardiotoxicity and nephrotoxicity. *Free Radical Biology & Medicine, 65*, 117–130. doi:10.1016/j.freeradbiomed.2013.05.041 PMID:23792276

Jang, E., Kim, B.-J., Lee, K.-T., Inn, K.-S., & Lee, J.-H. (2015). A survey of therapeutic effects of Artemisia capillaris in liver diseases. *Evidence-Based Complementary and Alternative Medicine.* PMID:26366183

Janisch, K. M., Williamson, G., Needs, P., & Plumb, G. W. (2004). Properties of quercetin conjugates: Modulation of LDL oxidation and binding to human serum albumin. *Free Radical Research, 38*(8), 877–884. doi:10.1080/10715760410001728415 PMID:15493462

Jayaseelan, C., Ramkumar, R., Rahuman, A. A., & Perumal, P. (2013). Green synthesis of gold nanoparticles using seed aqueous extract of *Abelmoschus esculentus* and its antifungal activity. *Industrial Crops and Products, 45*, 423–429. doi:10.1016/j.indcrop.2012.12.019

Jayawardena, R., Sooriyaarachchi, P., Chourdakis, M., Jeewandara, C., & Ranasinghef, P. (2020). Enhancing immunity in viral infections, with special emphasis on COVID-19: A review. *Diabetes & Metabolic Syndrome: Clinical Research & Reviews*, 1-54.

Je, J. Y., & Kim, S. K. (2012). Chitosan as potential marine nutraceutical. *Advances in Food and Nutrition Research, 65*, 121–135. doi:10.1016/B978-0-12-416003-3.00007-X PMID:22361183

Jenaa, J., Pradhana, N., Dashb, B. P., Suklaa, L. B., & Pandaa, P. K. (2013). Biosynthesis and characterization of silver nanoparticles using microalga *Chlorococcum humicola* and its antibacterial activity. *International Journal of Nanomaterials and Biostructures., 3*, 1–8.

Jena, J., Pradhan, N., Nayak, R. R., Dash, B. P., Sukla, L. B., Panda, P. K., & Mishra, B. K. (2014). Microalga *Scenedesmus* sp.: A Potential Low-Cost Green Machine for Silver Nanoparticle Synthesis. *Journal of Microbiology and Biotechnology, 24*(4), 522–533. doi:10.4014/jmb.1306.06014 PMID:24394192

Jha, A. K., & Prasad, K. (2010). Green synthesis of silver nanoparticles using Cycas leaf. *International Journal of Green Nanotechnology: Physical Chemistry, 1*, 110–117.

Jha, S. K., & Dey, S. (2011). Microemulsions-potential carrier for improved drug delivery. *Asian J. Biomed PharmSci, 1*, 5–9.

Jiang, H. L., Cui, Y. L., & Qi, Y. (2013). Microencapsulation of rutin in chitosan-coated alginate microspheres through internal gelation technique. *Advanced Materials Research, 716*, 433–458. doi:10.4028/www.scientific.net/AMR.716.455

Jiang, S., Han, J., Li, T., Xin, Z., Ma, Z., Di, W., Hu, W., Gong, B., Di, S., Wang, D., & Yang, Y. (2017). Curcumin as a potential protective compound against cardiac diseases. *Pharmacological Research, 119*, 373–383. doi:10.1016/j.phrs.2017.03.001 PMID:28274852

Jiang, T., Wang, T., Li, T., Ma, Y., Shen, S., He, B., & Mo, R. (2018). Enhanced Transdermal Drug Delivery by Transfersome-Embedded Oligopeptide Hydrogel for Topical Chemotherapy of Melanoma. *ACS Nano, 12*(10), 9693–9701. doi:10.1021/acsnano.8b03800 PMID:30183253

Jiang, Y., You, X.-Y., Fu, K.-L., & Yin, W.-L. (2012). Effects of extract from Mangifera indica leaf on monosodium urate crystal-induced gouty arthritis in rats. *Evidence-Based Complementary and Alternative Medicine*. PMID:23304232

Jin, J., Sklar, G. E., Min Sen Oh, V., & Chuen Li, S. (2008). Factors affecting therapeutic compliance: A review from the patient"s perspective. *Therapeutics and Clinical Risk Management, 4*(1), 269–286. doi:10.2147/TCRM.S1458 PMID:18728716

Joerger, R., Klaus, T., & Granqvist, C. G. (2000). Biologically Produced Silver-Carbon Composite Materials for Optically Functional Thin-Film Coatings. *Advanced Materials, 12*(6), 407–409. doi:10.1002/(SICI)1521-4095(200003)12:6<407::AID-ADMA407>3.0.CO;2-O

Johansson, E. M., Dubois, J., Darbre, T., & Reymond, J. L. (2010). Glycopeptide dendrimer colchicine conjugates targeting cancer cells. *Bioorganic & Medicinal Chemistry, 18*(17), 6589–6597. doi:10.1016/j.bmc.2010.04.026 PMID:20674369

John, D. N., Franklin, C. K., Anthony, A. A., & Salome, A. C. (2012). Different approaches to formulation of herbal extracts/ phytopharmaceuticals/ bioactive phytoconstituents- A review. *International Journal of Pharmaceutical Sciences Review and Research, 16*(1), 1–8.

Johnson, I. T. (2007). Phytochemicals and cancer. *The Proceedings of the Nutrition Society*, *66*(2), 207–215. doi:10.1017/S0029665107005459 PMID:17466103

Joshi, A., Chaturvedi, S., Kumar, V., & Pathak, A. (2008). *Phytosomes: A revolution in herbal drugs. The Pharma Review*. Kongposh Publications Pvt. Ltd.

Kadari, A., Gudem, S., Kulhari, H., Bhandi, M. M., Borkar, R. M., Kolapalli, V. R. M., & Sistla, R. (2017). Enhanced oral bioavailability and anticancer efficacy of fisetin by encapsulating as inclusion complex with HPβCD in polymeric nanoparticles. *Drug Delivery*, *24*(1), 224–232. doi:10.1080/10717544.2016.1245366 PMID:28156161

Kalabegishvili, T., Kirkesali, E., Frontasyeva, M. V., & Pavlov, S. S. (2012). Synthesis of Gold Nanoparticles by Blue-Green Algae *Spirulina Platensis. Proceedings of the international conference nanomaterials: applications and properties.*

Kalia, A. N. (2005). *Text Book of Industrial Pharmacognosy*. Oscar Publication.

Kalinovskaya, N. I., Ivanova, E. P., Alexeeva, Y. V., Gorshkova, N. M., Kuznetsova, T. A., Dmitronek, A. D., & Nicolau, D. V. (2004). Low-molecular-weight, biologically active compounds from marine *Pseudoalteromonas* species. *Current Microbiology*, *48*(6), 441–446. doi:10.100700284-003-4240-0 PMID:15170241

Kalita, B., Das, K. M., & Sharma, K. A. (2013). Novel phytosome formulation making herbal extract more effective. *The Journal of Pharmacy Technology*, *6*(11), 1295.

Kamble, B., Talreja, S., Gupta, A., Patil, D., Pathak, D., Moothedath, I., & Duraiswamy, B. (2013). Development and biological evaluation of Gymnema sylvestre extract-loaded nonionic surfactant-based niosomes. *Nanomedicine (London)*, *8*(8), 1295–1305. doi:10.2217/nnm.12.162 PMID:23259778

Kang, E. H., Kown, T. Y., Oh, G. T., Park, W. F., Park, S. I., Park, S. K., & Lee, Y. I. (2006). The flavonoid ellagic acid from a medicinal herb inhibits host immune tolerance induced by the hepatitis B virus-e antigen. *Antiviral Research*, *72*(2), 100–106. doi:10.1016/j.antiviral.2006.04.006 PMID:16720052

Kannan, B., & Narayanan, N. S. (2010). Biological synthesis of metal nanoparticles by microbes. *Advances in Colloid and Interface Science*, *156*(1-2), 1–13. doi:10.1016/j.cis.2010.02.001 PMID:20181326

Karak, P. (2019). Biological activities of flavonoids: An overview. *International Journal of Pharmaceutical Sciences and Research*, *10*(4), 1567–1574.

Karaś, M., Jakubczyk, A., Szymanowska, U., Złotek, U., & Zielińska, E. (2017). Digestion and bioavailability of bioactive phytochemicals. *International Journal of Food Science & Technology*, *52*(2), 291–305. doi:10.1111/ijfs.13323

Karimi, N., Ghanbarzadeh, B., Hamishehkar, H., Keyvani, F., Pezeshki, A., & Gholian, M. M. (2015). Phytosome and liposome: the beneficial encapsulation systems in drug delivery and food application. *Applied Food Biotechnology,* 17-27.

Karwa, A., Gaikwad, S., & Rai, M. (2011). Mycosynthesis of Silver Nanoparticles Using Lingzhi or Reishi Medicinal Mushroom, *Ganoderma lucidum* (W. Curt.:Fr.) P. Karst. and their Role as Antimicrobials and Antibiotic Activity Enhancers. *International Journal of Medicinal Mushrooms*, *13*(5), 483–491. doi:10.1615/IntJMedMushr.v13.i5.80 PMID:22324414

Kasthuri, J., Kathiravan, K., & Rajendiran, N. (2009). Phyllanthin-assisted biosynthesis of silver and gold nanoparticles: A novel biological approach. *Journal of Nanoparticle Research*, *11*(5), 1075–1085. doi:10.100711051-008-9494-9

Kastorini, C. M., Milionis, H. J., Esposito, K., Giugliano, D., Goudevenos, J. A., & Panagiotakos, D. B. (2011). The effect of mediterranean diet on metabolic syndrome and its components: A meta-analysis of 50 studies and 534,906 individuals. *Journal of the American College of Cardiology*, *57*(11), 1299–1313. doi:10.1016/j.jacc.2010.09.073 PMID:21392646

Kausar, H., Mujeeb, M., Ahad, A., Moolakkadath, T., Aqil, M., Ahmad, A., & Akhter, M. H. (2019). Optimization of ethosomes for topical thymoquinone delivery for the treatment of skin acne. *Journal of Drug Delivery Science and Technology*, *49*, 177–187. doi:10.1016/j.jddst.2018.11.016

Kavithaa, K., Sumathi, S., & Padma, P. R. (2017). Intracellular uptake of PEG-funtionalized baicalein loaded iron oxide nanoparticles regulates apoptotic genes in triple negative breast cancer cells: Mitochondrial pathway targeted therapy for breast cancer. *Journal of Cluster Science*, *28*(4), 2057–2073. doi:10.100710876-017-1204-2

Kavitha, D., Naga, S. J., & Panaganti, S. (2010). Pharmacosomes: An emerging vesicular system. *International Journal of Pharmaceutical Sciences Review and Research*, *5*(3), 168–171.

Kaviya, S., Santhanalakshmi, J., Viswanathan, B., Muthumary, J., & Srinivasan, K. (2011b). Biosynthesis of silver nanoparticles using Citrus sinensis peel extract and its antibacterial activity. *Spectrochimica Acta. Part A: Molecular and Biomolecular Spectroscopy*, *79*(3), 594–598. doi:10.1016/j.saa.2011.03.040 PMID:21536485

Keservani, R., Sharma, A., & Kesharwani, R. (Eds.). (2017). Drug Delivery Approaches and Nanosystems, Volume 1 (Novel Drug Carriers). CRC Press.

Keservani, R. K., Kesharwani, R. K., Sharma, A. K., & Jarouliya, U. (2015). Dietary supplements, nutraceutical, and functional foods in immune response (immunomodulators). In D. Bagchi, A. Swaroop, & H. G. Preuss (Eds.), *Nutraceutical and Functional Foods in Human Life and Disease Prevention* (pp. 343–360). CRC Press, Taylor and Francis.

Keservani, R. K., Sharma, A. K., & Kesharwani, R. K. (2017). An overview and therapeutic applications of nutraceutical and functional foods. In *Recent Advances in Drug Delivery Technology* (pp. 160–201). IGI Global.

Keservani, Sharma, & Kesharwani, Vyas, & Chadoker. (2010). Nutritional Supplements: An Overview. *International Journal of Current Pharmaceutical Review and Research*, *1*(1), 59–75.

Kesharwani & Misra. (2011). Prediction of binding site for Curcuminoids at human Topoisomerase II α protein; an in silico approach. *Current Science*, *101*(8), 1060–1064.

Kesharwani & Misra. (2021). *Biotechnology in the Modern Medicinal System: Advances in Gene Therapy, Immunotherapy, and Targeted Drug Delivery*. Apple Academic Press.

Kesharwani, J., Yoon, K. Y., Hwang, J., & Rai, M. (2009). Phytofabrication of silver nanoparticles by leaf extract of Datura metel: Hypothetical mechanism involved in synthesis. *Journal of Bionanoscience.*, *3*(1), 39–44. doi:10.1166/jbns.2009.1008

Kesharwani, R. K., & Misra, K. (2011). Prediction of binding site for curcuminoids at human topoisomerase II α protein; an in silico approach. *Current Science*, 1060–1065.

Kesharwani, R. K., Misra, K., & Singh, D. B. (2019). Perspectives and challenges of tropical medicinal herbs and modern drug discovery in the current scenario. *Asian Pacific Journal of Tropical Medicine*, *12*(1), 1–7. doi:10.4103/1995-7645.250337

Kesharwani, R. K., Srivastava, V., Singh, P., Rizvi, S. I., Adeppa, K., & Misra, K. (2015). A novel approach for overcoming drug resistance in breast cancer chemotherapy by targeting new synthetic curcumin analogues against Aldehyde Dehydrogenase 1 (ALDH1A1) and Glycogen Synthase Kinase-3 β (GSK-3β). *Applied Biochemistry and Biotechnology*, *176*(7), 1996–2017. doi:10.100712010-015-1696-x PMID:26113217

Kesharwani, S., & Singh, R. Adeppa, & Misra. (2015). A novel approach for overcoming drug resistance in breast cancer chemotherapy by targeting new synthetic curcumin analogues against Aldehyde Dehydrogenase 1 (ALDH1A1) and Glycogen Synthase Kinase-3 β (GSK-3β). *Applied Biochemistry and Biotechnology*. Advance online publication. doi:10.100712010- 015-1696-x

Khajuria, A., Zutshi, U., & Bedi, K. L. (1998). Permeability characteristics of piperine on oral absorption-an active alkaloid from peppers and a bioavailability enhancer. *Indian Journal of Experimental Biology*, *36*, 46–50. PMID:9536651

Khalil, M. M. H., Ismail, E. H., El-Baghdady, K. Z., & Mohamed, D. (2013). Green synthesis of silver nanoparticles using olive leaf extract and its antibacterial activity. *Arabian Journal of Chemistry*, *7*(6), 1131–1139. doi:10.1016/j.arabjc.2013.04.007

Khandare, J. N., Madhavi, G., & Tamhankar, B. M. (1994). Niosomes-novel drug Delivery system. *Eastern Pharmacist*, *37*, 61–61.

Kharat, A. (2014). Novel drug delivery system in herbal's. *International Journal of Pharma and Bio Sciences*, *4*(4), 910–930.

Kharat, A., & Pawar, P. (2014). Novel drug delivery system in Herbal's. *International Journal of Pharmaceutical, Chemical and Biological Sciences*, *4*(4), 910–930.

Kharisov, B. I., Dias, H. V. R., Kharissova, O. V., Vázquez, A., Peña, Y., & Gómez, I. (2014). Solubilization, dispersion and stabilization of magnetic Nanoparticles in water and non aqueous solvent: Recent trends. *RSC Advances*, *4*(85), 45354–45381. doi:10.1039/C4RA06902A

Khemani, M., Sharon, M., & Sharon, M. (2012). Encapsulation of berberine in nano-sized PLGA synthesized by emulsification method. *ISRN Nanotechnol.*, *34*, 12–21. doi:10.5402/2012/187354

Khopade, A.J., Jain, S., & Jain, N.K. (1996). The Microsponge. *Eastern Pharmacist*, 49-53.

Kidd, P. M. (1997). Glutathione: Systemic protectant against oxidative and free radical damage. *Alternative Medicine Review*, *2*(3), 155–176.

Kidd, P. M. (2009). Bioavailability and activity of phytosome complexes from botanical polyphenols: The silymarin, curcumin, green tea, and grape seed extracts. *Alternative Medicine Review*, *14*(3), 226–246. PMID:19803548

Kim, J. H. (2006). *Nanoparticle composition for prevention of hair loss and promotion of hair growth.* (US20100104646A1).

Kim, J. H. (2010). *Nanoparticle composition for prevention of hair loss and promotion of hair growth.* US patent (US 20100104646 A1).

Kim, E. Y., Kim, D. G., Kim, Y. R., Hwang, H. J., Nam, T. J., & Kong, I. S. (2011). An improved method of protein isolation and proteome analysis with *Saccharina japonica* (Laminariales) incubated under different pH conditions. *Journal of Applied Phycology*, *23*(1), 123–130. doi:10.100710811-010-9550-6

Kim, H. J., Yoo, H. S., Kim, J. C., Park, C. S., Choi, M. S., Kim, M., ... Yoon, S. W. (2009). Antiviral effect of Curcuma longa Linn extract against hepatitis B virus replication. *Journal of Ethnopharmacology*, *124*(2), 189–196. doi:10.1016/j.jep.2009.04.046 PMID:19409970

Kim, H. S., Kwon, H. K., Lee, D. H., Le, T. N., Park, H. J., & Kim, M. I. (2019). Poly(γ-Glutamic Acid)/Chitosan Hydrogel Nanoparticles For Effective Preservation And Delivery Of Fermented Herbal Extract For Enlarging Hair Bulb And Enhancing Hair Growth. *International Journal of Nanomedicine*, *14*, 8409–8419. doi:10.2147/IJN.S227514 PMID:31695374

Kim, J. T., Barua, S., Kim, H., Hong, S. C., Yoo, S. Y., Jeon, H., Cho, Y., Gil, S., Oh, K., & Lee, J. (2017). Absorption study of genistein using solid lipid microparticles and nanoparticles: Control of oral bioavailability by particle sizes. *Biomolecules & Therapeutics*, *25*(4), 452–459. doi:10.4062/biomolther.2017.095 PMID:28605834

Kim, J., Ha, H.-L., Moon, H.-B., Lee, Y.-W., Cho, C.-K., Yoo, H.-S., & Yu, D.-Y. (2011). Chemopreventive effect of Curcuma longa Linn on liver pathology in HBx transgenic mice. *Integrative Cancer Therapies*, *10*(2), 168–177. doi:10.1177/1534735410380613 PMID:21190953

Kim, K. I., Yoon, Y. H., & Baek, Y. J. (1996). Effects of rehydration media and immobilization in Ca-alginate on the survival of Lactobacillus casei and Bifido bacterium bifidum. *Korean J Dairy Sci*, *18*, 193–198.

Kim, S. K. (2012). Marine Medical Foods: Implications and Applications, Animals and microbes. *Advances in Food and Nutrition Research*, 65.

Kim, T. I., Lee, Y. K., Park, S. G., Choi, I. S., Ban, J. O., Park, H. K., Nam, S.-Y., Yun, Y. W., Han, S. B., Oh, K. W., & Hong, J. T. (2009). l-Theanine, an amino acid in green tea, attenuates b-amyloid-induced cognitive dysfunction and neurotoxicity: Reduction in oxidative damage and inactivation of ERK/p38 kinase and NF-kB pathways. *Free Radical Biology & Medicine*, *47*(11), 1601–1610. doi:10.1016/j.freeradbiomed.2009.09.008 PMID:19766184

Kızılbey, K. (2019). Optimization of rutin-loaded PLGA nanoparticles synthesized by single-emulsion solvent evaporation method. *ACS Omega*, *4*(1), 555–562. doi:10.1021/acsomega.8b02767

Kjer, J., Debbab, A., Aly, A. H., & Proksch, P. (2010). Methods for isolation of marine-derived endophytic fungi and their bioactive secondary products. *Nature Protocols*, *5*(3), 479–490. doi:10.1038/nprot.2009.233 PMID:20203665

Kokate, C. K., Purohit, A. P., & Gokhale, S. B. (2003). *Textbook of Pharmacognosy*. Nirali Prakashan.

Komal, R., & Arya, V. (2013). Biosynthesis and characterization of silver nanoparticles from aqueous leaf extracts of *Carica papaya* and its antibacterial activity. *International Journal of Nanomaterials and Biostructures.*, *3*, 17–20.

Kondratenko, R. M., Baltina, L. A., Mustafina, S. R., Vasil'eva, E. V., Pompei, R., Deidda, D., Plyasunova, O. A., Pokrovskii, A. G., & Tolstikov, G. A. (2004). The Synthesis and antiviral activity of glycyrrhizic acid conjugates with α-d-glucosamine and some glycosylamines. *Russian Journal of Bioorganic Chemistry*, *30*(3), 275–282. doi:10.1023/B:RUBI.0000030135.97089.37 PMID:15344661

Kong, L., Cai, Y., Huang, W., Cheng, C. H., & Tan, R. (2000). Inhibition of xanthine oxidase by some Chinese medicinal plants used to treat gout. *Journal of Ethnopharmacology*, *73*(1-2), 199–207. doi:10.1016/S0378-8741(00)00305-6 PMID:11025157

König, G., Kehraus, S., Seibert, S., Abdel-Lateff, A., & Müller, D. (2006). Natural products from marine organisms and their associated microbes. *ChemBioChem*, *7*(2), 229–238. doi:10.1002/cbic.200500087 PMID:16247831

Koo, O. M., Rubinstein, I., & Onyuksel, H. (2005). Role of nanotechnology in targeted drug delivery and imaging: A concise review. *Nanomedicine; Nanotechnology, Biology, and Medicine*, *1*(3), 193–212. doi:10.1016/j.nano.2005.06.004 PMID:17292079

Kopustinskiene, D. M., Jakstas, V., Savickas, A., & Bernatoniene, J. (2020). Flavonoids as anticancer agents. *Nutrients*, *12*(2), 457. doi:10.3390/nu12020457 PMID:32059369

Krishnan, G., Subramaniyan, J., Subramani, P. C., Muralidharan, B., & Thiruvengadam, D. (2017). Hesperetin conjugated PEGylated gold nanoparticles exploring the potential role in anti-inflammation and anti-proliferation during diethylnitrosamine-induced hepatocarcinogenesis in rats. *Asian Journal of Pharmaceutical Sciences*, *12*(5), 442-455.

Kulkarni, V., & Waghulde, S. (2010). Nanomedicine: The newer generation fusion molecular nanotechnology. *RJPBCS*, *1*(3), 551–557.

Kulkarni, P. R., & Yadav, J. D. (2011). Liposomes: A novel drug delivery system. *International Journal of Current Pharmaceutical Research*, *3*(2), 10–18.

Kumar, A., Naidu, P., Seghal, N., & Padi, S. (2006). Neuroprotective effects of resveratrol against intracerebroventricular colchicine-induced cognitive impairment and oxidative stress in rats. *Pharmacology*, *79*(1), 17–26. doi:10.1159/000097511 PMID:17135773

Kumar, A., Yadev, S. K., Pakade, Y. B., Singh, B., & Yadev, S. C. (2010). Development of biodegradable nanoparticles for delivery of quercetin. *Colloids and Surfaces. B, Biointerfaces*, *15*(2), 184–192. doi:10.1016/j.colsurfb.2010.06.002 PMID:20598513

Kumar, B., Smita, K., Cumbal, L., & Debut, A. (2014). Biogenic synthesis of iron oxide nanoparticles for 2-arylbenzimidazole fabrication. *Journal of Saudi Chemical Society*, *18*(4), 364–369. doi:10.1016/j.jscs.2014.01.003

Kumari, P., Singh, N., & Cheriyan, P., & Neelam. (2011). Phytosome: A novel approach for phytomedicine. *International Journal of Institutional Pharmacy and Life Sciences*, *1*, 89–100.

Kumar, K. P. S., & Bhowmik, D. (2010). Transdermal drug delivery system-A novel drug delivery system and its market scope and opportunities. *International Journal of Pharmacy and Biological Sciences*, *1*, 1–21.

Kumar, K., & Rai, A. (2012). Miraculous therapeutic effect of herbal drug using novel drug delivery system. *IRJP*, *3*(2), 27–30.

Kumar, P. R., Vivekanandhan, S., Misra, M., Mohanty, A., & Satyanarayana, N. (2012). Soybean (*Glycine max*) leaf extract based green synthesis of palladium nanoparticles. *Journal of Biomaterials and Nanobiotechnology*, *3*(01), 14–19. doi:10.4236/jbnb.2012.31003

Kumar, P., Yadav, S., Agarwal, A., & Kumar, N. (2010). Phytosomes a novel phyto- phospholipid carrier: An overview. *Int J Pharm Res Dev*, *2*(6), 1–7.

Kumar, R. P., & Abraham, A. (2016). PVP-coated naringenin nanoparticles for biomedical applications–In vivo toxicological evaluations. *Chemico-Biological Interactions*, *257*, 110–118. doi:10.1016/j.cbi.2016.07.012 PMID:27417253

Kumar, R., & Kumar, M. S. (2012). Multiple emulsions: A review. *International Journal of Advances in Pharmaceutical Research*, *2*, 9–19.

Kumar, V., & Kesari, A. (2011). Herbosome a novel carrier for herbal drug delivery. *International Journal of Current Pharmaceutical Research*, *3*(3), 36–41.

Kumar, V., & Yadav, S. K. (2011). Synthesis of Stable, Polyshaped Silver and Gold Nanoparticles Using Leaf Extract of *Lonicera japonica* (L.). *International Journal of Green Nanotechnology.*, *3*(4), 281–291. doi:10.1080/19430892.2011.633474

Kuo, C.-Y., Kao, E.-S., Chan, K.-C., Lee, H.-J., Huang, T.-F., & Wang, C.-J. (2012). Hibiscus sabdariffa L. extracts reduce serum uric acid levels in oxonate-induced rats. *Journal of Functional Foods*, *4*(1), 375–381. doi:10.1016/j.jff.2012.01.007

Kurepa, J., Nakabayashi, R., Paunesku, T., Suzuki, M., Saito, K., Woloschak, G. E., & Smalle, J. A. (2014). Direct isolation of flavonoids from plants using ultra-small anatase TiO 2 nanoparticles. *The Plant Journal*, *77*(3), 443–453. doi:10.1111/tpj.12361 PMID:24147867

Kurniawansyah, F., Mammucari, R., & Foster, N. (2015). Inhalable curcumin formulations by supercritical technology. *Powder Technology, 284*, 289–298. doi:10.1016/j.powtec.2015.04.083

Kurzrock, R., & Li, L. (2011). *Liposomal formulation of curcumin for the treatment of cancer.* US patent (US 20070042062 A1).

Kushwaha, S., Rastogi, A., Rai, A., & Singh, S. (2012). Novel drug delivery system for anticancer drug: A review. *International Journal of Pharm Tech Research, 4*(2), 542–553.

Kwong, T. F., Miao, L., Li, X., & Qian, P. Y. (2006). Novel Antifouling and Antimicrobial Compound from a Marine-Derived Fungus *Ampelomyces* sp. *Marine Biotechnology (New York, N.Y.), 8*(6), 634–640. doi:10.100710126-005-6146-2 PMID:16924374

Kwon, S. H., Kim, S. Y., Ha, K. W., Kang, M. J., Huh, J. S., Kim, Y. M., ... Lee, J. (2007). Pharmaceutical evaluation of genistein-loaded pluronic micelles for oral delivery. *Archives of Pharmacal Research, 30*(9), 1138–1143. doi:10.1007/BF02980249 PMID:17958332

Lachman, L., Lieberman, H., & Kanig, J. (1996). *The Theory and Practice of Industrial Pharmacy* (3rd ed.). Lea & Febiger.

Lai, C.-L., Gane, E., Liaw, Y.-F., Hsu, C.-W., Thongsawat, S., Wang, Y., ... Bzowej, N. (2007). Telbivudine versus lamivudine in patients with chronic hepatitis B. *The New England Journal of Medicine, 357*(25), 2576–2588. doi:10.1056/NEJMoa066422 PMID:18094378

Lapenna, S., Bilia, A., Morris, G., & Nilsson, M. (2009). Novel artemisinin and curcumin micellar formulation: Drug solubility studies by NMR spectroscopy. *Journal of Pharmaceutical Sciences, 98*(10), 3666–3675. doi:10.1002/jps.21685 PMID:19199296

Latheeshjlal, L., & Phanitejaswini, P. (2011). Transdermal drug delivery systems: An overview. *International Journal of Pharm Tech Research, 3*(4), 2140–2148.

Lavasanifar, A., Samuel, J., & Kwon, G. (2002). Poly (ethylene oxide)-block-poly (L-amino acid) micelles for drug delivery. *Advanced Drug Delivery Reviews, 54*(2), 169–190. doi:10.1016/S0169-409X(02)00015-7 PMID:11897144

Lawrence, M. J., & Rees, G. D. (2012). Microemulsion-based media as novel drug delivery systems. *Advanced Drug Delivery Reviews, 64*, 175–193. doi:10.1016/j.addr.2012.09.018 PMID:11104900

Lee, D., Ko, W. K., Hwang, D. S., Heo, D. N., Lee, S. J., Heo, M., Lee, K.-S., Ahn, J.-Y., Jo, J., & Kwon, I. K. (2016). Use of baicalin-conjugated gold nanoparticles for apoptotic induction of breast cancer cells. *Nanoscale Research Letters, 11*(1), 381. doi:10.118611671-016-1586-3 PMID:27576521

Lee, G. H., Lee, S. J., Jeong, S. W., Kim, H. C., Park, G. Y., Lee, S. G., & Choi, J. H. (2016). Antioxidative and antiinflammatory activities of quercetin-loaded silica nanoparticles. *Colloids and Surfaces. B, Biointerfaces, 143*, 511–517. doi:10.1016/j.colsurfb.2016.03.060 PMID:27038916

Lee, H. E., Yang, G., Park, Y. B., Kang, H. C., Cho, Y.-Y., Lee, H. S., & Lee, J. Y. (2019). Epigallocatechin-3-gallate prevents acute gout by suppressing NLRP3 inflammasome activation and mitochondrial DNA synthesis. *Molecules (Basel, Switzerland), 24*(11), 2138. doi:10.3390/molecules24112138 PMID:31174271

Lee, H. J., Lee, G., Jang, N. R., Yun, J. H., Song, J. Y., & Kim, B. S. (2011). Biological synthesis of copper nanoparticles using plant extract. *Nanotechnology, 1*, 371–374.

Lee, K. S., Lee, B. S., Semnani, S., Avanesian, A., Um, C.-Y., Jeon, H.-J., Seong, K.-M., Yu, K., Min, K.-J., & Jafari, M. (2010). Curcumin extends life span, improves health span, and modulates the expression of age-associated aging genes in Drosophila melanogaster. *Rejuvenation Research, 13*(5), 561–570. doi:10.1089/rej.2010.1031 PMID:20645870

Lee, S.-I., Lee, Y.-K., Kim, S.-D., Cheng, J., Yang, S. H., & Suh, J.-W. (2014). Xanthine and aldehyde oxidase inhibitory activities, and antihyperuricemic effects of fermented Smilax china L. Leaf extracts and fractions. *Journal of Applied Biological Chemistry*, *57*(1), 53–59. doi:10.3839/jabc.2014.009

Lee, Y.-S., Son, E., Kim, S.-H., Lee, Y. M., Kim, O. S., & Kim, D.-S. (2017). Synergistic uric acid-lowering effects of the combination of Chrysanthemum indicum linne flower and Cinnamomum cassia (L.) J. Persl Bark Extracts. *Evidence-Based Complementary and Alternative Medicine*, *2017*, 2017. doi:10.1155/2017/9764843 PMID:28769989

Lemoine, M., Eholié, S., & Lacombe, K. (2015). Reducing the neglected burden of viral hepatitis in Africa: Strategies for a global approach. *Journal of Hepatology*, *62*(2), 469–476. doi:10.1016/j.jhep.2014.10.008 PMID:25457207

Lengke, M., Ravel, B., Fleet, M. E., Wanger, G., Gordon, R. A., & Southam, G. (2006). Mechanisms of gold bioaccumulation by filamentous cyanobacteria from gold(III)-chloride complex. *Environmental Science & Technology*, *40*(20), 6304–6309. doi:10.1021/es061040r PMID:17120557

Lenhoff, R. J., & Summers, J. (1994a). Construction of avian hepadnavirus variants with enhanced replication and cytopathicity in primary hepatocytes. *Journal of Virology*, *68*(9), 5706–5713. doi:10.1128/JVI.68.9.5706-5713.1994 PMID:8057452

Lenhoff, R. J., & Summers, J. (1994b). Coordinate regulation of replication and virus assembly by the large envelope protein of an avian hepadnavirus. *Journal of Virology*, *68*(7), 4565–4571. doi:10.1128/JVI.68.7.4565-4571.1994 PMID:8207830

Leonard, K., Ahmmad, B., Okamura, H., & Kurawaki, J. (2011). In situ green synthesis of biocompatible ginseng capped gold nanoparticles with remarkable stability. *Colloids and Surfaces. B, Biointerfaces*, *82*(2), 391–396. doi:10.1016/j.colsurfb.2010.09.020 PMID:20980131

Leung, A. W., Amador, C., Wang, L. C., Mody, U. V., & Bally, M. B. (2019). What Drives Innovation: The Canadian Touch on Liposomal Therapeutics. *Pharmaceutics*, *11*(3), 124. doi:10.3390/pharmaceutics11030124 PMID:30884782

Li, L., Wang, D. K., Li, L. S., Jia, J., Chang, D., & Ai, L. (2007). Preparation of docetaxel submicron emulsion for intravenous administration. *Journal of Shenyang Pharmaceutical University*, *12*, 736–739.

Liao, V. H., Yu, C. W., Chu, Y. J., Li, W. H., Hsieh, Y. C., & Wang, T. T. (2011). Curcumin-mediated lifespan extension in Caenorhabditiselegans. *Mechanisms of Ageing and Development*, *132*(10), 480–487. doi:10.1016/j.mad.2011.07.008 PMID:21855561

Li, B., Gao, B., Ye, L., Han, X., Wang, W., Kong, L., ... Li, S. (2007). Hepatitis B virus X protein (HBx) activates ATF6 and IRE1-XBP1 pathways of unfolded protein response. *Virus Research*, *124*(1-2), 44–49. doi:10.1016/j.virusres.2006.09.011 PMID:17092596

Lieberman, H., Rieger, M., & Banker, G. (1998). Pharmaceutical Dosage Forms: Disperse systems. New York: Marcel Dekker Inc.

Li, F., Gong, Q., Dong, H., & Shi, J. (2012). Resveratrol, a neuroprotective supplement for Alzheimer's disease. *Current Pharmaceutical Design*, *18*(1), 27–33. doi:10.2174/138161212798919075 PMID:22211686

Li, F., Liu, Y., Xie, Y., Liu, Z., & Zou, G. (2020). Epigallocatechin gallate reduces uric acid levels by regulating xanthine oxidase activity and uric acid excretion in vitro and in vivo. *Annals of Palliative Medicine*, *9*(2), 331–338. doi:10.21037/apm.2019.11.28 PMID:32008337

Li, H., Ou, G., He, Y., Ren, L., Yang, X., & Zeng, M. (2019). Resveratrol attenuates the MSU crystal-induced inflammatory response through the inhibition of TAK1 activity. *International Immunopharmacology*, *67*, 62–68. doi:10.1016/j.intimp.2018.12.004 PMID:30537632

Li, J., Wang, X., & Zhang, T. (2014). phytosome-A-and-major-difference-between phytosome and liposome. *Asian Journal of Pharmaceutical Sciences, 10*(2). Advance online publication. doi:10.1016/j.ajps.2014.09.004

Li, K., Zhang, H., Gao, L., Zhai, Y., Shi, M., Li, J., Xiu, C., Cao, J., Cheng, S., Jiang, L., & Di, H. (2016). Preparation and Characterization of Baicalein-Loaded Nanoliposomes for Antitumor Therapy. *Journal of Nanomaterials, 2016*, 2016. doi:10.1155/2016/2861915

Li, L., Braiteh, F. S., & Kurzrock, R. (2005). Liposome-encapsulated curcumin: In vitro and in vivo effects on proliferation, apoptosis, signaling, and angiogenesis. *Cancer, 104*(6), 1322–1331. doi:10.1002/cncr.21300 PMID:16092118

Li, L., Wang, D., Li, L., Jia, J., Chang, D., & Ai, L. (2007). Preparation of docetaxel submicron emulsion formation for intravenous administration. *Journal of Shenyang Pharmaceutical University, 7*(12), 736–739.

Li, N., Han, Z., Li, L., Zhang, B., Liu, Z., & Li, J. (2018). The anti-cataract molecular mechanism study in selenium cataract rats for baicalin ophthalmic nanoparticles. *Drug Design, Development and Therapy, 12*, 1399–1411. doi:10.2147/DDDT.S160524 PMID:29872263

Lin, H.-Y., Chang, T.-C., & Chang, S.-T. (2018). A review of antioxidant and pharmacological properties of phenolic compounds in Acacia confusa. *Journal of Traditional and Complementary Medicine, 8*(4), 443–450. doi:10.1016/j.jtcme.2018.05.002 PMID:30302324

Lin, Y., Liu, P.-G., Liang, W.-Q., Hu, Y.-J., Xu, P., Zhou, J., Pu, J.-B., & Zhang, H.-J. (2018). Luteolin-4′-O-glucoside and its aglycone, two major flavones of Gnaphalium affine D. Don, resist hyperuricemia and acute gouty arthritis activity in animal models. *Phytomedicine, 41*, 54–61. doi:10.1016/j.phymed.2018.02.002 PMID:29519319

Lipinski, C. A., Lombardo, F., Dominy, B. W., & Feeney, P. J. (1997). Experimental and computational approaches to estimate solubility and permeability in drug discovery and development settings. *Advanced Drug Delivery Reviews, 23*(1-3), 3–25. doi:10.1016/S0169-409X(96)00423-1 PMID:11259830

Lira, M. C., Ferraz, M. S., da Silva, D. G., Cortes, M. E., Teixeira, K. I., Caetano, N. P., ... Santos-Magalhaes, N. S. (2009). Inclusion complex of usnic acid with β-cyclodextrin: Characterization and nanoencapsulation into liposomes. *Journal of Inclusion Phenomena and Macrocyclic Chemistry, 64*(3-4), 215–224. doi:10.100710847-009-9554-5

Li, S. K., Shen, Y. H., Xie, A. J., Yu, X. R., Zhang, X. Z., Yang, L. B., & Li, C. H. (2007). Rapid, room-temperature synthesis of amorphous selenium/protein composites using *Capsicum annuum* L. extract. *Nanotechnology, 18*(40), 405101–405109. doi:10.1088/0957-4484/18/40/405101

Liu, B., Wang, Y., Yu, Q., Li, D., & Li, F. (2018). Synthesis, characterization of catechin-loaded folate-conjugated chitosan nanoparticles and their anti-proliferative effect. *CYTA: Journal of Food, 16*(1), 868–876. doi:10.1080/19476337.2018.1491625

Liu, J. R., Chen, G. F., Shih, H. N., & Kuo, P. C. (2008). Enhanced antioxidant bioactivity of Salvia miltiorrhiza (Danshen) products prepared using nanotechnology. *Phytomedicine, 15*(1-2), 23–30. doi:10.1016/j.phymed.2007.11.012 PMID:18077145

Liu, J., Lin, H., & McIntosh, H. (2001). Genus Phyllanthus for chronic hepatitis B virus infection: A systematic review. *Journal of Viral Hepatitis, 8*(5), 358–366. doi:10.1046/j.1365-2893.2001.00307.x PMID:11555193

Liu, M., Hong, C., Li, G., Ma, P., & Xie, Y. (2016). The generation of myricetin-nicotinamide nanococrystals by top down and bottom up technologies. *Nanotechnology, 27*(39), 395601–395601. doi:10.1088/0957-4484/27/39/395601 PMID:27535365

Liu, Q., Liu, H., Yuan, Z., Wei, D., & Ye, Y. (2012). Evaluation of antioxidant activity of chrysanthemum extracts and tea beverages by gold nanoparticles-based assay. *Colloids and Surfaces. B, Biointerfaces*, *92*, 348–352. doi:10.1016/j.colsurfb.2011.12.007 PMID:22221458

Liu, S., Wei, W., Shi, K., Cao, X., Zhou, M., & Liu, Z. (2014). In vitro and in vivo anti-hepatitis B virus activities of the lignan niranthin isolated from Phyllanthus niruri L. *Journal of Ethnopharmacology*, *155*(2), 1061–1067. doi:10.1016/j.jep.2014.05.064 PMID:25009077

Liu, X., Chen, R., Shang, Y., Jiao, B., & Huang, C. (2009). Superoxide radicals scavenging and xanthine oxidase inhibitory activity of magnesium lithospermate B from Salvia miltiorrhiza. *Journal of Enzyme Inhibition and Medicinal Chemistry*, *24*(3), 663–668. doi:10.1080/14756360802323829 PMID:18686136

Liu, X., Li, S., & Meng, D. (2016). Anti-gout nor-oleanane triterpenoids from the leaves of Stauntonia brachyanthera. *Bioorganic & Medicinal Chemistry Letters*, *26*(12), 2874–2879. doi:10.1016/j.bmcl.2016.04.048 PMID:27133595

Li, W., Yi, S., Wang, Z., Chen, S., Xin, S., Xie, J., & Zhao, C. (2011). Self-nanoemulsifying drug delivery system of persimmon leaf extract: Optimization and bioavailability studies. *International Journal of Pharmaceutics*, *420*(1), 161–171. doi:10.1016/j.ijpharm.2011.08.024 PMID:21884770

Li, X., Kim, S. K., Nam, K. W., Kang, J. S., Choi, H. D., & Son, B. W. (2006). A new antibacterial dioxopiperazine alkaloid related to gliotoxin from a marine isolate of the fungus *Pseudallescheria. The Journal of Antibiotics*, *59*(4), 248–250. doi:10.1038/ja.2006.35 PMID:16830893

Li, X., Xu, H., Chen, Z. S., & Chen, G. (2011). Biosynthesis of nanoparticles by microorganisms and their applications. *Journal of Nanomaterials*, *2011*, 16. doi:10.1155/2011/270974

Li, Y., Fang, H., & Xu, W. (2007). Recent advance in the research of flavonoids as anticancer agents. *Mini-Reviews in Medicinal Chemistry*, *7*(7), 663–678. doi:10.2174/138955707781024463 PMID:17627579

Li, Y., Guo, M., Lin, Z., Zhao, M., Xia, Y., Wang, C., Xu, T., & Zhu, B. (2018). Multifunctional selenium nanoparticles with Galangin-induced HepG2 cell apoptosis through p38 and AKT signalling pathway. *Royal Society Open Science*, *5*(11), 180509. doi:10.1098/rsos.180509 PMID:30564384

Li, Y., & Jiang, J.-G. (2018). Health functions and structure–activity relationships of natural anthraquinones from plants. *Food & Function*, *9*(12), 6063–6080. doi:10.1039/C8FO01569D PMID:30484455

Li, Z., Li, L., Sun, Y., & Li, J. (2007). Identification of natural compounds with anti-hepatitis B virus activity from Rheum palmatum L. ethanol extract. *Chemotherapy*, *53*(5), 320–326. doi:10.1159/000107690 PMID:17785969

Logeswari, P., Silambarasan, S., & Abraham, J. (2013). Ecofriendly synthesis of silver nanoparticles from commercially available plant powders and their antibacterial properties. *Scientia Iranica F.*, *20*, 1049–1054.

Lopes, V. R., Fernández, N., Martins, R. F., & Vasconcelos, V. (2010). Primary screening of the bioactivity of brackish water cyanobacteria: Toxicity of crude extracts to *Artemia salina* larvae and *Paracentrotus lividus* embryos. *Marine Drugs*, *8*(3), 471–482. doi:10.3390/md8030471 PMID:20411110

Lübtow, M. M., Nelke, L. C., Seifert, J., Kühnemundt, J., Sahay, G., Dandekar, G., Nietzer, S. L., & Luxenhofer, R. (2019). Drug induced micellization into ultra-high capacity and stable curcumin nanoformulations: Physico-chemical characterization and evaluation in 2D and 3D in vitro models. *Journal of Controlled Release*, *303*, 162–180. doi:10.1016/j.jconrel.2019.04.014 PMID:30981815

Luesch, H., Harrigan, G. G., Goetz, G., & Horgen, F. D. (2002). The cyanobacterial origin of potent anticancer agents originally isolated from sea hares. *Current Medicinal Chemistry*, *9*(20), 1791–1806. doi:10.2174/0929867023369051 PMID:12369878

Lu, M. F., Cheng, Y. Q., Li, L. J., & Wu, J. J. (2005). Progress of study on passive targeting of drug delivery system. *Mater Rev*, *19*(9), 108–110.

Luo, D., Carter, K. A., Molins, E. A., Straubinger, N. L., Geng, J., Shao, S., Jusko, W. J., Straubinger, R. M., & Lovell, J. F. (2019). Pharmacokinetics and pharmacodynamics of liposomal chemophototherapy with short drug-light intervals. *Journal of Controlled Release*, *297*, 39–47. doi:10.1016/j.jconrel.2019.01.030 PMID:30684512

Luo, H., Jiang, B., Li, B., Li, Z., Jiang, B. H., & Chen, Y. C. (2012). Kaempferol nanoparticles achieve strong and selective inhibition of ovarian cancer cell viability. *International Journal of Nanomedicine*, *7*, 3951–3959. doi:10.2147/IJN.S33670 PMID:22866004

Luque-Alcaraz, A. G., Lizardi, J., Goycoolea, F. M., Valdez, M. A., Acosta, A. L., Iloki-Assanga, S. B., ... Argüelles-Monal, W. (2012). Characterization and antiproliferative activity of nobiletin-loaded chitosan nanoparticles. *Journal of Nanomaterials*.

Lu, Y., Hou, S. X., Chen, T., Sun, Y. Y., Yang, B. X., & Yuan, Z. Y. (2005). Preparation of transfersomes of vincristine sulfate and study on its prcutaneous penetration. Zhongguo Zhong yao za zhi, Zhongguo zhongyao zazhi. *Zhongguo Zhongyao Zazhi*, *30*(12), 900–903. PMID:16124605

Lu, Y., Hou, S. X., Zhang, L. K., Li, Y., He, J. Y., & Guo, D. D. (2007). Transdermal and lymph targeting transfersomes of vincristine. *Yao Xue Xue Bao*, *42*(10), 1097–1101. PMID:18229621

Ma, B., Duan, X., & Wang, Z. (2000). Clinical and experimental study on Shuanghua aerosol in treating infantile upper respiratory tract infection. *Chinese Journal of Integrated Traditional and Western Medicine*, *20*(9), 653–655. PMID:11789167

Machida, Y., Onishi, H., Kurita, A., Hata, H., Morikawa, A., & Machida, Y. (2000). Pharmacokinetics of prolonged-release CPT-11-loaded microspheres in rats. *Journal of Controlled Release*, *66*(2-3), 159–175. doi:10.1016/S0168-3659(99)00267-9 PMID:10742577

MacRedmond, R., Singhera, G., Attridge, S., Bahzad, M., Fava, C., Lai, Y., Hallstrand, T. S., & Dorscheid, D. (2010). Conjugated linoleic acid improves airway hyper-reactivity in overweight mild asthmatics. *Clinical and Experimental Allergy*, *40*(7), 1071–1078. doi:10.1111/j.1365-2222.2010.03531.x PMID:20642580

Maensiria, S., Laokula, P., Klinkaewnaronga, J., Phokhaa, S., Promarakc, V., & Seraphin, S. (2008). Indium oxide (In2O3) nanoparticles using*Aloe vera*plant extract: Synthesis and optical properties. *Journal of Optoelectronics and Advanced Materials*, *10*, 161–165.

Maffei Facino, R., Carini, M., Aldini, G., Bombardelli, E., & Morazzoni, P. (1994). Free radicals scavenging action and anti-enzyme activities of procyanidins from Vitisvinifera. A mechanism for their capillary protective action. *Arzneimittel-Forschung*, *44*, 592–601. PMID:8024628

Magdi, H. M., Mourad, M. H., Abd, E., & El-Aziz, M. M. (2014). Biosynthesis of silver nanoparticles using fungi and biological evaluation of mycosynthesized silver nanoparticles. *Egyptian Journal of Experimental Biology. (Bot.)*, *10*(1), 1–12.

Mahdavi, M., Namvar, F., Ahmad, M. B., & Mohamad, R. (2013). Green Biosynthesis and Characterization of Magnetic Iron Oxide (Fe_3O_4) Nanoparticles Using Seaweed (*Sargassum muticum*) Aqueous Extract. *Molecules (Basel, Switzerland)*, *18*(5), 5954–5964. doi:10.3390/molecules18055954 PMID:23698048

Mahdieha, M., Zolanvari, A., Azimeea, A. S., & Mahdiehc, M. (2012). Green biosynthesis of silver nanoparticles by *Spirulina platensis. Scientia Iranica F., 19*(3), 926–929. doi:10.1016/j.scient.2012.01.010

Mainardes, R. M., Gremião, M. P., & Evangelista, R. C. (2006). Thermoanalytical study of praziquatel-loaded PLGA nanoparticles. *Brazilian Journal of Pharmaceutical Sciences, 42*, 523–530.

Maiti, K., Mukherjee, K., Gantait, A., Ahamed, H., Saha, B., & Mukherjee, P. (2005). Enhanced therapeutic benefit of quercetin-phospholipid complex in carbon tetrachloride induced acute liver injury in rats: A comparative study. *Int J Pharm Technol, 4*, 84–90.

Maiti, K., Mukherjee, K., Gantait, A., Bishnu, P., & Mukherjee, P. (2006). Enhanced therapeutic potential of naringenin-phospholipid complex in rats. *The Journal of Pharmacy and Pharmacology, 58*(9), 1227–1233. doi:10.1211/jpp.58.9.0009 PMID:16945181

Maiti, K., Mukherjee, K., Gantait, A., Saha, B. P., & Mukherjee, P. K. (2007). Curcumin-phospholipid complex: Preparation, therapeutic evaluation and pharmacokinetic study in rats. *International Journal of Pharmaceutics, 330*, 155–163.

Majumdar, D., Jung, K. H., Zhang, H., Nannapaneni, S., Wang, X., Amin, A. R., ... Shin, D. M. (2014). Luteolin nanoparticle in chemoprevention: In vitro and in vivo anticancer activity. *Cancer Prevention Research (Philadelphia, Pa.), 7*(1), 65–73.

Makarov, V. V., Love, A. J., Sinitsyna, O. V., Makarova, S. S., Yaminsky, I. V., Taliansky, M. E., & Kalinina, N. O. (2014). Green. *Nanotechnologies: Synthesis of Metal Nanoparticles Using Plants. Acta Naturae., 6*(1), 35–44. PMID:24772325

Maloney, K. N., Macmillan, J. B., Kauffman, C. A., Jensen, P. R., Dipasquale, A. G., Rheingold, A. L., & Fenical, W. (2009). Lodopyridone, a structurally unprecedented alkaloid from a marine actinomycete. *Organic Letters, 11*(23), 5422–5424. doi:10.1021/ol901997k PMID:19883103

Mamillapalli, V. (2016). Nanoparticles for Herbal Extracts. *Asian Journal of Pharmaceutics, 10*(2), S54–S60.

Manach, C., Scalbert, A., Morand, C., Rémésy, C., & Jiménez, L. (2004). Polyphenols: Foodsources and bioavailability. *The American Journal of Clinical Nutrition, 79*(5), 727–747. doi:10.1093/ajcn/79.5.727 PMID:15113710

Mandal, S. C., & Mandal, M. (2010). Current status and future prospects of new drug delivery system. *Pharmacy Times, 42*(4), 13–16.

Manju, S., & Sreenivasan, K. (2011). Conjugation of curcumin onto hyaluronic acid enhances its aqueous solubility and stability. *Journal of Colloid and Interface Science, 359*(1), 318–325. doi:10.1016/j.jcis.2011.03.071 PMID:21492865

Manmode, A. S., Sakarkar, D. M., & Mahajan, N. M. (2009). Nanoparticles-tremendous therapeutic potential: A review. *International Journal of Pharm Tech Research, 1*(4), 1020–1027.

Mansoori, M. A., & Agrawal, S. (2012). A review on liposome. *IJARPB, 2*(4), 453–464.

Manu, C., & Vijay, N. (2012). *Topical micro-emulsions for the treatment of rheumatic disorders.* (EP 2437725 A1)

Marchiol, L., Mattiello, A., Poscic, F., Giordano, C., & Musetti, R. (2014). In vivo synthesis of nanomaterials in plants: Location of silver nanoparticles and plant metabolism. *Nanoscale Research Letters, 9*(1), 101. doi:10.1186/1556-276X-9-101 PMID:24581279

Marconi, B., Mancini, F., Colombo, P., Allegra, F., Giordano, F., Gazzaniga, A., Orecchia, G., & Santi, P. (1999). Distribution of khellin in excised human skin following iontophoresis and passive dermal transport. *Journal of Controlled Release, 60*(2–3), 261–268. doi:10.1016/S0168-3659(99)00080-2 PMID:10425331

Marechal, D., & Wg, Y. (2006). *Sustained-release microgranules containing gingko biloba extract and the process for manufacturing these.* United States Patent 7569236.

Marotta, F., Chui, D. H., Jain, S., Polimeni, A., Koike, K., Zhou, L., Lorenzetti, A., Shimizu, H., & Yang, H. (2011). Effect of a fermented nutraceutical on thioredoxin level and TNF-alpha signaling in cirrhotic patients. *Journal of Biological Regulators and Homeostatic Agents*, *25*, 37–45. PMID:21382272

Maryana, W., Rahma, A., Mudhakir, D., & Rachmawati, H. (2015). Phytosome containing silymarin for oral administration: Formulation and physical evaluation. *Journal of Biomedical Science and Engineering*, *25*, 56.

Maskey, R. P., Helmke, E., Kayser, O., Fiebig, H. H., Maier, A., Busche, A., & Laatsch, H. (2004). Anti-cancer and antibacterial trioxacarcins with high anti-malaria activity from a marine *Streptomycete* and their absolute stereochemistry. *The Journal of Antibiotics*, *57*(12), 771–779. doi:10.7164/antibiotics.57.771 PMID:15745111

Massiot, J., Rosilio, V., & Makky, A. (2019). Photo-triggerable liposomal drug delivery systems: From simple porphyrin insertion in the lipid bilayer towards supramolecular assemblies of lipid–porphyrin conjugates. *Journal of Materials Chemistry. B, Materials for Biology and Medicine*, *7*(11), 1805–1823. doi:10.1039/C9TB00015A PMID:32255044

Mathur, M. (2013). Approaches for improving the pharmacological and pharmacokinetic properties of herbal drugs. *Int. Res. J Pharm. App. Sci.*, *3*(4), 40–50.

Mayer, A. M. S., & Lehmann, V. K. B. (2000). Marine pharmacology. *The Pharmacologist*, *42*, 62–69. PMID:16901686

Mbah, C. C., Builders, P. F., & Attama, A. A. (2014). Nanovesicular carriers as alternative drug delivery systems: Ethosomes in focus. *Expert Opinion on Drug Delivery*, *11*(1), 45–59. doi:10.1517/17425247.2013.860130 PMID:24294974

McArthur, K. A., Mitchell, S. S., Tsueng, G., Rheingold, A., White, D. J., Grodberg, J., Lam, K. S., & Potts, B. C. (2008). Lynamicins A-E, chlorinated bisindole pyrrole antibiotics from a novel marine actinomycete. *Journal of Natural Products*, *71*(10), 1732–1737. doi:10.1021/np800286d PMID:18842058

McCarty, M., & DiNicolantonio, J. (2020). Nutraceuticals have potential for boosting the type 1 interferon response to RNA viruses including influenza and coronavirus. *Progress in Cardiovascular Diseases*, *63*(3), 1–8. doi:10.1016/j.pcad.2020.02.007 PMID:32061635

Medina, O. P., Zhu, Y., & Kairemo, K. (2004). Targeted liposomal drug delivery in cancer. *Current Pharmaceutical Design*, *10*(24), 2981–2989. doi:10.2174/1381612043383467 PMID:15379663

Meena, K., Dangi, J., Samal, P., & Namdeo, K. (2011). Recent advances in microspheres manufacturing technology. *Int J Pharm Technol*, *3*, 854–893.

Mehdinezhad, N., Ghannadi, A., & Yegdaneh, A. (2016). Phytochemical and biological evaluation of some *Sargassum* species from Persian Gulf. *Research in Pharmaceutical Sciences*, *11*(3), 243–249. PMID:27499794

Mei, Z., Chen, H., Weng, T., Yang, Y., & Yang, X. (2003). Solid lipid nanoparticle and microemulsion for topical delivery of triptolide. *European Journal of Pharmaceutics and Biopharmaceutics*, *56*(2), 189–196. doi:10.1016/S0939-6411(03)00067-5 PMID:12957632

Mei, Z., Li, X., Wu, Q., Hu, S., & Yang, X. (2005). The research on the anti-inflammatory activity and hepatotoxicity of triptolide-loaded solid lipid nanoparticle. *Pharmacological Research*, *51*(4), 345–351. doi:10.1016/j.phrs.2004.10.007 PMID:15683748

Mekjaruskul, C., & Sripanidkulchai, B. (2020). Kaempferia parviflora Nanosuspension Formulation for Scalability and Improvement of Dissolution Profiles and Intestinal Absorption. *AAPS PharmSciTech*, *21*(2), 52. doi:10.120812249-019-1588-4 PMID:31900735

Mekjaruskul, C., Yang, Y. T., Leed, M. G., Sadgrove, M. P., Jay, M., & Sripanidkulchai, B. (2013). Novel formulation strategies for enhancing oral delivery of methoxyflavones in Kaempferia parviflora by SMEDDS or complexation with 2-hydroxypropyl-β-cyclodextrin. *International Journal of Pharmaceutics, 445*(1-2), 1–11. doi:10.1016/j.ijpharm.2013.01.052 PMID:23376503

Merin, D. D., Prakash, S., & Bhimba, B. V. (2010). Antibacterial screening of silver nanoparticles synthesized by marine micro algae. *Asian Pacific Journal of Tropical Medicine, 3*(10), 797–799. doi:10.1016/S1995-7645(10)60191-5

Metuku, R. P., Pabba, S., Burra, S., Bindu, S. V., Gudikandula, K., & Charya, M. A. S. (2013). Biosynthesis of silver nanoparticles from *Schizophyllum radiatum* HE 863742.1: Their characterization and antimicrobial activity. *Biotechnology.*, 3. PMID:28324427

Meyers, M. A., Mishra, A., & Benson, D. J. (2006). Mechanical properties of nanocrystalline materials. *Progress in Materials Science, 51*(4), 427–556. doi:10.1016/j.pmatsci.2005.08.003

Milanovic, J., Manojlovic, V., Levic, S., Rajic, N., Nedovic, V., & Bugarski, B. (2010). Microencapsulation of flavors in carnauba wax. *Sensors (Basel), 10*(1), 901–912. doi:10.3390100100901 PMID:22315575

Miraj, S. (2016). Therapeutic effects of Rheum palmatum L.(Dahuang): A systematic review. *Der Pharma Chemica, 8*(13), 50–54.

Mishra, D., & Panda, G. (2012). Novel drug delivery system for herbal formulation in cancer treatment. *World Journal of Pharmaceutical Research, 6*(15), 341–353.

Mishra, H., Kesharwani, R., Singh, D., Tripathi, S., Dubey, S., & Misra, K. (2018). Computational study of curcumin, retinoic acid and its conjugates against GSK-3 beta. *Network Modeling and Analysis in Health Informatics and Bioinformatics, 8*, 3. doi:10.100713721-018-0177-x

Mittal, A. K., Chisti, Y., & Banerjee, U. C. (2013). Synthesis of metallic nanoparticles using plant extracts. *Journal of Biotechnology Advances, 31*(2), 346–356. doi:10.1016/j.biotechadv.2013.01.003 PMID:23318667

Miyashita, K., Nishikawa, S., Beppu, F., Tsukui, T., Abe, M., & Hosokawa, M. (2011). The allenic carotenoid fucoxanthin, a novel marine nutraceutical from brown seaweeds. *Journal of the Science of Food and Agriculture, 91*(7), 1166–1174. doi:10.1002/jsfa.4353 PMID:21433011

Modak, M., Dixit, P., Londhe, J., Ghaskadbi, S., & Devasagayam, T. P. A. (2007). Indian herbs & herbal drugs used for the treatment of diabetes. *Journal of Clinical Biochemistry and Nutrition, 40*(3), 163–173. doi:10.3164/jcbn.40.163 PMID:18398493

Mohamadkhani, A., Sayemiri, K., Ghanbari, R., Elahi, E., Poustchi, H., & Montazeri, G. (2010). The inverse association of serum HBV DNA level with HDL and adiponectin in chronic hepatitis B infection. *Virology Journal, 7*(1), 228. doi:10.1186/1743-422X-7-228 PMID:20840785

Mohamed, S., & El-Ridy, A. (2012). Niosomes as A novel pharmaceutical formulation encapsulating the hepatoprotective drug silymarin. *International Journal of Pharmacy and Pharmaceutical Sciences, 4*(1), 549–559.

Mohammadinejad, S., Akbarzadeh, A., Rahmati-Yamchi, M., Hatam, S., Kachalaki, S., Zohreh, S., & Zarghami, N. (2015). Preparation and evaluation of chrysin encapsulated in PLGA-PEG nanoparticles in the T47-D breast cancer cell line. *Asian Pacific Journal of Cancer Prevention, 16*(9), 3753–3758.

Mohan, A., Nair, S. V., & Lakshmanan, V. K. (2017). Leucas aspera nanomedicine shows superior toxicity and cell migration retarded in prostate cancer cells. *Applied Biochemistry and Biotechnology, 181*(4), 1388–1400. doi:10.100712010-016-2291-5 PMID:27812900

Mohanraj, K., Karthikeyan, B. S., Vivek-Ananth, R. P., Chand, R. B., Aparna, S. R., Mangalapandi, P., & Samal, A. (2018). IMPPAT: A curated database of I ndian M edicinal P lants, P hytochemistry A nd T herapeutics. *Scientific Reports*, *8*(1), 1–17.

Moharrer, S., Mohammadi, B., Gharamohammadi, R. A., & Yargoli, M. (2012). Biological synthesis of silver nanoparticles by *Aspergillus flavus*, isolated from soil of Ahar copper mine. *Indian Journal of Science and Technology*, *5*(3), 2443–2444. doi:10.17485/ijst/2012/v5i3.41

Mohnaraj, V. J., & Chen, Y. (2016). Nanoparticles-A review. *Tropical Journal of Pharmaceutical Research*, *5*(1), 561–573.

Mollazade, M., Nejati-Koshki, K., Akbarzadeh, A., Zarghami, N., Nasiri, M., Jahanban-Esfahlan, R., & Alibakhshi, A. (2013). PAMAM dendrimers augment inhibitory effects of curcumin on cancer cell proliferation: Possible inhibition of telomerase. *Asian Pacific Journal of Cancer Prevention*, *14*(11), 6925–6928. doi:10.7314/APJCP.2013.14.11.6925 PMID:24377627

Moolakkadath, T., Aqil, M., Ahad, A., Imam, S. S., Praveen, A., Sultana, Y., Mujeeb, M., & Iqbal, Z. (2019). Fisetin loaded binary ethosomes for management of skin cancer by dermal application on UV exposed mice. *International Journal of Pharmaceutics*, *560*, 78–91. doi:10.1016/j.ijpharm.2019.01.067 PMID:30742987

Moscarella, S., Giusti, A., Marra, F., Marena, C., Lampertico, M., Relli, P., Gentilini, P., & Buzzelli, G. (1993). Therapeutic and anti lipoperoxidant effect of silybin phosphatidylcholine complex in chronic liver disease: Preliminary result. *Current Therapeutic Research, Clinical and Experimental*, *53*(1), 98–102. doi:10.1016/S0011-393X(05)80160-2

Mueller, R. H., Maeder, K., & Gohla, S. (2000). Solid lipid nanoparticles (SLN) for controlled drug delivery – a review of the state of the art. *European Journal of Pharmaceutics and Biopharmaceutics*, *50*, 161–177. doi:10.1016/S0939-6411(00)00087-4 PMID:10840199

Mujaffar, F., & Singh, U. K. (2013). Review of microemulsion as futuristic drug delivery. *International Journal of Pharmacy and Pharmaceutical Sciences*, *5*, 39–51.

Mujoriya, R. Z., Dhamande, K., & Bodla, R. B. (2011). Niosomal drug delivery system—A review. *Int J Appl Pharm*, *3*(3), 7–10.

Mujoriya, R. Z., Dhamande, K., & Bodla, R. B. (2011). Niosomal drug delivery system—A review. *International Journal of Applied Pharmaceutics*, *3*(3), 7–10.

Mukerjee, A., & Vishwanatha, J. (2009). Formulation, characterization and evaluation of curcumin-loaded PLGA nanospheres for cancer therapy. *Anticancer Research*, *29*(10), 3867–3875. PMID:19846921

Mukerjee, A., & Vishwanatha, J. K. (2009). Formulation, characterization and evaluation of curcumin loaded PLGA nanospheres for cancer therapy. *Anticancer Research*, *29*(10), 3867–3875. PMID:19846921

Mukheriee, P. K., & Wahile, A. (2006). Integrated approaches towards drug development from Ayurveda and other Indian system of medicines. *Journal of Ethnopharmacology*, *103*(1), 25–35. doi:10.1016/j.jep.2005.09.024 PMID:16271286

Mukherjee, P., Harwansh, R., & Bhattacharyya, S. (2015). Bioavailability of herbal products: approach toward improved pharmacokinetics. In Evidence-Based Validation of Herbal Medicine. Elsevier Inc. doi:10.1016/B978-0-12-800874-4.00010-6

Mukherjee, P., Ahmad, A., Mandal, D., Senapati, S., Sainkar, S. R., Khan, M. I., Parishcha, R., Ajaykumar, P. V., Alam, M., Kumar, R., & Sastry, M. (2001). Fungus mediated synthesis of silver nanoparticles and their immobilization in the mycelia matrix: A novel biological approach to nanoparticle synthesis. *Nano Letters*, *1*(10), 515–519. doi:10.1021/nl0155274

Mukherjee, P., Ahmad, A., Mandal, D., Senapati, S., Sainkar, S. R., Khan, M. I., Ramani, R., Parischa, R., Ajayakumar, P. V., Alam, M., Sastry, M., & Kumar, R. (2001). Bioreduction of AuCl4 - ions by the fungus, *Verticillium* sp. and surface trapping of the gold nanoparticles formed. *Angewandte Chemie International Edition*, *40*(19), 3585–3588. doi:10.1002/1521-3773(20011001)40:19<3585::AID-ANIE3585>3.0.CO;2-K PMID:11592189

Mukherjee, P., Senapati, S., Mandal, D., Ahmad, A., Khan, M. I., Kumar, R., & Sastry, M. (2002). Extracellular synthesis of gold nanoparticles by the fungus *Fusarium oxysporum*. *ChemBioChem*, *3*(5), 461–463. doi:10.1002/1439-7633(20020503)3:5<461::AID-CBIC461>3.0.CO;2-X PMID:12007181

Mukherjee, S., Chowdhury, D., Kotcherlakota, R., Patra, S., & Vinothkumar, B. (2014). Potential Theranostics Application of Bio-Synthesized Silver Nanoparticles (4-in-1 System). *Theranostics*, *4*(3), 316–335. doi:10.7150/thno.7819 PMID:24505239

Mukunthan, K., & Balaji, S. (2012). Cashew apple juice (Anacardium occidentale L.) speeds up the synthesis of silver nanoparticles. *International Journal of Green Nanotechnology.*, *4*(2), 71–79. doi:10.1080/19430892.2012.676900

Muley, S., Nandgude, T., & Poddar, S. (2016). Extrusion–spheronization a promising pelletization technique: In-depth review. *Asian Journal of Pharmaceutical Sciences, 11*(6), 684-699.

Murray, D. (2008). *Phytosomes-Increase the absorption of herbal extract.* Available at: www.doctormurray.com/articles/silybin.htm

Murugaiyah, V., & Chan, K.-L. (2006). Antihyperuricemic lignans from the leaves of Phyllanthus niruri. *Planta Medica*, *72*(14), 1262–1267. doi:10.1055-2006-947224 PMID:16953466

Murugaiyah, V., & Chan, K.-L. (2009). Mechanisms of antihyperuricemic effect of Phyllanthus niruri and its lignan constituents. *Journal of Ethnopharmacology*, *124*(2), 233–239. doi:10.1016/j.jep.2009.04.026 PMID:19397979

Mustafa Kiyani, M., Sohail, M. F., Shahnaz, G., Rehman, H., Akhtar, M. F., Nawaz, I., ... Imran Bokhari, S. A. (2019). Evaluation of turmeric nanoparticles as anti-gout agent: Modernization of a traditional drug. *Medicina*, *55*(1), 10. doi:10.3390/medicina55010010 PMID:30642012

Musthaba, S. M., Baboota, S., Ahmed, S., Ahuja, A., & Ali, J. (2009). Status of novel drug delivery technology for phytotherapeutics. *Expert Opinion on Drug Delivery*, *6*(6), 625–637. doi:10.1517/17425240902980154 PMID:19505192

Nagarajan, S., & Kuppusamy, K. A. (2013). Extracellular synthesis of zinc oxide nanoparticle using seaweeds of gulf of Mannar, India. *Journal of Nanobiotechnology*, *11*(1), 39. doi:10.1186/1477-3155-11-39 PMID:24298944

Nagpal, N., Arora, M., & Swami, G., Rageeb, & Kapoor, R. (2016). Designing of a phytosome dosage form with *Tecomellaundulata*as a noveldrug delivery for better utilization. *Pakistan Journal of Pharmaceutical Sciences*, *29*(4), 1231–1235. PMID:27393436

Naik, S. R., Pilgaonkar, V. W., & Panda, V. S. (2006). Evaluation of antioxidant activity of Ginkgo biloba phytosomes in rat brain. *Phytotherapy Research*, *20*(11), 1013–1016. doi:10.1002/ptr.1976 PMID:16909446

Naksuriya, O., Okonogi, S., Schielers, R., & Hennink, W. (2014). Curcumin nanoformulations: A review of pharmaceutical properties and preclinical studies and clinical data related to cancer treatment. *Biomaterials*, *35*(10), 3365–3383. doi:10.1016/j.biomaterials.2013.12.090 PMID:24439402

Nalla, A., & Chinnala, K. (2017). Novel herbal drug delivery system - An overview. *World Journal of Pharmacy and Pharmaceutical Sciences*, *6*(8), 369–395. doi:10.20959/wjpps20178-9712

Nandre, B., Bakliwal, S., Rane, B., & Pawar, S. (2012). Traditional fermented formulations- Asava and arishta. *International Journal of Pharmaceutical and Biological Archives*, *3*(6), 1313–1319.

Narayanan, K. B., & Sakthivel, N. (2008). Coriander leaf mediated biosynthesis of gold nanoparticles. *Materials Letters, 62*(30), 4588–4590. doi:10.1016/j.matlet.2008.08.044

Natarajan, E., Purushothaman, B., Palanisamy, P., Somasundaram, D., & And Subathra, S. (2012). Studies on morphological characterization and antimicrobial activity of silver nanoparticles synthesized by bio and chemoreductive methods. *International Journal of Pharma and Bio Sciences, 3*, 264–273.

Natarajan, V., Krithica, N., Madhan, B., & Sehgal, P. K. (2011). Formulation and evaluation of quercetin polycaprolactone microspheres for the treatment of rheumatoid arthritis. *Journal of Pharmaceutical Sciences, 100*(1), 195–205. doi:10.1002/jps.22266 PMID:20607810

Natrajan, V., Madhan, B., & Sehgal, P. (2010). Formulation and evalution of qucertin polycaprolactone microsphere for the treatment of Rheumatoid arthritis. *J Pharm Sophora Alopecuroides Sci, 100*, 195-205.

Nenkep, V. N., Yun, K., Li, Y., Choi, H. D., Kang, J. S., & Son, B. W. (2010). New production of haloquinones, bromochlorogentisylquinones A and B, by a halide salt from a marine isolate of the fungus *Phoma herbarum. The Journal of Antibiotics, 63*(4), 199–201. doi:10.1038/ja.2010.15 PMID:20224602

Neto, C. (2007). Cranberry and blueberry: Evidence for protective effects against cancer and vascular diseases. *Molecular Nutrition & Food Research, 51*(6), 652–664. doi:10.1002/mnfr.200600279 PMID:17533651

Neveu, V., Perez-Jiménez, J., Vos, F., Crespy, V., Du Chaffaut, L., Mennen, L., & Scalbert, A. (2010). *Phenol-Explorer: an online comprehensive database on polyphenol contents in foods. Database. Journal of Biological Database Biocuration.*

Newman, D. J., & Hill, R. T. (2006). New drugs from marine microbes: The tide is turning. *Journal of Industrial Microbiology & Biotechnology, 33*(7), 539–544. doi:10.100710295-006-0115-2 PMID:16598493

Nguyen, M. T. T., Awale, S., Tezuka, Y., Le Tran, Q., Watanabe, H., & Kadota, S. (2004). Xanthine oxidase inhibitory activity of Vietnamese medicinal plants. *Biological & Pharmaceutical Bulletin, 27*(9), 1414–1421. doi:10.1248/bpb.27.1414 PMID:15340229

Nikalje, A. P., & Tiwari, S. (2012). Ethosomes: A Novel Tool for Transdermal Drug Delivery. *IJRPS, 2*(1), 1–20.

Nikalje, A., & Tiwari, S. (2012). Ethosomes: A novel tool for transdermal drug delivery. *International Journal of Current Pharmaceutical Research, 2*(1), 1–20.

Ninganagouda, S., Rathod, V., Jyoti, H., Singh, D., & Prema, K. & Manzoor-Ul-Haq. (2013). Extracellular biosynthesis of silver nanoparticles using *Aspergillus flavus* and their antimicrobial activity against gram negative mdr strains. *International Journal of Pharma and Bio Sciences, 4*, 222–229.

Nishizawa, M., Menon, V. P., & Martin, C. R. (1995). Metal nanotubule membranes with electrochemically switchable ion-transport selectivity. *Science, 268*(5211), 700–702. doi:10.1126cience.268.5211.700 PMID:17832383

Norman, G. B. (2001). A handbook for practice on a scientific basis (2nd ed). Stuttgart: Medpharm Scientific Publishers and CRC Press.

Norton, P. A., Gong, Q., Mehta, A. S., Lu, X., & Block, T. M. (2003). Hepatitis B virus-mediated changes of apolipoprotein mRNA abundance in cultured hepatoma cells. *Journal of Virology, 77*(9), 5503–5506. doi:10.1128/JVI.77.9.5503-5506.2003 PMID:12692252

Novoa-Carballal, R., Fernandez-Megia, E., Jimenez, C., & Riguera, R. (2011). NMR methods for unravelling the spectra of complex mixtures. *Natural Product Reports, 28*(1), 78–98. doi:10.1039/C005320C PMID:20936238

O'Hara, G. A., McNaughton, A. L., Maponga, T., Jooste, P., Ocama, P., Chilengi, R., ... Gikungi, D. M. (2017). Hepatitis B virus infection as a neglected tropical disease. *PLoS Neglected Tropical Diseases*, *11*(10), e0005842. doi:10.1371/journal.pntd.0005842 PMID:28981505

Ohishi, T., Goto, S., Monira, P., Isemura, M., & Nakamura, Y. (2016). Anti-inflammatory action of green tea. *Anti-Inflammatory & Anti-Allergy Agents in Medicinal Chemistry (Formerly Current Medicinal Chemistry-Anti-Inflammatory and Anti-Allergy Agents)*, *15*(2), 74-90.

Ojha, R., Singh, J., Ojha, A., Singh, H., Sharma, S., & Nepali, K. (2017). An updated patent review: Xanthine oxidase inhibitors for the treatment of hyperuricemia and gout (2011-2015). *Expert Opinion on Therapeutic Patents*, *27*(3), 311–345. doi:10.1080/13543776.2017.1261111 PMID:27841045

Okami, Y. J. (1993). The search for bioactive metabolites form marine bacteria. *Marine Biotechnology (New York, N.Y.)*, *1*, 59–65.

Okonogai, S., Sirithunyalang, J., & Chen, U. (2008). Nanoencapsulation of Centella asiatica bioactive extract. *XVIth International Conference on Bioencapsulation*, *4*(6), 1-4.

Okore, V. C., Attama, A. A., Ofokansi, K. C., Esimone, C. O., & Onuigbo, E. B. (2011). Formulation and evaluation of niosomes. *Indian Journal of Pharmaceutical Sciences*, *73*(3), 323. PMID:22457561

Olano, C., Méndez, C., & Salas, J. A. (2009). Antitumor compounds from marine actinomycetes. *Marine Drugs*, *7*(2), 210–248. doi:10.3390/md7020210 PMID:19597582

Organization, W. H. (2017). *Global hepatitis report 2017*. World Health Organization.

Osvelia, E. R., Rene, H. D., Rosa, I. S., Gabriel, A. M., Nereyda, N., María del Carmen, S. N., Facundo, R., & Claudio, C. R. (2016). Green Synthesis of Silver Nanoparticles and Their Bactericidal and Antimycotic Activities against Oral Microbes. *Journal of Nanomaterials*.

Ott, M., Thyagarajan, S., & Gupta, S. (1997). Phyllanthus amarus suppresses hepatitis B virus by interrupting interactions between HBV enhancer I and cellular transcription factors. *European Journal of Clinical Investigation*, *27*(11), 908–915. doi:10.1046/j.1365-2362.1997.2020749.x PMID:9395786

Ouyang, Y., Chen, L., Qian, L., Lin, X., Fan, X., Teng, H., & Cao, H. (2020). Fabrication of caseins nanoparticles to improve the stability of cyanidin 3-O-glucoside. *Food Chemistry*, *317*, 126418.

Owen, P. L., & Johns, T. (1999). Xanthine oxidase inhibitory activity of northeastern North American plant remedies used for gout. *Journal of Ethnopharmacology*, *64*(2), 149–160. doi:10.1016/S0378-8741(98)00119-6 PMID:10197750

Oza, G., Pandey, S., Shah, R., & Sharon, M. (2012). A Mechanistic Approach for Biological Fabrication of Crystalline Gold Nanoparticles Using Marine Algae, *Sargassum wightii. European Journal of Experimental Biology*, *2*, 505–512.

Pal, D., Sahu, C., & Haldar, A. (2014). Bhasma: The ancient Indian nanomedicine. *Journal of Advanced Pharmaceutical Technology & Research*, *5*(1), 4–12. doi:10.4103/2231-4040.126980 PMID:24696811

Palliyaguru, D. L., Singh, S. V., & Kensler, T. W. (2016). Withania somnifera: From prevention to treatment of cancer. *Molecular Nutrition & Food Research*, *60*(6), 1342–1353. doi:10.1002/mnfr.201500756 PMID:26718910

Palu, A., Deng, S., West, B., & Jensen, J. (2009). Xanthine oxidase inhibiting effects of noni (Morinda citrifolia) fruit juice. *Phytotherapy Research*, *23*(12), 1790–1791. doi:10.1002/ptr.2842 PMID:19434757

Panda, K. K., Achary, V. M. M., Krishnaveni, R., Padhi, B. K., Sarangi, S. N., Sahu, S. N., & Panda, B. B. (2011). *In vitro* biosynthesis and genotoxicity bioassay of silver nanoparticles using plants. *Toxicology In Vitro, 25*(5), 1097–1105. doi:10.1016/j.tiv.2011.03.008 PMID:21419840

Pandey, M., Verma, R., & Sara, S. (2010). Nutraceuticals: new era of medicine and health. *AJPCR, 3*(1).

Pandey, N., Prasad, M., Rai, S., & Rai, S. (2011). Medicinal plants derived nutraceuticals: A re-emerging health aid. *Int J Pharm Bio Sci, 2*(4), 20–41.

Pandey, S., Oza, G., Mewada, A., & Sharon, M. (2012). Green Synthesis of Highly Stable Gold Nanoparticles using *Momordica charantia* as Nano fabricator. *Archives of Applied Science Research, 4*, 1135–1141.

Pandita, A., & Sharma, P. (2013). Pharmacosomes: An Emerging Novel Vesicular Drug Delivery System for Poorly Soluble Synthetic and Herbal Drugs. *ISRN Pharmaceutics, 2013*, 1–10. doi:10.1155/2013/348186 PMID:24106615

Pang, X., Lu, Z., Du, H., Yang, X., & Zhai, G. (2014). Hyaluronic acid-quercetin conjugate micelles: Synthesis, characterization, in vitro and in vivo evaluation. *Colloids and Surfaces. B, Biointerfaces, 123*, 778–786. doi:10.1016/j.colsurfb.2014.10.025 PMID:25454664

Paolino, D., Lucania, G., Mardente, D., Alhaique, F., & Fresta, M. (2005). Ethosomes for skin delivery of ammonium glycyrrhizinate: In vitro percutaneous permeation through human skin and in vivo anti-inflammatory activity on human volunteers. *Journal of Controlled Release, 106*(1-2), 99–110. doi:10.1016/j.jconrel.2005.04.007 PMID:15935505

Parakh, S. R., & Gothoskar, A. V. (2003). Review of mouth dissolving tablet technologies. Pharmaceutical Technology. Duluth, MN: Advanstar Communications, ETATS-UNIS.

Parashar, P., Rathor, M., Dwivedi, M., & Saraf, S. A. (2018). Hyaluronic acid decorated naringenin nanoparticles: Appraisal of chemopreventive and curative potential for lung cancer. *Pharmaceutics, 10*(1), 33.

Parasuram, R., Rawat, B., & Thangvel, S. (2011). Nutraceuticals: An area of tremendous scope. *International Journal of Research in Ayurveda and Pharmacy, 2*(4), 10–15.

Parida, K., Panda, S., Ravanan, P., & Roy, H. (2013). Microparticles Based Drug Delivery Systems: Preparation and Application in Cancer Therapeutics. *IAAST, 4*(3), 68–75.

Park, K. (2014). Controlled drug delivery systems: Past forward and future back. *Journal of Controlled Release, 190*, 3–8. doi:10.1016/j.jconrel.2014.03.054 PMID:24794901

Paroha, S., Chandel, A. K. S., & Dubey, R. D. (2017). *Nanotechnology Delivery Systems of Coenzyme Q10: Pharmacokinetic and Clinical Implications. In Nanoscience in Food and Agriculture 4.* Springer.

Paroha, S., Chandel, A. K. S., & Dubey, R. D. (2018). Nanosystems for drug delivery of coenzyme Q10. *Environmental Chemistry Letters, 16*(1), 71–77. doi:10.100710311-017-0664-9

Parris, N., Cooke, P., & Hicks, K. (2005). Encapsulation of essential oils in zeinnano spherical particles. *Journal of Agricultural and Food Chemistry, 53*(12), 4788–4792. doi:10.1021/jf040492p PMID:15941317

Parth, S., & Surajpal, V. (2016). Global need for novel herbal drug formulations. *International Journal of Pharmacognosy and Phytochemical Research, 8*(9), 1535–1544.

Pasca, R. D., Mocanu, A., Cobzac, S. C., Petean, I., Horovitz, O., & Tomoaia-Cotisel, M. (2014). Biogenic syntheses of gold nanoparticles using plant extracts. *Particulate Science and Technology: An International Journal., 32*(2), 131–137. doi:10.1080/02726351.2013.839589

Pastore, M. N., Kalia, Y. N., Horstmann, M., & Roberts, M. S. (2015). Transdermal patches: History, development and pharmacology. *British Journal of Pharmacology*, *172*(9), 2179–2209. doi:10.1111/bph.13059 PMID:25560046

Patel, E. K., & Oswal, R. J. (2012). Nanosponge and Microsponges: A Novel Drug Delivery System. *IJRP2*.

Patel, R., Singh, S. K., Singh, S., Sheth, N. R., & Gendle, R. (2009). Development and characterization of curcumin loaded transfersome for transdermal delivery. *Journal of Pharmaceutical Sciences and Research*, *1*(4), 71.

Patela, J., & Patelb, R. (2009). An overview of phytosomes as an advanced herbal drug delivery system. *Asian Journal of Pharmaceutical Sciences*, *4*(6), 363–371.

Patel, J., Patel, R., Khambolja, K., & Patel, N. (2009). An overview of phytosomes as an advanced herbal drug delivery system. *Asian J Pharm Sci*, *4*(6), 363–371.

Patel, R., & Singh, S. K. (2009). Development and characterization of curcumin loaded transferosomes for transdermal delivery. *Journal of Pharmaceutical Sciences*, *1*, 71–80.

Patel, R., Singh, S., Singh, S., Sheth, N., & Gendle, R. (2009). Development and characterization of curcumin loaded transfer some for transdermal delivery. *J Pharm Sci Res*, *1*, 71–80.

Pathan, R., & Bhandari, U. (2011). Preparation and characterization of embelin- phospholipid complex as effective drug delivery tool. *Journal of Inclusion Phenomena and Macrocyclic Chemistry*, *9*, 139–147.

Patil, A. G., & Jobanputra, A. H. (2015). Rutin-chitosan nanoparticles: Fabrication, characterization and application in dental disorders. *Polymer-Plastics Technology and Engineering*, *54*(2), 202–208.

Patil, P. M., & Chaudhari, P. D. (2012). Recent trend in challenges and opportunities of transdermal drug delivery system. *International Journal of Drug Development and Research*, *4*, 39–50.

Patil, P., Salunkhe, V., Magdum, C., & Mohite, S. (2016). Phytosomes: Increasing bioavailability of phytoconstituents. *International Journal of Universal Pharmacy and Bio Sciences*, *5*(4), 81–94.

Patil, R. Y., Patil, S. A., Chivate, N. D., & Patil, Y. N. (2018). Herbal Drug Nanoparticles: Advancements in Herbal Treatment. *Research Journal of Pharmacy and Technology*, *11*(1), 421–426. doi:10.5958/0974-360X.2018.00078.1

Patra, J. K., & Beak, K. H. (2017). Antibacterial Activity and Synergistic Antibacterial Potential of Biosynthesized Silver Nanoparticles against Foodborne Pathogenic Bacteria along with its Anticandidal and Antioxidant Effects. *Frontiers in Microbiology*, *8*. Advance online publication. doi:10.3389/fmicb.2017.00167 PMID:28261161

Pattni, B. S., Chupin, V. V., & Torchilin, V. P. (2015). New developments in liposomal drug delivery. *Chemical Reviews*, *115*(19), 10938–10966. doi:10.1021/acs.chemrev.5b00046 PMID:26010257

Patwardhan, B., Vaidya, A. D., & Chorghade, M. (2004). Ayurveda and natural products drug discovery. *Current Science*, *86*, 789.

Paulkumar, K., Gnanajobitha, G., Vanaja, M., & Rajeshkumar, S. (2014). *Piper nigrum.* Leaf and Stem Assisted Green Synthesis of Silver Nanoparticles and Evaluation of Its Antibacterial Activity Against Agricultural Plant Pathogens. Scientific World Journal.

Pawar, H. A., & Bhangale, B. D. (2015). Phytosome as a Novel Biomedicine: A Microencapsulated. *Drug Delivery System*, *7*(1), 6–12.

Pawar, H., & Bhangale, B. (2015). Phytosome as a novel biomedicine: A microencapsulated drug delivery system. *Journal of Bioanalysis & Biomedicine*, *7*(1), 6–12.

Pawar, P., & Kalamkar, R. (2015). Ethosomes: A novel tool for herbal drug delivery. *Ijppr. Human*, *3*(4), 191–202.

Pawlus, A. D., & Kinghorn, A. D. (2007). Review of the ethnobotany, chemistry, biological activity and safety of the botanical dietary supplement Morinda citrifolia (noni). *The Journal of Pharmacy and Pharmacology*, *59*(12), 1587–1609. doi:10.1211/jpp.59.12.0001 PMID:18053321

Pegg, R., & Shahidi, F. (2007). Encapsulation, stabilization, and controlled release of food ingredients and bioactives. In M. S. Rahman (Ed.), *Handbook of food preservation* (2nd ed., pp. 1–1088). CRC Press.

Peng, Q., Tao, G., Jiao, Z., Jie, L., Dong, Z., & Zhirong, Z. (2008). Enhanced the oral bioavailability of savianolic acid B by phospholipid complex loaded nanoparticles. *Die Pharmazie*, *63*, 661–666. PMID:18819519

Peng, W., Qin, R., Li, X., & Zhou, H. (2013). Botany, phytochemistry, pharmacology, and potential application of Polygonum cuspidatum Sieb. et Zucc.: A review. *Journal of Ethnopharmacology*, *148*(3), 729–745. doi:10.1016/j.jep.2013.05.007 PMID:23707210

Pentel, P. R., Malin, D. H., Ennifar, S., Hieda, Y., Keyler, D. E., Lake, J. R., ... Naso, R. (2000). A nicotine conjugate vaccine reduces nicotine distribution to brain and attenuates its behavioral and cardiovascular effects in rats. *Pharmacology, Biochemistry, and Behavior*, *65*(1), 191–198. doi:10.1016/S0091-3057(99)00206-3 PMID:10638653

Pérez, M., Crespo, C., Schleissner, C., Rodríguez, P., Zúñiga, P., & Reyes, F. (2009). Tartrolon D, a cytotoxic macrodiolide from the marine-derived actinomycete *Streptomyces* sp. MDG-04-17-069. *Journal of Natural Products*, *72*, 2192–2194. doi:10.1021/np9006603 PMID:19968258

Peterson, D. L. (1981). Isolation and characterization of the major protein and glycoprotein of hepatitis B surface antigen. *The Journal of Biological Chemistry*, *256*(13), 6975–6983. PMID:7240257

Philip, D. (2011). *Mangifera Indica* leaf-assisted biosynthesis of well-dispersed silver nanoparticles. *Spectrochimica Acta Part A.*, *78*(1), 327–331. doi:10.1016/j.saa.2010.10.015 PMID:21030295

Philip, D., Unnib, S., & Aswathy, A. V. K. (2011). *Murraya Koenigii* leaf-assisted rapid green synthesis of silver and gold nanoparticles. *Spectrochimica Acta Part A.*, *78*(2), 899–904. doi:10.1016/j.saa.2010.12.060 PMID:21215687

Pickering, T. D., Posa, S., & Reuben, J. S. (2007). Intentional introductions of commercially harvested alien seaweeds. *Botanica Marina*, *50*(5/6), 338–350. doi:10.1515/BOT.2007.039

Pinto, J. F. (2010). Site specific drug delivery systems within gastro intestinal tract: From the mouth to the colon. *International Journal of Pharmaceutics*, *395*(1-2), 44–52. doi:10.1016/j.ijpharm.2010.05.003 PMID:20546856

Pinto, J. F. (2010). Site-specific drug delivery systems within the gastro-intestinal tract: From the mouth to the colon. *International Journal of Pharmaceutics*, *395*, 44–52.

Pires, A. M., & Araújo, P. S. (2012). Percepção de risco e conceitos sobre plantas medicinais, fitoterápicos e medicamentos alopáticos entre gestantes. *Revista baiana de saúde pública*, *35*(2), 320.

Piyush, M., Bothiraja, C., Kakasaheb, M., Shivajirao, K., & Atmaram, P. (2018). Phytoconstituent based dry powder inhalers as biomedicine for the management of pulmonary disease. *Biomedicine and Pharmacotherapy*, *108*, 828–837. doi:10.1016/j.biopha.2018.09.094 PMID:30372894

Plaza, M., Cifuentes, A., & Ibanez, E. (2008). In the search of new functional food ingredients from algae. *Trends in Food Science & Technology*, *19*(1), 31–39. doi:10.1016/j.tifs.2007.07.012

Politi, M., Zloh, M., Pintado, M., Castro, P., Heinrich, M., & Prieto, J. M. (2009). Direct metabolic fingerprinting of commercial herbal tinctures by nuclear magnetic resonance spectroscopy and mass spectrometry. *Phytochem Anal: PCA, 20*(4), 328–334. doi:10.1002/pca.1131 PMID:19405164

Pool, H., Campos-Vega, R., Herrera-Hernández, M. G., García-Solis, P., García-Gasca, T., Sánchez, I. C., ... Vergara-Castañeda, H. (2018). Development of genistein-PEGylated silica hybrid nanomaterials with enhanced antioxidant and antiproliferative properties on HT29 human colon cancer cells. *American Journal of Translational Research, 10*(8), 2306.

Porkert, M. (1974). *The theoretical foundations of Chinese medicine: Systems of correspondence* (Vol. 3). MIT Press.

Porres, J. C., Carreño, V., Ruíz, M., Marrón, J., & Bartolomé, J. (1989). Interferon antibodies in patients with chronic HBV infection treated with recombinant interferon. *Journal of Hepatology, 8*(3), 351–357. doi:10.1016/0168-8278(89)90034-2 PMID:2732449

Pouton, C. W. (1985). Self-emulsifying drug delivery systems: Assessment of the efficiency of emulsification. *International Journal of Pharmaceutics, 27*(2-3), 335–348. doi:10.1016/0378-5173(85)90081-X

Pouton, C. W. (2000). Lipid formulations for oral administration of drugs: Non-emulsifying, self-emulsifying and 'self-microemulsifying'drug delivery systems. *European Journal of Pharmaceutical Sciences, 11*, S93–S98. doi:10.1016/S0928-0987(00)00167-6 PMID:11033431

Pouton, C. W., & Porter, C. J. (2008). Formulation of lipid-based delivery systems for oral administration: Materials, methods and strategies. *Advanced Drug Delivery Reviews, 60*(6), 625–637. doi:10.1016/j.addr.2007.10.010 PMID:18068260

Prajapati, B. G., & Patel, M. M. (2007). Conventional and alternative pharmaceutical methods to improve oral bioavailability of lipophilic drugs. *Asian Journal of Pharmaceutics, 1*(1), 1–8.

Prakash, D., & Gupta, C. (2014). Phytochemicals of nutraceutical importance from Curcuma longa L. and their role in human health. In Phytochemicals of Nutraceutical Importance. Wallingford: CABI.

Prasad, T. N. V. K. V., & Elumalai, E. K. (2011). Biofabrication of Ag nanoparticles using *Moringa oleifera* leaf extract and their antimicrobial activity. *Asian Pacific Journal of Tropical Biomedicine, 1*(6), 439–442. doi:10.1016/S2221-1691(11)60096-8 PMID:23569809

Prasongwatana, V., Woottisin, S., Sriboonlue, P., & Kukongviriyapan, V. (2008). Uricosuric effect of Roselle (Hibiscus sabdariffa) in normal and renal-stone former subjects. *Journal of Ethnopharmacology, 117*(3), 491–495. doi:10.1016/j.jep.2008.02.036 PMID:18423919

Prathna, T. C., Chandrasekaran, N., Raichur, A. M., & Mukherjee, A. (2011a). Kinetic evolution studies of silver nanoparticles in a bio-based green synthesis process. *Colloids and Surfaces. A, Physicochemical and Engineering Aspects, 377*(1-3), 212–216. doi:10.1016/j.colsurfa.2010.12.047

Prathna, T. C., Raichur, A. M., Chandrasekaran, N., & Mukherjee, A. (2011b). Biomimetic synthesis of silver nanoparticles by Citrus limon (lemon) aqueous extract and theoretical prediction of particle size. *Colloids and Surfaces. B, Biointerfaces, 82*(1), 152–159. doi:10.1016/j.colsurfb.2010.08.036 PMID:20833002

Prausnitz, M. R., & Langer, R. (2008). Transdermal drug delivery. *Nature Biotechnology, 26*(11), 1261–1268. doi:10.1038/nbt.1504 PMID:18997767

Prausnitz, M. R., Mitragotri, S., & Langer, R. (2004). Current status and future potential of transdermal drug delivery. *Nature Reviews. Drug Discovery, 3*(2), 115–124. doi:10.1038/nrd1304 PMID:15040576

Price, W. S., Nara, M., & Arata, Y. (1997). A pulsed field gradient NMR study of the aggregation and hydration of parvalbumin. *Biophysical Chemistry, 65*(2–3), 179–187. doi:10.1016/S0301-4622(97)00003-3 PMID:17029854

Priprem, A., Sutthiparinyanont, S., Na, H.-K., Surh, Y.-J., & Chulasiri, M. (2015). Effect of formulations of nano-sized quercetin liposomes on COX-2 and NF-kB in MCF-10A cells. *Pharmaceutical Nanotechnology, 1*(1), 26–34. doi:10.2174/2211738511301010026

Priprem, A., Watanatorn, J., Sutthiparinyanont, S., Phachonpai, W., & Muchimapura, S. (2008). Anxiety and cognitive effects of quercetin liposomes in rats. *Nanomedicine; Nanotechnology, Biology, and Medicine, 4*(1), 70–78. doi:10.1016/j.nano.2007.12.001 PMID:18249157

Proksch, P., Proksch, P., Edrada, R. A., & Ebel, R. (2002). Drugs from the sea – current status and microbiological implications. *Applied Microbiology and Biotechnology, 59*(2-3), 125–134. doi:10.100700253-002-1006-8 PMID:12111137

Prudhomme, J., McDaniel, E., Ponts, N., Bertani, S., Fenical, W., Jensen, P., & Le Roch, K. (2008). Marine actinomycetes: A new source of compounds against the human malaria parasite. *PLoS One, 3*(6), e2335. doi:10.1371/journal.pone.0002335 PMID:18523554

Pushpangadan, P., & Rao, C. (2007). *Novel antidiabetic herbal formulation.* US Patent (US 20070042062 A1).

Qi, F., Wang, Z., Cai, P., Zhao, L., Gao, J., Kokudo, N., ... Tang, W. (2013). Traditional Chinese medicine and related active compounds: A review of their role on hepatitis B virus infection. *Drug Discoveries & Therapeutics, 7*(6), 212–224. doi:10.5582/ddt.2013.v7.6.212 PMID:24423652

Qing, W., Wang, Y., Li, H., Ma, F., Zhu, J., & Liu, X. (2017). Preparation and characterization of copolymer micelles for the solubilization and in vitro release of luteolin and luteoloside. *AAPS PharmSciTech, 18*(6), 2095–2101.

Radjasa, O. K. (2004). Marine invertebrate-associated bacteria in coral reef ecosystems as a new source of bioactive compounds. *J. Coast. Dev., 7*, 65–70.

Rafe, M. R. (2018). Liposomal Drug Delivery Systems Have Opened a New Window in Pharmaceutical Sciences: A Literature-based Review. *Asian Journal of Pharmaceutics, 11*(04).

Rahimpour, Y. & Hamishehkar, H. (2012). Niosomes as carrier in dermal drug delivery. *Recent Advances in Novel Drug Carrier Systems*, 141-164.

Rahimpour, Y., & Hamishehkar, H. (2012). Niosomes as carrier in dermal drug delivery. In *Recent Advances in Novel Drug Carrier Systems*. IntechOpen. doi:10.5772/51729

Rahman, A., Ismail, A., Jumbianti, D., Magdalena, S., & Sudrajat, H. (2009). Synthesis of copper oxide nano particles by using *Phormidium* cyanobacterium. *Indonesian Journal of Chemistry., 9*(3), 355–360. doi:10.22146/ijc.21498

Rahmanian, N., Hamishehkar, H., Dolatabadi, J. E. N., & Arsalani, N. (2014). Nano graphene oxide: A novel carrier for oral delivery of flavonoids. *Colloids and Surfaces. B, Biointerfaces, 123*, 331–338.

Rahmani, Z., Huh, K.-W., Lasher, R., & Siddiqui, A. (2000). Hepatitis B virus X protein colocalizes to mitochondria with a human voltage-dependent anion channel, HVDAC3, and alters its transmembrane potential. *Journal of Virology, 74*(6), 2840–2846. doi:10.1128/JVI.74.6.2840-2846.2000 PMID:10684300

Raja, K., Ukken, J. P., Athul, P. V., Tamizharasi, S., & Sivakumar, T. (2011). Formulation and evaluation of maltodextrin based proniosomal drug delivery system containing anti-diabetic (glipizide) drug. *International Journal of Pharm Tech Research, 3*, 471–477.

Raja, K., Ukken, J., Athul, P., Tamizharasi, S., & Sivakumar, T. (2011). Formulation and evaluation of maltodextrin based proniosomal drug delivery system containing antidiabetic (glipizide) drug. *International Journal of Pharm Tech Research, 3*, 471–477.

Rajakumar, R., & Allwin Prem Singh, Y. (2017). Preliminary Phytochemical and Antimicrobial studies on the crude extract of red algae *Gracilaria edulis* against clinical isolates. *European Journal Pharmaceutical and Medical Research, 4*(07), 763–766.

Rajasekaran, A., Sivagnanam, G., & Xavier, R. (2008). Nutraceuticals as therapeutic agents: A review. *Res J Pharm Tech, 3*, 28–40.

Rajendran, N., Selvan, K., Sobana, P., & Logeswar, V., Kathiresan, T., & Vennison, J. (2014). Phytochemicals, Antimicrobial and Antioxidant Screening From Five Different Marine Microalgae. *Journal of Chemical and Pharmaceutical Sciences, 2*, 78–85.

Rajesh, K. (2019). Kesharwani, K Misra, DB Singh, Perspectives and challenges of tropical medicinal herbs and modern drug discovery in the current scenario. *Asian Pacific Journal of Tropical Medicine, 12*(1), 1–7.

Rajeshkumar, S., Kannan, C., & Annadurai, G. (2012). Green synthesis of silver nanoparticles using marine brown algae *Turbinaria conoides* and its antibacterial activity. *International Journal of Pharma and Bio Sciences, 3*, 502–510.

Rajesh, W. R., Jaya, R. J., Niranjan, S. K., Vijay, D. M., & Sahebrao, K. B. (2009). Phytosynthesis of Silver Nanoparticle Using *Gliricidia sepium* (Jacq.). *Current Nanoscience, 5*(1), 117–122. doi:10.2174/157341309787314674

Raliya, R., Biswas, P., & Tarafdar, J. C. (2015). TiO_2 nanoparticle biosynthesis and its physiological effect on mung bean (Vigna radiata L.). *Biotechnology Reports (Amsterdam, Netherlands), 5*, 22–26. doi:10.1016/j.btre.2014.10.009 PMID:28626678

Ramaprasad, C., & Sirsi, M. (1956). Indian medicinal plants: Curcuma longa; in vitro antibacterial activity of curcumin and the essential oil. *Journal of Scientific and Industrial Research, C*, 15, 239–241.

Ramshankar, Y. V., Suresh, S., & Devi, K. (2008). Novel self-emulsifying formulation of curcumin with improved dissolution, antiangiogenic and anti-inflammatory activity. *Clinical Research and Regulatory Affairs, 25*(4), 213–234. doi:10.1080/10601330802600893

Rane, B., & Kesarwani, R. (2020). *Introduction to nutraceuticals and dietary supplements*. CRC Press. doi:10.1201/9780367821517-4

Rane, S., & Prabhakar, B. (2009). Formulation and Evaluation of pH-Sensitive, Long circulating Liposomes for Paclitaxel Delivery. *International Journal of Pharm Tech Research, 1*, 914–917.

Rao, D. S., Sekhara, N. C., Satyanarayana, M. N., & Srinivasan, M. (1970). Effect of curcumin on serum and liver cholesterol levels in the rat. *The Journal of Nutrition, 100*(11), 1307–1315. doi:10.1093/jn/100.11.1307 PMID:5476433

Raposo, M. F. D., de Morais, R., & de Morais, A. (2013). Health applications of bioactive compounds from marine microalgae. *Life Sciences, 93*(15), 479–486. doi:10.1016/j.lfs.2013.08.002 PMID:23994664

Rasaie, S., & Ghanbarzadeh, S. (2014). Nano phytosomes of quercetin: A promising formulation for fortification of food products with antioxidants. *Pharmaceutical Sciences, 20*, 96–101.

Rasheed, A., Sravya, R. & Roja, C. (2012). A Review on standardization of herbal formulation. *International Journal of Phytotherapy, 2*, 74-88.

Rasheed, S. H., & Haribabu, R. (2011). Transdermal drug delivery system. Simplified medication regimen- A review. *Research Journal of Pharmaceutical, Biological and Chemical Sciences, 2*, 223–238.

Ravi, G., Chandur, V., Shabaraya, A., & Sanjay, K. (2015). Phytosomes: An advanced herbal drug delivery system. *International Journal of Pharmaceutical Research and Bio-Science, 4*(3), 415–432.

Rayapu, L., Makkar, F., Chakraborty, K., & Valluru, L. (2017). Phytochemical Evaluation and Antimicrobial Activity of *Gracilaria Opuntia*: An Important Anti-Diabetic Red Marine Macroalgae. *International Journal of Current Pharmaceutical Research, 9*(6), 37–41. doi:10.22159/ijcpr.2017v9i6.23426

Rechtman, M. M., Har-Noy, O., Bar-Yishay, I., Fishman, S., Adamovich, Y., Shaul, Y., ... Shlomai, A. (2010). Curcumin inhibits hepatitis B virus via down-regulation of the metabolic coactivator PGC-1α. *FEBS Letters, 584*(11), 2485–2490. doi:10.1016/j.febslet.2010.04.067 PMID:20434445

Reddy, J. A., Dorton, R., Westrick, E., Dawson, A., Smith, T., Xu, L. C., Vetzel, M., Kleindl, P., Vlahov, I. R., & Leamon, C. P. (2007). Preclinical evaluation of EC145, a folate-vinca alkaloid conjugate. *Cancer Research, 67*(9), 4434–4442. doi:10.1158/0008-5472.CAN-07-0033 PMID:17483358

Rees, F., Hui, M., & Doherty, M. (2014). Optimizing current treatment of gout. *Nature Reviews. Rheumatology, 10*(5), 271–283. doi:10.1038/nrrheum.2014.32 PMID:24614592

Reichard, P., Nielsen, O. S., Bauer, S., Hartmann, J. T., Schoffski, P., & Christensen, T. B. (2007). Exatecan in pretreated adult patients with advanced soft tissue sarcoma: Result of a phase-II. A study of EORTC soft tissue and bone sarcoma group. *Euro J Cnacer., 43*(6), 1017–1022. doi:10.1016/j.ejca.2007.01.014

Reiss, H. (1975). Entropy-induced dispersion of bulk liquids. *Journal of Colloid and Interface Science, 53*(1), 61–70. doi:10.1016/0021-9797(75)90035-1

Re, M. I. (1998). Microencapsulation by spray drying. *Drying Technology, 16*(6), 1195–1236. doi:10.1080/07373939808917460

Riaz, G., & Chopra, R. (2018). A review on phytochemistry and therapeutic uses of Hibiscus sabdariffa L. *Biomedicine and Pharmacotherapy, 102*, 575–586. doi:10.1016/j.biopha.2018.03.023 PMID:29597091

Riches, P. L., Wright, A. F., & Ralston, S. H. (2009). Recent insights into the pathogenesis of hyperuricaemia and gout. *Human Molecular Genetics, 18*(R2), R177–R184. doi:10.1093/hmg/ddp369 PMID:19808794

Rios, J., & Waterman, P. (1997). A review of the pharmacology and toxicology of Astragalus. *Phytotherapy Research: An International Journal Devoted to Medical and Scientific Research on Plants and Plant Products, 11*(6), 411–418. doi:10.1002/(SICI)1099-1573(199709)11:6<411::AID-PTR132>3.0.CO;2-6

Riva, A., Ronchi, M., Petrangolini, G., Bosisio, S., & Allegrini, P. (2019). Improved Oral Absorption of Quercetin from Quercetin Phytosome®, a New Delivery System Based on Food Grade Lecithin. *European Journal of Drug Metabolism and Pharmacokinetics, 44*(2), 169–177. doi:10.100713318-018-0517-3 PMID:30328058

Robinson, J. R. (1996). Introduction: semi-solid formulations of oral drug delivery. *Bulletin Technique-Gattefosse*, 11-14.

Romanenko, L. A., Uchino, M., Kalinovskaya, N. I., & Mikhailov, V. V. (2008a). Isolation, phylogenetic analysis and screening of marine mollusc-associated bacteria for antimicrobial, hemolytic and surface activities. *Microbiological Research, 163*(6), 633–644. doi:10.1016/j.micres.2006.10.001 PMID:19216104

Romanenko, L. A., Uchino, M., Tanaka, N., Frolova, G. M., Slinkina, N. N., & Mikhailov, V. V. (2008b). Occurrence and antagonistic potential of *Stenotrophomonas* strains isolated from deep-sea invertebrates. *Archives of Microbiology, 189*(4), 337–344. doi:10.100700203-007-0324-8 PMID:18034228

Romanenko, L. A., Uchino, M., Tebo, B. M., Tanaka, N., Frolova, G. M., & Mikhailov, V. V. (2008c). *Pseudomonas marincola* sp. nov., isolated from marine environments. *International Journal of Systematic and Evolutionary Microbiology, 58*(3), 706–710. doi:10.1099/ijs.0.65406-0 PMID:18319482

Rothwell, J. A., Perez-Jimenez, J., Neveu, V., Medina-Remon, A., M'Hiri, N., García-Lobato, P., ... Scalbert, A. (2013). Phenol-Explorer 3.0: A major update of the Phenol-Explorer database to incorporate data on the effects of food processing on polyphenol content. *Database (Oxford).*

Rothwell, J. A., Urpi-Sarda, M., Boto-Ordonez, M., Knox, C., Llorach, R., Eisner, R., ... Andres-Lacueva, C. (2012). Phenol-Explorer 2.0: A major update of the Phenol-Explorer database integrating data on polyphenol metabolism and pharmacokinetics in humans and experimental animals. *Database (Oxford), •••*, 2012.

Rowland, I. (1999). Optimal nutrition: Fibre and phytochemicals. *The Proceedings of the Nutrition Society, 58*(2), 415–419. doi:10.1017/S0029665199000543 PMID:10466185

Roy, M., Pal, R., & Chakraborti, A. S. (2017). Pelargonidin-PLGA nanoparticles: Fabrication, characterization, and their effect on streptozotocin induced diabetic rats. *Indian Journal of Experimental Biology, 55*, 819–830.

Ruby, A. J., Kuttan, G., Babu, K. D., Rajasekharan, K. N., & Kuttan, R. (1995). Anti-tumour and antioxidant activity of natural curcuminoids. *Cancer Letters, 94*(1), 79–83. doi:10.1016/0304-3835(95)03827-J PMID:7621448

Ruiz-Miyazawa, K. W., Staurengo-Ferrari, L., Mizokami, S. S., Domiciano, T. P., Vicentini, F. T., Camilios-Neto, D., ... Teixeira, M. M. (2017). Quercetin inhibits gout arthritis in mice: Induction of an opioid-dependent regulation of inflammasome. *Inflammopharmacology, 25*(5), 555–570. doi:10.100710787-017-0356-x PMID:28508104

Sacco, S. M., Horcajada, M. N., & Offord, E. (2013). Phytonutrients for bone health during ageing. *British Journal of Clinical Pharmacology, 75*(3), 697–707.

Sachan, K., & Gupta, A. (2015). A review on nanotized herbal drugs. *International Journal of Pharmaceutical Sciences and Research, 6*(3), 961–970.

Sachan, R., & Parashar, T. (2013). Drug carrier Transfersomes: A novel tool for transdermal drug delivery system. *Int. J. Res. Dev. Pharm. Lex et Scientia, 2*(2), 309–316.

Sachan, R., Parashar, T., Singh, S., Singh, G., Tyagi, S., Patel, C., & Gupta, A. (2013). A drug carrier transferosomes: A novel tool for transdermal drug delivery system. *International Journal of Research and Development in Pharmacy and Life Sciences, 2*(2), 309–316.

Safaepour, M., Shahverdi, A. R., Shahverdi, H. R., Khorramizadeh, M. R., & Gohari, A. R. (2009). Green synthesis of small silver nanoparticles using geraniol and its cytotoxicity against Fibrosarcoma–Wehi 164. *Avicenna Journal of Medical Biotechnology, 1*, 111–115. PMID:23407598

Sagar, S., Yance, D., & Wong, R. (2006). Natural health products that inhibit angiogenesis: A potential source for investigational new agents to treat cancer-part 1. *Current Oncology (Toronto, Ont.), 13*, 14–26. PMID:17576437

Saha, S., Sarma, A., Saikia, P., & Chakraarty, T. (2013). Phytosome: A brief overview. *Scholars Academic Journal of Pharmacy, 2*, 12–20.

Sahni, J., Baboota, S., & Ali, J. (2011). Promising Role of Nanopharmaceuticals in Drug Delivery. *Pharmacy Times, 43*, 16–18.

Sahoo, S. K., & Labhasetwar, V. (2003). Nanotech approaches to drug delivery and imaging. *Drug Discovery Today, 8*(24), 1112–1120. doi:10.1016/S1359-6446(03)02903-9 PMID:14678737

Sahu, N., Soni, D., Chandrashekhar, B., Satpute, D. B., Saravanadevi, S., Sarangi, B. K., & Pandey, R. A. (2016). Synthesis of silver nanoparticles using flavonoids: Hesperidin, naringin and diosmin, and their antibacterial effects and cytotoxicity. *International Nano Letters, 6*(3), 173–181.

Sak, K. (2014). Cytotoxicity of dietary flavonoids on different human cancer types. *Pharmacognosy Reviews*, *8*(16), 122.

Saklani, A., & Kutty, S. K. (2008). Plant derived compounds in clinical trials. *Drug Discovery Today*, *13*(3–4), 161–171. doi:10.1016/j.drudis.2007.10.010 PMID:18275914

Sakthivel, L., Timmakondu, N., Chellappan, D., & Subramaniam, S. (2012). Nutraceuticals and their medicinial importance. *IJHAS*, *1*(2), 47–53.

Salvia-Trujillo, L., Olga, M., & McClements, D. (2016). Excipient Nanoemulsions for Improving Oral Bioavailability of Bioactives. *Nanomaterials MDPI*, *6*(17), 1–16. doi:10.3390/nano6010017 PMID:28344274

Sangeetha, K. S. S., Umamaheswari, S., Reddy, C. U. M., & Kalkura, S. N. (2017). Chrysin loaded chitosan nanoparticle: Formulation and in-vitro characterization. *International Journal of Pharmaceutical Sciences and Research*, *8*(3), 1102–1109. doi:10.13040/IJPSR.0975-8232.8(3).1102-09

Sanghi, R., & Verma, P. (2008). Biomimetic synthesis and characterization of protein capped silver nanoparticles. *Bioresource Technology*, *100*(1), 501–504. doi:10.1016/j.biortech.2008.05.048 PMID:18625550

Sanli, O., Karaca, I., & Isiklan, N. (2009). Preparation, characterization, and salicylic acid release behaviour of chitosan/poly (vinyl alcohol) blend microspheres. *Journal of Applied Polymer Science*, *111*(6), 2731–2740. doi:10.1002/app.29319

Santos, E. L., Maia, B. H. L. N. S., Ferriani, A. P., & Teixeira, S. D. (2017). *Flavonoids: Classification, biosynthesis and chemical ecology* (Vol. 6). InTech.

Sapkale, A., Thorat, M., VirPrasad, R., & Singh, M. (2012). Nutraceuticals –Global status and applications: A review. *IJPCS*, *1*(3).

Saraf, S., Jeswani, G., Kaur, C. D., & Saraf, S. (2011). Development of novel herbal cosmetic cream with Curcuma longa extract loaded transfersomes for antiwrinkle effect. *The Journal of Pharmacy and Pharmacology*, *5*(8), 1054–1062.

Saraf, S., & Kaur, C. D. (2010). Phytoconstituents as photoprotective novel cosmetic formulations. *Pharmacognosy Reviews*, *4*(7), 1–11. doi:10.4103/0973-7847.65319 PMID:22228936

Sarangi, M., & Padhi, S. (2018). Novel herbal drug delivery system: an overview. *Arch Med Health Sci*, *6*, 171-9.

Sarawate, C. A., Brewer, K. K., Yang, W., Patel, P. A., Schumacher, H. R., Saag, K. G., & Bakst, A. W. (2006). Gout medication treatment patterns and adherence to standards of care from a managed care perspective. *Mayo Clinic Proceedings*. 10.4065/81.7.925

Sarin, B., Verma, N., Martín, J. P., & Mohanty, A. (2014). An overview of important ethnomedicinal herbs of Phyllanthus species: Present status and future prospects. *TheScientificWorldJournal*. PMID:24672382

Sarin, R., Sharma, M., Singh, R., & Kumar, S. (2012). Nutraceuticals: A review. *Int Res J Pharm*, *3*, 95–99.

Sarwa, K. K., Mazumder, B., Rudrapal, M., & Verma, V. K. (2015). Potential of capsaicin-loaded transfersomes in arthritic rats. *Drug Delivery*, *22*(5), 638–646. doi:10.3109/10717544.2013.871601 PMID:24471764

Sathishkumar, M., Sneha, K., Won, W. S., Cho, C. W., Kim, S., & Yun, Y. S. (2009). *Cynamon zeylanicum* bark extract and powder mediated green synthesis of nanocrystallinesilver particles and its bactericidal activity. *Colloids and Surfaces. B, Biointerfaces*, *73*(2), 332–338. doi:10.1016/j.colsurfb.2009.06.005 PMID:19576733

Sathishkumar, P., Li, Z., Huang, B., Guo, X., Zhan, Q., Wang, C., & Gu, F. L. (2019). Understanding the surface functionalization of myricetin-mediated gold nanoparticles: Experimental and theoretical approaches. *Applied Surface Science*, *493*, 634–644.

Sathyavathi, R., Balamurali, K. M., Venugopal, R. S., Saritha, R., & Narayana, R. D. (2010). Biosynthesis of Silver Nanoparticles Using *Coriandrum Sativum* Leaf Extract and Their Application in Nonlinear Optics. *Advanced Science Letters*, *3*(2), 1–6. doi:10.1166/asl.2010.1099

Sato, V. H., Sungthong, B., Rinthong, P.-O., Nuamnaichati, N., Mangmool, S., Chewchida, S., & Sato, H. (2018). Pharmacological effects of Chatuphalatika in hyperuricemia of gout. *Pharmaceutical Biology*, *56*(1), 76–85. doi:10.1080/13880209.2017.1421235 PMID:29298537

Satpute, S. K., Banat, I. M., Dhakephalkar, P. K., Banpurkar, A. G., & Chopade, B. A. (2007). Biosurfactants, bioemulsifiers and exopolysaccharides from marine microorganisms. *Biotechnology Advances*, *28*(4), 436–450. doi:10.1016/j.biotechadv.2010.02.006 PMID:20172021

Satyan, K. S., Jaiswal, A. K., Ghosal, S., & Bhattacharya, S. K. (1998). Anxiolytic activity of ginkgolic acid conjugates from Indian Ginkgo biloba. *Psychopharmacology*, *136*(2), 148–152. doi:10.1007002130050550 PMID:9551771

Savithramma, N., Linga, R. M., Ankanna, S., & Venkateswarlu, P. (2012). Screening of medicinal plants for effective biogenesis of silver nano particles and efficient anti-microbial activity. *International Journal of Pharmaceutical Sciences and Research*, *3*, 1141–1148.

Scarfato, P., Avallone, E., Iannelli, P., Aquino, R. P., Lauro, M. R., Rossi, A., & Acierno, D. (2008). Quercetin microspheres by solvent evaporation: Preparation, characterization and release behavior. *Journal of Applied Polymer Science*, *109*(5), 2994–3001. doi:10.1002/app.28365

Schmid, G. (2011). *Nanoparticles: From theory to application*. John Wiley & Sons.

Schreier, H., & Bouwstra, J. (1994). Liposomes and niosomes as topical drug carriers: Dermal and transdermal drug delivery. *Journal of Controlled Release*, *30*(1), 1–15. doi:10.1016/0168-3659(94)90039-6

Schulz, V., Hansel, R., & Tyler, V. E. (2000). *A physicians guide to herbal medicine. In Rational phytotherapy*. Springer.

Schwarz, C., Mehnert, M., Lucks, J., & Muller, R. (1994). Solid lipid nanoparticles (SLN) for controlled drug delivery: I. Production, characterization and sterilization. *Journal of Controlled Release*, *30*(1), 83–96. doi:10.1016/0168-3659(94)90047-7

Schwarz, J. A. (2004). *Dekker encyclopedia of Nanoscienceand nanotechnology*. Marcel Dekker.

Sebastian, M., Ninan, N., & Haghi, A. K. (Eds.). (2012). *Nanomedicine and drug delivery*. CRC Press. doi:10.1201/b13119

Seema, A. (2014). Recent development of herbal formulation- a novel drug. *Int. Ayur Med J.*, *2*(6), 952–958.

Selby-Pham, S. N., Miller, R. B., Howell, K., Dunshea, F., & Bennett, L. E. (2017). Physicochemical properties of dietary phytochemicals can predict their passive absorption in the human small intestine. *Scientific Reports*, *7*(1), 1–15.

Selvam, R. P., & Singh, A. K. (2010). Transdermal drugdelivery systems for antihypertensive drugs-A review. *International Journal of Pharmaceutical and Biomedical Research*, *1*(1), 1–8.

Selvin, J., Shanmughapriya, S., Gandhimathi, S., Kiran, G. S., Ravji, T. R., Natarajaseenivasan, K., & Hema, T. A. (2009). Optimization and production of novel antimicrobial agents from sponge associated marine actinomycetes *Nocardiopsis dassonvillei* MAD08. *Applied Microbiology and Biotechnology*, *83*(3), 435–445. doi:10.100700253-009-1878-y PMID:19190903

Semalty, A., Semalty, M., Rawat, B. S., Singh, D., & Rawat, M. S. (2009). Pharmacosomes: The lipid-based new drug delivery system. *Expert Opinion on Drug Delivery*, *6*(6), 599–612. doi:10.1517/17425240902967607 PMID:19519287

Semalty, A., Semalty, M., Rawat, M. S., & Franceschim, F. (2010). Supramolecular phospholipids-polyphenolics interactions: The phytosome strategy toimprove the bioavailability of phytochemicals. *Fitoterapia*, *81*(5), 306–314. doi:10.1016/j.fitote.2009.11.001 PMID:19919847

Sepeur, S., Laryea, N., Goedicke, S., & Groß, F. (2013). Nanotechnology: technical basics and applications. Hannover: Vincentz. 168. doi:10.1515/9783748602347

Setthacheewakul, S., Kedjinda, W., Maneenuan, D., & Wiwattanapatapee, R. (2011). Controlled release of oral tetrahydrocurcumin from a novel self-emulsifying floating drug delivery system (SEFDDS). *AAPS PharmSciTech*, *12*(1), 152–164. doi:10.120812249-010-9568-8 PMID:21181511

Shah, M., Fawcett, D., Sharma, S., Tripathy, S. K., & Poinern, G. E. J. (2015). Green synthesis of metallic nanoparticles via biological entities. *Material.*, *8*(11), 7278–7308. doi:10.3390/ma8115377 PMID:28793638

Shah, P., Halodia, D., & Shelat, P. (2010). Nanoemulsion: A pharmaceutical review. *Systematic Reviews in Pharmacy*, *1*(1), 24–32. doi:10.4103/0975-8453.59509

Shaji, J., & Joshi, V. (2005). Self-micro emulsifying drug delivery system (SMEDDS) for improving bioavailability of hydrophobic drugs and its potential to give sustain release dosage form. *Indian Journal of Pharmaceutical Education*, *39*(3), 130.

Shankar, S. S., Rai, S. A., Ahmad, A., & Sastry, M. (2004). Rapid synthesis of Au, Ag,and bimetallic Au core–Ag shell nanoparticles using Neem (*Azadirachta indica*) leaf broth. *Journal of Colloid and Interface Science*, *275*(2), 496–502. doi:10.1016/j.jcis.2004.03.003 PMID:15178278

Shanmugam, B., Shanmugam, K. R., Ravi, S., Subbaiah, G. V., Ramakrishana, C., Mallikarjuna, K., & Reddy, K. S. (2017). Exploratory studies of (-)-Epicatechin, a bioactive compound of Phyllanthus niruri, on the antioxidant enzymes and oxidative stress markers in D-galactosamine-induced hepatitis in rats: A study with reference to clinical prospective. *Pharmacognosy Magazine*, *13*(49, Suppl 1), S56. doi:10.4103/0973-1296.203973 PMID:28479727

Shanmugam, S., Baskaran, R., Balakrishnan, P., Thapa, P., Yong, C. S., & Yoo, B. K. (2011). Solid self-nanoemulsifying drug delivery system (S-SNEDDS) containing phosphatidylcholine for enhanced bioavailability of highly lipophilic bioactive carotenoid lutein. *European Journal of Pharmaceutics and Biopharmaceutics*, *79*(2), 250–257. doi:10.1016/j.ejpb.2011.04.012 PMID:21550401

Shao, B., Tang, J., Ji, H., Liu, H., Liu, Y., Zhu, D., & Wu, L. (2010). Enhanced oral bioavailability of Wurenchun (Fructus Schisandrae Chinensis extracts) by self-emulsifying drug delivery systems. *Drug Development and Industrial Pharmacy*, *36*(11), 1356–1363. doi:10.3109/03639045.2010.480975 PMID:20849350

Sharma, M. (2014). Applications of nanotechnology based dosage forms for delivery of herbal drugs. *Research and Reviews: Journal of Pharmaceutics and Nanotechnology, 2*(1), 23-30.

Sharma, A. (2012). Transdermal approach of antidiabetic drug glibenclamide: A review. *Int. J. Pharm. Res. Dev.*, *3*, 25–32.

Sharma, A. K. (2003). Panchkarma Therapy in Ayurvedic Medicine. In L. C. Mishra (Ed.), *Scientific Basis for Ayurvedic Therapies*. CRC Press. doi:10.1201/9780203498583.ch4

Sharma, A. T., Mitkare, S. S., & Moon, R. S. (2011). Multicomponent herbal therapy: A review. *International Journal of Pharmaceutical Sciences Review and Research*, *6*, 185–187.

Sharma, A., Keservani, R., & Kesharwani, R. (Eds.). (2018). *Nanobiomaterials: applications in drug delivery*. CRC Press. doi:10.1201/9781315204918

Sharma, D., Ali, A. A. E., & Aate, J. R. (2018). Niosomes as novel drug delivery system: Review article. *Pharmatutor, 6*(3), 58–65. doi:10.29161/PT.v6.i3.2018.58

Sharma, G., Anabousi, S., Ehrhardt, C., & Ravi Kumar, M. N. V. (2006). Liposomes as targeted drug delivery systems in the treatment of breast cancer. *Journal of Drug Targeting, 14*(5), 301–310. doi:10.1080/10611860600809112 PMID:16882550

Sharma, G., Jasuja, N. D., Ali, M. I., & Joshi, S. C. (2014). A Review on Nanomedicinal and Nanosensing Potential of Nanoparticles. *International Journal of Biological Chemistry., 8*(2), 58–54. doi:10.3923/ijbc.2014.58.84

Sharma, G., Sharma, A. R., Bhavesh, R., Park, J., Ganbold, B., Nam, J.-S., & Lee, S.-S. (2014). Biomolecule-Mediated Synthesis of Selenium Nanoparticles using Dried *Vitis vinifera* (Raisin) Extract. *Molecules (Basel, Switzerland), 19*(3), 2761–2770. doi:10.3390/molecules19032761 PMID:24583881

Sharma, K., Agrawal, S. S., & Gupta, M. (2015). Development and validation of uv spectrophotometric method for the estimation of curcumin in bulk drug and pharmaceutical dosage forms. *International Journal of Drug Development and Research., 4*(2), 375–380.

Sharma, M. (2014). Application of nanotechnology based dosage form for delivery of herbal drugs. *Research and Reviews: Journal of Pharmaceutics and Nanotechnology, 2*(1), 23–30.

Sharma, N. C., Sahi, S. V., Nath, S., Parsons, J. G., Gardea-Torresdey, J. L., & Pal, T. (2007). Synthesis of plant-mediated gold nanoparticles and catalytic role of biomatrix-embedded nanomaterials. *Environmental Science & Technology, 41*(14), 5137–5142. doi:10.1021/es062929a PMID:17711235

Sharma, N., Singh, A. K., & Sodhi, S. S., Zhang, J. J., Mongre, R. K., Ghosh, M., ... Jeong, D. K. (2017). Anti-tumor activity of wogonin, an extract from Scutellaria baicalensis, through regulating different signaling pathways. *Chinese Journal of Natural Medicines, 15*(1), 15–40.

Sharma, P. K., Saxena, P., Jaswanth, A., Chalamaiah, M., Tekade, K. R., & Balasubramaniam, A. (2016). Novel encapsulation of lycopene in niosomes and assessment of its anticancer activity. *Journal of Bioequivalence & Bioavailability, 8*(5), 224–232.

Sharma, R. A., Gescher, A. J., & Steward, W. P. (2005). Curcumin: The story so far. *European Journal of Cancer, 41*(13), 1955–1968. doi:10.1016/j.ejca.2005.05.009 PMID:16081279

Sharma, R. A., McLelland, H. R., Hill, K. A., Ireson, C. R., Euden, S. A., Manson, M. M., ... Steward, W. P. (2001). Pharmacodynamic and pharmacokinetic study of oral Curcuma extract in patients with colorectal cancer. *Clinical Cancer Research, 7*(7), 1894–1900. PMID:11448902

Sharma, R., Kaur, A., Thakur, S., Bhardwaj, K., & Bose, S. (2017). Role of nutraceuticals in health care. *IJGP, 11*(3), S385.

Sharma, R., & Singh, R. B. (2013). Bioactive foods and nutraceutical supplementation criteria in cardiovascular protection. *The Open Nutraceuticals Journal, 3*, 141–153.

Sheena, I. P., Singh, U. V., Kamath, R., Devi, P. U., & Udupa, N. (1998). Niosomal withaferin A with better antitumor efficacy. *Indian Journal of Pharmaceutical Sciences, 60*(1), 45–48.

Shen, Q., Wang, Y., & Zhang, Y. (2011). Improvement of colchicine oral bioavailability by incorporating eugenol in the nanoemulsion as an oil excipient and enhancer. *International Journal of Nanomedicine, 6*, 1237. doi:10.2147/IJN.S20903 PMID:21753875

Shen, R.-M., Zhong, L.-B., & Li, G.-Q. (2019). Anti-inflammatory effect of luteolin in acute gouty arthritis rat model. *Hainan Yixueyuan Xuebao, 25*(17), 20–24.

Shen, Y. J., Zhang, Z. W., Luo, X. G., Wang, X. F., & Wang, H. L. (2008). Nanoparticles of traditional Chinese herbs inhibit thrombosis *in vivo*. *Haematologica*, *93*, 1457.

Sheu, S.-Y., Fu, Y.-T., Huang, W.-D., Chen, Y.-A., Lei, Y.-C., Yao, C.-H., ... Kuo, T.-F. (2016). Evaluation of xanthine oxidase inhibitory potential and in vivo hypouricemic activity of Dimocarpus longan Lour. extracts. *Pharmacognosy Magazine*, *12*(46, Suppl 2), S206. doi:10.4103/0973-1296.182176 PMID:27279708

Shibamoto, T., Kanazawa, K., Shahidi, F., & Ho, C. (2008). Functional food and health: an overview. In T. Shibamoto, K. Kanazawa, F. Shahidi, & C.-T. Ho (Eds.), ACS symposium series: Vol. 993. *Functional food and health* (pp. 1–6). Oxford Univ. Press. doi:10.1021/bk-2008-0993.ch001

Shi, J., Votruba, A. R., Farokhzad, O. C., & Langer, R. (2010). Nanotechnology in drug delivery and tissue engineering: From discovery to applications. *Nano Letters*, *10*(9), 3223–3230. doi:10.1021/nl102184c PMID:20726522

Shimada, S. (2008). Composition comprising nanoparticle Ginkgo biloba extract with the effect of brain function activation IPC8 Class-AA61K914FI, USPC Class-424489.

Shin, M. S., Kang, E. H., & Lee, Y. I. (2005). A flavonoid from medicinal plants blocks hepatitis B virus-e antigen secretion in HBV-infected hepatocytes. *Antiviral Research*, *67*(3), 163–168. doi:10.1016/j.antiviral.2005.06.005 PMID:16118024

Shin, W.-Y., Shim, D.-W., Kim, M.-K., Sun, X., Koppula, S., Yu, S. H., Kim, H.-B., Kim, T.-J., Kang, T.-B., & Lee, K.-H. (2017). Protective effects of Cinnamomum cassia (Lamaceae) against gout and septic responses via attenuation of inflammasome activation in experimental models. *Journal of Ethnopharmacology*, *205*, 173–177. doi:10.1016/j.jep.2017.03.043 PMID:28347828

Shiny, P. J., Mukherjee, A., & Chandrasekaran, N. (2013). Marine algae mediated synthesis of the silver nanoparticles and its antibacterial efficiency. *International Journal of Pharmacy and Pharmaceutical Sciences*, *5*, 239–241.

Shi, Y. W., Wang, C. P., Liu, L., Liu, Y. L., Wang, X., Hong, Y., Li, Z., & Kong, L. D. (2012). Antihyperuricemic and nephroprotective effects of resveratrol and its analogues in hyperuricemic mice. *Molecular Nutrition & Food Research*, *56*(9), 1433–1444. doi:10.1002/mnfr.201100828 PMID:22865646

Shi, Y., & Williamson, G. (2016). Quercetin lowers plasma uric acid in pre-hyperuricaemic males: A randomised, double-blinded, placebo-controlled, cross-over trial. *British Journal of Nutrition*, *115*(5), 800–806. doi:10.1017/S0007114515005310 PMID:26785820

Shrivastava, D. (2012). Transdermal approach of antidiabetic drug glibenclamide: A review. *World Journal of Pharmacy and Pharmaceutical Sciences*, *1*, 532–544.

Shukla, G., Kumari, S., Maguddayao, A., Prashar, S., & Kumar, C. (2014). Nutraceuticals: The future therapeutics. *Int J Pharm Technol*, *4*(1), 46–50.

Shukla, N., & Tiwari, M. (2011). Proniosomal drug delivery systems – Clinical applications. *International Journal of Research in Pharmaceutical and Biomedical Sciences*, *2*, 880–887.

Siddiqui, I. A., Adhami, V., Bharali, D., Hafeez, B., Asim, M., Khwaja, S., Ahmad, N., Cui, H., Mousa, S. A., & Mukhtar, H. (2009). Introducing nanochemoprevention as a novel approach for cancer control: Proof of principle with green tea polyphenol epigallocatechin-3-gallate. *Cancer Research*, *2*(7), 1712–1716. doi:10.1158/0008-5472.CAN-08-3978 PMID:19223530

Sikarwar, M. S., Sharma, S., Jain, A. K., & Parial, S. D. (2008). Preparation, characterization and evaluation of marsupsin phospholipid complex. *AAPS PharmSciTech*, *9*(1), 129–137. doi:10.120812249-007-9020-x PMID:18446473

Silva, A. P., Nunes, B. R., De Oliveira, M. C., Koester, L. S., Mayorga, P., Bassani, V. L., & Teixeira, H. F. (2009). Development of topical nanoemulsions containing the isoflavone genistein. Die Pharmazie-An. *International Journal of Pharma Sciences*, *64*(1), 32–35. PMID:19216228

Silva, C. R., Fröhlich, J. K., Oliveira, S. M., Cabreira, T. N., Rossato, M. F., Trevisan, G., ... Athayde, M. L. (2013). The antinociceptive and anti-inflammatory effects of the crude extract of Jatropha isabellei in a rat gout model. *Journal of Ethnopharmacology*, *145*(1), 205–213. doi:10.1016/j.jep.2012.10.054 PMID:23127654

Simmons, T. L., Engene, N., Ureña, L. D., Romero, L. I., Ortega-Barría, E., Gerwick, L., & Gerwick, W. H. (2008). Viridamides A and B, lipodepsipeptides with antiprotozoal activity from the marine cyanobacterium *Oscillatoria nigro*-Viridis. *Journal of Natural Products*, *71*(9), 1544–1550. doi:10.1021/np800110e PMID:18715036

Singer, J. W., Bhatt, R., Tulinsky, J., Buhler, K. R., Heasley, E., Klein, P., & de Vries, P. (2001). Water-soluble poly-(l-glutamic acid)–Gly-camptothecin conjugates enhance camptothecin stability and efficacy in vivo. *Journal of Controlled Release*, *74*(1-3), 243–247. doi:10.1016/S0168-3659(01)00323-6 PMID:11489501

Singh, A., Chaudhary, M., & Sastry, M. (2006). Construction of conductive multilayer films of biogenic triangular gold nanoparticles and their application in chemical vapour sensing. *Nanotechnology*, *17*(9), 2399–2405. doi:10.1088/0957-4484/17/9/055

Singh, Agarwal, Kesharwani, & Misra. (2013). Atom based QSAR and pharmacophore study of curcuminoids and curcumin analogs: Interaction with thioredoxin reductase. *Interdisciplinary Sciences, Computational Life Sciences*, *5*, 286–295.

Singhal, G., Bhavesh, R., Kasariya, K., Sharma, A. R., & Singh, R. P. (2011). Biosynthesis of silver nanoparticles using Ocimum sanctum (Tulsi) leaf extract and screening its antimicrobial activity. *Journal of Nanoparticle Research*, *13*(7), 2981–2988. doi:10.100711051-010-0193-y

Singh, D. V., Agarwal, S., Kesharwani, R. K., & Misra, K. (2013). 3D QSAR and pharmacophore study of curcuminoids and curcumin analogs: Interaction with thioredoxin reductase. *Interdisciplinary Sciences, Computational Life Sciences*, *5*(4), 286–295. doi:10.100712539-013-0177-6 PMID:24402822

Singh, Gupta, Kesharwani, & Misra. (n.d.). Comparative docking and ADMET study of some curcumin derivatives and herbal congeners targeting β-amyloid. *Network Modeling and Analysis in Health Informatics and Bioinformatics*. Advance online publication. doi:10.100713721-012-0021-7

Singh, H., Utreja, P., Tiwari, A., & Jain, S. (2009). Elastic Liposomal formulation for sustained delivery of colchicine: In vitro Characterization and in vivo evaluation of anti-gout activity. *AAPS*, *11*(1), 54–64. doi:10.120812248-008-9078-8 PMID:19191031

Singh, J., & Sinha, S. (2012). Classification and regulatory acts and applications of nutraceuticals for health. *IJPBS*, *2*(1), 177–187.

Singh, K. P., Crane, M., Audsley, J., Avihingsanon, A., Sasadeusz, J., & Lewin, S. R. (2017). HIV-hepatitis B virus coinfection: Epidemiology, pathogenesis, and treatment. *AIDS (London, England)*, *31*(15), 2035–2052. doi:10.1097/QAD.0000000000001574 PMID:28692539

Singh, R. P., Gangadharappa, V. H., & Mruthunjaya, K. (2016). Phytosome loaded novel herbal drug delivery system: A review. *Int Res J Pharm*, *7*(6), 15–21. doi:10.7897/2230-8407.07656

Singh, R. P., Shukla, V. K., Yadav, R. S., Sharma, P. K., Singh, P. K., & Pandey, A. C. (2011). Biological approach of zinc oxide nanoparticles formation and its characterization. *Advanced Materials Letters*, *2*(4), 313–317. doi:10.5185/amlett.indias.204

Singh, R. P., Singh, S. G., Naik, H., Jain, D., & Bisla, S. (2011). Herbal excipients in novel drug delivery system. *Int J ComprPharm, 2*, 1–7.

Singh, Y., Meher, J. G., Raval, K., Khan, F. A., Chaurasia, M., Jain, N. K., & Chourasia, M. K. (2017). Nanoemulsion: Concepts, development and applications in drug delivery. *Journal of Controlled Release, 252*, 28–49. doi:10.1016/j.jconrel.2017.03.008 PMID:28279798

Sinico, C., De Logu, A., Lai, F., Valenti, D., Manconi, M., Loy, G., Bonsignore, L., & Fadda, A. M. (2005). Liposomal incorporation of Artemisia arborescens L. essential oil and in vitro antiviral activity. *European Journal of Pharmaceutics and Biopharmaceutics, 59*(1), 161–168. doi:10.1016/j.ejpb.2004.06.005 PMID:15567314

Sintov, A. C. (2015). Transdermal delivery of curcumin via microemulsion. *International Journal of Pharmaceutics, 481*(1–2), 97–103. doi:10.1016/j.ijpharm.2015.02.005

Sivakranth, M., Anjuma, A., Krishnaveni, C., & Venkatesh, E. (2012). Ethosomes: A novel vesicular drug delivery system. *Int J Adv Pharm, 2*(1), 16–27.

Sivaraj, R., Rahman, P. K., Rajiv, P., Narendhran, S., & Venckatesh, R. (2014). Biosynthesis and characterization of Acalypha indica mediated copper oxide nanoparticles and evaluation of its antimicrobial and anticancer activity. *Spectrochimica Acta. Part A: Molecular and Biomolecular Spectroscopy, 129*, 255–258. doi:10.1016/j.saa.2014.03.027 PMID:24747845

Sivonen, K., Leikoski, N., Fewer, D. P., & Jokela, J. (2010). Cyanobactins-ribosomal cyclic peptides produced by cyanobacteria. *Applied Microbiology and Biotechnology, 86*(5), 1213–1225. doi:10.100700253-010-2482-x PMID:20195859

Smith, A. (2009). *The benefits of natural medicine*. Retrieved from http://ezinearticles.com/?expert=Alden_Smith

Sohn, B. H., & Cohen, R. E. (1991). *Chem Mater. Processible optically transparent block copolymer films containing super paramagnetic iron oxide nano preparation*. Academic Press.

Solans, C., Izquierdo, P., Nolla, J., Azemar, N., & Garcia-Celma, M. J. (2005). Nano-emulsions. *Curr Opin Colloid In, 10*(3–4), 102–110. doi:10.1016/j.cocis.2005.06.004

Solecki, R. S., & Shanidar, I. V. (1975). A neanderrhal flower burial in northern Iraq. *Science, 190*, 880–881.

Soman, A. G., Gloer, J. B., Angawi, R. F., Wicklow, D. T., & Dowd, P. F. (2001). Vertilecanins: New Phenopicolinic Acid Analogs from *Verticillium lecanii*. *Journal of Natural Products, 64*(2), 189–192. doi:10.1021/np000094q PMID:11429997

Song, J. Y., Kwon, E. Y., & Kim, B. S. (2010). Biological synthesis of platinum nanoparticles using *Diopyros kaki* leaf extract. *Bioprocess and Biosystems Engineering, 33*(1), 159–164. doi:10.100700449-009-0373-2 PMID:19701776

Song, Y., Ping, Q., & Wu, Z. (2005). Preparation of silybin nanoemulsion and its pharmacokinetics in rabbits. *Zhongguo Yaoke Daxue Xuebao, 36*(5), 427.

Song, Y., Ping, Q., & Wu, Z. H. (2005). Preparation of silybin nano emulsion and its pharmacokinetics in rabbits. *J Chin Pharm Univ, 5*, 427–431.

Spanou, C., Veskoukis, A. S., Kerasioti, T., Kontou, M., Angelis, A., Aligiannis, N., Skaltsounis, A.-L., & Kouretas, D. (2012). Flavonoid glycosides isolated from unique legume plant extracts as novel inhibitors of xanthine oxidase. *PLoS One, 7*(3), e32214. doi:10.1371/journal.pone.0032214 PMID:22396752

Sri, S. N., Thiagarajan, R., Manikandan, R., & Arumugam, M. (2019). Curcumin-Based Food Supplements: Challenges and Future Prospects. In Nonvitamin and Nonmineral Nutritional Supplements. Academic Press.

Srikanth, P., & Raju, N. (2013). A review on oral controlled drug delivery. *Int. J. Adv. Pharm., 3*, 51–58.

Srinivas, P., Philbert, M., Vu, T., Huang, Q., Kokini, J., Saltos, E., Chen, H., & Ross, S. (2009). Nanotechnology research: Applications in nutrition sciences. *The Journal of Nutrition*, *140*(1), 119–124. doi:10.3945/jn.109.115048 PMID:19939997

Stadler, M., Anke, H., & Sterner, O. (1995). Metabolites with nematicidal and antimicrobial activities from the ascomycete *Lachnum papyraceum* (Karst.) Karst. III. production of novel isocoumarin derivatives, isolation and biological activities. *The Journal of Antibiotics*, *48*(3), 261–266. doi:10.7164/antibiotics.48.261 PMID:7730162

Sterer, N., Nuas, S., Mizrahi, B., Goldenberg, C., Weiss, E. I., Domb, A., & Davidi, M. P. (2008). Oral malodor reduction by a palatal mucoadhesive tablet containing herbal formulation. *Journal of Dentistry*, *36*(7), 535–539. doi:10.1016/j.jdent.2008.04.001

Subramanian, A. P., Jaganathan, S. K., Manikandan, A., Pandiaraj, K. N., Gomathi, N., & Supriyanto, E. (2016). Recent trends in nano-based drug delivery systems for efficient delivery of phytochemicals in chemotherapy. *RSC Advances*, *6*(54), 48294–48314. doi:10.1039/C6RA07802H

Sudhakar, C. K., Upadhyay, N., Verma, A., Jain, A., Charyulu, R. N., & Jain, S. (2015). Nanomedicine and tissue engineering. In *Nanotechnology Applications for Tissue Engineering* (pp. 1–19). William Andrew Publishing. doi:10.1016/B978-0-323-32889-0.00001-7

Sukirtha, R., Priyanka, K. M., Antony, J. J., Kamalakkannan, S., Ramar, T., & Palani, G. (2011). Cytotoxic effect of green synthesized silver nanoparticles using Meliaazedarach against in vitro HeLa cell lines and lymphoma mice model. *Process Biochemistry*, *47*(2), 273–279. doi:10.1016/j.procbio.2011.11.003

Suleria, H. A. R., Osborne, S., Masci, P., & Gobe, G. (2015). Marine-Based Nutraceuticals: An Innovative Trend in the Food and Supplement Industries. *Marine Drugs*, *13*(10), 6336–6351. doi:10.3390/md13106336 PMID:26473889

Summers, J., Smith, P. M., & Horwich, A. L. (1990). Hepadnavirus envelope proteins regulate covalently closed circular DNA amplification. *Journal of Virology*, *64*(6), 2819–2824. doi:10.1128/JVI.64.6.2819-2824.1990 PMID:2335817

Summers, J., Smith, P. M., Huang, M., & Yu, M. (1991). Morphogenetic and regulatory effects of mutations in the envelope proteins of an avian hepadnavirus. *Journal of Virology*, *65*(3), 1310–1317. doi:10.1128/JVI.65.3.1310-1317.1991 PMID:1995945

Sun, H. W., & Ouyang, W. Q. (2007). Preparation, Quality and Safety Evaluation of Berberine Nanoemulsion for Oral Application. *Shanghai Jiaotong Daxue Xuebao. Nongye Kexueban*, 1.

Sungthongjeen, S., Pitaksuteepong, T., Somsiri, A., & Sriamornsak, P. (1999). Studies on pectins as potential hydrogelmatrices for controlled-release drug delivery. *Drug Development and Industrial Pharmacy*, *25*(12), 1271–1276. doi:10.1081/DDC-100102298 PMID:10612023

Sungthongjeen, S., Puttipipatkhachorn, S., Paeratakul, O., Dashevsky, A., & Bodmeier, R. (2004). Development of pulsatile release tablets with swelling and rupturable layers. *Journal of Controlled Release*, *95*(2), 147–159. doi:10.1016/j.jconrel.2003.10.023

Sun, H. W., & Ouyang, W. Q. (2007). The preparation of neem oil microemulsion (Azdirachta Indica) and the comparission of acaricidal time between neemoil microemulsion and other formulation in vitro. [Agric Sci]. *J Shanghai Jiao Tong Univy*, *1*, 60–65.

Sun, H., & Ouyang, W. (2007). Preparation, quality and safety evaluation of berbarinenano emulsion for oral application. *Journal of Shanghai Jiaotong University*, *1*, 60–65.

Sun, Y., Li, L., Li, J., & Li, Z. (2007). Inhibition of hepatitis B virus replication by Rheum palmatum L. ethanol extract in a stable HBV-producing cell line. *Virologica Sinica*, *22*(1), 14–20. doi:10.100712250-007-0056-6

Su, Y. L., Fu, Z. Y., Zhang, J. Y., Wang, W. M., Wang, H., Wang, Y. C., & Zhang, Q. J. (2008). Microencapsulation of Radix salvia miltiorrhiza nanoparticles by spray-drying. *Powder Technology, 184*(1), 114–121. doi:10.1016/j.powtec.2007.08.014

Synytsia, I. (2016). Evaluation of using quercetin in patients with gout and hypertension. *Ukrainian Scientific Medical Youth Journal*, (4 (98)), 54–58.

Tacar, O., Sriamornsak, P., & Dass, C. R. (2013). Doxorubicin: An update on anticancer molecular action, toxicity and novel drug delivery systems. *The Journal of Pharmacy and Pharmacology, 65*(2), 157–170. doi:10.1111/j.2042-7158.2012.01567.x PMID:23278683

Tai, M. C., Tsang, S. Y., Chang, L. Y., & Xue, H. (2005). Therapeutic potential of wogonin: A naturally occurring flavonoid. *CNS Drug Reviews, 11*(2), 141–150. doi:10.1111/j.1527-3458.2005.tb00266.x PMID:16007236

Takahashi, Y., & Omura, S. (2003). Isolation of new actinomycete strains for the screening of new bioactive compounds. *The Journal of General and Applied Microbiology, 49*(3), 141–154. doi:10.2323/jgam.49.141 PMID:12949697

Taki, M., Tagami, T., Fukushige, K., & Ozeki, T. (2016). Fabrication of nanocomposite particles using a two-solution mixing-type spray nozzle for use in an inhaled curcumin formulation. *International Journal of Pharmaceutics, 511*(1), 104–110. doi:10.1016/j.ijpharm.2016.06.134 PMID:27374204

Talele & Gudsoorkar. (n.d.). Novel approaches for solidification of SEDDS. *Int. J Pharm and Bio., 4*(15), 90-101.

Talele, S. G. (2017). Response Surface Methodology as a Tool for Optimization of self-nanoemulsified Drug Delivery System of Quetiapine Fumarate. *Asian Journal of Pharmaceutics (AJP), 11*(4).

Talele, S. G., & Gudsoorkar, V. R. (2016). Novel approaches for solidification of SMEDDS. *Int J Pharm Biosci, 15*, 90–101.

Tandon, V. R. (2005). Medicinal uses and biological activities of Vitex negundo. *Natural Product Radiance, 4*(3), 162–165.

Tang, D. W., Yu, S. H., Ho, Y. C., Huang, B. Q., Tsai, G. J., Hsieh, H. Y., ... Mi, F. L. (2013). Characterization of tea catechins-loaded nanoparticles prepared from chitosan and an edible polypeptide. *Food Hydrocolloids, 30*(1), 33–41.

Tang, H., Yang, L., Li, W., Li, J., & Chen, J. (2016). Exploring the interaction between Salvia miltiorrhiza and xanthine oxidase: Insights from computational analysis and experimental studies combined with enzyme channel blocking. *RSC Advances, 6*(114), 113527–113537. doi:10.1039/C6RA24396G

Tang, J., Sun, J., Cui, F., Zhang, T., Liu, X., & He, Z. (2008). Self-emulsifying drug delivery systems for improving oral absorption of ginkgo biloba extracts. *Drug Delivery, 15*(8), 477–484. doi:10.1080/10717540802039089 PMID:18720135

Tang, J., Xu, N., Ji, H., Liu, H., Wang, Z., & Wu, L. (2011). Eudragit Nanoparticles containing genistein: Formulation, development and bioavailability assessment. *International Journal of Nanomedicine, 6*, 2429–2435. PMID:22072878

Tangri, P., & Khurana, S. (2011). Niosomes: Formulation and evaluation. *Int J Biopharm, 2*, 47–53.

Tank, D., Gandhi, S., & Shah, M. (2010). Nutraceuticals-portmanteau of science and nature. *IJPSR, 5*(3), 33–38.

Tan, W.-J., Xu, J.-C., Li, L., & Chen, K.-L. (2009). Bioactive compounds of inhibiting xanthine oxidase from Selaginella labordei. *Natural Product Research, 23*(4), 393–398. doi:10.1080/14786410802228736 PMID:19296380

Tanwar, Y. S., Gupta, G. D., & Ramawa, K. G. (2006). *Development and evaluation of microparticles of Gugulipid. The PharmaReview*. Kongposh Publications Pvt., Ltd.

Tarafdar, A., Raliya, R., Wang, W. N., Biswas, P., & Tarafdar, J. C. (2013). Green synthesis of TiO2 Nanoparticle using *Aspergillus tubingensis. Advanced Science, Engineering and Medicine, 5*(9), 1–7. doi:10.1166/asem.2013.1376

Tarun, P., & Soniya. (2013). Ethosomes: A recent vesicle of transdermal drug delivery system. *International Journal of Research and Development in Pharmacy and Life Sciences*, *2*(2), 285–292.

Taylor, L. (2004). *The healing power of rainforest herbs: A Guide to Understanding and Using Herbal Medicinals*. Square One Publishers Inc.

Tennesen, H. H., & Greenhill, J. V. (1992). Studies on curcumin and curcuminoids. XXII: Curcumin as a reducing agent and as a radical scavenger. *International Journal of Pharmaceutics*, *87*(1-3), 79–87. doi:10.1016/0378-5173(92)90230-Y

Tedesco, D., Steidler, S., Galletti, S., Tameni, M., Sonzogni, O., & Ravarotto, L. (2004). Efficacy of silymarin-phospholipid complex in reducing the toxicity of aflatoxin B1 in broiler chicks. *Poultry Science*, *83*(11), 1839–1843. doi:10.1093/ps/83.11.1839 PMID:15554059

Teng, C.-F., Yu, C.-H., Chang, H.-Y., Hsieh, W.-C., Wu, T.-H., Lin, J.-H., Wu, H.-C., Jeng, L.-B., & Su, I.-J. (2019). Chemopreventive effect of phytosomal curcumin on hepatitis b virus-related hepatocellular carcinoma in a transgenic mouse model. *Scientific Reports*, *9*(1), 1–13. doi:10.103841598-019-46891-5 PMID:31316146

Terreno, E., Delli Castelli, D., Cabella, C., Dastrù, W., Sanino, A., Stancanello, J., Tei, L., & Aime, S. (2008). Paramagnetic liposomes as innovative contrast agents for magnetic resonance (MR) molecular imaging applications. *Chemistry & Biodiversity*, *5*(10), 1901–1912. doi:10.1002/cbdv.200890178 PMID:18972531

Thakkar, K. N., Mhatre, S. S., & Parikh, R. Y. (2010). Biological synthesis of metallic nanoparticles. *Nanomedicine; Nanotechnology, Biology, and Medicine*, *6*(2), 257–262. doi:10.1016/j.nano.2009.07.002 PMID:19616126

Thapa, R. K., & Khan, G. M. (2013). Herbal Medicine Incorporated nanoparticles: Advancements in herbal treatment. *Asian Journal of Biomedical and Pharmaceutical Sciences*, *3*(24), 7–14.

Thomas, R. G., Moon, M., Lee, S., & Jeong, Y. Y. (2015). Paclitaxel loaded hyaluronic acid nanoparticles for targeted cancer therapy: In vitro and in vivo analysis. *International Journal of Biological Macromolecules*, *72*, 510–518. doi:10.1016/j.ijbiomac.2014.08.054 PMID:25224289

Thomas, T. R. A., Kavlekar, D. P., & LokaBharathi, P. A. (2010). Marine Drugs from Sponge-Microbe Association–A Review. *Marine Drugs*, *8*(4), 1417–1468. doi:10.3390/md8041417 PMID:20479984

Tian, Q., Wang, W., He, X., Zhu, X., Huang, W., Zhang, C., & Chen, X. (2009). Glycyrrhetinic acid-modified nanoparticles for drug delivery: Preparation and characterization. *Chinese Science Bulletin*, *54*(18), 3121–3126. doi:10.100711434-009-0249-5

Tian, Y., Chen, W., & Ou, J.-J. (2011). Effects of interferon-α/β on HBV replication determined by viral load. *PLoS Pathogens*, *7*(7), e1002159. doi:10.1371/journal.ppat.1002159 PMID:21829354

Tiwari, A., Mishra, M., Nayak, K., Yadav, S., & Shukla, A. (2016). Ethosomes: A novel vesicular carrier system for therapeutic applications. *IOSR Journal of Pharmacy*, *6*(9), 1, 25–33.

Tiwari, R., Kumar, A., & Singh, K. (2019). Nutraceuticals Inspiring the Current Therapy for Lifestyle Diseases. *Advances in Pharmacological Sciences*, 1–5. PMID:30755770

Tong, W., Wang, L., & D'Souza, M. J. (2003). Evaluation of PLGA microspheres as delivery system for antitumor agentcamptothecin. *Drug Development and Industrial Pharmacy*, *29*(7), 745–756. doi:10.1081/ddc-120021774

Touitou, E. (2010). *Terbinafine compositions for onchomycosis treatment*. WPO Patent application WO/2010/086723.

Touitou, E., Dayan, N., Bergelson, L., Godin, B., & Eliaz, M. (2000). Ethosomes-novel vesicular carriers for enhanced delivery: Characterization and skin penetration properties. *Journal of Controlled Release*, *65*(3), 403–418. doi:10.1016/S0168-3659(99)00222-9 PMID:10699298

Tripathy, S., Patel, D., Baro, L., & Nair, S. (2013). A review on phytosomes, their characterization, advancement and potential for transdermal application. *Journal of Drug Delivery and Therapeutics*, *3*(3), 147–152. doi:10.22270/jddt.v3i3.508

Trischman, J. A., Tapiolas, D. M., Jensen, P. R., Dwight, R., McKee, T. C., Ireland, C. M., Stout, T. J., & Clardy, J. (1994). Salinamides A and B: Anti-inflammatory depsipeptides from a marine *Streptomycete*. *Journal of the American Chemical Society*, *116*(2), 757–758. doi:10.1021/ja00081a042

Tseng, C. K. (2001). Algal biotechnology industries and research activities in China. *Journal of Applied Phycology*, *13*(4), 375–380. doi:10.1023/A:1017972812576

Tseng, Y. P., Wu, Y. C., Leu, Y. L., Yeh, S. F., & Chou, C. K. (2010). Scutellariae radix suppresses hepatitis B virus production in human hepatoma cells. *Frontiers in Bioscience (Elite Edition)*, *2*, 1538–1547. PMID:20515825

Tsibakhashvili, N. Y., Kirkesali, E. I., Dodo, T., Pataraya, D. T., & Gurielidze, M. A. (2011). Microbial synthesis of silver nanoparticles by Streptomyces glaucus and Spirulina platensis. *Nanomaterials: Applications and Properties*, *2*, 306–310.

Tung, Y.-T., & Chang, S.-T. (2010). Inhibition of xanthine oxidase by Acacia confusa extracts and their phytochemicals. *Journal of Agricultural and Food Chemistry*, *58*(2), 781–786. doi:10.1021/jf901498q PMID:20047272

Tung, Y.-T., Hsu, C.-A., Chen, C.-S., Yang, S. C., Huang, C.-C., & Chang, S.-T. (2010). Phytochemicals from Acacia confusa heartwood extracts reduce serum uric acid levels in oxonate-induced mice: Their potential use as xanthine oxidase inhibitors. *Journal of Agricultural and Food Chemistry*, *58*(18), 9936–9941. doi:10.1021/jf102689k PMID:20806936

Tzeng, C. W., Yen, F. L., Wu, T. H., Ko, H. H., Lee, C. W., Tzeng, W. S., & Lin, C. C. (2011). Enhancement of dissolution and antioxidant activity of kaempferol using a nanoparticle engineering process. *Journal of Agricultural and Food Chemistry*, *59*(9), 5073–5080.

Uhumwangho, M. U., & Okor, R. S. (2005). Current trends in the production and biomedical applications of liposomes: A review. *Journal of Medicine and Biomedical Research*, *4*(1), 9–21. doi:10.4314/jmbr.v4i1.10663

Ukil, A., Maity, S., Karmakar, S., Datta, N., Vedasiromoni, J. R., & Das, P. K. (2003). Curcumin, the major component of food flavour turmeric, reduces mucosal injury in trinitrobenzene sulphonic acid-induced colitis. *British Journal of Pharmacology*, *139*(2), 209–218. doi:10.1038j.bjp.0705241 PMID:12770926

Umamaheswari, M., Asokkumar, K., Sudalaivelmurugiah, M., Sivashnmugam, A., & Subhadradevi, V. (2009). Hypouricaemic and antioxidant activities of the fractions of Vitex negundo L. leaf extract. *Phytopharmacology and Therapeutic Values V*, 59-70.

Upadhyaya, J., Kesharwani, R. K., & Misra, K. (2009). Metabolism, Pharmacokinetics and Bioavailability of Ascorbic Acid; Synergistic Effect in presence of Tocopherols and Curcumin. *J Comput Intel Bioinform*, *2*(1), 77–84.

Upadhyaya, J., Kesharwani, R. K., & Misra, K. (2009). Metabolism, pharmacokinetics and bioavailability of ascorbic acid; synergistic effect with tocopherols and curcumin. *J Comput Intell Bioinform*, *2*(1), 77–84.

Upadhyaya, Kesharwani, & Misra. (2009). Metabolism, Pharmacokinetics and Bioavailability of Ascorbic Acid; Synergistic Effect in presence of Tocopherols and Curcumin. *Journal of Computational Intelligence in Bioinformatics*, *2*(1), 77–84.

Upadhyay, N., Mandal, S., Bhatia, L., Shailesh, S., & Chauhan, P. (2011). A review on ethosomes: An emerging approach for drug delivery through the skin. *Rec Res Sci Tec*, *3*(7), 19–24.

Vahabi, K., Mansoori, G. A., & Karimi, S. (2011). Biosynthesis of Silver Nanoparticles by Fungus *Trichoderma Reesei. Insciences Journal, 1*, 65–79. doi:10.5640/insc.010165

Vaidya, A. D. B., & Devasagayam, T. P. A. (2007). Recent advances in Indian herbal drug research guest editor: Thomas Paul Asir Devasagayam current status of herbal drugs in India: an overview. Academic Press.

Valenzuela, A., Aspillaga, M., Vial, S., & Guerra, R. (1989). Selectivity of silymarin on the increase of the glutathione content in different tissues of the rat. *Planta Medica, 55*(05), 420–422. doi:10.1055-2006-962056 PMID:2813578

Varde, N., Mehta, N., Thakor, N., Shah, V., & Upadhyay, U. (2012). Phytosomes a potential phospholipid nanoparticulate carrier for the bioavailability enhancement of herbal extracts. *International Journal of Comprehensive Pharmacy, 10*, 1-7.

Varde, N. K., & Pack, D. W. (2004). Microspheres for controlled release drug delivery. *Expert Opinion on Biological Therapy, 4*(1), 35–51. doi:10.1517/14712598.4.1.35

Vasir, J. K., Tambwekar, K., & Garg, S. (2003). Bioadhesive microspheres as a controlled drug delivery system. *International Journal of Pharmaceutics, 255*(1–2), 13–32. doi:10.10160378-5173(03)00087-5

Veeramuthu, D., Raja, W. R. T., Al-Dhabi, N. A., & Savarimuthu, I. (2017). Flavonoids: anticancer properties. *Flavonoids: From Biosynthesis to Human Health, 287.*

Venkatesan, N., Babu, B. S., & Vyas, S. P. (2000). Protected particulate drug carriers for prolonged systemic circulation. *Indian Journal of Pharmaceutical Sciences, 62*, 327–333.

Venkateswaran, P., Millman, I., & Blumberg, B. S. (1987). Effects of an extract from Phyllanthus niruri on hepatitis B and woodchuck hepatitis viruses: In vitro and in vivo studies. *Proceedings of the National Academy of Sciences of the United States of America, 84*(1), 274–278. doi:10.1073/pnas.84.1.274 PMID:3467354

Venugopal, J., Prabhakaran, M. P., Low, S., Choon, A. T., Deepika, G., & Dev, V. R. (2009). Continuous nanostructures for the controlled release of drugs. *Current Pharmaceutical Design, 15*(15), 1799–1808. doi:10.2174/138161209788186344 PMID:19442191

Vergote, G. J., Vervaet, C., Van Driessche, I., Hoste, S., De Smedt, S., Demeester, J., Jain, R. A., Ruddy, S., & Remon, J. P. (2001). An oral controlled release matrix pellet formulation containing nanocrystalline ketoprofen. *International Journal of Pharmaceutics, 219*(1-2), 81–87. doi:10.1016/S0378-5173(01)00628-7 PMID:11337168

Verma, H., & Prasad, S. B. (2013). Herbal drug delivery system: A modern era prospective. *International Journal of Current Pharmaceutical Review and Research, 4*, 88–101.

Verma, H., Prasad, S. B., & Yashwant, S. H. (2013). Herbal drug delivery system: A modern era prospective. *Int J Current Pharma Rev Res, 4*, 88–101.

Verma, M., & Gupta, P. K. (2007). Development of transdermal drug dosage formulation for the anti-rheumatic ayurvedic medicinal plants. *Ancient Science of Life, 11*, 66–69.

Verma, N. K., Crosbie-Staunton, K., Satti, A., Gallagher, S., Ryan, K. B., Doody, T., ... Volkov, Y. (2013). Magnetic core-shell nanoparticles for drug delivery by nebulization. *Journal of Nanobiotechnology, 11*(1), 1.

Verma, P., & Pathak, K. (2010). Therapeutic and cosmeceutical potential of ethosomes: An overview. *Journal of Advanced Pharmaceutical Technology & Research, 1*(3), 274. doi:10.4103/0110-5558.72415 PMID:22247858

Vicentini, F. T., Simi, T. R., Del Ciampo, J. O., Wolga, N. O., Pitol, D. L., Iyomasa, M. M., Bentley, M., & Fonseca, M. J. (2008). Quercetin in w/o microemulsion: In vitro and in vivo skin penetration and efficacy against UVB-induced skin damages evaluated in vivo. *European Journal of Pharmaceutics and Biopharmaceutics*, *69*(3), 948–957. doi:10.1016/j.ejpb.2008.01.012 PMID:18304790

Vidya, C., Hirematha, S., Chandraprabhab, M. N., Antonyraja, M. A. L. & Gopala, I. V. (2013). Green synthesis of ZnO nanoparticles by *Calotropis Gigantea. International Journal of Current Engineering and Technology*, 1.

Vigneshwaran, N., Ashtaputre, N. M., Varadarajan, P. V., Nachane, R. P., Paralikarand, K. M., & Balasubramanya, R. H. (2007). Biological synthesis of silver nanoparticles using the fungus *Aspergillus flavus. Materials Letters*, *61*(6), 1413–1418. doi:10.1016/j.matlet.2006.07.042

Vijayan, V., & Shaik, A. (2013). Formulation and characterization of solid lipid nanoparticles loaded neem oil for topical treatment of acne. *Journal of Acute Disease*, *2*(4), 282–286. doi:10.1016/S2221-6189(13)60144-4

Vijayaraghavan, K., Nalini, S., Prakash, N. U., & Madhankumar, D. (2012). One step green synthesis of silver nano/microparticles using extracts of Trachyspermum ammi and Papaver somniferum. *Colloids and Surfaces. B, Biointerfaces*, *94*, 114–117. doi:10.1016/j.colsurfb.2012.01.026 PMID:22348989

Vivekanandan, K. E., Rajb, K. G., Kumaresana, S., & Pandib, M. (2012). Biosynthesis of silver nanoparticle activity against bacterial strain, cephalexin antibiotic synergistic activity. *International Journal of Current Science*, *4*, 1–7.

Voilley, A., & Etievant, P. (2006). *Flavorin food.* Woodhead Publishing Limited. doi:10.1533/9781845691400

Volkman, J. K. (2003). Sterols in microorganisms. *Applied Microbiology and Biotechnology*, *60*(5), 495–506. doi:10.100700253-002-1172-8 PMID:12536248

Vos, P., Faas, M., Spasojevic, M., & Sikkema, J. (2010). Review: Encapsulation for preservation of functionality and targeted delivery of bioactive food components. *International Dairy Journal*, *20*(4), 292–302. doi:10.1016/j.idairyj.2009.11.008

Vue, B., Zhang, S., & Chen, Q. (2015). Synergistic effects of dietary natural products as anti-prostate cancer agents. *Natural Product Communications*, *10*(12), 2179–2188. doi:10.1177/1934578X1501001241 PMID:26882694

Vyas, A., Saraf, S., & Saraf, S. (2008). Cyclodextrin based novel drug delivery systems. *Journal of Inclusion Phenomena and Macrocyclic Chemistry*, *62*(1-2), 23–42. doi:10.100710847-008-9456-y

Vyas, S. P., & Khar, R. K. (2002). *Targeted and controlled drug delivery novel carrier systems* (1st ed.). CBS Publishers.

Vyas, S., & Khar, R. (2004). Targeted and controlled drug delivery. *CBS Publisher and Distributors, New Delhi India*, *1*, 420–445.

Wadhwa, J., Nair, A., & Kumria, R. (2012). Emulsion forming drug delivery system for lipophilic drugs. *Acta Poloniae Pharmaceutica*, *69*(2), 179–191. PMID:22568032

Waghmare, S. S., Deshmukh, A. M., Kulkarni, S. W., & Oswaldo, L. A. (2011). Biosynthesis and Characterization of Manganese and Zinc Nanoparticles. *Universal Journal of Environmental Research and Technology*, *1*, 64–69.

Waghulde, S., & Naik, P. (2013). Development, recent inventions and evaluation techniques of transdermal drug delivery system—A review. *International Journal of Pharmaceutical and Phytopharmacological Research*, *3*(2), 152–160.

Waghulde, S., & Naik, P. (2017). An overview of therapeutic applications. *Advances in Medical Technologies and Clinical Practice*, •••, 1–25. doi:10.4018/978-1-5225-0751-2.ch001

Wahab, B., & Abd, S. (2012). Ginkgo biloba protects against intermittent hypoxia-induced memory deficits and hippocampal DNA damage in rats. *Phytomedicine*, *19*(5), 444–450. doi:10.1016/j.phymed.2011.11.011 PMID:22265820

Wahyuningsih, S., & Sukandar, E. (2016). In vitro xanthine oxidase inhibitor activity of ethanol extract and fraction roselle calyx (Hibiscus sabdariffa L.). *Int. J. Pharma. Clin. Res.*, *94*, 5–35.

Wahyuningsih, S., Sukandar, E. Y., & Sukrasno, L. D. (2016). Antihyperuricemia activity of the ethanol extract of Roselle calyx and its fraction (Hibiscus sabdariffa Linn) on male wistar rats. *International Journal of Pharmacy and Pharmaceutical Sciences*, *8*, 278–280.

Walve, J. R., & Bakliwal, S. R. (2011). Transfersomes: A surrogated carrier for transdermal drug delivery system. *International Journal of Applied Biology and Pharmaceutical Technology*, *2*(1), 204–213.

Walve, J., Bakliwal, S., Rane, B., & Pawar, S. (2011). Transfersomes: A surrogated carrier for transdermal drug delivery system. *International Journal of Applied Biology and Pharmaceutical Technology*, *2*(1), 204–213.

Wandrey, C., Bartkowiak, A., & Harding, S. (2009). Materials for Encapsulation. In N. J. Zuidam & V. A. Nedovic (Eds.), Encapsulation Technologies for Food Active Ingredients and Food Processing, Springer: Dordrecht (pp. 31–100). Academic Press.

Wang, W. (2008). *Why is a novel drug delivery system important for herbal or ayurvedic medicines*. Retrieved from http://www.articlealley.com/article_673669_17.html

Wang, B. E. (2000). Treatment of chronic liver diseases with traditional Chinese medicine. *Journal of Gastroenterology and Hepatology*, *15*(5 (Suppl.)), E67–E70. doi:10.1046/j.1440-1746.2000.02100.x PMID:10921385

Wang, B.-Q. (2010). Salvia miltiorrhiza: Chemical and pharmacological review of a medicinal plant. *Journal of Medicinal Plants Research*, *4*(25), 2813–2820.

Wang, L., Li, X., Zhang, G., Dong, J., & Eastoe, J. (2007). Oil-in-water nanoemulsions for pesticide formulations. *Journal of Colloid and Interface Science*, *314*(1), 230–235. doi:10.1016/j.jcis.2007.04.079 PMID:17612555

Wang, L., Zhang, D. Z., & Wang, Y. X. (2017). Bioflavonoid fisetin loaded α-tocopherol-poly (lactic acid)-based polymeric micelles for enhanced anticancer efficacy in breast cancers. *Pharmaceutical Research*, *34*(2), 453–461.

Wang, L., Zhang, H., Chen, B., Xia, G., Wang, S., Cheng, J., ... Ren, Y. (2012). Effect of magnetic nanoparticles on apoptosis and cell cycle induced by wogonin in Raji cells. *International Journal of Nanomedicine*, *7*, 789.

Wang, L., Zhu, L., Duan, C., Li, L., & Chen, G. (2020). Total saponin of Dioscorea collettii attenuates MSU crystal-induced inflammation via inhibiting the activation of the NALP3 inflammasome and caspase-1 in THP-1 macrophages. *Molecular Medicine Reports*, *21*(6), 2466–2474. doi:10.3892/mmr.2020.11035 PMID:32236574

Wang, P., Ren, D., Chen, Y., Jiang, M., Wang, R., & Wang, Y.-G. (2015). Effect of sodium alginate addition to resveratrol on acute gouty arthritis. *Cellular Physiology and Biochemistry*, *36*(1), 201–207. doi:10.1159/000374064 PMID:25967960

Wang, S., Yang, C., Liao, J., Zhen, W., Chu, F., & Chang, S. (2008). Essential oil from leaves of Cinnamomum osmophloeum acts as a xanthine oxidase inhibitor and reduces the serum uric acid levels in oxonate-induced mice. *Phytomedicine*, *15*(11), 940–945. doi:10.1016/j.phymed.2008.06.002 PMID:18693097

Wang, T. Y., Li, Q., & Bi, K. S. (2018). Bioactive flavonoids in medicinal plants: Structure, activity and biological fate. *Asian Journal of Pharmaceutical Sciences*, *13*(1), 12–23.

Wang, X., Chen, Y., Dahmani, F. Z., Yin, L., Zhou, J., & Yao, J. (2014). Amphiphilic carboxymethyl chitosan-quercetin conjugate with P-gp inhibitory properties for oral delivery of paclitaxel. *Biomaterials*, *35*(26), 7654–7665. doi:10.1016/j.biomaterials.2014.05.053 PMID:24927684

Wang, X., Jiang, Y., Wang, Y., Huang, M., Ho, C., & Huang, Q. (2008). Enhancing anti inflammation activity of curcumin through o/w nanoemulsions. *Food Chemistry*, *108*(2), 419–424. doi:10.1016/j.foodchem.2007.10.086 PMID:26059118

Wang, Y.-P., Zhao, W., Xue, R., Zhou, Z.-X., Liu, F., Han, Y.-X., ... Chen, H.-S. (2011). Oxymatrine inhibits hepatitis B infection with an advantage of overcoming drug-resistance. *Antiviral Research*, *89*(3), 227–231. doi:10.1016/j.antiviral.2011.01.005 PMID:21277330

Waris, G., Huh, K.-W., & Siddiqui, A. (2001). Mitochondrially associated hepatitis B virus X protein constitutively activates transcription factors STAT-3 and NF-κB via oxidative stress. *Molecular and Cellular Biology*, *21*(22), 7721–7730. doi:10.1128/MCB.21.22.7721-7730.2001 PMID:11604508

War, P. A., Bhang, A. H., & Ale, D. B. (2015). Phytsome as a novel biomedicine: A microencapsulated drug delivery system. *Journal of Bioanalysis & Biomedicine*, *7*(1), 8.

Weissmann, G., Bloomgarden, D., Kaplan, R., Cohen, C., Hoffstein, S., Collins, T., Gotlieb, A., & Nagle, D. (1975). A general method for the introduction of enzymes, by means of immunoglobulin-coated liposomes, into lysosomes of deficient cells. *Proceedings of the National Academy of Sciences of the United States of America*, *72*(1), 88–92. doi:10.1073/pnas.72.1.88 PMID:1054517

Wei, Z.-Q., Zhang, Y.-H., Ke, C.-Z., Chen, H.-X., Ren, P., He, Y.-L., Hu, P., Ma, D.-Q., Luo, J., & Meng, Z.-J. (2017). Curcumin inhibits hepatitis B virus infection by down-regulating cccDNA-bound histone acetylation. *World Journal of Gastroenterology*, *23*(34), 6252. doi:10.3748/wjg.v23.i34.6252 PMID:28974891

Wen, Z., Liu, B., Zheng, Z., You, X., Pu, Y., & Li, Q. (2010). Preparation of liposomes entrapping essential oil from Atractylodes macrocephala Koidz by modified RESS technique. *Chemical Engineering Research & Design*, *88*(8), 1102–1107. doi:10.1016/j.cherd.2010.01.020

Wen, Z., Liu, B., Zheng, Z., You, X., Pu, Y., & Li, Q. (2010). Preparation of Liposomes entrapping essential oil from AtractylodesmacrocephalaKoidz by modified RESS technique. *Chemical Engineering Research & Design*, *88*, 1102–1107.

Winters, M. (2006). Ancient medicine, modern use: Withania somnifera and its potential role in integrative oncology. *Alternative Medicine Review*, *11*, 269–277. PMID:17176166

Wu, P. S., Li, Y. S., Kuo, Y. C., Tsai, S. J. J., & Lin, C. C. (2019). Preparation and Evaluation of Novel Transfersomes Combined with the Natural Antioxidant Resveratrol. *Molecules (Basel, Switzerland)*, *24*(3), 600. doi:10.3390/molecules24030600 PMID:30743989

Wu, S. J., Don, T. M., Lin, C. W., & Mi, F. L. (2014). Delivery of berberine using chitosan/fucoidan-taurine conjugate nanoparticles for treatment of defective intestinal epithelial tight junction barrier. *Marine Drugs*, *12*(11), 5677–5697. doi:10.3390/md12115677 PMID:25421323

Wu, X.-H., Ruan, J.-L., Zhang, J., Wang, S.-Q., & Zhang, Y.-W. (2014). Pallidifloside D, a saponin glycoside constituent from Smilax riparia, resist to hyperuricemia based on URAT1 and GLUT9 in hyperuricemic mice. *Journal of Ethnopharmacology*, *157*, 201–205. doi:10.1016/j.jep.2014.09.034 PMID:25267580

Wu, X.-H., Wang, C.-Z., Wang, S.-Q., Mi, C., He, Y., Zhang, J., Zhang, Y.-W., Anderson, S., & Yuan, C.-S. (2015). Anti-hyperuricemia effects of allopurinol are improved by Smilax riparia, a traditional Chinese herbal medicine. *Journal of Ethnopharmacology*, *162*, 362–368. doi:10.1016/j.jep.2015.01.012 PMID:25617746

Wu, X.-H., Yu, C.-H., Zhang, C.-F., Anderson, S., & Zhang, Y.-W. (2014). Smilax riparia reduces hyperuricemia in mice as a potential treatment of gout. *The American Journal of Chinese Medicine*, *42*(01), 257–259. doi:10.1142/S0192415X14200018 PMID:24467548

Wu, X., Liu, L., Xie, H., Liao, J., Zhou, X., Wan, J., Yu, K., Li, J., & Zhang, Y. (2012). Tanshinone IIA prevents uric acid nephropathy in rats through NF-κB inhibition. *Planta Medica*, *78*(09), 866–873. doi:10.1055-0031-1298487 PMID:22588836

Wu, Y.-H. (2016). Naturally derived anti-hepatitis B virus agents and their mechanism of action. *World Journal of Gastroenterology*, *22*(1), 188. doi:10.3748/wjg.v22.i1.188 PMID:26755870

Wu, Y., Lu, Y., Li, S.-y., Song, Y., Hao, Y., & Wang, Q. (2015). Extract from Phyllanthus urinaria L. inhibits hepatitis B virus replication and expression in hepatitis B virus transfection model in vitro. *Chinese Journal of Integrative Medicine*, *21*(12), 938–943. doi:10.100711655-015-2076-7 PMID:25869593

Xiao, L., Zhang, Y., Jianchen, X. U., & Jin, X. (1994). Preparation of floating rutin-alginate-chitosan microcapsule. *Chinese Traditional and Herbal Drugs*, (2).

Xiao, J., Cao, Y., & Huang, Q. (2017). Edible nanoencapsulation vehicles for oral delivery of phytochemicals: A perspective paper. *Journal of Agricultural and Food Chemistry*, *65*(32), 6727–6735.

Xiao, J., Shen, X., Wu, M., & Lu, R. (2002). Epidemiologic survey on the association between green tea intake and fatty liver disease. *China Public Health*, *18*, 385–387.

Xiao, Y. L., & Li, B. (2002). Chine. *Trad. Herb. Drugs*, *33*, 385–388.

Xiao, Y., Song, Y., Chen, Z., & Ping, Q. (2006). The preparation of silybin–phospholipid complex and the study on its pharmacokinetics in rats. *International Journal of Pharmaceutics*, *37*, 77–82. PMID:16300915

Xiao-Ying, L., Luo, J. B., Yan, Z. H., Rong, H. S., & Huang, W. M. (2006). Preparation and in vitro and in vivo evaluations of topically applied capsaicin transfersomes. *Yao Xue Xue Bao*, *41*(5), 461–466.

Xi, J., Chang, Q., Chan, C. K., Meng, Z. Y., Wang, G. N., Sun, J. B., Wang, Y. T., Tong, H. H. Y., & Zheng, Y. (2009). Formulation development and bioavailability evaluation of a self-nanoemulsified drug delivery system of oleanolic acid. *AAPS PharmSciTech*, *10*(1), 172–182. doi:10.120812249-009-9190-9 PMID:19224372

Xi, J., & Guo, R. (2007). Interactions between flavonoids and hemoglobin in lecithin liposomes. *International Journal of Biological Macromolecules*, *40*(4), 305–311. doi:10.1016/j.ijbiomac.2006.08.011 PMID:16997370

Xiong, L. (1993). Therapeutic effect of combined therapy of Salvia miltiorrhizae and Polyporus umbellatus polysaccharide in the treatment of chronic hepatitis B. *Zhongguo Zhong xi yi jie he za zhi Zhongguo Zhongxiyi jiehe zazhi= Chinese journal of integrated traditional and Western medicine*, *13*(9), 533.

Xiong, H., Qi, S., Xu, Y., Li, M., & Qian, P.-Y. (2009). Antibiotic and antifouling compound production by the marine-derived fungus *Cladosporium* sp. F14. *J. Hydro-. Environmental Research*, *2*, 264–270.

Xue, B., He, D., Gao, S., Wang, D., Yokoyama, K., & Wang, L. (2016). Biosynthesis of silver nanoparticles by the fungus Arthroderma fulvum and its antifungal activity against genera of Candida, Aspergillus and Fusarium. *International Journal of Nanomedicine*, *11*, 1899–1906. PMID:27217752

Xu, H., Fang, Q., Wang, J., & Wang, P. (2008). Study on preparation of paclitaxel loaded PEG-PLGA nanoparticles in vitro experiment. *China Hospital Pharmacy Journal*, *28*, 11–14.

Xu, X., & Burgess, D. J. (2011). Liposomes as carriers for controlled drug delivery. *Advances in Delivery Science and Technology*, *3*, 195–220.

Xu, Y. Q., Chen, W. R., Tsosie, J. K., Xie, X., Li, P., Wan, J. B., He, C.-W., & Chen, M. W. (2016). Niosome encapsulation of curcumin: Characterization and cytotoxic effect on ovarian cancer cells. *Journal of Nanomaterials, 2016*, 2016. doi:10.1155/2016/6365295

Xu, Y., He, H., Schulz, S., Liu, X., Fusetani, N., Xiong, H., Xiao, X., & Qian, P. Y. (2010). Potent antifouling compounds produced by marine *Streptomyces. Bioresource Technology, 101*(4), 1331–1336. doi:10.1016/j.biortech.2009.09.046 PMID:19818601

Yadav, D., & Suri, S. (2011). Novel Approach: Herbal Remedies And Natural Products In Pharmaceutical Science As Nano Drug Delivery Systems. *IJPT, 3*(3), 3092–3116.

Yadav, D., Suri, S., Choudhary, A. A., Sikender, M., Hemant, K., & Beg, N. M. (2011). Novel approach: Herbal remedies and natural products in pharmaceutical science as nano drug delivery systems. *Int J Pharmtech, 3*, 3092–3116.

Yadav, D., Suri, S., Choudhary, A., Sikender, M., & Hemant, N. (2011). Novel approach: Herbal remedies and natural products in pharmaceutical science as nano drug delivery systems. *Int J Pharm Tech, 3*, 3092–3116.

Yadav, M., Bhatia, V., Doshi, G., & Shastri, K. (2014). Novel techniques in herbal drug delivery systems. *International Journal of Pharmaceutical Sciences Review and Research, 28*(2), 83–89.

Yaddalapudi, S., Palla, G., & Krishnaiah, D. (2015). Solid lipid Nanoparticles. *J Compr Phar, 2*(4), 128–144. doi:10.37483/JCP.2015.2404

Yadev, D., Suri, S., Choudhary, A. A., & Sikender, M., & Heman, B. M. N. (2011). Novel approach, herbal remedies and natural products in pharmaceutical science as nano drug delivery systems. *International Journal of Pharm Tech Research, 3*(3), 3092–3116.

Yallapu, M., Ebeling, M., Khan, S., Sundram, V., Chauhan, N., Gupta, B., Puumala, S., Jaggi, M., & Chauhan, S. (2013). Novel curcumin-loaded magnetic nanoparticles for or pancreatic cancer treatment. *NIH Public Access, 12*(8), 1471–1480. doi:10.1158/1535-7163.MCT-12-1227 PMID:23704793

Yang, H., Gao, L., Niu, Y., Zhou, Y., Lin, H., Jiang, J., Kong, X., Liu, X., & Li, L. (2015). Mangiferin inhibits renal urate reabsorption by modulating urate transporters in experimental hyperuricemia. *Biological & Pharmaceutical Bulletin, 38*(10), b15–b00402. doi:10.1248/bpb.b15-00402 PMID:26228630

Yang, H., Zhou, Z., He, L., Ma, H., Qu, W., Yin, J., Jia, M., Zhao, X., Shan, J., & Gao, Y. (2018). Hepatoprotective and inhibiting HBV effects of polysaccharides from roots of Sophora flavescens. *International Journal of Biological Macromolecules, 108*, 744–752. doi:10.1016/j.ijbiomac.2017.10.171 PMID:29111266

Yang, K., Lin, L., Tseng, T., Wang, S., & Tsai, T. (2007). Oral bioavailability of curcumin in rat and the herbal analysis from Curcuma longa by LC-MS/MS. *Journal of Chromatography. B, Analytical Technologies in the Biomedical and Life Sciences, 853*(1-2), 183–189. doi:10.1016/j.jchromb.2007.03.010 PMID:17400527

Yang, Q.-B., He, Y.-L., Zhong, X.-W., Xie, W.-G., & Zhou, J.-G. (2019). Resveratrol ameliorates gouty inflammation via upregulation of sirtuin 1 to promote autophagy in gout patients. *Inflammopharmacology, 27*(1), 47–56. doi:10.100710787-018-00555-4 PMID:30600470

Yang, S., Kim, H., Lefeber, A., Erkelens, C., Angelova, N., Choi, Y., & Verpoorte, R. (2006). Application of two-dimensional nuclear magnetic resonance spectroscopy to quality control of ginseng commercial products. *Planta Medica, 72*(4), 364–369. doi:10.1055-2005-916240 PMID:16557479

Yang, T., Cui, F. D., Choi, M. K., Lin, H., Chung, S. J., Shim, C. K., & Kim, D. D. (2007). Liposome formulation of paclitaxel with enhanced solubility and stability. *Drug Delivery, 14*(5), 301–308. doi:10.1080/10717540601098799

Yan, J., Zhang, G., Hu, Y., & Ma, Y. (2013). Effect of luteolin on xanthine oxidase: Inhibition kinetics and interaction mechanism merging with docking simulation. *Food Chemistry*, *141*(4), 3766–3773. doi:10.1016/j.foodchem.2013.06.092 PMID:23993547

Yan, Z., Yuhui, W., Huanxiang, L., Guoqiang, Z., & Xinan, W. (2010). Preparation and In vitro Evaluation of EthosomalTotal Alkaloids of Sophoraalopecuroides loaded by Transmembrane pH-Gradient Method. *AAPS PharmSciTech*, *1*, 1–9.

Yao, H., Lu, H., Zhang, J., Xue, X., Yin, C., Hu, J., ... Xu, H. (2019). Preparation of Prolonged-Circulating Galangin-Loaded Liposomes and Evaluation of Antitumor Efficacy In Vitro and Pharmacokinetics In Vivo. *Journal of Nanomaterials*.

Yari, A., & Rashnoo, S. (2017). Optimization of a new method for extraction of cyanidin chloride and pelargonidin chloride anthocyanins with magnetic solid phase extraction and determination in fruit samples by HPLC with central composite design. *Journal of Chromatography. B, Analytical Technologies in the Biomedical and Life Sciences*, *1067*, 38–44.

Yarnell, E., & Abascal, K. (2010). Herbal medicine for viral hepatitis. *Alternative and Complementary Therapies*, *16*(3), 151–157. doi:10.1089/act.2010.16308

Yasam, V. R., Jakki, S. L., Natarajan, J., & Kuppusamy, G. (2014). A review on novel vesicular drug delivery. *Proniosomes. Drug Deliv*, *21*, 243–249.

Ye, G., Zhu, H. Y., Li, Z. X., Ma, C. H., Fan, M. S., Sun, Z. L., & Huang, C. G. (2007). LC-MS characterization of efficacy substances in serum of experimental animals treated with Sophora flavescens extracts. *Biomedical Chromatography*, *21*(6), 655–660. doi:10.1002/bmc.805 PMID:17370298

Yen, F. L., Wu, T. H., Lin, L. T., Cham, T. M., & Lin, C. C. (2008). Nanoparticles formulation of Cuscuta chinensis prevents acetaminophen-induced hepatotoxicity in rats. *Food and Chemical Toxicology*, *46*(5), 1771–1777. doi:10.1016/j.fct.2008.01.021 PMID:18308443

Yin, Y., Cui, F., Mu, C., Choi, M., Kim, J., Chung, S., Shim, C., & Kim, D. (2009). Docetaxel microemulsion for enhanced oral bioavailability: Preparation and in vitro and in vivo evaluation. *Journal of Controlled Release*, *140*(2), 86–94. doi:10.1016/j.jconrel.2009.08.015 PMID:19709639

Yi, Z., Sun, Z., Chen, G., Zhang, H., Ma, X., Su, W., ... Li, X. (2018). Size-controlled, colloidally stable and functional nanoparticles based on the molecular assembly of green tea polyphenols and keratins for cancer therapy. *Journal of Materials Chemistry. B, Materials for Biology and Medicine*, *6*(9), 1373–1386.

Yoo, J. H., Shanmugam, S., Thapa, P., Lee, E. S., Balakrishnan, P., Baskaran, R., Yoon, S.-K., Choi, H.-G., Yong, C. S., Yoo, B. K., & Han, K. (2010). Novel self-nanoemulsifying drug delivery system for enhanced solubility and dissolution of lutein. *Archives of Pharmacal Research*, *33*(3), 417–426. doi:10.100712272-010-0311-5 PMID:20361307

You, J., Cui, F., Han, X., Wang, Y., Yang, L., Yu, Y., & Li, Q. (2006). Study of the preparation of sustained-release microspheres containing zedoary turmeric oil by the emulsion-solvent-diffusion method and evaluation of the self-emulsification and bioavailability of the oil colloids. *Surf B*, *48*(1), 35–41. doi:10.1016/j.colsurfb.2005.12.011 PMID:16480856

Yu, A. H., & Zhai, G. X. (2006). Preparation and quality evaluation of puerarin microemulsion. *Chinese Journal of Pharmaceuticals*, *7*, 471-473.

Yuan, D. F., & Yi, Y. M. (2003). Her. *El Medico*, *22*, 113–114.

Yukuyama, M. N., Ghisleni, D. D. M., Pinto, T. D. J. A., & Bou-Chacra, N. A. (2016). Nanoemulsion: Process selection and application in cosmetics–a review. *International Journal of Cosmetic Science*, *38*(1), 13–24. doi:10.1111/ics.12260 PMID:26171789

Yumita, A., Suganda, A. G., & Sukandar, E. Y. (2013). Xanthine oxidase inhibitory activity of some Indonesian medicinal plants and active fraction of selected plants. *International Journal of Pharmacy and Pharmaceutical Sciences*, *5*, 293–296.

Zacharakis, G., Koskinas, J., Kotsiou, S., Papoutselis, M., Tzara, F., Vafeiadis, N., Archimandritis, A. J., & Papoutselis, K. (2005). Natural history of chronic HBV infection: A cohort study with up to 12 years follow-up in North Greece (part of the Interreg I-II/EC-project). *Journal of Medical Virology*, *77*(2), 173–179. doi:10.1002/jmv.20434 PMID:16121378

Zare, B., Babaie, S., Setayesh, N., & Shahverdi, A. R. (2013). Isolation and characterization of a fungus for extracellular synthesis of small selenium nanoparticles. *Nanomedicine Journal*, *1*, 13–19.

Zarse, K., Jabin, S., & Ristow, M. L. (2012). Theanine extends lifespan of adult Caenorhabditis elegans. *European Journal of Nutrition*, *51*(6), 765–768. doi:10.100700394-012-0341-5 PMID:22422488

Zaveri, N. T. (2006). Green tea and its polyphenolic catechins: Medicinal uses in cancer and non-cancer applications. *Life Sciences*, *78*(18), 2073–2080. doi:10.1016/j.lfs.2005.12.006 PMID:16445946

Zeeb, B., Saberi, A., Weiss, J., & McClements, D. (2015). Formation and characterization of filled hydrogel beads based on calcium alginate: Factors influencing nanoemulsion retention and release. *Food Hydrocolloids*, *50*, 27–36. doi:10.1016/j.foodhyd.2015.02.041

Zeisser-Labouèbe, M., Lange, N., Gurny, R., & Delie, F. (2006). Hypericin-loaded nanoparticles for the photodynamic treatment of ovarian cancer. *International Journal of Pharmaceutics*, *326*(1–2), 174–181. doi:10.1016/j.ijpharm.2006.07.012

Zeng, F., & Zimmerman, S. C. (1997). Dendrimers in Supramolecular Chemistry: From Molecular Recognition to Self-Assembly. *Chemical Reviews*, *97*(5), 1681–1712. doi:10.1021/cr9603892

Zhai, Y., Guo, S., Liu, C., Yang, C., Dou, J., Li, L., & Zhai, G. (2013). Preparation and in vitro evaluation of apigenin-loaded polymeric micelles. *Colloids and Surfaces. A, Physicochemical and Engineering Aspects*, *429*, 24–30.

Zhang, D., & Guan, L. I. (2008). *Preparation and characterization of biodegradable polylactide (PLA) microspheres encapsulating ginsenoside Rg3, 24*. Chem Res. Chin. University.

Zhang, Y. (1994). Advances in research on target-oriented drug delivery system of Chinese materia medica. *Chinese Traditional and Herbal Drugs*, (5).

Zhang, C., Wang, R., Zhang, G., & Gong, D. (2018). Mechanistic insights into the inhibition of quercetin on xanthine oxidase. *International Journal of Biological Macromolecules*, *112*, 405–412. doi:10.1016/j.ijbiomac.2018.01.190 PMID:29410028

Zhang, D., Yang, X., Kang, J. S., Choi, H. D., & Son, B. W. (2008). Chlorohydroaspyrones A and B, antibacterial aspyrone derivatives from the marine-derived fungus *Exophiala* sp. *Journal of Natural Products*, *71*(8), 1458–1460. doi:10.1021/np800107c PMID:18661951

Zhang, G., & Zhang, J. (2018). Enhanced oral bioavailability of EGCG using pH-sensitive polymeric nanoparticles: Characterization and in vivo investigation on nephrotic syndrome rats. *Drug Design, Development and Therapy*, *12*, 2509.

Zhang, H., Cui, Y., Zhu, S., Feng, F., & Zheng, X. (2010). Characterization and antimicrobial activity of a pharmaceutical microemulsion. *International Journal of Pharmaceutics*, *395*(1-2), 154–160. doi:10.1016/j.ijpharm.2010.05.022 PMID:20580790

Zhang, H., Li, C., Kwok, S.-T., Zhang, Q.-W., & Chan, S.-W. (2013). A review of the pharmacological effects of the dried root of Polygonum cuspidatum (Hu Zhang) and its constituents. *Evidence-Based Complementary and Alternative Medicine*. PMID:24194779

Zhang, H., Yu, C.-H., Jiang, Y.-P., Peng, C., He, K., Tang, J.-Y., & Xin, H.-L. (2012). Protective effects of polydatin from Polygonum cuspidatum against carbon tetrachloride-induced liver injury in mice. *PLoS One*, *7*(9), e46574. doi:10.1371/journal.pone.0046574 PMID:23029551

Zhang, J., Hou, S., & Liu, H. (2007). Comparison of preparing two polylactide nanoparticles loaded lipophilic anti-cancer herb drug by nanoprecipitation method. *Zhongguo Zhongyao Zazhi*, *32*, 303–306. PMID:17455462

Zhang, J., Peng, Q., Shi, S., Zhang, Q., Sun, X., Gong, T., & Zhang, Z. (2011). Preparation, characterization, and in vivo evaluation of a self-nanoemulsifying drug delivery system (SNEDDS) loaded with morin-phospholipid complex. *International Journal of Nanomedicine*, *6*, 3405. PMID:22267925

Zhang, J., Tang, Q., Xu, X., & Li, N. (2013). Development and evaluation of a novel phytosome-loaded chitosan microsphere system for curcumin delivery. *International Journal of Pharmaceutics*, *448*(1), 168–174. doi:10.1016/j.ijpharm.2013.03.021

Zhang, L., Pornpattananangkul, D., Hu, C. M., & Huang, C. M. (2010). Development of nanoparticles for antimicrobial drug delivery. *Current Medicinal Chemistry*, *17*(6), 585–594. doi:10.2174/092986710790416290 PMID:20015030

Zhang, L., Wang, G., Hou, W., Li, P., Dulin, A., & Bonkovsky, H. L. (2010). Contemporary clinical research of traditional Chinese medicines for chronic hepatitis B in China: An analytical review. *Hepatology (Baltimore, Md.)*, *51*(2), 690–698. doi:10.1002/hep.23384 PMID:20101751

Zhang, L., Zhu, W., Yang, C., Guo, H., Yu, A., Ji, J., ... Zhai, G. (2012). A novel folate-modified self-microemulsifying drug delivery system of curcumin for colon targeting. *International Journal of Nanomedicine*, *7*, 151. PMID:22275831

Zhang, S., Wang, J., & Pan, J. (2016). Baicalin-loaded PEGylated lipid nanoparticles: Characterization, pharmacokinetics, and protective effects on acute myocardial ischemia in rats. *Drug Delivery*, *23*(9), 3696–3703.

Zhang, Y. Y., & Hu, K. Q. (2015). Rethinking the pathogenesis of hepatitis B virus (HBV) infection. *Journal of Medical Virology*, *87*(12), 1989–1999. doi:10.1002/jmv.24270 PMID:25989114

Zhang, Y.-B., Luo, D., Yang, L., Cheng, W., He, L.-J., Kuang, G.-K., Li, M.-M., Li, Y.-L., & Wang, G.-C. (2018). Matrine-type alkaloids from the roots of Sophora flavescens and their antiviral activities against the hepatitis B virus. *Journal of Natural Products*, *81*(10), 2259–2265. doi:10.1021/acs.jnatprod.8b00576 PMID:30298740

Zhang, Y.-B., Zhan, L.-Q., Li, G.-Q., Wang, F., Wang, Y., Li, Y.-L., Ye, W.-C., & Wang, G.-C. (2016). Dimeric matrine-type alkaloids from the roots of Sophora flavescens and their anti-hepatitis B virus activities. *The Journal of Organic Chemistry*, *81*(15), 6273–6280. doi:10.1021/acs.joc.6b00804 PMID:27352066

Zhang, Y., Xia, Q., Li, Y., He, Z., Li, Z., Guo, T., Wu, Z., & Feng, N. (2019). CD44 Assists the Topical Anti-Psoriatic Efficacy of Curcumin-Loaded Hyaluronan-Modified Ethosomes: A New Strategy for Clustering Drug in Inflammatory Skin. *Theranostics*, *9*(1), 48–64. doi:10.7150/thno.29715 PMID:30662553

Zhang, Z., Huang, Y., Gao, F., Gao, Z., Bu, H., Gu, W., & Li, Y. (2011). A self-assembled nanodelivery system enhances the oral bioavailability of daidzein: In vitro characteristics and in vivo performance. *Nanomedicine (London)*, *6*(8), 1365–1379.

Zhang, Z., Zhang, R., Zou, L., Chen, L., Ahmed, Y., Bisri, W., Balamash, K., & McClements, D. (2016). Encapsulation of curcumin in polysaccharide-based hydrogel beads: Impact of bead type on lipid digestion and curcum in bioaccesibility. *Food Hydrocolloids*, *58*, 160–170. doi:10.1016/j.foodhyd.2016.02.036

Zhao, H. R., Wang, K., Zhao, Y., & Pan, L. Q. (2002). Novel sustained-release implant of herb extract using chitosan. *Biomaterials*, *23*, 4459–4462.

Zhao, H., Wang, K., Zhao, Y., & Pan, L. (2002). Novel sustained release implant of herbal extract using chitosan. *Biomaterials, 23*(23), 4459–4462. doi:10.1016/S0142-9612(02)00162-X PMID:12322964

Zhao, P., Chen, K., Zhang, G., Deng, G., & Li, J. (2017). Pharmacological basis for use of Selaginella moellendorffii in gouty arthritis: Antihyperuricemic, anti-inflammatory, and xanthine oxidase inhibition. *Evidence-Based Complementary and Alternative Medicine, 2017*, 2017. doi:10.1155/2017/2103254 PMID:28250791

Zhao, Q., Chen, X.-Y., & Martin, C. (2016). Scutellaria baicalensis, the golden herb from the garden of Chinese medicinal plants. *Science Bulletin, 61*(18), 1391–1398. doi:10.100711434-016-1136-5 PMID:27730005

Zhao, T., Tang, H., Xie, L., Zheng, Y., Ma, Z., Sun, Q., & Li, X. (2019). Scutellaria baicalensis Georgi.(Lamiaceae): A review of its traditional uses, botany, phytochemistry, pharmacology and toxicology. *The Journal of Pharmacy and Pharmacology, 71*(9), 1353–1369. doi:10.1111/jphp.13129 PMID:31236960

Zhaowu, Z., Xiaoli, W., Yangde, Z., & Nianfeng, L. (2009). Preparation of matrine ethosome, its percutaneous permeation in vitro and anti-inflammatory activity in vivo in rats. *Journal of Liposome Research, 19*(2), 155–162. doi:10.1080/08982100902722381

Zhao, Y., Geng, C.-A., Chen, H., Ma, Y.-B., Huang, X.-Y., Cao, T.-W., He, K., Wang, H., Zhang, X.-M., & Chen, J.-J. (2015). Isolation, synthesis and anti-hepatitis B virus evaluation of p-hydroxyacetophenone derivatives from Artemisia capillaris. *Bioorganic & Medicinal Chemistry Letters, 25*(7), 1509–1514. doi:10.1016/j.bmcl.2015.02.024 PMID:25737008

Zhao, Y., Geng, C.-A., Ma, Y.-B., Huang, X.-Y., Chen, H., Cao, T.-W., He, K., Wang, H., Zhang, X.-M., & Chen, J.-J. (2014). UFLC/MS-IT-TOF guided isolation of anti-HBV active chlorogenic acid analogues from Artemisia capillaris as a traditional Chinese herb for the treatment of hepatitis. *Journal of Ethnopharmacology, 156*, 147–154. doi:10.1016/j.jep.2014.08.043 PMID:25219603

Zhao, Y., Geng, C.-A., Sun, C.-L., Ma, Y.-B., Huang, X.-Y., Cao, T.-W., He, K., Wang, H., Zhang, X.-M., & Chen, J.-J. (2014). Polyacetylenes and anti-hepatitis B virus active constituents from Artemisia capillaris. *Fitoterapia, 95*, 187–193. doi:10.1016/j.fitote.2014.03.017 PMID:24685503

Zhao, Y., Wang, C., Chow, A. H., Ren, K., Gong, T., Zhang, Z., & Zheng, Y. (2010). Self-nanoemulsifying drug delivery system (SNEDDS) for oral delivery of Zedoary essential oil: Formulation and bioavailability studies. *International Journal of Pharmaceutics, 383*(1-2), 170–177. doi:10.1016/j.ijpharm.2009.08.035 PMID:19732813

Zheng, G., Zheng, M., Yang, B., Fu, H., & Li, Y. (2019). Improving breast cancer therapy using doxorubicin loaded solid lipid nanoparticles: Synthesis of a novel arginine-glycine-aspartic tripeptide conjugated, pH sensitive lipid and evaluation of the nanomedicine in vitro and in vivo. *Biomedicine and Pharmacotherapy, 116.*

Zheng, L., Han, X., Chen, H., Lin, W., & Yan, X. (2005). Marine bacteria associated with marine macro-organisms: The potential antimicrobial resources. *Annals of Microbiology, 55*, 119–124.

Zheng, Y., Hou, S. X., Chen, T., & Lu, Y. (2006). Preparation and characterization of transfersomes of three drugs in vitro. Zhongguo Zhong yao za zhi, Zhongguo zhongyao zazhi. *Zhongguo Zhongyao Zazhi, 31*(9), 728–731. PMID:17048677

Zheng, Y., Hou, S., Chen, T., & Lu, Y. (2006). Preparation and characterization of transfersomes of three drugs *in vitro. Zhongguo Zhongyao Zazhi, 31*, 728–731. PMID:17048677

Zhigaltsev, I. V., Maurer, N., Akhong, Q. F., Leone, R., Leng, E., Wang, J., ... Cullis, P. R. (2005). Liposome-encapsulated vincristine, vinblastine and vinorelbine: A comparative study of drug loading and retention. *Journal of Controlled Release, 104*(1), 103–111. doi:10.1016/j.jconrel.2005.01.010

Zhiguo, P., Yanpei, W., & Peizheng, G. (1999). Observation on Effects of Combined Treatment of Chinese Toad Bufotoxin and Salvia Miltiorrhiza in Patients Suffering from Chronic Hepatitis B. *Modern Diagnosis & Treatment, 3*.

Zhong, H., Deng, Y., Wang, X., & Yang, B. (2005). Multivesicular liposome formulation for the sustained delivery of breviscapine. *International Journal of Pharmaceutics*, *301*(1-2), 15–24. doi:10.1016/j.ijpharm.2005.04.001 PMID:16023316

Zhong, L., Hu, J., Shu, W., Gao, B., & Xiong, S. (2015). Epigallocatechin-3-gallate opposes HBV-induced incomplete autophagy by enhancing lysosomal acidification, which is unfavorable for HBV replication. *Cell Death & Disease*, *6*(5), e1770–e1770. doi:10.1038/cddis.2015.136 PMID:25996297

Zhou, L., Chow, M., & Zhou, Z. (2006). Improved quality control method for Danshen products – consideration of both hydrophilic and lipophilic active componenets. *Journal of Pharmaceutical and Biomedical Analysis*, *41*(3), 744–750. doi:10.1016/j.jpba.2005.12.032 PMID:16458472

Zhou, Y., Wei, Y. H., Zhang, G. Q., & Wu, X. A. (2010). Synergistic penetration of ethosomes and lipophilic prodrug on the transdermal delivery of acyclovir. *Archives of Pharmacal Research*, *33*(4), 567–574. doi:10.100712272-010-0411-2 PMID:20422366

Zhou, Y., Wei, Y., Liu, H., Zhang, G., & Wu, X. A. (2010). Preparation and in vitro evaluation of ethosomal total alkaloids of Sophora alopecuroides loaded by a transmembrane pH-gradient method. *AAPS PharmSciTech*, *11*(3), 1350–1358. doi:10.120812249-010-9509-6 PMID:20740333

Zhou, Z., Zhang, Y., Ding, X.-R., Chen, S.-H., Yang, J., Wang, X.-J., Jia, G.-L., Chen, H.-S., Bo, X.-C., & Wang, S.-Q. (2007). Protocatechuic aldehyde inhibits hepatitis B virus replication both in vitro and in vivo. *Antiviral Research*, *74*(1), 59–64. doi:10.1016/j.antiviral.2006.12.005 PMID:17298850

Zhu, C., Xu, Y., Liu, Z.-H., Wan, X.-C., Li, D.-X., & Tai, L.-L. (2018). The anti-hyperuricemic effect of epigallocatechin-3-gallate (EGCG) on hyperuricemic mice. *Biomedicine and Pharmacotherapy*, *97*, 168–173. doi:10.1016/j.biopha.2017.10.013 PMID:29091862

Zhu, J. X., Wang, Y., Kong, L. D., Yang, C., & Zhang, X. (2004). Effects of Biota orientalis extract and its flavonoid constituents, quercetin and rutin on serum uric acid levels in oxonate-induced mice and xanthine dehydrogenase and xanthine oxidase activities in mouse liver. *Journal of Ethnopharmacology*, *93*(1), 133–140. doi:10.1016/j.jep.2004.03.037 PMID:15182918

Zou, S., Carey, J., Liedo, P., Ingram, D., Yu, B., & Ghaedian, R. (2010). Prolongevity effects of an oregano and cranberry extract are diet dependent in the Mexican fruit fly (Anastrephaludens). *Journal of Gerontology*, *65*, 41–50. PMID:19906819

Zou, S., Carey, J., Liedo, P., Ingram, D., Yu, B., & Ghaedian, R. (2012). Prolongevity effects of a botanical with oregano and cranberry extracts in Mexican fruit flies: Examining interactions of diet restriction and age. *Age Jordor*, *34*(2), 269–279. doi:10.100711357-011-9230-8 PMID:21455602

Zuidam, N., & Heinrich, J. (2009). Encapsulation of aroma. In N. Zuidam & V. Nedovic (Eds.), Encapsulation technologies for food active ingredients and food processing; Springer: Dordrecht (pp. 127–160). Academic Press.

About the Contributors

Rajesh Kumar Kesharwani, PhD, has more than 10 years of research and 10years of teaching experience in various institutes of India, imparting bioinformatics and biotechnology education. He has received several awards, including the NASI-Swarna Jayanti Puruskar by The National Academy of Sciences of India. He has supervised 01 Ph.D., and more than 20 UG, PG students for their research work, has authored over 43 peer reviewed articles, 20 book chapters and 12 edited Books with international publishers. He has been a member of many scientific communities as well as a reviewer for many international journals. He has presented many papers in various national and international seminars/ conferences. Dr. Kesharwani received his Ph.D. from the Indian Institute of Information Technology, Allahabad and worked at NIT Warangal for two-semester. He has been a recipient of Ministry of Human Resource recipient of Development (India) Fellowship and Senior Research Fellowship from the Indian Council of Medical Research, India. His research fields of interest are Medical Informatics, Protein Structure and Function Prediction, Computer-Aided Drug Designing, Structural Biology, Drug Delivery, Cancer Biology, Nano-Biotechnology and Biomedical Sciences.

Raj K. Keservani, MPharm, Faculty of B. Pharmacy, CSM Group of Institutions, Allahabad, India. He has more than 10 years of academic experience from various institutes of India in pharmaceutical education. He has published 30 peer-reviewed papers in the field of pharmaceutical sciences in national and international journals, thirty book chapters, 2 co-authored books, and 15 edited books. He is also active as a reviewer for several international scientific journals. Mr. Keservani graduated with a pharmacy degree from the Department of Pharmacy, Kumaun University, Nainital (UA), India. He received his Master of Pharmacy (MPharm) (specialization in pharmaceutics) from the School of Pharmaceutical Sciences, Rajiv Gandhi Proudyogiki Vishwavidyalaya, Bhopal, India. His research interests include nutraceutical and functional foods, novel drug delivery systems (NDDS), transdermal drug delivery/ drug delivery, health science, cancer biology, and neurobiology.

Anil K. Sharma is an expert in the area of pharmaceutics with a background in drug delivery. He has taught these subjects for nearly 10 years at universities such as the Delhi Institute of Pharmaceutical Sciences and Research, University of Delhi, and School of Medical and Allied Sciences, G D Goenka University. Prior to taking up the current role in 2018, Anil Kumar Sharma served in academic position such as Lecturer (Pharmaceutics), Delhi Institute of Pharmaceutical Sciences and Research, University of Delhi. Anil Kumar Sharma holds a PhD (Pharmaceutical Sciences) from the University of Delhi; M. Pharmacy (Pharmaceutics) from the Rajiv Gandhi Proudyogiki Vishwavidyalaya; and B. Pharmacy from the University of Rajasthan.

* * *

Eknath D. Ahire, Assistant Professor in the Department of Pharmaceutics at Shrishakti Shaikshanik Sanstha's, Divine college of Pharmacy, Satana, Nashik (Savitribai Phule Pune University, Pune). He has obtained his graduation (B. Pharm) degree from Savitribai Phule Pune University in 2016. He obtained his master's degree (M. S. Pharm) in Pharmaceutics in 2018 from National Institute of Pharmaceutical Education and Research-Ahmedabad (NIPER-A) with 2 years of research work.

Mohammad Irfan Ali, Assistant Professor, School of Applied Sciences, Suresh Gyan Vihar University Jaipur, Rajasthan, India. He has more than ten years of teaching and research experience in various national organizations and authored nine research papers in various national and international peer-review referral journals.

Akshada Atul Bakliwal is working as Asst. professor in dept. of pharmaceutics at Sandip Institute of Pharmaceutical Sciences, Mahiravani, Nashik since last 2 years. she has completed her M. Pharmacy (Pharmaceutics) at SPPU, Pune university and have more than 5 research and review articles on her credit.

Anamika Basu is currently working as the HOD and Lecturer in Dept. of Biochemistry, Gurudas College (Affiliated to University of Calcutta, India) in Kolkata. She received her M.Sc. degree in Biochemistry from Kalyani University and M. Tech in Biotechnology from Jadavpur University. She has completed her PhD on Computational biology from Jadavpur University. She has 16 years of teaching experience and 11 years of research experience. She teaches Immunology, Molecular biology, Cell Biology and Clinical Biochemistry in graduate and Bioinformatics in post-graduate level. She is a co-author of seven book chapters and several journal papers and conference papers. Her research interest includes Computational Biology, Bioinformatics, Molecular modeling, Molecular docking, Molecular Biology and Plant Biology.

Mounika Bharath is currently a Research Scholar at Department of Pharmaceutics, Shri D. D. Vispute, College of Pharmacy & Research Center, New Panvel affiliated to University of Mumbai. Her area of research interest is formulation development and evaluation of various microparticulate and vesicles based gel systems.

Arvind K. Singh Chandel has completed his Ph.D. from CSIR CSMCRI Bhavnagar Gujarat. He completed his M.S. Pharm from NIPER Hajipur. His research area of interest are interdisciplinary Pharmaceutical Biotechnology and Drug delivery system, Biopolymers for biomedical applications. He has published more than 20 international peer reviews research articles, several patents, and more than ten book chapters in various renowned publications. He has awarded several national and international awards and fellowships.

Jyotsna Dayma received her Master's degree in Agriculture with specialization in Agricultural Biotechnology from Himachal Pradesh Agriculture University in 2009. Following that she worked as a Project Assistant from the Institute of Himalayan Bioresource Technology, CSIR where she acquainted herself with advanced techniques in Biotechnological research. In 2016, she had joined as an Assistant Professor at Suresh Gyan Vihar University and displayed commendable expertise in the area of teaching, guiding students and research. Presently, she is a research fellow and working on hostplant- pathogen interaction.

Deelip V. Derle is working as Professor at M. V. P. College of Pharmacy, Nasik Maharashtra, India. He has published 35 Paper, 5 books and presented more than 40 Papers in different national and international conferences.

Nilesh Gorde is currently working as an HOD & Assistant Professor in Department of Pharmaceutics with Konkan Gyanpeeth Rahul Dharkar College of Pharmacy & Research Institute, Karjat (Affiliated to University of Mumbai, India). He has 11 years of teaching experience. He has 4 patents to his credits(1 granted and 3 published) and published more than 20 research and review articles in various national / international journals. He has also presented various research papers in national / international conference, seminars, symposia and workshops.

Charu Gupta (Gold Medalist; NET, GATE qualified), Associate Professor, Amity Institute of Herbal Research & Studies, Amity University Uttar Pradesh carries with over 13 years of experience in teaching and research at University level. She has published around 60 research and review papers in SCI journals, authored 5 books, 30 chapters in books, around 17 most popular articles in both English & Hindi languages and around 100 abstracts in both national and international conferences. During her tenure at Amity, she has filed several patents and related to the medicinal plants and microbiology. Her research interests are in probiotics & utilization of agro-industrial wastes for production of value added products.

Ta Thi Thu Hang, Research Scholar, University of Medicine and Pharmacy, Viet Nam National University Ha Noi. She uses the in silico method to screen to find out the lead compounds and then develop to therapeutic drugs. Furthermore, she focuses on pharmacokinetics, pharmacology and toxicology studies of natural product compounds.

Ashish Jain is currently Principal, Shri D. D. Vispute, College of Pharmacy & Research Center, New Panvel affiliated to University of Mumbai. He has more than 14 years of teaching experience at UG & PG level till date. He has authored more than 40 research and review articles in UGC approved national & international journals. He has contributed in many international books as an author. He received grant from Mumbai University for minor research project His area of research interest are herbal formulation development and evaluation.

Nilofer Khan is currently working as an Assistant Professor in Department of Pharmacognosy and Phytochemistry at Konkan Gyanpeeth Rahul Dharkar College of Pharmacy & Research Institute, Karjat (Affiliated to University of Mumbai, India). She has 8 years of teaching experience. She has published more than 20 research and review articles in various national / international journals.

Vu Khanh Linh, Research Scholar, University of Medicine and Pharmacy, Viet Nam National University Ha Noi. Her interest in studying about medicinal plants and to find its bioactive compounds for the treatment of diseases.

Sarmad Moin is an Assistant Dean (Research) at School of Applied Sciences, Suresh Gyan Vihar University, Jaipur, India, where he has been on faculty since 2016 and has more than seven years of Post - Ph. D. teaching and research experience in plant biotechnology, proteomics, and bioprospecting. He completed a funded project from DST-Rajasthan on "ovicidal and larvicidal activity of medicinal plant". Dr. Sarmad Moin also serving as Editor of the journal Suresh Gyan Vihar University, International Journal of Environment, Science, and Technology. He published many research papers in international peer-reviewed journals.

Nguyen Hong Nhung, Research Scholar, University of Medicine and Pharmacy, Viet Nam National University Ha Noi. She is interested in researching medicinal plants, especially its pharmacology and bioactive compounds.

Rutuja Patil is a currently Research Scholar at Department of Pharmaceutics, Shri D. D. Vispute, College of Pharmacy & Research Centre, New Panvel affiliated to University of Mumbai. Her area of research interest is formulation development and evaluation of various microparticulate and vesicles based gel systems.

Dhan Prakash has over 43 years of research experience in life sciences, worked as guest scientist at GSF-Munich (Germany), Freiburg University (Germany), and Ecole Normale Superieur, Lyon (France); guided more than 25 Ph. D. thesis, published 160 research papers in SCI journals, 35 book chapters, 210 abstracts in conferences, filed 40 patents and edited 5 books. He is leading a team at Amity University Noida for advance research in Chemical & Pharmaceutical Sciences for techniques and methodology used in basic & applied research for biotechnology, drug design, development of different formulations, their scientific validation for safety, efficacy etc. through recent scientific tools.

Bhushan Rajendra Rane is at present Associate Professor and Head at Department of Pharmaceutics, Shri. D. D. Vispute, College of Pharmacy and Research Center, New Panvel affiliated to Mumbai University. He has over 13 years of teaching experience at UG and PG Levels. Till date, he has guided more than 40 students for M. Pharm. He has published more than 60 peer reviewed research and review articles in national and international journals. He has co-authored 5 books at National level and 8 book chapters at international level. He is a reviewer for several scientific and international journals. He received grant upto Rs. 20 Lakhs from various apex bodies for research.

Gokul Shravan Talele, Professor & Principal, Matoshri College of Pharmacy, Odhagaon, Eklahare, Nashik, Maharashtra, India He is member of Board of studies of Savitribai Phule Pune university, Pune and Kavayitri Bahinabai Chaudhari North Maharashtra University, Jalgaon He has taught Pharmaceutical Analysis at both the undergraduate and postgraduate levels and has guided eight Ph. D. students and 30 postgraduate students. His area of interest includes development of analytical methods, drug delivery systems, and Phytochemistry. He has published several research papers, book chapters, reviews, in various reputed journals. Presently, he is serving as a reviewer and editorial board member for several journals of international repute. He is a member of a number of professional and scientific societies, such as the Indian Pharmaceutical Association (IPA), All India Pharmaceutical Teachers association (APTI).

Swati G. Talele is currently serving as an Assistant Professor, Department of Pharmaceutics, at Sandip Institute of Pharmaceutical Sciences. She has 18 years experience in research along with teaching. She has published more than 21 research papers in various reputed international and national journals. She has supervised many M.Pharm students and currently associated with many research projects. She has published more than 30 review papers and presented research work at several conferences and received awards by Universities. She has also authored the book titled Natural excipients and many chapters and books is in progress. Her interest are in field of Nanotechnology, Natural Polymers, herbal formulations and radiolabelling based bio distribution studies.

Bui Thanh Tung received his PhD in Pharmacology from the Seville University, Spain in 2014. Then he worked in University of Medicine and Pharmacy, Vietnam National University Ha Noi as lecturer. In 2018 he was pointed as Associate professor. His main research focuses on medicinal plants for the treatment of various diseases such as diabetes, Alzheimer, cancer. His special interest is on the development of new drugs from Vietnamese natural resources. He writes and presents widely on issues of natural products, bioactive compounds and their pharmacological activities.

Sandeep O. Waghulde is currently working as an HOD & Assistant Professor in Department of Pharmaceutical Chemistry, at Konkan Gyanpeeth Rahul Dharkar College of Pharmacy & Research Institute, Karjat (Affiliated to University of Mumbai, India). He has 13 years of teaching experience & 8 years of Research experience. He has 2 patents to his credits and published more than 25 research and review articles in various national / international journals. He has also presented various research papers in national / international conference, seminars, symposia and workshops.

Index

N

P

S

T

U

V

X

www.ingramcontent.com/pod-product-compliance
Lightning Source LLC
LaVergne TN
LVHW060302011026
849161LV00011B/2760
* 9 7 8 1 7 9 9 8 4 4 5 3 2 *